# Clinical Judgment
# USMLE Step 3 Review

# Clinical Judgment
# USMLE Step 3 Review

**George P. Lee, MD**
*Chicago, Illinois*

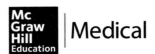

New York • Chicago • San Francisco • Athens • London • Madrid • Mexico City
Milan • New Delhi • Singapore • Sydney • Toronto

1 2 3 4 5 6 7 8 9 0   QVS/QVS   19 18 17 16 15 14

ISBN-13: 978-0-07-173908-5
MHID: 0-07-173908-4


This book was set in Minion Pro Regular by MPS Limited.
The editors were Catherine A. Johnson and Karen G. Edmonson.
The production supervisor was Richard Ruzycka.
Project management was provided by Vipra Fauzdar at MPS Limited.
The cover designer was Thomas De Pierro.
Image credit: Biddiboo/Getty Images.
Quad Graphics Versailles was printer and binder.


This book is printed on acid-free paper.


**Library of Congress Cataloging-in-Publication Data**

Lee, George P. (George Park), 1972- author.
  Clinical judgment USMLE Step 3 review / George P. Lee.
      p. ; cm.
  Includes index.
  ISBN 978-0-07-173908-5 (pbk. : alk. paper)—ISBN 0-07-173908-4 (pbk. : alk. paper)
  I. Title.
  [DNLM: 1. Diagnosis—Examination Questions. 2. Diagnosis—Outlines. 3. Clinical Medicine—methods—Examination Questions. 4. Clinical Medicine—methods—Outlines. 5. Decision Making—Examination Questions. 6. Decision Making—Outlines. 7. Decision Making, Computer-Assisted—Examination Questions. 8. Decision Making, Computer-Assisted—Outlines. 9. Judgment—Examination Questions. 10. Judgment—Outlines. WB 18.2]
  RB38.25
  616.07'5076—dc23

2014014055

McGraw-Hill books are available at special quantity discounts to use as premiums and sales promotions, or for use in corporate training programs. To contact a representative, please visit the Contact Us pages at www.mhprofessional.com.

*To my mother and father for their support, encouragement,
and most importantly, for their unconditional (agape) love.*

# Contents

# Preface

Medical information is constantly growing and changing, and the nature of the USMLE Step 3 is no exception. It is nearly impossible to know every single fact and concept in medicine, hence the reason for specialties and subspecialties. Therefore, the concept of this book is not to necessarily memorize every single fact and concept, but rather to attain a certain skill: clinical judgment. Once you develop and nurture your clinical judgment skills, you can position yourself at a higher percentage of answering exam questions correctly, and you will also make good decisions in your daily patient care.

The next question you have to consider is, "How do I know I've reached sound clinical judgment?" It is just like when the boiling point of water is reached at 100°C, the water starts to bubble. You may be at 86°C or 98°C in your preparation now, but if you continue to work hard, digest and integrate the information, and think with a critical lens, then at one point, the water will boil and you will notice that you are making good decisions on the majority of your practice questions. Remember that developing your clinical judgment skills does not come overnight. It is a process that takes time like any developing skill. Therefore, it is important to start early in your exam preparation.

The design of this book will enable you to see typical and atypical presentations in the Clinical Features and Pattern Recognition sections. Basic science concepts (foundational science) are correlated with the clinical topics. The goal of the basic science concepts is to help you understand the disease in a broader context. In addition, medical information from different specialties is interrelated by the Connecting Point feature of this book. At this stage of your medical journey, you should know the basic flow of patient care: history and physical → diagnostic tests → treatment. The Next Step section of this book will shift your thinking about patient management helping you prioritize your thoughts. (For example, in tension pneumothorax it is important to perform an immediate decompression of the lung before ordering a chest x-ray.) Finally, it is imperative to start your computer-based case simulations (CCS) preparation early, and therefore the CCS component is integrated in the majority of the chapters.

A successful outcome on Step 3 is largely determined by your preparation and attitude. Remember, by the closure of your exam preparation you may still feel that you do not know enough, but the point of this book is to develop your clinical judgment skills. It is my hope that once you achieve sound clinical judgment, you will be able to pass the exam and carry over this lifelong skill into your field of practice. Good luck on the USMLE Step 3 exam!

George P. Lee, M.D.
Chicago, Illinois

# Acknowledgments

I would like to take this opportunity to thank my editor, Catherine Johnson, for all her encouragement and for believing in this project. I would also like to recognize my other editor, Karen G. Edmonson, for her counsel and her editorial skills in preparing the manuscript for production. I want to thank my production supervisor, Richard Ruzycka, for his invaluable assistance in preparation of the book. I am also grateful to Vipra Fauzdar at MPS for her professionalism and remarkable talents for overseeing the composition of the book. Finally, I am indebted to my publisher, McGraw-Hill, for providing me a platform to make a contribution to medicine and for their strong commitment to high quality publishing in the healthcare field.

# Introduction

## EXAM LOGISTICS

### ▌ PURPOSE

The purpose of the USMLE Step 3 exam is to assess the examinee's ability to understand and apply medical knowledge that is considered essential for the unsupervised practice of medicine. In other words, this can be a challenging test.

### ▌ GENERAL INFORMATION

For a detailed description of the USMLE Step 3 exam, including physician tasks, objectives, content, and CCS overview, please review the *USMLE Step 3 Content Description and General Information*. It is also recommended to review the *USMLE Bulletin of Information* to understand eligibility, scoring, and score reporting. Finally, it is essential to review the *USMLE Step 3 practice materials* that are provided to you upon registration, or you can download the information by visiting www.usmle.org.

### ▌ REGISTRATION

To apply for the Step 3 exam, please follow the instructions on the Federation of State Medical Boards (FSMB) website at www.fsmb.org. Starting August 2014, the state board sponsorship for Step 3 will be discontinued.

### ▌ EXAM BREAKDOWN

The USMLE Step 3 is a 2-day examination that comprises a total of 480 multiple-choice questions and 12 CCS cases.

**Day 1**
- Total of 336 multiple-choice questions.
- Total of 7 blocks.
- 48 questions per block.
- 60 minutes per block. If you finish any block early, any remaining time may be added to your total break time.
- Total of 7 hours of testing.

- A minimum of 45 minutes break time.
- 15 minute optional tutorial. It is highly recommended to do an audio calibration and to adjust the monitor resolution to a minimum of $1024 \times 768$. If you finish the tutorial early, any remaining time may be added to your total break time.
- Expect the day to last ≤8 hours for day 1.

**Day 2**
- Total of 144 multiple-choice questions.
- Total of 4 blocks.
- 36 questions per block.
- 45 minutes per block. If you finish any block early, any remaining time may be added to your total break time.
- Total of 3 hours for the first four blocks.
- 12 CCS cases follow the multiple-choice questions with a total of 4 hours to complete all the cases.
- A minimum of 45 minutes break time.
- 15 minute optional tutorial for the CCS. If you finish the tutorial early, any remaining time may be added to your total break time.
- Expect the day to last ≤8 hours for day 2.

### ▌ PASSING USMLE STEP 3

Passing the Step 3 exam is imperative. Consider three reasons: (1) if you fail the exam, you might compromise your eligibility to be reappointed to the next postgraduate year position, (2) you might compromise your eligibility for state licensure based on the number of USMLE attempts and time limit for completing all Steps, and (3) "Do you really want to take another two grueling days of examinations?" For the initial medical licensure process, the following table lists the maximum number of USMLE attempts for each state. Additional postgraduate training may be required in certain states if the maximum attempts are exceeded for medical licensure. For further information regarding state-specific requirements for medical licensure, please visit www.fsmb.org.

### Maximum Number of USMLE Attempts by State

| State | USMLE Attempts | State | USMLE Attempts | State | USMLE Attempts |
|---|---|---|---|---|---|
| **Alabama** | 10 total at all Steps | **Louisiana** | No limit at Step 1; 4 at Step 2; 4 at Step 3 | **Oklahoma** | 3 per Step |
| **Alaska** | 2 per Step | **Maine** | 3 at Step 3 | **Oregon** | 3 at Step 3 |
| **Arizona** | No limit | **Maryland** | 4 per Step | **Pennsylvania** | No limit |
| **Arkansas** | 3 per Step | **Massachusetts** | 3 at Step 3 | **Puerto Rico** | No limit |
| **California** | 4 at Step 3 | **Michigan** | No limit | **Rhode Island** | 3 per Step |
| **Colorado** | No limit | **Minnesota** | 3 per Step | **South Carolina** | 4 per Step |
| **Connecticut** | No limit | **Mississippi** | 3 at Step 3 | **South Dakota** | 3 per Step |
| **Delaware** | 6 per Step | **Missouri** | 3 at Step 3 | **Tennessee** | No limit |
| **Washington, DC** | 3 at Step 3 | **Montana** | 3 at Step 3 | **Texas** | 3 per Step |
| **Florida** | No limit | **Nebraska** | 4 per Step | **Utah** | 3 at Step 3 |
| **Georgia** | 3 per Step | **Nevada** | 9 total at all Steps with Step 3 in no more than 3 attempts | **Vermont** | 3 at Step 3 |
| **Hawaii** | No limit | **New Hampshire** | 3 per Step | **Virginia** | No limit |
| **Idaho** | 2 per Step | **New Jersey** | 5 at Step 3 | **Washington** | 3 at Step 3 |
| **Illinois** | 5 total at all Steps | **New Mexico** | 6 per Step | **West Virginia** | 6 per Step |
| **Indiana** | 3 per Step | **New York** | No limit | **Wisconsin** | 3 per Step |
| **Iowa** | 6 at Step 1; 6 at Step 2; 3 at Step 3 | **North Carolina** | 3 per Step | **Wyoming** | 7 total at all Steps |
| **Kansas** | No limit | **North Dakota** | 3 per Step | | |
| **Kentucky** | 4 per Step | **Ohio** | 4 per Step | | |

# EXAM PREPARATION

## INTRODUCTION

Physicians are trained to become highly evolved creatures of learning. Learning has transitioned from the lectures in the classroom to the clinical wards during medical school. Once a resident, he or she has to learn under time constraints and is expected to pass Step 3 and show overall improvement in the in-training exams. Once residency is over, the practicing physician has to pass his or her specialty board, continue with lifelong learning through the Maintenance of Certification (MOC), and learn in a different setting (eg, academics, private sector). Throughout each stage of learning, the only constant is the physician's ability to understand, extract information, and apply medical knowledge. At this stage of your training and onward, time is valuable and self-learning is imperative. Therefore, use your time wisely and carefully select materials that will maximize your learning potential.

## STRATEGY

From day 1 of your preparation to the last exam question, you need to take control of your destiny, which is to pass Step 3. In general, a systematic approach to your preparation will usually result in a successful outcome, therefore, it is important to start early. You may have your own strategy, but make it methodical and take ownership of your valuable time and efforts. The following is a recommended approach, and if you follow these 3 basic principles, then I believe that you have a higher percentage of passing Step 3.

**Stage I: Strengthen Your Knowledge Base**

- The bottom line is that you have to put in the time, there are no tricks.

- Make sure that the time you put in is **efficient**, **effective**, and **exciting** ("Triple E's").

  - **Efficient time** means mastering a chapter or section of a chapter that is related to the rotation you are on, for example, mastering the cardiology chapter by the end of the cardiology rotation. If you have a lot of time on an elective rotation, then you should master 2 to 3 chapters. If you are on a hard rotation like ICU, then do parts of a chapter such as the "EKG Review" section. If you find pockets of time during your schedule, master another section. Remember that the time you put in will all add up. You don't have to go in order, but you do have to take control of your preparation, and be sure to monitor your progress.

- **Effective time** means being extremely focused. For example, after coming home from work, give your undivided attention for 1 complete hour of Step 3. On the way to work in the morning, try to remember, recite, and repeat what you learned the night before.

- The time you put in should be **exciting**, don't look at it like "work." Examples may include personalizing your preparation, summarizing tables, photocopying a table and carrying it with you during the day, or after seeing a patient with a certain disease making sure you read about that disease the same day.

- It is important to have good momentum in your preparation. During your preparation you want to keep pushing forward with good velocity. You can remember this concept from the fact that momentum is proportional to the velocity from the equation: momentum (p) = mass (m) × velocity (v). If you find that some sections are harder than others, then move on and take a break from that section and come back with a renewed sense of purpose and finish the section in pieces in order to maintain good momentum.

**Stage II: Transition into Questions**

- After beefing up your knowledge base, it is important to apply your knowledge with questions.

- After reading all the chapters and the appendices, it is important to get your mind frame into a question mode style of thinking. It is also important to assess your timing. You have 1 minute and 15 seconds per question.

- Remember that you don't have to do 1,000 practice questions to be successful on the exam.

- It is highly recommended to do the *USMLE practice questions* with the timing on. The practice questions will be similar to the actual format of the exam.

**Stage III: Final Review**

- It is important to leave enough time for your final review.

- All the information must be consolidated, assimilated, and integrated.

- At this point, it is important to start firing those neurons to make hardwire connections because everything must stick.

## THE PEDAGOGY

The following features will enhance and nurture your clinical judgment skills and maximize your ability to interrelate medical information. Once you embrace all the features of this book you will be able to have a deeper understanding of the material and ultimately success on Step 3.

### Keywords Review:

At the beginning of each chapter is a description of medical terms. Some of the terms may not be seen in the chapter, but they will be mentioned to highlight the specialty.

### Introduction:

When appropriate, the introduction of each topic discusses the etiology and pathophysiology of the disease.

### Clinical Features:

Typical and atypical presentations are presented in this section. Because systemic diseases can present in a disarrayed fashion, the Clinical Features section incorporates a relative head-to-toe presentation to help you organize your thoughts.

### Next Step:

A strong focus on patient management is presented in this section. The Next Step section provides a logical sequential approach that will help you prioritize your thoughts. By having an organized thought process, you can tackle any clinical situation in a systematic approach. During your review process, you may find steps within steps in this section, but this entire section should be viewed as a working paradigm that ultimately incorporates the standard of care. Just like in the real world, having a working paradigm as part of your mental framework allows you to account for other factors in patient management (eg, comorbidities, available resources, insurance). Once you train your thoughts to figure out what the most important steps are in management, then you develop sharper clinical judgment skills.

### Option-based Management:

The option-based management is described in the Next Step section and provides alternatives to patient management. Remember that there is more than one way to appropriately treat a patient.

### Short- and Long-term Management:

Short- and long-term management are described in the Next Step section and mentioned in the CCS tips. By integrating this type of management, you begin to understand how to "bridge your therapy" by addressing any acute issues (eg, pain) along with long-term issues (eg, prevention). With this approach, you become more comprehensive in patient management. In addition, this style of approach will help prioritize your thoughts for the CCS cases.

### Follow-Up/Disposition:

The Follow-up section describes the follow-up care for patients for topics that would most likely be seen in the office. The Disposition section describes the placement of the patient that is typically seen in the emergency department. This section should engage you to think about topics that are emergent or office-based during the exam.

### Pearls:

This section provides "pearls of wisdom" for the particular topic in addition to serving as an umbrella for other features that are considered pearls (eg, caveats, foundational points, CCS tips, clinical judgments, connecting points). Once you have read through the Introduction, Clinical Features, Next Step, Follow-up/Disposition, and Pearls section for each topic, then you begin to have a broader perspective of the disease. This is where your clinical judgment begins to be refined.

### Caveats:

Caveats are presented in the Pearls section and serve to give precautions or warnings for that particular topic.

### Foundational Points:

Foundational points are presented in the Pearls section and describe a basic science concept in reference to that particular clinical topic. Foundational science concepts may also be found in the Keywords Review (eg, Allergy and Immunology).

### Connecting Points:

The beauty of medicine is that everything truly is interconnected. By connecting one seemingly unlikely piece of knowledge to another piece of medical knowledge, you begin to see the symphony or orchestration of the human body as a whole. One of the goals of connecting points is to strengthen your memory of one topic to another topic by "neuronal wiring." Each connecting point will have a reference for you to make another medical connection. By the end of your final review (Stage III), you should be able to move quickly and interrelate all the connecting points without hesitation.

### Clinical Judgments (CJ):

CJ questions are presented in the Pearls section. Initially, try to answer the CJ without looking at the answer.

### CCS Tips:

CCS tips are presented in the Pearls section and offer you tips on that particular topic.

### CCS Cases:

At the end of each chapter, some CCS cases will be offered. This is an opportunity for you to understand and integrate your CCS preparation early. Do not wait until the last minute to prepare the CCS component of the exam. Try to get your hands on a computer and practice the CCS software with each chapter review so that you can become proficient.

### Pattern Recognition:

A special section on Pattern Recognition appears as Appendix A. Both typical and atypical presentations are described, and the concept of this section is to develop your gut instinct about a disease. Although it is not recommended to memorize every feature of each disease (you might drive yourself crazy!), begin incorporating this section in Stage I of your preparation.

### Rapid-fire Clinical Judgments:

Rapid-fire clinical judgment questions appear in Appendix B. Begin incorporating this section into Stage I and Stage II of your preparation.

### Factoids:

Factoids are pure medical facts, and appear in Appendix C. This section should serve to strengthen your knowledge base, and you should begin incorporating this section during Stage I of your exam preparation.

### Key Lab Values:

In your last 1 to 2 days prior to the exam, you should know some basic lab values. These are presented in Appendix D. It is recommended to take this extra step in learning some basic lab values to improve your efficiency with exam questions and to maintain a good rhythm during the course of each exam block.

### Final Pearls:

This section appears as Appendix E and should serve as your last piece of review prior to your examination.

# EXAM EXECUTION

## ▌ THE QUARTER METHOD

It is important to be conscious about your timing during the exam. You may be a naturally slow reader or you may be a relatively fast reader, but you might get stuck on time because you spent too much time on a question or you are just plain tired. Therefore, it is essential to have landmarks. Just as a surgeon needs anatomic landmarks for surgery, you need to have time landmarks for the exam. The quarter method takes the time and number of questions per block and divides it by 4. Therefore, you have 4 quarters or 4 intervals for which you should be on target or may need to catch up. Every quarter should serve as a reference point. This method can be applied to any exam, and it works well if you answer the questions in sequential order. It is recommended not to skip more than 5 questions because you have to take into account the time that you did not spend on the skipped questions. For example, if you skip 5 questions and do them at the end of the block, then you have to account for 6 minutes and 15 seconds since you have 1 minute and 15 seconds per question. If you apply the quarter method on the exam you will have a sense of control during each block. Remember, do not let the exam control you, you control the exam. The following depiction is a clock with landmarks that encompass the time remaining (Tr) and the target question (Tq). If the landmarks are hard to remember, you can always draw this picture on the dry-erase board provided on the exam. Try the quarter method during Stage II of your preparation.

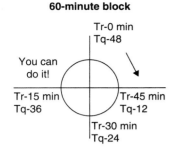

**60-minute block**

Tr-0 min
Tq-48

You can do it!

Tr-15 min
Tq-36

Tr-30 min
Tq-24

Tr-45 min
Tq-12

**45-minute block**

Tr-0 min
Tq-36

Push it!

Tr-11 min
Tq-27

Tr-22 min
Tq-18

Tr-33 min
Tq-9

## THE AUDIBLE PLAN

Prior to the exam, you should devise your own plan on how to tackle the blocks and allocate your break time. Sometimes during the exam day you have to make adjustments with your break time and the number of consecutive blocks you want to attack. It is important to have at least 2 to 3 different audible plans going into the exam. In American football, the term *audible* refers to a change in playing tactics that is usually called by the quarterback as an adjustment to the playing situation. Similarly, you may have to adjust your tactics during the examination. By having an audible plan, you control the exam day, the day does not control you. The following are examples of an audible plan, and you may be able to allocate more time to your breaks if you finish any block or tutorial earlier.

Option 1:

| **Day 1** | **Day 2** |
| --- | --- |
| Block 1 | Block 1 |
| Block 2 | Block 2 |
| 10-minute break | 10-minute break |
| Block 3 | Block 3 |
| Block 4 | Block 4 |
| 25-minute lunch break | 10-minute break |
| Block 5 | CCS Cases 1-3 |
| Block 6 | 20-minute lunch break |
| 10-minute break | CCS Cases 4-6 |
| Block 7 | CCS Cases 7-9 |
| | 5-minute break |
| | CCS-Cases 10-12 |

Option 2:

| **Day 1** | **Day 2** |
| --- | --- |
| Block 1 | Block 1 |
| 5-minute break | 5-minute break |
| Block 2 | Block 2 |
| 5-minute break | 5-minute break |
| Block 3 | Block 3 |
| 5-minute break | 5-minute break |
| Block 4 | Block 4 |
| 20-minute lunch break | 5-minute break |
| Block 5 | CCS Cases 1-2 |
| Block 6 | 10-minute lunch break |
| 10-minute break | CCS Cases 3-6 |
| Block 7 | 10-minute break |
| | CCS Cases 7-10 |
| | 5-minute break |
| | Cases 11-12 |

Option 3:

| **Day 1** | **Day 2** |
| --- | --- |
| Block 1 | Block 1 |
| Block 2 | Block 2 |
| Block 3 | Block 3 |
| 10-minute break | 10-minute break |
| Block 4 | Block 4 |
| 25-minute lunch break | CCS Cases 1-2 |
| Block 5 | 20-minute lunch break |
| Block 6 | CCS Cases 3-6 |
| 10-minute break | 10-minute break |
| Block 7 | CCS Cases 7-10 |
| | 5-minute break |
| | CCS-Cases 11-12 |

## FUEL

The best way to achieve optimal mental capacity is to have a basal level of glucose throughout the exam day. Consider munching on snacks throughout the day rather than having a big lunch. Instead of eating a full sandwich at lunch, try eating half the sandwich at lunch and the rest of the sandwich during your breaks. In this approach you should feel relatively light rather than bloated and still maintain a good level of glucose throughout the day. It is still crucial to stay alert and focused toward the end of the day because the last block could potentially determine your destiny. If you feel a little tired at the end of the day, then consider an extra boost of energy during your break time (eg, caffeinated beverage, chocolate-covered coffee beans).

# Allergy and Immunology

## CHAPTER OUTLINE

## KEYWORDS REVIEW

CD4—CD4 is a surface marker on T cells. The CD4 molecule is closely associated with the components of the T-cell receptor (TCR), and hence, they are sometimes referred to as co-receptors. Lck tyrosine kinase is also closely associated with the CD4 co-receptor, but on the cytoplasmic side of the T cell. The CD4 marker is necessary for interacting with cells that express MHC class II molecules that present the antigen to the T cells. Naive CD4 T cells can differentiate into T helper subsets of $T_H1$ or $T_H2$ cells (see below).

CD8—CD8 is a surface marker on T cells. The T cells are often referred to as cytotoxic T cells, and like CD4, they are associated with the TCR and Lck tyrosine kinase. The CD8 marker is necessary for interacting with cells that express MHC class I molecules that present the antigen to the T cells. Cytotoxicity occurs by two mechanisms. First, cytotoxic T cells that have the Fas ligand (CD95L) will target cells that express the Fas molecule (CD95) and trigger apoptosis. Second, granules are delivered into the target cell via perforin-induced pores.

Cytokines—Proteins secreted by cells that act as signals to other cells. Consider the following:

**IL-1**—Mediates inflammation; the major source is from macrophages.

**IL-2**—Involved in T cell proliferation.

**IL-3**—Enhances growth of blood cells made by the bone marrow.

**IL-4**—Enhances IgE switching, enhances B-cell proliferation, and ↓ inflammatory cytokines.

**IL-5**—Enhances IgA switching and enhances eosinophil growth.

**IL-6**—Enhances B and T cell proliferation and acute phase protein production.

**IL-7**—Enhances pre-B and pre-T cell growth.

**IL-8**—Induces neutrophil chemotaxis.

**IL-9**—Enhances mast cell activity.

**IL-10**—Inhibits $T_H1$ cell development and suppresses macrophage function.

**IL-12**—Enhances T$_H$1 cell development.

**IL-13**—Similar effects to IL-4.

**IFN-gamma**—Activates macrophages and increases MHC expression.

**TNF (α and β)**—Mediates inflammation.

**Endotoxin**—A toxin that is not secreted, but rather released during bacterial cell lysis. Endotoxin is present only in gram-negative bacteria except for *Listeria monocytogenes* (gram-positive). The term *endotoxin* is used interchangeably with *lipopolysaccharide* (LPS). LPS is part of the outer membrane of the gram-negative cell envelope. LPS is made of three components, which include O-antigen, core polysaccharide, and **lipid A** (ie, lipid A is the toxic component of the LPS).

**Exotoxin**—A toxin that is secreted by both gram-negative and gram-positive (except *Listeria monocytogenes*) bacteria. Exotoxins that act on the CNS or GI tract are referred to as neurotoxin and enterotoxin, respectively. Some exotoxins can act as superantigens (eg, TSST-1, streptococcal pyogenic exotoxins) that can bind to the MHC class II and T-cell receptor simultaneously (ie, without processing of the toxin by an antigen-presenting cell) and thereby stimulate a subset of T cells.

**Fab (fragment antigen binding)**—The "arms" of the antibody that contain both heavy and light chains. It is involved in antigen binding.

**Fc (fragment crystallizable) region**—The "tail" portion of an antibody that contains only heavy chains and is involved in binding to cell receptors and complement proteins.

**HIV glycoproteins**—The HIV viral envelop is studded with glycoprotein (gp)120 that is attached to transmembrane gp-41. GP-120 has high affinity to CD4 molecules. Once binding occurs between gp-120 and CD4, a conformational change occurs in the gp-41, which now mediates the fusion between the viral envelope and the target cell.

**Lck tyrosine kinase**—Lck tyrosine kinase is found on the cytoplasmic side of the T cell and is closely associated with the CD4 and CD8 co-receptors. Once an antigen binds to the T cell receptor, Lck tyrosine kinase is activated and initiates intracellular signaling. Lck tyrosine kinase is important for the development and function of the T cell.

**Opsonization**—The process of enhancing phagocytosis by having opsonins (eg, antibodies or complement fragments) bind onto antigens, marking them for an immune response.

**Sphingosine kinase**—An enzyme that catalyzes sphingosine to sphingosine-1-phosphate (S1P). S1P is implicated in many physiological processes such as cell survival, cellular adhesion, motility, angiogenesis, immunity, and inflammation.

**T$_H$1 cells**—T$_H$1 cells are primarily involved in immunity to intracellular pathogens, autoimmunity, pro-inflammatory response, and delayed hypersensitivity reactions. The major cytokines produced by T$_H$1 cells include IL-2, IFN-gamma, and TNF.

**T$_H$2 cells**—T$_H$2 cells are involved in allergic diseases (IgE response) and immunity to parasitic infections. The major cytokines produced by T$_H$2 cells include IL-4, IL-5, IL-9, IL-10, and IL-13.

# HUMORAL-MEDIATED IMMUNODEFICIENCY

## SELECTIVE IgA DEFICIENCY

Selective IgA deficiency is the most common primary immunodeficiency. IgA is normally found in mucosal secretions such as in the saliva, tears, GI tract, GU tract, breast milk, and nasal and pulmonary secretions. The majority of patients are asymptomatic, and it is thought that the lack of symptoms may be compensated by IgM, which may perform some of the same functions as IgA. The pathogenesis of selective IgA deficiency is unknown.

**Clinical Features:**

Selective IgA deficiency can occur sporadically or by familial inheritance. The majority of patients with selective IgA deficiency are **asymptomatic**. The remainder of patients that do have clinical symptoms may present with any of the following:

**Recurrent infections**—Sinopulmonary infections such as sinusitis, otitis media, bronchitis, or pneumonia may be recurrent. GI infections due to *Giardia lamblia* may also be recurrent.

**Autoimmune diseases**—Patients can develop SLE, ITP, RA, type 1 diabetes, or Graves' disease.

**Atopic diseases**—Patients can develop atopic dermatitis (eczema), allergic conjunctivitis, allergic rhinitis, asthma, or food allergies.

**Anaphylactic reactions**—Patients can develop an anaphylactic reaction (type 1 hypersensitivity) to blood products that contain IgA such as platelets, packed RBCs, whole blood, cryoprecipitate, FFP, IVIG, or granulocytes.

**GI diseases**—Crohn's disease, ulcerative colitis, celiac disease, and nodular lymphoid hyperplasia are associated with selective IgA deficiency.

## Next Step:

**Step 1)** Selective IgA deficiency is a diagnosis of exclusion, particularly of other types of primary humoral immune deficiencies. The diagnosis may not be readily apparent, but a pattern of recurrent infections, chronic diarrhea, autoimmune disease, atopic disease, anaphylactic reactions to blood products, family history, or a combination of these problems may provide insight to a possible diagnosis of selective IgA deficiency. The best test to confirm a clinical suspicion is to obtain serum immunoglobulins of IgA, IgG, and IgM levels. Patients with selective IgA deficiency will have **low IgA, normal IgG,** and **normal IgM levels.** In addition, patients must be older than 4 years of age, since children younger than 4 years old may still be able to normalize their IgA levels.

**Step 2)** Further evaluation may be indicated in patients with coexisting diseases such as SLE (eg, ANA, dsDNA antibodies), ITP (eg, CBC with peripheral smear), RA (eg, anti-CCP or rheumatoid factor), type 1 diabetes (eg, Hb A1C), Graves' disease (eg, TSH), asthma (eg, spirometry), celiac disease (eg, IgG-antigliadin antibodies or IgG-based anti-tissue transglutaminase antibodies), Crohn's disease or ulcerative colitis (eg, colonoscopy).

**Step 3)** There is no therapeutic intervention to replace IgA. Patients should be educated and counseled about other associated conditions, and treatment should be offered for the coexisting diseases. In cases of recurrent infections, prophylactic antibiotics may be considered in select cases to reduce the frequency of infections. The use of IVIG in patients with isolated IgA deficiency (ie, without coexisting IgG subclass deficiency) is controversial and is not routinely recommended.

## Follow-Up:

There are two important elements in the follow-up care. First, children younger than 4 years old should be monitored periodically to see if their IgA levels normalize. Second, patients diagnosed with selective IgA deficiency should be periodically reevaluated to assess the frequency of infections and to remain vigilant about the development of associated disorders.

## Pearls:

- Medications can cause a reduction in immunoglobulins, including IgA. These medications include anticonvulsants (eg, carbamazepine, phenytoin, valproic acid), cyclosporine, captopril, sulfasalazine, D-penicillamine, and thyroxine.
- It is unlikely that children with immune defects will present with recurrent infections before the age of 6 months since maternal immunoglobulins (IgG) are still present until that age.
- Patients that require transfusions should receive "washed" blood products to remove as much of the IgA and thereby reduce the risk of anaphylaxis.
- Patients diagnosed with selective IgA deficiency may have a family history of either IgA deficiency or common variable immunodeficiency (CVID).
- In a subset of patients, selective IgA deficiency can progress to common variable immunodeficiency (CVID).

- **Foundational point**—The five antibody isotypes include IgG, IgA, IgM, IgE, and IgD. Consider the main features of each type:

  **IgG**—Most abundant isotype; only isotype that can cross the placenta; major player in the secondary response to an antigen.

  **IgA**—Principally found in secretions and a major player in mucosal immunity.

  **IgM**—Major player in the primary response to an antigen (ie, the first antibody to appear).

  **IgE**—Major player in type 1 hypersensitivity. Allergen-specific IgE binds to the cell surface of mast cells and basophils. Upon re-exposure to the allergen, cross-linking of the IgE results in degranulation and secretion of the inflammatory mediators.

  **IgD**—Function is unclear, but is usually coexpressed with IgM on the cell surface of mature B cells.

- **On the CCS,** obtaining serum IgA, IgG, and IgM measurements will provide you with the actual value and the normal value in the practice CCS.

- **On the CCS,** "counsel family/patient" is available in the practice CCS.

- **On the CCS,** you will be evaluated on your diagnostic work-ups, appropriate treatments, monitoring the patient, sequence of actions, timing, and appropriately locating the patient to the right setting.

# ▌ COMMON VARIABLE IMMUNODEFICIENCY

Common variable immunodeficiency (CVID) is characterized by the inability of B cells to differentiate into plasma cells that are capable of producing the various immunoglobulin isotypes (ie, hypogammaglobulinemia). The pathogenesis of CVID is unknown.

## Clinical Features:

CVID can occur sporadically or by familial inheritance. Males and females are equally affected, and the peak of onset appears to have a bimodal distribution affecting children 1 to 5 years old and individuals 16 to 25 years old. Common **variable** immunodeficiency is truly **variable** in its clinical manifestations, which can make this disease hard to detect. Consider the following features:

**Recurrent infections**—Sinopulmonary infections such as sinusitis, otitis media, bronchitis, pneumonia, or conjunctivitis may be recurrent. GI infections due to *Giardia lamblia*, cryptosporidium, or CMV. Other possible infections may include meningitis, septic arthritis, or enterovirus infections.

**Autoimmune diseases**—Possible autoimmune disorders include SLE, ITP, RA, diabetes, psoriasis, vitiligo, alopecia totalis, autoimmune hemolytic anemia, autoimmune neutropenia, pernicious anemia, or thyroid diseases.

**Granulomatous diseases**—Noncaseating granulomas may be found in the lungs, liver, lymph nodes, spleen, intestine, brain, skin, or conjunctivae.

**Growth**—Failure to thrive (FTT) may be seen in children.

**Malignancy**—There is an increased risk of developing non-Hodgkin's lymphoma (NHL) and gastric cancers.

CVID can also affect specific organ systems, and it may be helpful to consider them in a relative head to toe fashion:

**Pulmonary**—Bronchiectasis may be the result of repeated infections.

**GI**—Crohn's disease, ulcerative colitis, sprue-like disorder, malabsorption, and nodular lymphoid hyperplasia are associated with CVID.

**Hepatobiliary**—Primary biliary cirrhosis (PBC) may be seen.

**Spleen**—Splenomegaly is a relatively common finding.

**Lymph nodes**—Lymphadenopathy may be seen in the neck, chest, or abdomen.

## Next Step:

**Step 1)** CVID is a diagnosis of exclusion. The diagnosis may not be straightforward early in the course of the disease, but a combination of problems may point you in that direction. The best initial test is to obtain serum immunoglobulins of IgG, IgA, and IgM levels. Patients with CVID will have **low IgG** in addition to a **low IgA and/or low IgM levels**. Patients should also be older than 4 years of age to make the diagnosis.

**Step 2)** The next best step in patients with low levels of immunoglobulins is to assess an antibody response to vaccines. The diagnosis can be established if the patient has a poor or absent response to the vaccines.

**Step 3)** Patients should be counseled and educated about the disease, especially younger individuals since they may be more inclined to withdraw from social activities.

**Step 4)** Management approach in patients with CVID is to treat any coexisting diseases and treatment with **immune globulin replacement** either intravenously (IVIG) or subcutaneously (SCIG). The subcutaneous route of administration may offer more convenience (ie, self-administration at home) than the intravenous route.

## Follow-Up:

Patients receiving immune globulin replacement should have trough levels of IgG every several months. Children suspected of having CVID should be monitored periodically to see if their immunoglobulin levels improve and to assess antibody titers.

## Pearls:

- **Common** variable immunodeficiency is a relatively **common** primary immunodeficiency, but not as frequent as selective IgA deficiency.
- Soon after birth, maternal IgG declines and reaches a low point at approximately 3 to 6 months of life. Meanwhile, the infant's own endogenous IgG production begins to rise. There is a point when the infant normally has low immunoglobulin levels that is referred to as normal physiologic hypogammaglobulinemia. Prolongation of this physiologic phenomenon is referred to as **transient**

**hypogammaglobulinemia of infancy (THI)** and is usually present after the sixth month of life. THI can be characterized by low IgG, with or without diminished values of the other isotypes. However, the IgG levels should normalize by 2 to 4 years of age. In addition, patients with THI will have adequate antibody response to vaccines, usually before the immunoglobulin levels become normal.

- The overall B cell numbers in patients with CVID is normal or slightly reduced.
- In a subset of patients with CVID, a low CD4/CD8 T cell ratio can be observed.
- Patients diagnosed with CVID should receive age-appropriate cancer screening.
- **On the CCS**, "IVIG" is available in the practice CCS, but not "SCIG."
- **On the CCS**, you can advance the clock by selecting "On," "In," "With next available result," or "Call/see me as needed."
- **On the CCS**, early in your CCS preparation, you might want to stick with a particular routine that is familiar with you when you advance the clock.

# X-LINKED AGAMMAGLOBULINEMIA

X-linked agammaglobulinemia (XLA), also referred to as Bruton's agammaglobulinemia, is caused by a mutation in a gene that codes for Bruton's tyrosine kinase (BTK). BTK is a signal transduction molecule that is important in B cell development. Failure of B cell development results in diminished levels of mature B lymphocytes that can no longer generate antibody producing plasma cells.

## Clinical Features:

The clinical manifestations of XLA typically present after 3 months of age since the maternal IgG is protecting the newborn before that time. XLA primarily affects **males** because the disease is an X-linked recessive trait. On physical exam, most patients will have very small tonsils, adenoids, lymph nodes, or spleen. The main feature of XLA is recurrent infections:

**Recurrent infections**—Patients with XLA are susceptible to encapsulated bacteria such as *Streptococcus pneumoniae*, *Haemophilus influenzae*, and *Pseudomonas* species. Other common bacteria include staphylococcus. Infection with specific viruses such as enteroviruses can also occur. The possible types of infection vary, and they may include sinusitis, otitis media, bronchitis, pneumonia, conjunctivitis, osteomyelitis, septic arthritis, sepsis, hepatitis, CNS infections, skin infections, respiratory infections, or GI infections (eg, giardia, campylobacter, shigella, or salmonella).

## Next Step:

**Step 1)** The best initial step in a patient with suspected XLA (ie, male, family history, recurrent infections) is to obtain serum immunoglobulins of IgG, IgA, and IgM levels. Patients with XLA will have **low IgG, IgA, and IgM levels**.

**Step 2)** If the serum immunoglobulins are low, the next best step is obtain measurement of the B cell numbers. Patients with XLA will demonstrate less than 2% of circulating CD19$^+$ B cells.

**Step 3)** If the B cell numbers are low from Step 2, XLA can be confirmed with molecular studies (ie, analysis of DNA, RNA, or protein), which will identify the mutation in the BTK gene.

**Step 4)** Genetic counseling should be offered to the family since the patient's female family members may be carriers.

**Step 5)** Unfortunately, there is no cure for XLA. However, patients should be treated for any coexisting diseases (eg, infections) and treatment with **immune globulin replacement** via intravenously (IVIG) or subcutaneously (SCIG).

### Follow-Up:

Patients on immune globulin replacement will require trough levels. Overall, patients can live a relatively normal life with immune globulin therapy.

### Pearls:

- In X-linked recessive disorders, males only require one bad copy of the X chromosome to be affected, while females require two bad copies of the X chromosome.

- All female offspring of patients diagnosed with XLA will be carriers.

- All female carriers will be asymptomatic, but they have a 50% chance of transmitting the disease to each of their sons and a 50% chance that each of their daughters will be carriers.

- There is no male-to-male transmission in X-linked recessive inheritance.

- When a male patient is diagnosed with XLA and his mother as a carrier, look closely at the maternal uncles since they may be affected as well.

- XLA patients will have very low numbers of B cells, while CVID patients will have close to normal B cell numbers.

- XLA patients will have a poor response to vaccines (ie, low antibody titers to immunizations).

- **Foundational point**—CD19 and CD20 are proteins that are found on the cell surface of mature B cells.

- **Foundational point**—Tyrosine kinases are intracellular signaling proteins that function as molecular switches turning on and off various cellular functions.

- **Connecting point** (pg. 163)—Know the pattern of X-linked recessive genes.

- **On the CCS,** "B cell count" is available in the practice CCS.

- **On the CCS,** "Genetic counseling" is available in the practice CCS.

- **On the CCS,** you are expected to know the routes of administration and frequency (ie, one time/bolus or continuous), but not the dosages or fluid rates of the medication.

- **On the CCS,** when you order something during the case, the "clerk" will recognize the first three characters of the order, even abbreviations (eg, CXR for chest x-ray). Be sure to try different abbreviations in the practice CCS software.

# CCS: ANAPHYLAXIS CASE INTRODUCTION

Day 1 @ 14:30
Emergency Room

A 12-year-old white boy is rushed to the emergency room by his mother because of generalized urticaria, crampy abdominal pain, and lightheadedness for the past 45 minutes. He appears to be in mild distress.

**Initial Vital Signs:**
Temperature: 37.0°C (98.6°F)
Pulse: 102 beats/min
Respiratory: 32/min
Blood pressure: 88/68 mm Hg
Height: 162.6 cm (64.0 inches)
Weight: 65.8 kg (145 lb; >95th percentile)
BMI: 24.9 kg/m$^2$

**Initial History:**
Reason(s) for visit: Urticaria, abdominal pain, lightheadedness.

**HPI:**
A 12-year-old child is brought to the ED by his mother because of itchy "hives" distributed throughout his body, crampy abdominal pain, and lightheadedness that started 45 minutes ago. They were both at a birthday party when the symptoms started to appear. The mother recalls that her son was interacting very well with his friends at the party, but the symptoms appeared after he finished his hot dog and birthday cake with yellow frosting. The patient felt a crampy pain in his abdomen approximately 10 minutes after ingesting his food, and at the same time his friends noticed skin lesions appearing over his neck, face, and arms. His friends called his mother, who was in an adjacent room, to see him. The patient was sitting on the floor with friends by the time his mother arrived. He told his mother, "I feel a little weak and lightheaded."

**Past Medical History:** None. No history of anaphylactic reactions.

**Past Surgical History:** Tonsillectomy at age 5.

**Medications:** None.

**Allergies:** Ragweed causes sneezing, runny nose, and itchy eyes.

**Vaccinations:** Up to date.

**Development History:** Patient's height has been in the 90th percentile since 2 years old. His weight has been above the 95th percentile for the past 3 years. He is considered obese for his age group. He likes to play video games nonstop while eating chips and soda. He also likes to ride his bike with his father on the weekends.

**Family History:** Father, age 38, has seasonal allergies. Mother, age 37, is healthy.

**Review of Systems:**

General: See HPI
Skin: See HPI
HEENT: Negative
Musculoskeletal: Negative
Cardiorespiratory: Negative
Gastrointestinal: See HPI
Genitourinary: Negative
Neuropsychiatric: See HPI

Day 1 @ 14:35

**Physical Examination:**

HEENT/Neck: No swelling of the lips, tongue, or uvula.

Chest/Lungs: Tachypnea. Chest wall normal. Diaphragm and chest moving equally and symmetrically with respiration. No expiratory wheezes. No audible stridor.

Heart/Cardiovascular: Tachycardia. S1, S2 normal. No murmurs, rubs, gallops, or extra sounds. No JVD.

Skin: Discrete wheals located over the face and neck. White-to-pink color annular lesions over the arms. Erythematous serpiginous lesions over the legs. White oval round lesions over the trunk and back.

**First Order Sheet:**

1) Epinephrine, IM, one time    **Note:** Epinephrine injected in the upper thigh.

**Second Order Sheet:**

1) IV access
2) Continuous cardiac monitor, stat    **Result:** Sinus tachycardia

3) Continuous blood pressure cuff, stat    **Result:** 88/68 mm Hg
4) Pulse oximetry, stat    **Result:** 97%
5) EKG, 12-lead, stat    **Result:** Sinus tachycardia. Other findings: WNL

**Third Order Sheet:**

1) Normal saline solution, 0.9% NaCl, IV, one time/bolus
2) Urine output, stat, q1 hour
3) Diphenhydramine, IV, one time
4) Methylprednisolone, IV, one time

**Physical Examination:**

Abdomen: Normal bowel sounds; no bruits. No tenderness. No masses. No hepatosplenomegaly.

Extremities/Spine: No joint deformity or warmth. No cyanosis or clubbing. No edema. Peripheral pulses 1+ (diminished). Spine exam normal.

Neuro/Psych: Alert; normal neurologic exam.

**Fourth Order Sheet:**

1) Vital signs, stat    **Result:** 37°C, HR: 100, RR: 30, BP: 90/70 mm Hg

**Note:** Approximately 15 minutes has elapsed since the last dose of epinephrine.

**Fifth Order Sheet:**

1) Epinephrine, IM, one time    **Note:** Epinephrine injected in the lower thigh.

**Actions:**

1) Reevaluate case: In 10 minutes

**Sixth Order Sheet:**

1) Vital signs, stat    **Result:** 37°C, HR: 92, RR: 26, BP: 115/74 mm Hg

**Seventh Order Sheet:**

1) Normal saline solution, 0.9% NaCl, IV, continuous
2) Pediatric allergy medicine consult    **Reason:** Anaphylactic reaction to unknown substance, please evaluate with skin testing.

**Urine output is now available**    **Result:** 135 mL/hr

**Physical Examination:**

1) **Skin:**    Resolving skin lesions.
2) **Extremities/Spine:**    Peripheral pulses 2+ (normal).

**Follow-Up History:**
Patient feels better. No more lightheadedness or abdominal pain.

**Actions:**
1) Change location to ICU

**Note:** Vitals are automatically ordered as q4 hrs in the practice CCS.

**This case will end in the next few minutes of "real time."**
You may **add** or **delete** orders at this time,
then enter a diagnosis on the following screen.

**Eighth Order Sheet:**
1) Counsel patient on using epi pen
2) Advise patient, exercise
3) Allergy skin test, routine

Future date: In 30 days

**Result:** Cutaneous reaction to Yellow 5 Lake

**Please enter your diagnosis:**

Anaphylaxis

**DISCUSSION:**
**Anaphylaxis is a medical emergency.** It is typically caused by re-exposure to an allergen that results in cross-linking of the IgE on presensitized mast cells and basophils, with subsequent release of various substances (eg, histamine, tryptase, chymase, heparin, platelet-activating factor, leukotrienes, prostaglandins, IL-4, IL-13).

**Anaphylactic Triggers:**

Food (nuts, egg, milk, shellfish, fish, soybeans, seeds, wheat, sulfites), food additives (coloring, emulsifiers, enhancers), Hymenoptera stings, bugs, latex, venom, vaccines, meds (NSAIDs, beta-lactam antibiotics, TMP-SMX, hormones), radiocontrast materials

**Clinical Features:**

The signs and symptoms of anaphylaxis are usually sudden, with manifestations appearing within minutes to <1 hour, although a delayed presentation (several hours) can sometimes be seen. The course of anaphylaxis is typically uniphasic (occurs only once), although a biphasic course (occurring again after the initial event) or protracted course (a prolonged event of hours to days) can occur. In some cases, a fatal reaction can occur with symptoms appearing within 25 minutes and death within the first hour. The clinical manifestations can vary, and it may be helpful to consider them in a relative head to toe fashion:

**Neurologic**—Anxiety (feeling of impending doom), dizziness, or headache

**Eyes**—Swelling (angioedema), tearing, conjunctival injection or pruritus

**Oral**—Metallic taste, swelling of the lips, tongue, or uvula

**Respiratory**—Dyspnea, cough, hoarseness, wheezing, audible stridor, feeling of throat closure, rhinorrhea, nasal congestion, sneezing, or shortness of breath

**Cardiovascular**—Hypotension, lightheadedness (secondary to low BP), syncope, weakness, chest tightness, chest pain, palpitations, dysrhythmia, or tachycardia

**GI**—Nausea, vomiting, abdominal cramps, bloating, or diarrhea

**GU**—Urinary incontinence, cramps

**Skin**—Flushing, angioedema (soft-tissue swelling), warmth, pruritus, or urticaria, which can take different shapes due to the confluence and resolution of the lesions, which are intensely pruritic.

**Next Step Summary:**

**Step 1)** Anaphylaxis is a true medical emergency, and you need to act quickly because fatalities do occur. The best initial step is to assess the **A**irway, **B**reathing, and **C**irculation. Securing the airway should be the top priority, and intubation should be performed immediately if there is audible stridor or respiratory distress or arrest. In our case, the physical exam revealed no tongue swelling or stridor on the initial assessment. If the skin exam reveals an inciting antigen (eg, stinger), remove it right away or remove the offending substance. Notice that we did not need to do the full exam in the beginning of the case. You can do the rest of the exam while you're waiting to see if the patient responds to the epinephrine. The patient should also be in the supine position with the legs elevated (unless the patient is vomiting or in respiratory distress) to facilitate perfusion of the vital organs.

**Step 2)** Anaphylaxis is a clinical diagnosis. Look for a history of exposure to an inciting substance. Also, patients may have a combination of organ-system involvement (eg, respiratory, cutaneous, cardiovascular, or GI). Patients with food-induced anaphylaxis tend to have more GI involvement as in this case. Since anaphylaxis is a clinical diagnosis, laboratory studies are usually not required.

**Step 3)** Treatment of anaphylaxis can be broken down to first-line and second-line treatments. Consider the following:

**First-line Treatments**

**Epinephrine**—Rapid administration of epinephrine should be one of the first things you do. Epinephrine can be given subcutaneously (SubQ) or intramuscularly (IM). The preferred route of administration is **intramuscularly** because it provides faster absorption compared to SubQ. The way to think about anaphylaxis and an easy way to remember this is to "Stick it in **IM**!" The ideal injection site is the mid-outer thigh rather than the deltoid because it provides more effective peak levels of the drug. In our case, the injection site was in the upper thigh where you have to penetrate through more fat to get to the muscle, especially in an obese patient. Therefore, the patient partially responded to the first injection. Ideally, in an obese patient, the injection site should be in the lower half of the thigh or even in the calf muscle where there is better access to muscular tissue. Epinephrine injections can be given every 5 to 15 minutes. Epinephrine infusion should be considered in patients that do not respond adequately (usually after the third injection) to IM epinephrine.

**Oxygen**—Provide oxygen to maintain an $SaO_2$ of >90%.

**Fluids**—Isotonic (0.9% NaCl) saline solution should be given as a bolus and repeated as necessary. Massive fluid shifts from intravascular to the extravascular space do occur in anaphylaxis. Be sure to monitor the urine output when giving fluids. In our case, the patient was producing an adequate amount of urine. Children with oliguria will typically make less than 1 to 2 mL/kg/hr.

### Second-line Treatments

**Glucocorticoids**—IV methylprednisolone, IV hydrocortisone, or PO prednisone are acceptable choices. Glucocorticoids do not have an immediate effect on anaphylaxis, but the rationale for giving steroids is to prevent a biphasic or protracted anaphylactic course. Tapering is usually not required.

**Antihistamines**—Antihistamines are considered adjunctive therapy to epinephrine. $H_1$ antihistamines (eg, diphenhydramine, cetirizine, hydroxyzine, promethazine) relieve itching and urticaria. $H_2$ antihistamines (eg, ranitidine, cimetidine) can be given in conjunction with an $H_1$ antihistamine, but it is not required.

**Bronchodilators**—Nebulized albuterol is typically given to patients who are wheezing. It is considered an adjunctive therapy to epinephrine.

**Step 4)** Prior to discharge, the patient and family members should be educated on how to administer self-injectable epinephrine and when to inject the medication (ie, emergency action plan).

**Step 5)** Patients should have allergy skin testing 4 to 6 weeks following the episode. In our case, the inciting antigen was the yellow food coloring in the cake, Yellow 5 Lake (also known as tartrazine).

### Disposition:

Patients who had airway intervention, severe anaphylaxis (ie, cardiovascular or respiratory issues), or patients who do not respond promptly to epinephrine should be transferred to the ICU for further monitoring. However, patients who initially respond immediately to epinephrine can be observed in the ED for several hours and then safely discharged home.

### Pearls:

- Approximately 90% of patients with anaphylaxis will have some type of skin manifestations, while 10% of patients may not have any skin findings at all.

- A reference for low systolic blood pressure in children that are 11 to 17 years old is a systolic blood pressure (SBP) <90 mm Hg.

- **Caveat 1**—Care must be taken when administering vaccines in patients with egg allergies. Vaccines that are egg protein based are influenza, yellow fever, MMR, and rabies.

- **Caveat 2**—Care must be taken when giving the appropriate diluted epinephrine solution. When giving epinephrine as IM or SubQ, the diluted solution should be 1:1000. When giving epinephrine as IV, the diluted solution should be more diluted to 1:10,000 which makes sense because you are injecting it directly into the blood. If you give a 1:1000 solution in the IV form, the patient may have arrhythmias, chest pain, MI, sharp rise in BP, and even a cerebral hemorrhage.

- **Caveat 3**—Patients may require a second vasopressor (eg, dobutamine) to support the blood pressure, but remember to have continuous monitoring.

- **Caveat 4**—Patients who are on beta-blocker therapy may have a reduced bronchodilator response to the beta-adrenergic effects of epinephrine (ie, beta$_2$ agonist effects).

- **Caveat 5**—Caution is warranted in two types of patients that are taking beta-blockers. First, patients that are given epinephrine can develop **hypertension** secondarily to an unopposed alpha-adrenergic effect of epinephrine (ie, alpha$_1$ agonist effect). Second, patients may have refractory anaphylaxis that is poorly responsive to epinephrine and fluids. In such cases, patients will actually be **hypotensive** and the next best step is to give IV glucagon as a bolus (over 3 to 5 minutes). If there is no response, another dose can be given as a bolus or followed by an IV infusion. Glucagon provides chronotropic and inotropic effects on the heart.

- Serum sickness is a type III hypersensitivity reaction that results from exposure to a foreign antigen or serum. One to two weeks after exposure to the inciting agent (eg, medications), patients can develop fever (which usually precedes skin findings), malaise, skin manifestations (eg, rash, edema, papules, palpable purpura), polyarthralgias, headaches, blurred vision, lymphadenopathy, or GI complaints (eg, nausea, vomiting, cramps, abdominal pain, diarrhea, bloating). Once the causative agent is removed, symptoms usually resolve within two weeks.

- Arthus reaction is a type III hypersensitivity reaction that results from local intradermal injection of foreign antigen into the skin. Several hours later, patients can develop swelling, induration, and hemorrhage followed occasionally by necrosis. On light microscope, fibrinoid necrosis of a vessel can sometimes be seen.

- **Foundational point**—The effects of epinephrine include alpha1 agonist (vasoconstriction, ↓ mucosal edema), beta$_1$ agonist (↑ heart rate, ↑ cardiac contractility), and beta$_2$ agonist (bronchodilation) effects.

- **Foundational point**—The four types of hypersensitivity reactions can be remembered by the mnemonic **ACID**:

**Type I**—**A**naphylaxis or **A**llergy

    **Mediator:** Antibody (IgE)

    **Antigen:** Soluble (exogenous)

    **MOA:** Antigen binds to IgE on presensitized mast cells and basophils

    **End result:** Release of vasoactive substances

    **Reaction onset:** Immediate

**Examples:** Asthma, anaphylaxis, allergic rhinitis, allergic conjunctivitis, urticaria, food allergy, drug allergies (eg. urticarial rash), atopic dermatitis

### Type II—Cytotoxic

**Mediator:** Antibody (IgG, IgM)

**Antigen:** Cell surface (Note: Drugs can bind to cell surfaces and act as antigens.)

**MOA:** Antibodies bind to antigens on cell surfaces

**End result:** Cell lysis (via MAC) or susceptible to phagocytosis (via opsonization)

**Reaction onset:** Minutes to days

**Examples:** Hemolytic anemia, Rh incompatibility (erythroblastosis fetalis), ITP, blood transfusion reactions, Grave's disease, Goodpasture's syndrome, drug reactions (eg, hemolytic anemia, thrombocytopenia, neutropenia), rheumatic fever, myasthenia gravis, pernicious anemia, pemphigus vulgaris, bullous pemphigoid, vasculitides

### Type III—Immune Complex

**Mediator:** Antibody (IgG, IgM)

**Antigen:** Soluble (exogenous or endogenous)

**MOA:** If antigen circulates in blood, an antibody-antigen complex can form, resulting in immune complex deposition into vessel walls or tissues with subsequent complement activation leading to an inflammatory reaction. If antigen is locally injected into tissue, an antibody-antigen complex can form, resulting in complement activation and an ensuing local inflammatory response.

**End result:** Inflammatory reaction. A systemic inflammatory response can result in **serum sickness**, while a local inflammatory response results in the **Arthus reaction**.

**Reaction onset:** Serum sickness occurs within weeks, but earlier (within days) if the patient was previously exposed to the inciting agent. Arthus reaction occurs within hours (peaks at 4 to 10 hours).

**Examples:** SLE, rheumatoid arthritis, post-streptococcal glomerulonephritis, infective endocarditis, polyarteritis nodosa, Farmer's lung, serum sickness, Arthus reaction, drug reactions (eg, drug fever), Henoch-Schönlein purpura, arthritis, glomerulonephritis, vasculitides

### Type IV—Delayed Hypersensitivity

**Mediators:** Not antibody mediated, but rather CD4 T cells (mainly $T_H1$ cells) and CD8 T cells (also known as cytotoxic T cells)

**Antigen:** Antigen presented by antigen-presenting cells (APC) on MHC class II molecules or on MHC class I molecules

**MOA:** CD4 T cells interact with MHC class II molecules that stimulate T cells to secrete cytokines and chemokines. CD8 T cells interact with MHC class I molecules that triggers the T cell to directly kill the target cell. (Note: MHC molecules are encoded by the **HLA** [Human Leukocyte Antigen] genes.)

**End result:** CD4 T cells trigger an inflammatory response with macrophages as the dominant cell type recruited to the site. CD8 T cells directly cause tissue damage.

**Reaction onset:** Delayed, usually after many hours to even weeks after exposure. PPD reaction peaks 48 to 72 hours after injection.

**Examples:** PPD reaction, type 1 diabetes, contact dermatitis (eg, poison ivy), Hashimoto's thyroiditis morbilliform/maculopapular eruptions, Steven-Johnson syndrome, toxic epidermal necrolysis, drug reactions (eg, drug rash), allograft rejection, graft versus host disease, granulomatous inflammation (eg, Crohn's disease, sarcoidosis, schistosomiasis, leprosy, TB)

- **On the CCS,** do not assume that any orders will be written for you (eg, vitals) during the CCS cases.
- **On the CCS,** "allergy skin test" is available in the practice CCS.
- **On the CCS,** "counsel patient, use of epi pen" is available in the practice CCS.
- **On the CCS,** you cannot order fluids as a bolus in the practice CCS, but rather in the continuous mode of frequency.
- **On the CCS,** timing is very important in anaphylaxis. Suboptimal management would include delaying treatment (eg, ordering an ABG if the patient really needs to be intubated or ordering a chest x-ray when the patient really needs epinephrine, STAT).
- **On the CCS,** poor management would include failure to monitor the patient (eg, urine output, pulse oximetry, physical exams, cardiac monitor, BP, HR, RR, or locate to a monitored setting).
- **On the CCS,** remember to "bridge" your therapy by addressing any acute issues (eg, securing airway, anaphylaxis) with the long-term management of anaphylaxis (eg, allergy skin testing, instructions on how and when to use epinephrine).

# 2

# Biostatistics

# MEASURES OF DIAGNOSTIC TEST PERFORMANCE

## SENSITIVITY

Sensitivity is the ability of a test to detect disease. The higher the sensitivity of a diagnostic test (eg, 99%), the more likely it will test positive for the disease with fewer false negative results (see Table 2-1).

$$\frac{\text{True Positives (a)}}{\text{True Positives (a)} + \text{False Negatives (c)}}$$

Table 2-1 • Measures of Diagnostic Test Performance

|  | Disease | No Disease |  |
|---|---|---|---|
| Positive Test | True positives (a) | False positives (b) | → PPV = a/a + b |
| Negative Test | False negatives (c) | True negatives (d) | → NPV = d/d + c |
|  | ↓ Sensitivity = a/a + c | ↓ Specificity = d/d + b |  |

## SPECIFICITY

Specificity is the ability of a test to detect the absence of disease. The higher the specificity of a diagnostic test (eg, 99%), the more likely it will test negative for the disease with fewer false positive results (see Table 2-1).

$$\frac{\text{True Negatives (d)}}{\text{True Negatives (d)} + \text{False Positives (b)}}$$

## POSITIVE PREDICTIVE VALUE

The positive predictive value (PPV) is the probability or likelihood that a person who tested positive for the disease truly does have the disease. The higher the PPV, the more likely the person has the disease (see Table 2-1).

$$\frac{\text{True Positives (a)}}{\text{True Positives (a)} + \text{False Positives (b)}}$$

## NEGATIVE PREDICTIVE VALUE

The negative predictive value (NPV) is the probability or likelihood that a person who tested negative for the disease truly does not have the disease. The higher the NPV, the more likely the person does not have the disease (see Table 2-1).

$$\frac{\text{True Negatives (d)}}{\text{True Negatives (d)} + \text{False Negatives (c)}}$$

# MEASURES OF DISEASE FREQUENCY

## INCIDENCE

The number of new cases of disease in a population at risk within a specified time period.

$$\frac{\text{Number of \textbf{new} cases in a specified time period}}{\text{Number of people at risk during that time period}}$$

## PREVALENCE

Prevalence is the total number of cases, including new and old, at a given point of time or a specified time period in a population at risk during that time.

$$\frac{\text{Number of \textbf{all} cases at a specific point of time or interval of time}}{\text{Number of people at risk during that time}}$$

# MEASURES OF QUALITY

## RELIABILITY

Reliability (ie, reproducibility) refers to a test's ability to measure something consistently. In other words, can a test reproduce the same result repeatedly?

## VALIDITY

Validity (ie, trueness) refers to a test's ability to measure the true intended goal. In other words, did a test measure what it claimed to measure?

# STUDY DESIGN

## ▌PROSPECTIVE STUDY

Prospective studies are forward-looking studies that follow subjects over time to look for a particular outcome.

## ▌RETROSPECTIVE STUDY

Retrospective studies are backward-looking studies in which researchers try to learn what factors may have been associated with the disease or condition.

## ▌DESCRIPTIVE STUDIES

Descriptive studies describe accounts of a particular situation, individual, or group (somewhat like a documentary). Descriptive studies do not try to answer a particular question (and therefore require no comparison groups) but rather to bring a particular event to attention in the medical literature.

### Case Report

A case report is a detailed report (with clinical presentation, diagnosis, treatment, and follow-up) that usually describes an unusual medical occurrence from a single clinical event. Case reports may be the first clue in identifying a new disease or adverse effect from a type of exposure.

### Case Series

A case series is a group or series of case reports that describe patients with an outcome of interest (eg, an aspect of a condition or reaction to a treatment). However, there are no comparative or control groups.

## ▌OBSERVATIONAL ANALYTIC STUDIES

Observational studies observe patients for a particular outcome, but no attempt is made to affect the outcome. Unlike descriptive studies, observational studies typically use comparison groups.

### Cohort Study

Cohort study observes a group of subjects (two or more) with a particular exposure of interest (eg, exposed vs. nonexposed) and follows these cohorts for a particular outcome of interest. Data can be collected **prospectively** or **retrospectively** (ie, from past medical records). **Relative risk** is used to calculate the risk.

### Case-Control Study

A case-control study compares a group of people with a specific disease (cases) with a group of people without the disease (control). Researchers look at the outcome of interest and then work backward to the exposure of interest (the opposite of cohort study). Case-control study is performed **retrospectively** and utilizes the **odds ratio** to provide an estimate of the risk.

### Cross-Sectional Study

Cross-sectional studies provide a "snapshot" or observation of a population at a given point in time. Both exposure and outcome of interest are determined simultaneously.

## ▌EXPERIMENTAL STUDIES

Experimental studies use comparison groups (experimental vs control group) and intervene in the studies to answer a particular question.

### Randomized Controlled Trial

A randomized controlled trial (RCT) is a prospective study that randomly assigns participants to a treatment group or placebo control group. In **single-blind studies**, only the researcher knows which group of subjects are "tested" but not the subjects. In **double-blind studies**, both researcher and subjects are unaware of which group the subjects are placed in. In this sense, a double-blind study provides a higher level of scientific rigor and is considered the gold standard among study design. In general, randomized controlled trials reduce confounding variables.

## ▌LITERATURE REVIEW

A literature review is the process of reviewing, analyzing, and summarizing the available medical literature. There are several kinds of literature review.

### Meta-Analysis

Meta-analysis is the process of pooling several studies (usually RCTs) about the same subject to draw a single conclusion based on all the statistical results of the studies, which would yield a greater statistical power when compared to a single study alone. Meta-analysis can be thought of as one large trial rather than several smaller studies.

### Systematic Review

A systematic review is a comprehensive review that pools all the relevant information (published and unpublished studies) about a particular subject and draws a summary based on the information. The main difference between a meta-analysis and a systematic review is that systematic reviews do not use statistical analysis to combine all the studies. In effect, a systematic review can be viewed as a "qualitative perspective," while meta-analysis can be viewed as a "quantitative perspective."

## ▌HIERARCHY OF EVIDENCE

The various types of study design can be listed in order of the level of evidence they provide for a conclusion as follows:

1) Systematic reviews and meta-analysis (highest level of evidence)
2) Randomized controlled trials (double-blind studies provide a higher level of evidence than single-blind)
3) Cohort studies
4) Case-control studies
5) Case series
6) Case reports
7) Editorials (lowest level of evidence)

# PRINCIPLES OF RISK

## RELATIVE RISK

Relative risk (RR), or risk ratio, tells us the probable risk of a certain event happening in one group exposed to a factor compared to another group that is not exposed to the factor. Relative risk can be expressed as the incidence among the exposed group divided by the incidence of the unexposed group. Mathematically, it can also be expressed as $[a/(a+b)]/[c/(c+d)]$. Relative risk is typically interpreted relative to the number one. If the relative risk is greater than one, it usually means that exposure to the factor increases the risk of that event happening. If the relative risk is less than one, it means that exposure to the factor decreases the risk of that event happening. If the relative risk equals one, there is no difference or association between the two groups in terms of that event happening. Relative risk is typically used in prospective studies (cohort or clinical studies). Consider the following examples:

**Example 1**—A cohort study of exposure to cigarette smoke and the development of lung cancer.

|  | Disease (Lung Cancer) | No Disease | Total |
| --- | --- | --- | --- |
| Exposure (Smoke) | a = 20 | b = 10 | 30 |
| No Exposure | c = 5 | d = 25 | 30 |

**RR calculation:** $(20/30)/(5/30) = 4.0$

**Bottom line:** RR is greater than 1, which indicates there is a risk of developing lung cancer with smoke exposure.

**Example 2**—A randomized controlled trial looking at the mortality when comparing a new medical therapy vs a control group for the same medical condition.

|  | Death | Survival | Total |
| --- | --- | --- | --- |
| New Medical Therapy | a = 25 | b = 50 | 75 |
| Control | c = 50 | d = 25 | 75 |

**RR calculation:** $(25/75)/(50/75) = 0.5$

**Bottom line:** The risk of dying from the new medical treatment is 33% (25/75) and the risk of dying in the control group is 66% (50/75). The RR is less than 1, which indicates there is a decrease risk of death in the group treated with the new medical therapy.

## ODDS RATIO

The odds ratio (OR) tells us the odds of a certain event happening in one group compared to the odds of it occurring in another group. Mathematically, it can be expressed as **(a/b)/(c/d)** or

**ad/bc**. Similar to relative risk, odds ratio is interpreted relative to the number one. However, the relative risk cannot be used in case-control studies (ie, retrospective study), rather the odds ratio is calculated, which provides an estimate of the relative risk.

**Example 3**—A case-control study of patients with breast cancer (cases) and non–breast cancer patients (control) with exposure to heavy alcohol drinking.

|  | Breast Cancer | No Disease |
| --- | --- | --- |
| Exposure (Heavy EtOH) | a = 12 | b = 3 |
| No Exposure | c = 20 | d = 5 |

**OR calculation:** $(12 \times 5)/(3 \times 20) = 1.0$

**Bottom line:** OR = 1, which indicates that there is no difference in the odds of an event happening (ie, breast cancer) when comparing the two groups (cases vs controls).

## ATTRIBUTABLE RISK

Attributable risk (AR) is the difference in the rate of disease in exposed compared to an unexposed population.

(Incidence of disease in exposed) − (Incidence of disease in nonexposed)

## ABSOLUTE RISK REDUCTION

Absolute risk reduction (ARR), which is also known as excess risk or risk difference, looks at the difference between the control group's event rate (CER) and the experimental group's event rate (EER). Absolute risk reduction can be expressed as **CER − EER**, which is the same as $[c/(c+d)] - [a/(a+b)]$. ARR is used in randomized control trials.

**Example 4**—Using the data from example 2, what is the ARR?

**ARR calculation:** $(50/75) - (25/75) = 0.666 - 0.333 = 0.333$

**Bottom line:** The absolute risk reduction in using the new medical therapy is 33.3%.

**Example 5**—A randomized clinical trial demonstrated that a new NSAID on the market has lowered the number of cardiovascular events in patients with coronary heart disease from 100 per 1000 patients to 20 per 1000 patients. What is the ARR?

**ARR calculation:** $(100/1000) - (20/1000) = 0.1 - 0.02 = 0.08$

**Bottom line:** The absolute risk reduction with the new NSAID is 8%.

## RELATIVE RISK REDUCTION

Relative risk reduction (RRR) can viewed as the percent reduction in events in the treated group compared to the control group. Relative risk reduction can be expressed as

CER − EER/CER, which is the same as $[c/(c + d) − a/(a + b)]/c/(c + d)$, which is the same as $1 − [a/(a + b)]/[c/(c + d)]$, which is the same as 1 − relative risk. For board purposes, it is not important to know every single formula, but rather to understand that there is a risk reduction in a specific event when comparing two groups (eg, treated vs control). RRR is typically used in randomized control trials.

**Example 6**—Using the data from example 2, what is the RRR?

> **RRR calculation:** 1 − Relative Risk = 1 − 0.5 = 0.5

> **Bottom line:** The relative risk reduction in using the new medical therapy is 50%. Be aware that the relative risk reduction appears to show a greater magnitude of risk reduction compared to the absolute risk reduction seen in example 4. Ads will sometimes use the relative risk reduction as opposed to the ARR. An easy way to remember the difference is that "absolute" will give you absolute real values while "relative" is really just relative.

## NUMBER NEEDED TO TREAT

Number needed to treat (NNT) tells us the number of patients who need to be treated in order to prevent one bad outcome. The ideal NNT is when it equals one because everyone benefits with the treatment and no one improves with the control.

A higher NNT suggests that the therapy in question is probably not that good. NNT can be expressed as 1/absolute risk reduction.

**Example 7**—If the absolute risk reduction between medical therapy vs a control group for a specific medical condition is 50%. What is the NNT?

> **NNT calculation:** 1/0.5 = 2

> **Bottom line:** Need to treat 2 patients to prevent one bad outcome (which is not too bad).

## NUMBER NEEDED TO HARM

Number needed to harm (NNH) can be calculated in a similar fashion to NNT, but instead we are looking at harm as the outcome rather than benefit. A higher NNH suggest that the therapy in question is good because adverse events are not common, while a lower NNH suggests that adverse events are common.

**Example 8**—If abatacept causes severe headaches in 3 of 100 patients (ie, 3%), what is the NNH?

> **NNH calculation:** 1/0.03 = 33

> **Bottom line:** Need to treat 33 patients to cause one patient to have a severe headache.

# DATA INFERENCES

## NULL HYPOTHESIS

When you think of the word *null*, you should think of such words as *void*, *empty*, *absent*, or *nullify*. Therefore the null hypothesis ($H_0$) tells us that there is **no difference**, **no association**, or a void between two measured phenomena (eg, drug A showed no difference between the treatment group and control group). In the statistical world, we have to decide whether we should or should not reject the null hypothesis. Once we reach a level of statistical significance, then we can decide to either reject or accept the null hypothesis.

## ALTERNATIVE HYPOTHESIS

The alternative hypothesis ($H_1$) states that there is a **difference** or **association** between the two measured phenomena.

## TYPE I ERROR

Type 1 error (also known as alpha or $\alpha$) is when the null hypothesis is rejected even though the null hypothesis is true. The bottom line is that there really is **no difference** or **no association**, but we mistakenly concluded that there was an effect.

## TYPE II ERROR

Type II error (also known as beta or $\beta$) is failure to reject the null hypothesis when in fact the null hypothesis is false. The bottom line is that there really is a **difference** or **association**, but we mistakenly concluded that there was no effect. Beta errors typically reflect a low power in the study.

## POWER

Power (which equals 1 − beta) is the ability of a study to reject the null hypothesis when the null hypothesis is actually false, thereby not committing a type II error. The bottom line is that you are trying to demonstrate an association if one exists. Increasing sample size will increase your power, but if the sample size is too small, the study will not be able to detect a true difference between the groups.

## P-VALUE

P-value is the probability that any particular outcome would have occurred by chance. In scientific practice, we arbitrarily set the $p < 0.05$ as "statistically significant." In other words, there is less than 5% or less than 1 in 20 probability that the findings have occurred by chance alone.

# CONFIDENCE INTERVAL

Confidence interval (CI) does not imply how confident your results are, but rather a boundary of values in which the true parameter actually lies (eg, relative risk, odds ratio, absolute difference, mean). Confidence interval can be reported at any level of confidence (eg, 80%, 90%), but we usually report a 95% CI as a high probability that the true value will be found within those boundaries. A wider confidence interval usually indicates a greater degree of uncertainty and typically reflects a smaller sample size. A narrower confidence interval narrows down the boundary levels and typically reflects a larger sample size. Whenever the confidence interval overlaps the null value (eg, RR = 1, OR = 1), you need to be more skeptical because it suggests that there might be no effect or that there is no statistically difference between the groups studied, and therefore you may not be able to reject the null hypothesis.

# CORRELATION COEFFICIENT

The correlation coefficient (r) expresses the association between two variables with regard to direction and magnitude (ie, $-1$ to $+1$). An r value of $-1$ indicates the strongest possible negative relationship, an r value equal to zero indicates no relationship, and an r value of $+1$ indicates the strongest possible positive relationship between two variables. For example, a study between lung cancer and cigarettes sales demonstrated an r value of $+0.98$, which signifies a strong positive relationship between lung cancer and cigarette sales.

# 3

# Cardiology

## CHAPTER OUTLINE

## KEY FINDINGS REVIEW

**Murmurs**

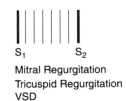

Mitral Stenosis
Tricuspid Stenosis

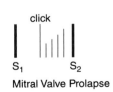

Mitral Regurgitation
Tricuspid Regurgitation
VSD

Mitral Valve Prolapse

Aortic Stenosis
Pulmonic Stenosis
HCM

Aortic Regurgitation
Pulmonic Regurgitation

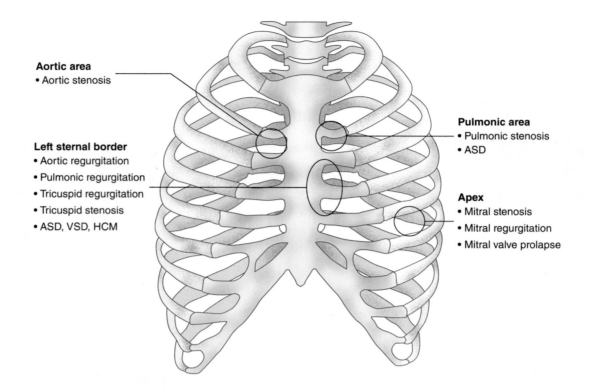

**Aortic area**
• Aortic stenosis

**Left sternal border**
• Aortic regurgitation
• Pulmonic regurgitation
• Tricuspid regurgitation
• Tricuspid stenosis
• ASD, VSD, HCM

**Pulmonic area**
• Pulmonic stenosis
• ASD

**Apex**
• Mitral stenosis
• Mitral regurgitation
• Mitral valve prolapse

### Heart Sounds

$S_1$—Normal mitral and tricuspid valve closure.

$S_2$—Normal aortic ($A_2$) and pulmonic ($P_2$) valve closure.

$S_3$—Rapid ventricular filling during early diastole. Normal in children and young adults, but suggestive of an enlarged ventricular chamber (eg, heart failure) in adults >40 years of age.

$S_4$—Late ventricular filling during late diastole, which corresponds to blood forced into a "stiffened" ventricle and can be seen in patients with HTN, aortic stenosis, or hypertrophic cardiomyopathy.

### $S_2$ Splits

Physiologic (normal) split—On inspiration, $A_2$ is separated from $P_2$. On expiration, $A_2$ and $P_2$ are fused as one sound.

Wide split—On inspiration, $A_2$ is more widely separated from $P_2$. On expiration, $A_2$ and $P_2$ are fused as one sound. This condition is seen in RBBB, WPW with preexcitation of the left ventricle, LV pacing, pulmonic stenosis, mitral regurgitation, pulmonary HTN with right-sided heart failure, VSD, and acute massive PE.

Fixed split—On inspiration and expiration, $A_2$ and $P_2$ are separated and unchanged throughout the respiratory cycle. This condition is commonly seen in ASD.

Paradoxical split—On inspiration, $A_2$ and $P_2$ are fused as one sound. On expiration, $P_2$ precedes $A_2$. This condition is seen in LBBB, WPW with preexcitation of the right ventricle, RV pacing, aortic stenosis, aortic regurgitation, HTN, PDA, and hypertrophic cardiomyopathy.

### Atrial Pressure Waveforms

a wave—An upward deflection produced by atrial contraction.

c wave—An upward deflection produced by mitral or tricuspid valve closure during ventricular contraction.

v wave—An upward deflection produced by atrial filling during ventricular contraction.

# PRESSURE DISORDER

## ▌HYPERTENSION

Hypertension can be categorized as either **primary (essential)** or **secondary hypertension**. Essential hypertension (no identifiable cause) accounts for approximately 95% of cases, and secondary hypertension (identifiable cause) accounts for 5%. In either case, hypertension is an important risk factor for the development of **strokes**, **heart attacks**, **heart failure**, and **kidney disease**.

Risk Factors for Essential HTN:

Obesity, weight gain, inactive lifestyle, excessive alcohol intake, high sodium intake, vitamin D deficiency, family history, older age, males, African Americans, stress, depression, dyslipidemia.

## Table 3-1 • Causes of Secondary Hypertension

| Disorder | Clinical Clues | Next Step Initial Approach |
|---|---|---|
| **Neurologic** | | |
| Sleep apnea | Loud snoring, fatigue, daytime somnolence | Sleep study |
| **Cardiovascular** | | |
| Coarctation of the aorta | **Coarctation after the left subclavian artery:**<br>• Elevated BP in the upper extremities compared to the lower extremities<br>• Radial-femoral pulse delay<br>**Coarctation before the left subclavian artery:**<br>• Elevated BP in the right arm compared to the left arm<br>• Delayed pulse in the left radial and femorals compared to the right radial artery | Transthoracic echocardiography (TTE) and a chest MRI or CT scan |
| **Renal** | | |
| Renovascular hypertension | Abdominal bruit, recurrent flash pulmonary edema, ↑ Cr levels after initiating an ACE inhibitor or ARB, atherosclerosis (older patients), fibromuscular dysplasia (young females), abrupt onset of severe HTN after 55 years of age, unexplained atrophic kidney, unprovoked hypokalemia | Since there is potential harm in radiologic testing, imaging studies are conducted only if there is a clinical suspicion for renovascular disease **and** a corrective procedure would be performed if renovascular disease was detected. **Renal arteriography** is considered the gold standard for diagnosis, but it is an invasive test. Less invasive testing may be considered prior to renal arteriography, and that may include any of the following:<br>• Duplex ultrasound<br>• CT angiography (CTA)<br>• MR angiography (MRA) |
| Primary renal disease | Elevated creatinine level, abnormal urinalysis | Evaluate for vascular disease (eg, vasculitis), glomerular disease (eg, infections, autoimmune disease), tubulointerstitial disease (eg, obstruction), cystic disease (eg, polycystic kidney disease), or chronic kidney disease (estimated GFR). |
| **Endocrine** | | |
| Cushing's syndrome | Moon facies, central obesity, buffalo hump, muscle weakness | Dexamethasone suppression test and a 24-hour urine free cortisol level |
| Pheochromocytoma | Diaphoresis, palpitations, headaches, sense of "impending doom" | 24-hour urinary metanephrine or catecholamine |
| Primary aldosteronism | Hypokalemia, metabolic alkalosis | Plasma renin level or activity (low)<br>Plasma aldosterone (high)<br>Aldosterone/renin ratio (high) |
| Hypothyroidism | Cold intolerance, weight gain, coarse hair | TSH (high) |
| Hyperthyroidism | Heat intolerance, weight loss, fine hair | TSH (low) |
| Primary hyperparathyroidism | "Bones, stones, abdominal groans, and psychic moans" | Serum calcium (high)<br>PTH (high) |

## Clinical Features:

The majority of hypertensive patients will be asymptomatic on routine screening. Patients with secondary HTN will have clinical features based on their specific etiology (see Table 3-1). At some point, chronic elevations in blood pressures can result in end-organ damage. The following are targets of end-organ damage (from head to toe):

**Neurologic**—Strokes, TIA, dementia

**Eyes**—Hemorrhages, microaneurysms, cotton-wool spots, exudates, papilledema, arteriovenous nicking, copper wiring

**Cardiac**—Heart failure, LVH, MI

**Renal**—Renal failure, nephrosclerosis

**Vascular**—Peripheral arterial disease, arteriosclerosis, aneurysm, dissection

## Next Step:

**Step 1)** After an initial blood pressure screen, patients should have ≥2 follow-up visits (spaced over one or more weeks) to obtain the average of ≥2 blood pressure readings to classify the blood pressure severity based on the JNC 7. The following are for adults 18 years and older. If there is a disparity between the systolic and diastolic pressures, the higher number is used to determine the severity of the hypertension.

>    **Normal BP:** systolic <120 Hg **and** diastolic <80 mm Hg
>
>    **Pre-HTN:** systolic 120 to 139 mm Hg **or** diastolic 80 to 89 mm Hg
>
>    **Stage 1 HTN:** systolic 140 to 159 mm Hg **or** diastolic 90 to 99 mm Hg
>
>    **Stage 2 HTN:** systolic ≥160 mm Hg **or** diastolic ≥100 mm Hg

**Step 2)** Patients with normal blood pressures can be followed up in 2 years, and patients that have prehypertension should be counseled about lifestyle modification (see step 4) and have a follow-up visit in 1 year. Patients diagnosed with hypertension should be evaluated for end-organ damage, to identify possible secondary causes of HTN (see Table 3-1), and to identify cardiovascular risk factors, which is based on the JNC 7:

- Age (men >55, women >65)
- Family history of premature cardiovascular disease (men <55, women <65)
- ↑ LDL (or total), or ↓ HDL
- Estimated GFR <60 mL/min
- Microalbuminuria
- Diabetes mellitus
- Obesity
- Weight gain
- Hypertension
- Tobacco use, particularly cigarettes

**Step 3)** Extensive testing for secondary hypertension is not recommended unless the clinical clues suggest the presence of secondary hypertension. However, the initial workup for all hypertensive patients should include the following:

- CBC (hematocrit)
- Blood chemistries ($K^+$, $Ca^{2+}$, Cr, or estimated GFR)
- Fasting blood glucose or A1c
- Lipid profile (LDL, HDL, triglycerides)
- Urinalysis
- Microalbuminuria (mainly for diabetics)
- EKG

**Step 4)** Target blood pressures should be **<140/90 mm Hg** in all hypertensive patients and **<130/80 mm Hg** in patients with diabetes or renal disease. The best initial treatment approach is with lifestyle modification (either alone or in concert with medications) for at least 3 to 6 months. **Lifestyle modifications** include the following:

- **Weight loss**—For every 1 kg lost, there is a 0.5 to 2.0 mm Hg reduction in BP.
- **Diet**—Reduce sodium intake, adopt DASH diet (↑ fruits, ↑ vegetables, low-fat dairy)
- **Exercise**—At least 30 min/dy for most days of the week
- **Alcohol**—Limit 2 drinks/dy in men and 1 drink/dy in women
- **Smoking cessation**—To reduce cardiovascular risk, not necessarily BP

**Step 5)** Pharmacologic therapy is the next best step when patients continue to have elevated blood pressures (systolic ≥140 and/or diastolic ≥90) despite attempts with lifestyle modification. Pharmacologic therapy can be easily remembered in four broad categories by their "**A, B, C, Ds**" (**A**CE inhibitors, **A**RBs, **B**eta-blocker, **C**alcium channel blocker, **D**iuretics). For most patients, thiazide diuretics are used as initial therapy, but under special conditions (see Table 3-2), the other classes of antihypertensive agents are used as initial therapy. The following is the initial pharmacologic management for stages 1 and 2 hypertension:

>    **Stage 1 HTN:** Thiazide-type diuretic (eg, chlorthalidone or HCTZ)
>
>    **Stage 2 HTN:** Thiazide-type diuretic + "**A, B, or C**"

**Step 6)** After initiation of lifestyle modification and drug therapy, suboptimal control of hypertension can occur. Consider four different clinical scenarios:

>    **Drug initiation:** In a patient that does not respond to an adequate dose of a drug, switching to another first-line agent should be attempted rather than adding another agent. In a patient that has a partial response with a drug but target blood pressure is not achieved, either the dose may be titrated up to the next step or a low-dose agent of another drug can be added. The goal of therapy is to maximize the response from a drug, but to minimize the side effects with lower dosages.
>
>    **Pseudoresistant hypertension:** Pseudoresistant hypertension refers to patients that have poorly controlled hypertension that appears to be resistant to medical treatment. However, the hypertension is usually due to the following:

- "White coat" hypertension or office hypertension
- Noncompliance
- Poor BP measurement technique

>    **Pseudohypertension:** Pseudohypertension refers to patients that have an overestimation of their blood pressure readings because of the inability of the blood pressure cuff to adequately compress against a calcified or stiffened brachial artery. The elderly are particularly prone to this condition and are inadvertently being overdosed on antihypertensive agents resulting in orthostatic hypotension and other side effects.
>
>    **Resistant hypertension:** Resistant hypertension refers to patients that cannot meet target blood pressures despite the use of three different classes of antihypertensives (one of which should be a diuretic), or blood pressure that is controlled with ≥4 drugs. Important aspects to consider are reversible factors that are associated with elevated blood pressures:

>    **Lifestyle**—Physical inactivity, high salt intake, or heavy alcohol intake
>
>    **Suboptimal therapy**—Ineffective drugs, inadequate dosing, or inappropriate combinations
>
>    **Secondary HTN**—Identifiable secondary causes of hypertension (see Table 3-1)
>
>    **Medications**—Glucocorticoids, NSAIDs, COX-2 inhibitors, OCPs (mainly estrogen), decongestants, diet pills, erythropoietin, tacrolimus, cyclosporine,

## Table 3-2 • Antihypertensive Drug Profiles

| Drugs | Side Effects | Avoid in These Conditions | Preferred Agents in These Conditions | Agents Shown to be Beneficial (Based on Clinical Trials) in These Conditions |
|---|---|---|---|---|
| **ACEIs**<br>• Benazepril<br>• Captopril<br>• Lisinopril | Cough, angioedema, hyperkalemia, worsening renal function with RAS | • Pregnancy<br>• Intolerable cough<br>• Hx of angioedema<br>• Hyperkalemia<br>• Poor renal function | • Diabetes<br>• Systolic HF<br>• Diastolic HF<br>• Stable angina<br>• UA/NSTEMI<br>• STEMI<br>• LV dysfunction | • Diabetes<br>• HF<br>• Post-MI<br>• High coronary disease risk<br>• CKD<br>• Recurrent stroke prevention |
| **ARBs**<br>• Candesartan<br>• Losartan<br>• Valsartan | Angioedema, hyperkalemia, worsening renal function with RAS | • Pregnancy<br>• Hx of angioedema<br>• Hyperkalemia<br>• Poor renal function | • Intolerable cough from using ACEIs | • Diabetes<br>• HF<br>• CKD |
| **Beta-blockers**<br>• Atenolol<br>• Metoprolol<br>• Propranolol | Bradycardia, bronchospasm, fatigue, Raynaud's syndrome, masking hypoglycemic symptoms, associated with new-onset diabetes | • Asthma<br>• COPD<br>• 2° or 3° AV blocks<br>• Sick sinus syndrome<br>• Severe bradycardia<br>• Severe PAD<br>• Depression<br>• Raynaud's syndrome<br>• Uncompensated HF | • Atrial fibrillation<br>• Stable angina<br>• UA/NSTEMI<br>• STEMI<br>• LV dysfunction<br>• Hyperthyroidism<br>• Essential tremor<br>• Migraine<br>• Compensated HF | • Diabetes<br>• HF<br>• Post-MI<br>• High coronary disease risk |
| **CCBs**<br>Dihydropyridines<br>• Amlodipine<br>• Nifedipine<br>Nondihydropyri-<br>dines<br>• Diltiazem<br>• Verapamil | Dihydropyridines<br>• Peripheral edema<br>• Reflex tachycardia<br>Nondihydropyridines<br>• Peripheral edema<br>• AV blocks<br>• Bradycardia | Dihydropyridines<br>• Hypotension<br>• Post MI<br>• Systolic HF<br>Nondihydropyridines<br>• Hypotension<br>• 2° or 3° AV blocks<br>• Sick sinus syndrome<br>• WPW syndrome<br>• Systolic HF | **In all CCBs:**<br>• Bronchospastic disease when BBs would be contraindicated.<br>• Raynaud's syndrome<br>• Migraine<br>• Atrial fibrillation (only nondihydropyridines) | **In all CCBs:**<br>• Diabetes<br>• High coronary disease risk |
| **Diuretics**<br>Thiazides<br>• Chlorthalidone<br>• HCTZ<br>Loops<br>• Furosemide<br>• Bumetanide | Hypokalemia, hyperuricemia, hyperglycemia, increase in cholesterol | • Hypokalemia<br>• Gout<br>• Cautious use in diabetics<br>• Severe dyslipidemia | • Systolic HF<br>• Osteoporosis (only thiazides)<br>• Edema | • Diabetes<br>• HF<br>• High coronary disease risk<br>• Recurrent stroke prevention |
| **Aldosterone antagonists**<br>• Spironolactone | Hyperkalemia, gynecomastia, irregular menses | • Hyperkalemia<br>• Renal failure | • Primary aldosteronism<br>• Hypokalemia | • HF<br>• Post-MI |

*ACEIs—angiotensin converting enzyme inhibitors, ARBs—angiotensin receptor blockers, AV—atrioventricular, BBs—beta-blockers, CCBs—calcium channel blockers, CKD—chronic kidney disease, HCTZ—hydrochlorothiazide, HF—heart failure, Hx—history, LV—left ventricular, MI—myocardial infarction, NSTEMI—non-ST segment elevation MI, PAD—peripheral arterial disease, RAS—renal artery stenosis, STEMI—ST segment elevation MI, UA—unstable angina, WPW—Wolff-Parkinson-White*

carbamazepine, clozapine, antidepressants, methylphenidate, metoclopramide

**Illicit drugs**—Cocaine, amphetamines, anabolic steroids, PCP, ketamine, narcotic withdrawal

**Natural compounds**—Ephedra, ma huang, licorice, bitter orange

**Follow-Up:**

Once antihypertensive agents are initiated, patients should be seen at monthly intervals or until blood pressure goals are achieved. Thereafter, patients can be seen every 3 to 6 months. Serum potassium and creatinine levels should be checked at least 1 or 2 times per year.

**Pearls:**

- Prehypertension is not considered a disease category, but rather identifies those that are at risk of developing hypertension.

- Reduction in blood pressure is the major determinant in reducing cardiovascular risk, not the type of medication.

- Under the age of 50, the diastolic blood pressure is a better predictor of cardiovascular risk.

- After the age of 50, the systolic blood pressure becomes the better predictor of cardiovascular risk.

- In the presence of microalbuminuria, diabetics have an increased risk of cardiovascular disease.

- Hypertension can result in left ventricular hypertrophy (LVH), which is usually characterized by **concentric hypertrophy**. LVH is associated with cardiovascular risk, and regression of LVH (via weight loss, salt restriction, and ↓ BP) can lower the risk of a cardiovascular event.

- Blood pressure can rise transiently with each cigarette, but habitual smokers generally have lower blood pressures compared to nonsmokers. Smoking cessation should be advised for cardiovascular risk reduction, not to lower the blood pressure.

- African Americans respond particularly well to thiazides and calcium channel blockers, but less so with ACEIs and beta-blockers. However, ACEIs and beta-blockers should still be used under specific indications (eg, diabetes/ACEIs, post-MI/beta-blockers).

- Elderly patients respond well to thiazides and calcium channel blockers, but they do not tolerate aggressive diuretic or beta-blocker therapy.

- Alpha-blockers (eg, doxazosin, prazosin, terazosin) are not considered first-line antihypertensive drugs, especially since they are associated with an increased risk of heart failure. However, alpha-blockers can be considered in older hypertensive men with concurrent prostatism that are not at high cardiovascular risk. Alpha-blockers should be discontinued in patients that have postural hypotension, which is a side effect of the medication.

- Calcium channel blockers (ie, verapamil, diltiazem, nifedipine) are generally avoided in patients with coexisting systolic heart failure because these agents have negative inotropic properties. Patients with **S**ystolic heart failure have a **"Sissy"** heart or a weakened floppy/dilated heart that can't pump well, and giving a negative inotropic agent will cause further clinical deterioration. However, amlodipine and felodipine are better tolerated and appear safer since they have almost no negative inotropic properties. In patients that have systolic heart failure with coexisting angina or hypertension, a

beta-blocker or ACE inhibitor would be the preferred agents since they have been shown to improve survival.

- Treatment options for renovascular hypertension include antihypertensive medications, percutaneous transluminal renal angioplasty (PTRA) ± stent, or surgical revascularization. Although ACEIs and ARBs can worsen renal function (↓ GFR, ↑ Cr) in patients with renal artery stenosis (RAS), it is not a contraindication to use in RAS as long as the renal function is carefully monitored. In fact, ACEIs and ARBs are fairly effective in controlling hypertension in these patients, but therapy should be discontinued if creatinine levels rise significantly.

- **Foundational point**—Hypertension is associated with two types of vascular pathology, (1) hyaline arteriolosclerosis, which is more common in the elderly and in diabetics (vessels consist of hyaline thickening), and (2) hyperplastic arteriolosclerosis, which is associated with acute or severe elevations in blood pressures (vessels consist of an onion-skin, concentric thickening).

- **Foundational point**—Sarcomeres are arranged in parallel instead of in series in concentric hypertrophy.

- **Connecting point** (pg. 76)—Know the management of Cushing's syndrome.

- **Connecting point** (pg. 78)—Know the management of pheochromocytoma.

- **Connecting point** (pg. 72)—Know the management of hypothyroidism.

- **Connecting point** (pg. 68)—Know the management of hyperthyroidism.

- **Connecting point** (pg. 73)—Know the management of primary hyperparathyroidism.

- **Connecting point** (pg. 58)—Know the pattern of LVH on EKG.

- **On the CCS**, remember to "counsel" all your hypertensive patients.

- **On the CCS**, remember to encourage lifestyle modifications. The practice CCS does have "weight loss diet," "low sodium diet," "advise patient exercise program," "advise patient limit alcohol intake," and "advise patient no smoking."

- **On the CCS**, when you place a patient on an antihypertensive medication, be sure to select the "continuous" mode of frequency, which takes into account the periodic administration (eg, q6 hours).

- **On the CCS**, office-based cases will usually require you to relocate patients back home, therefore become comfortable relocating patients prior to your Step 3 exam.

# LIPID METABOLISM DISORDER

## HYPERLIPIDEMIA

Hyperlipidemia is characterized by elevated lipoprotein particles in the plasma. Total serum cholesterol consists of LDL (60%-70%), HDL (20%-30%), and VLDL (10%-15%).

Chylomicrons (formed from dietary fat) and VLDL are both triglyceride-rich lipoproteins. An increase in cholesterol levels, particularly LDL, is a significant risk factor for coronary heart disease (CHD).

**Modifiable Risk Factors:**

Smoking, overweight, obesity, physical inactivity, high-fat diet, diabetes, hypertension.

## Clinical Features:

Hyperlipidemic patients will be asymptomatic on routine screening. Accumulation of cholesterol is usually deposited in the vascular system (atherosclerosis), eyes, tendons, joints, or skin. Consider the possible clinical manifestations of hyperlipidemia, which can be due to acquired or familial disorders:

1) **Arcus senilis**—An opaque ring-like deposit on the peripheral cornea.

2) **Lipemia retinalis**—Retinal blood vessels that take on a creamy appearance.

3) **Xanthomas**—Yellowish plaques or nodules that can be seen over skin, tendons (tendinous xanthoma), joints (tuberous xanthoma), or the inner canthus of the eyelids (xanthelasma).

## Next Step:

**Step 1)** Patients should be screened with a fasting lipid profile (ie, total cholesterol, LDL, HDL, triglyceride). There are two different recommendations on screening, so be aware of both:

**Adult Treatment Panel (ATP) III**—Screening should occur in all persons ≥20 years of age at least every 5 years.

**US Preventive Services Task Force (USPSTF)**—Screening should occur in men ≥35 years of age. Women should be screened ≥45 years of age who are at risk for coronary heart disease (eg, smokers, obese, HTN, DM, Hx of CHD, family Hx of heart disease).

**Step 2)** Patients should have a risk assessment to help guide management. The following major risk factors for CHD should be counted:

1) **Age:** Men ≥45 years, women ≥55 years

2) **Family Hx of premature CHD:** Male first-degree relative <55 years, female first-degree relative <65 years

3) **Cigarette smoking**

4) **Hypertension:** ≥140/90 mm Hg or on antihypertensive medication

5) **Low HDL:** <40 mg/dL, but if HDL is ≥60 mg/dL then one risk factor is negated from the total count of risk factors.

**Step 3)** Identify patients that have established CHD (eg, MI, stable angina, unstable angina, Hx of coronary procedures) or CHD risk equivalents that are **not** part of the total count of risk factors in step 2. The following are **CHD risk equivalents:**

- Diabetes
- Abdominal aortic aneurysm (AAA)
- Peripheral arterial disease
- Carotid artery disease (ie, >50% stenosis or symptomatic patients such as strokes or TIAs that originate from the carotids)
- Renal artery disease due to atherosclerosis
- Multiple risk factors that confer a >20% risk of a CHD event in 10 years (You won't be able to calculate this on the boards since you need the Framingham risk tables.)

**Step 4)** Determine the **risk category** (see Table 3-3), which is based on the ATP III.

**Step 5)** Initiate therapeutic lifestyle changes (either alone or in concert with medications) for at least 3 months in patients that are not at LDL goal (see Table 3-3). **Therapeutic lifestyle changes (TLC)** includes the following: ↓ saturated fats, ↓ cholesterol, consider plant stanols/sterols and viscous fiber, ↑ physical activity, weight control.

**Step 6)** Consider adding a **lipid-lowering agent** if LDL is not at goal despite TLC. Statins are the preferred agents because they are the only class of drugs to show improvements in mortality for primary prevention (ie, prevent new onset CHD) and secondary prevention (ie, prevent recurrent CHD in a person with established CHD). However, consider the other classes of lipid lowering drugs in Table 3-4.

**Step 7)** Concerns may arise during the clinical management of hyperlipidemia. Consider four different clinical scenarios:

**Myopathy**—Myopathy can occur after the initiation of statins. Manifestations of myopathy can range from myalgias (± creatine kinase elevations) to myositis or to rhabdomyolysis (± acute renal failure from the myoglobinuria). Patients that are susceptible to statin-induced myopathy are those with liver disease, renal disease, hypothyroidism, or concomitant use with other drugs (eg, azole antifungals,

### Table 3-3 • Clinical Management of the Different Risk Categories

| Risk Category | Goal LDL (mg/dL) | INITIATE TLC Based on the LDL Level | CONSIDER Drug Therapy Based on the LDL Level (After TLC) |
|---|---|---|---|
| 0-1 Risk factor | <160 | ≥160 | ≥190 |
| 2+ Risk factors | <130 | ≥130 | ≥160 (if 10-year risk <10%)[a] <br> ≥130 (if 10-year risk 10%-20%)[a] |
| CHD or CHD risk equivalent (10-year risk >20%)[a] | <100 <br> <70 (Optional for very high risk)[b] | ≥100 | ≥130 (**Initiate** drug therapy + TLC) <br> 100-129 (Consider drug therapy) |

[a]The percent risk of a CHD event in 10 years requires the Framingham risk tables, which you probably won't be able to calculate on the boards, but it is good to be aware of the LDL ranges.
[b]Very high risk patients include those that have coronary heart disease (CHD) + DM, CHD + acute coronary syndrome, CHD + metabolic syndrome, or CHD + poorly controlled risk factors (eg, persistent smoking)

**Table 3-4 • Lipid-lowering Drug Profiles**

| Drugs | Major Indications | Lipid Effects | Side Effects | Avoid in These Conditions |
|---|---|---|---|---|
| **HMG CoA reductase inhibitors (statins)**<br>• Atorvastatin<br>• Fluvastatin<br>• Simvastatin<br>• Rosuvastatin | To lower LDL (Considered first-line agents in LDL reduction) | LDL ↓↓<br>HDL ↑<br>TG ↓ | • Myopathy<br>• ↑ Transaminases | Pregnancy (Category X), breast-feeding, active or chronic liver disease, unexplained persistent ↑ in transaminases, or coadministration with macrolides (eg, erythromycin), antifungals (eg, itraconazole), HIV protease inhibitors (eg, telaprevir), or cyclosporine<br><br>**Precautions:**<br>• Caution with concomitant use with nicotinic acid or fibrates |
| **Bile acid sequestrants (resins)**<br>• Cholestyramine<br>• Colestipol<br>• Colesevelam | To lower LDL | LDL ↓<br>HDL ↑<br>TG ↑ or no effect | • Abdominal pain<br>• Bloating<br>• Nausea<br>• Constipation | Biliary obstruction, elevated triglycerides >200 mg/dL<br><br>**Precautions:**<br>• Resins can interfere with absorption of warfarin, digoxin, and fat-soluble vitamins; however, they can be taken 1 hour before or 4 hours after administration of the resin. |
| **Nicotinic acid (niacin)** | Favorable effects on all lipids, but long-term use is limited by side effects | LDL ↓<br>HDL ↑<br>TG ↓ | • Flushing<br>• Pruritus<br>• Acanthosis nigricans<br>• Hyperpigmentation<br>• Hyperglycemia<br>• Hyperuricemia<br>• Gout<br>• ↑ Transaminases<br>• ↓ Platelets<br>• Peptic ulcer | Active or chronic liver disease, severe gout, unexplained persistent ↑ in transaminases, arterial hemorrhage, or active peptic ulcer<br><br>**Precautions:**<br>• Cautious use in diabetics<br>• Caution with concomitant use with statins (rhabdomyolysis)<br>• Flushing and pruritus can be attenuated if aspirin or NSAID is taken 30 minutes before dosing |
| **Fibrates**<br>• Gemfibrozil<br>• Fenofibrate | To lower TG | LDL ↓<br>HDL ↑<br>TG ↓↓ | • Dyspepsia<br>• Cholelithiasis<br>• Myopathy<br>• Hepatitis | Severe renal or hepatic disease, gallbladder disease, PBC, and repaglinide should not be used concurrently with gemfibrozil<br><br>**Precautions:**<br>• Caution with concomitant use with statins (rhabdomyolysis)<br>• Caution with concomitant use with sulfonylureas (hypoglycemia)<br>• Caution with concomitant use with warfarin (↑ anticoagulation) |
| **Cholesterol inhibitor**<br>• Ezetimibe | To lower LDL | LDL ↓<br>HDL ↑<br>TG ↓ | • ↑ Transaminases<br>• Upper respiratory infections | Unexplained persistent ↑ in transaminases, or active liver disease plus coadministration with a statin |

*LDL—low density lipoprotein, HDL—high-density lipoprotein, PBC—primary biliary cirrhosis, TG—triglyceride*

macrolides, HIV protease inhibitors, cyclosporine, gemfibrozil). Patients that complain of muscle weakness, brown urine, or muscle pain should be advised to call their physician. A creatine kinase should be obtained to document the myopathy, and discontinuation of the statin is recommended if myopathy is suspected.

**Statin-induced transaminase elevations**—Patients should have a baseline LFT prior to initiating a statin. If patients develop an increase in transaminases after starting a statin, a repeat LFT should be obtained to confirm the elevation and then monitored frequently until the LFTs normalize. Statins should be discontinued if the AST/ALT is persistently elevated 3 times the upper limit of normal.

**Metabolic syndrome**—Patients with the metabolic syndrome are at risk of CHD. The first-line strategy is to change their lifestyle, particularly increasing physical activity and reducing weight. The components of the metabolic syndrome are as follows, and the ATP III criteria use the presence of any three of the five traits:

1) Abdominal obesity: Men >40 inches (102 cm), Women >35 inches (88 cm)

2) HDL: Men <40 mg/dL, Women <50 mg/dL

3) Triglycerides ≥150 mg/dL

4) Blood pressure ≥130/85 mm HG

5) Fasting glucose ≥110 mg/dL

**Elevated triglycerides**—Elevated triglycerides are associated with an increased risk for CHD. Acquired causes of elevated triglycerides include obesity, physical inactivity, smoking, excessive alcohol intake, high-carb diets, type 2 diabetes, hypothyroidism, renal failure, nephrotic syndrome, pregnancy, or drugs (eg, beta-blockers, glucocorticoids, cyclosporine, retinoids, protease inhibitors, estrogens, tamoxifen). The first-line strategy is to change the patients' lifestyle (eg, smoking cessation, ↑ physical activity, ↓ alcohol intake). Patients that have high triglycerides (≥500 mg/dL) are at risk of acute pancreatitis, in which case lifestyle changes plus drug therapy can be considered. Fibrates are the most effective, and bile acid sequestrants should be avoided.

### Follow-Up:

After initiating drug therapy, patients should be seen in 6 to 8 weeks for a repeat lipid profile. If there are any adjustments to the drug regimen, then the patient should be seen again in another 6 to 8 weeks. Once the patient is at goal, he or she can be seen every 4 to 6 months. Routine creatine kinase (CK) or LFTs are not necessary unless clinically indicated.

### Pearls:

- For every 10% reduction in cholesterol, there is an 11% reduction in total mortality risk and a 15% reduction in coronary heart disease mortality.

- An easy way to remember an ideal cholesterol level is to keep your "highs high" (ie, ↑ high-density lipoprotein) and your "lows low" (ie, ↓ low-density lipoprotein).

- Most statins can be taken at any time of day, but in particular, simvastatin should be taken in the evening because it has a relatively short half-life and most of the cholesterol synthesis occurs at night.

- Nicotinamide is also referred to as niacin, but it does not have any lipid lowering properties.

- Homocysteine appears to be associated with an increased risk for CHD, however it is not considered a "major" risk factor, and therefore, routine measurement or treatment of homocysteine levels is not recommended.

- Secondary causes of dyslipidemia include hypothyroidism, diabetes, nephrotic syndrome, chronic renal failure, obstructive biliary disease, and drugs (eg, corticosteroids, anabolic steroids, progestins, HIV protease inhibitors).

- If secondary dyslipidemia is suspected, a blood sample should also be sent for a TSH, A1c, UA (proteinuria), creatinine, and alkaline phosphatase.

- **Foundational point**—Statins inhibit the enzyme HMG CoA reductase, which plays a role in the rate-limiting step in cholesterol biosynthesis.

- **Foundational point**—Atherosclerotic plaques consists of a lipid-rich core within the intima covered by a fibrous cap.

- **Connecting point** (pg. 81)—Metabolic syndrome can be seen in type 2 diabetes.

- **Connecting point** (pg. 121)—Metabolic syndrome can be seen in PCOS.

- **On the CCS**, remember to "counsel" all your hyperlipidemic patients.

- **On the CCS**, remember to encourage therapeutic lifestyle changes. The practice CCS does have "diet low fat," "diet low cholesterol," "diet high fiber," "advise patient exercise program," and "weight loss diet" (recommend if patient is overweight).

# CORONARY HEART DISEASE—ACUTE CORONARY SYNDROMES

## ▌ STEMI, NSTEMI, AND UNSTABLE ANGINA

Acute coronary syndromes (ACS) represent a continuum of clinical presentations that ranges from unstable angina (**UA**) through non-ST elevation myocardial infarction (**NSTEMI**), and to ST elevation myocardial infarction (**STEMI**). There are varying degrees of coronary artery obstruction in which a complete occlusion is the typical cause for a STEMI, but a partial occlusion is the typical cause for UA and NSTEMI.

### Clinical Features:

**Unstable angina**—UA can present as either rest angina (>20 minutes), new-onset exertional angina, or previously diagnosed angina that takes on a crescendo pattern (increasing severity, frequency, or duration). Clinical manifestations are similar to those of a STEMI (see next).

**NSTEMI**—Symptoms typically present at rest and are characteristically more intense and prolonged. Clinical manifestations of a NSTEMI can also resemble those of a STEMI (see next).

**STEMI**—The classic presentation is retrosternal chest pain that radiates to the arms, neck, or back. Patients may not be able to precisely locate the pain, but may describe the pain as "heavy, pressure, aching, or discomfort," which reflects visceral pain (somatic pain is described as sharp with precise location). Patients can experience sympathetic (eg, cool, clammy hands and diaphoresis) and parasympathetic effects (eg, weakness, nausea, vomiting). If the MI results in LV dysfunction, patients may have pulmonary rales, tachypnea, hypotension (due to ventricular or valve dysfunction), $S_3$, $S_4$, paradoxical $S_2$ (LBBB), or a systolic murmur (ventral septal rupture, papillary muscle dysfunction, or a flail mitral leaflet). If the MI results in RV dysfunction, patients may have JVD, hypotension, right-sided $S_3$, or Kussmaul sign (↑ JVP with inspiration).

**Next Step:**

**Step 1)** Access and stabilize **A**irway, **B**reathing, and **C**irculation.

**Step 2)** Establish IV access.

**Step 3)** Place monitoring equipment on patient: pulse oximetry, continuous blood pressure cuff, continuous cardiac monitoring, 12-lead EKG. The EKG will give a clue to which anatomic part of the heart might be affected (see Table 3-5) and will help guide initial management of ACS (see step 7).

**Step 4)** Intervene with **MONA**:

> **M**orphine (IV)—Every 5 to 15 minutes (PRN) to alleviate chest pain or anxiety.
>
> **O**xygen—Maintain $O_2$ saturation >90%.
>
> **N**itroglycerin (sublingual)—Every 5 minutes for a maximum of 3 doses.
>
> **A**spirin (chewed and swallowed)—If unable to take orally, then rectal suppository.

**Step 5)** Perform a targeted history and physical. A focused physical exam may include general appearance, HEENT/neck, lung exam, heart exam, abdomen, and extremities.

**Step 6)** Obtain portable CXR (<30 minutes) and laboratory studies: CBC, electrolytes, cardiac enzymes (eg, troponin-I), coagulation studies (eg, PTT, PT/INR), lipid profile.

**Step 7)** In the early stages of management, your clinical suspicion for ACS and the initial 12-lead EKG will guide treatment approach. The cardiac enzymes are not useful in the early stages of patient care because in some patients it can take 4 to 6 hours (12 hours for all patients) for the cardiac enzymes to rise after an MI. However, for board purposes, you should be able to differentiate between unstable angina, NSTEMI, and STEMI.

> **Unstable angina**—No elevations in cardiac enzymes, and EKG may or may not show T wave inversions, ST depression, or transient ST elevation.
>
> **NSTEMI**—Elevation in cardiac enzymes, which distinguishes this condition from UA, and EKG may or may not show T-wave inversions, ST depression, or transient ST elevation.
>
> **STEMI**—Elevation in cardiac enzymes, and EKG will show new ST segment elevations in at least ≥2 contiguous leads or a new LBBB that is consistent with the presentation of ACS.

The ST segment elevations start at the J point with elevations ≥1 mm in all leads except $V_2$ and $V_3$, where elevations are ≥1.5 mm in all women, or ≥2 mm in men ≥40 years, or ≥2.5 mm in men <40 years.

**Step 8)** Therapeutic interventions consist of **reperfusion therapy** (PCI or fibrinolysis), **anti-ischemic therapy** (beta-blockers and nitrates) and **antithrombotic therapy** which consists of antiplatelets (eg, aspirin, thienopyridines [clopidogrel, prasugrel, ticlopidine], GPIIb/IIIa inhibitors [abciximab, eptifibatide, tirofiban]), and anticoagulation (eg, unfractionated heparin, LMWH, fondaparinux, bivalirudin). Consider the clinical management in the following three scenarios:

### Initial EKG Normal + Initial Enzymes Normal

1) Perform serial EKGs and serial cardiac enzymes.

2) If serial test results are negative and there is no further chest discomfort, then consider stress testing. If cardiac enzymes are positive or there is recurrent chest pain, then treat as UA/NSTEMI.

### STEMI

1) Select the reperfusion strategy without waiting for the results of the initial cardiac enzymes. Consider the 2 types of reperfusion therapies:

> **Percutaneous coronary intervention (PCI)**—PCI is the preferred approach if performed expeditiously (goal of door-to-balloon in <90 minutes). If long delays are anticipated (>120 minutes), then fibrinolytic therapy should be considered.
>
> **Fibrinolysis**—If fibrinolysis (eg, streptokinase, alteplase, reteplase) is the treatment of choice, therapy should be performed expeditiously (goal of door-to-needle in <30 minutes). Fibrinolysis is usually considered if symptom onset is <12 hours, PCI is unavailable, or no contraindications exist. **Absolute contraindications** to fibrinolysis include: active bleeding, Hx of intracranial hemorrhage, intracranial malignancy, ischemic stroke in the preceding 3 months, facial trauma/closed head injury in the preceding 3 months, cerebral vascular malformation, or suspected aortic dissection.

2) Start anti-ischemic therapy: IV nitroglycerin can be given if patient has persistent chest pain despite 3 doses of sublingual

| Table 3-5 • Wall Infarct-Artery-EKG Relationship | | |
|---|---|---|
| **Affected Wall** | **Affected Artery** | **Associated Leads** |
| Anteroseptal | LAD | $V_1$, $V_2$ |
| Anteroapical | LAD | $V_3$, $V_4$ |
| Anterolateral | Left circumflex | $V_5$, $V_6$, aVL, I |
| Inferior | RCA or left circumflex | II, III, aVF |
| Posterior | RCA or left circumflex | Tall R waves and/or ST depressions in $V_1$-$V_3$, ST elevations in $V_7$-$V_9$ (true posterior leads) |

*LAD—left anterior descending, RCA—right coronary artery (usually the posterior descending branch)*

nitroglycerin, and give a beta-blocker (eg, metoprolol) if the patient does not have bradycardia, AV blocks, overt heart failure, or reactive airway disease.

3) Start anticoagulation (eg, IV heparin).

4) Start antiplatelet therapy: Aspirin (add clopidogrel if PCI is planned).

5) Inititate reperfusion therapy.

**No ST Elevation (UA/NSTEMI)**

1) Start anti-ischemic therapy: IV nitroglycerin if there is persistent chest pain and a beta-blocker if not contraindicated.

2) Start anticoagulation (eg, IV heparin).

3) Start antiplatelet therapy:

Aspirin + clopidogrel (if noninvasive testing is selected), or

Aspirin + clopidogrel or GP IIb/IIIa inhibitor (if angiography is selected)

4) Decide which management strategy fits the patient. Consider the following:

**Immediate angiography**—Patients in this category usually have very high risk features such as cardiogenic shock, hemodynamic instability, sustained arrhythmias, heart failure, new mitral regurgitation, new ventricular septal rupture, or persistent chest pain despite optimal medical therapy.

**Early angiography**—Angiography is usually performed within a 24-hour period as the anti-ischemic and antithrombotic therapies are intensified. Patients in this category have high risk features, but they appear more stable. High risk features include elevated cardiac enzymes, prior CABG, prior PCI within 6 months, LVEF <40%, new ST segment depression on admission, or a high TIMI score.

**Noninvasive testing**—Patients in this category do not have high risk features. Patients can undergo stress testing (only if there is no recurrent chest pain and they have been clinically stable for 12 to 24 hours) or an echo to evaluate for LV function. If there are high risk findings on the stress test or echo (eg, LVEF <40%), patients should be referred for diagnostic angiography with intent to perform revascularization if needed.

**Step 9)** A predischarge assessment of the LV function with an echocardiography should be performed since there is an increase in mortality in the long-term with patients that have LV systolic dysfunction.

**Step 10)** Discharge medications in patients treated for a STEMI, UA, or NSTEMI include the following:

**Aspirin** is recommended indefinitely.

**Clopidogrel** for 1 month to 1 year.

**Beta-blocker** is recommended indefinitely, CCBs if beta-blockers are contraindicated.

**Statin** (eg, atorvastatin).

**ACEIs** (or ARB if ACEI intolerant) in patients with heart failure, LVEF ≤40%, diabetes, HTN, and anterior MI in STEMI patients.

**Disposition:**

Patients in the emergency room that are treated for a STEMI or UA/NSTEMI should be admitted to the hospital. Patients that are eventually released from the hospital should have close follow-up to reinforce secondary preventive measures. Low-risk patients can be seen in 2 to 6 weeks and higher-risk patients should be seen within 14 days.

**Pearls:**

• Women, elderly, and diabetic patients may present with "atypical" symptoms such as nausea, vomiting, weakness, syncope, palpitations, or dyspnea.

• Troponins can exist as I, T, or C. Only I and T are heart-specific, but C is expressed in heart and skeletal muscle.

• Troponins I or T is considered the marker of choice for the diagnosis of MI and much preferred over CK-MB because of their greater specificity and sensitivity.

• Creatine kinase (CK) can exist as MM, BB, or MB. All forms are distributed in different tissues, but there is more distribution of CK-MB in the heart. Specificity decreases in CK-MB in the setting of muscle injury, muscle disease, or surgery.

• Troponins (I or T) can rise as early as 2 to 3 hours after the onset of an acute MI and can persist for 10 to 14 days, permitting a late diagnosis.

• CK-MB can rise as early as 4 to 6 hours after the onset of an acute MI, but returns to baseline within 24 to 48 hours.

• Myoglobin and lactate dehydrogenase (LDH) are biomarkers for cardiac injury, but both lack specificity for the heart, and therefore, they are not routinely performed since troponins are more specific.

• Clopidogrel is an acceptable alternative to aspirin in patients that are intolerant to aspirin.

• A PPI should be given to patients with a history of GI bleeding that are concurrently taking aspirin or clopidogrel.

• **Caveat 1**—Nitrates can cause hypotension and therefore should be avoided in patients taking a phosphodiesterase-5 inhibitor (eg, sildenafil, tadalafil, vardenafil) for erectile dysfunction, severe aortic stenosis, low blood pressures, or right ventricular infarction (ie, patients rely on preload for cardiac output).

• **Caveat 2**—The initial EKG is often nondiagnostic in patients with ACS, therefore repeat EKGs at 10-minute intervals in patients with suspicion for ACS.

• **Caveat 3**—Fibrinolytic therapy is non-diagnostic recommended in patients with UA or NSTEMI.

• **Caveat 4**—Patients should avoid caffeine for 12 hours or theophylline for 48 hours if the vasodilator stress agents are used for stress testing since caffeine and theophylline can attenuate the effects of the vasodilatation.

• **Caveat 5**—All nonaspirin NSAIDs should be withheld in the management of ACS since there is an increased risk of cardiovascular events with its use.

• Stress (exercise or pharmacologic) testing can be assessed by EKG, echocardiography, or radionuclide imaging.

- Exercise EKG is often the initial test for patients that can exercise adequately and to risk-stratify patients with suspected coronary heart disease.

- Stress imaging (echocardiography or nuclear studies) is the preferred modality if the patient had a prior revascularization, is on digoxin, or the resting EKG shows a LBBB, LVH, ventricular preexcitation, paced ventricular rhythm, or a ST segment depression ≥1 mm.

- Pharmacologic stress agents include an adrenergic agonist (eg, dobutamine) or vasodilator stress agents (eg, adenosine, dipyridamole, regadenoson) that can increase coronary blood flow.

- Dobutamine should not be used in patients with severe hypertension, aortic dissection, significant LV outflow tract obstruction, unstable angina, recent MI, or ventricular arrhythmias.

- Adenosine, dipyridamole, and regadenoson should be avoided in patients with bronchospastic airway disease, sick sinus syndrome, high degree AV blocks, hypotension, or patients receiving oral dipyridamole for medical therapy.

- Stress (exercise or pharmacologic) nuclear studies require a radioactive tracer that uses either thallium or technetium (Tc) based agents.

- Benzodiazepines should be used early in the care of cocaine-related myocardial ischemia, but beta-blockers should be avoided because of concerns for unopposed alpha-adrenergic stimulation.

- Inferior MIs are frequently associated with right ventricular infarctions because they are usually supplied by the same right coronary artery. Patients may present with hypotension, and treatment consists of a fluid challenge with normal saline to maintain adequate right ventricular preload.

- UA/NSTEMI patients that have multivessel disease after diagnostic angiography can be considered for a CABG or multivessel PCI. In general, indications for a CABG in UA/NSTEMI patients are similar to those of stable angina, which include (1) left main coronary artery stenosis, (2) ≥70% stenosis of the proximal LAD and proximal left circumflex artery, (3) severe 3-vessel disease, (4) multivessel disease + DM, or (5) multivessel disease + poor LV function.

- CABG is infrequently performed in patients with a STEMI because of the relative quickness in reperfusion with either PCI or fibrinolysis; however, an urgent CABG can be considered in patients that are not candidates for PCI or fibrinolysis.

- Agents that reduce mortality include beta-blockers, ACEIs, aspirin, clopidogrel, prasugrel, and statins.

- There is no proven benefit (and there is potentially harm) in using fibrinolysis in patients with UA/NSTEMI.

- **On the CCS**, after the initial management in patients with a STEMI or UA/NSTEMI, remember to transfer the patient to the ICU setting for monitored care (ie, coronary care unit).

- **On the CCS**, remember to implement a course of action before a cardiology consultant is able to see your patient.

- **On the CCS**, if you want to order a stress test, type in "stress" in the order menu and then select your choice.

- **On the CCS**, be aware that a "PCI" is not the same as "coronary angiography" (mainly diagnostic) but rather the same terminology as a "coronary angioplasty" (ie, stent placement).

- **On the CCS**, you cannot order "fibrinolysis" or "thrombolytics" in the practice CCS, but rather the specific drugs (eg, streptokinase, alteplase, reteplase).

- **On the CCS**, with each CCS case you should be cognizant about monitoring the patient. Examples of monitoring parameters include repeat vital signs, physical exams, neuro checks, urine outputs, labs, pulse oximetry, cardiac monitoring, BP monitoring, fetal heart rate, or a monitored setting (eg, ICU).

- **On the CCS**, after managing a case on ACS, remember to "counsel family/patient," "advise patient, no smoking," "cardiac rehabilitation program," "advise patient, exercise program," "diet low fat," "diet low sodium," "advise patient, relaxation techniques," and "vaccination, influenza."

# VALVULAR DISORDERS

## ▌ MITRAL STENOSIS

Mitral stenosis is characterized by blood-flow obstruction from the left atrium to the left ventricle. The most common cause of mitral stenosis is **rheumatic fever**, and less commonly from congenital stenosis, mitral annular calcification, and large vegetations seen in endocarditis.

Clinical Features:

**Murmur Type:** Diastolic murmur (between $S_2$ and $S_1$).

**Heart Sounds:** A **loud $S_1$** can be heard after closure of the stenotic mitral value in systole. As the mitral value opens in $S_2$, an "**opening snap**" (OS) can be heard that is thought to represent tensing of the chordae tendineae in combination with opening of the stenotic leaflets. After the opening snap, a **mid to late diastolic, low-frequency decrescendo murmur** (ie, "diastolic rumble") can be best heard at the apex with the patient in the left lateral decubitus position in held expiration using the bell of the stethoscope. The diastolic rumble represents turbulent flow of blood through the stenotic valve. The intensity of the murmur will change upon different maneuvers (see Table 3-6).

**Clinical Progression:** As the left atrial pressures become higher due to the stenosis, the size of the left atrium can become large enough to compress the recurrent laryngeal nerve causing **hoarseness**. In addition, patients are more likely to develop **atrial fibrillation** due to left atrial enlargement. It should also be noted that an **embolic event** is often associated with atrial fibrillation. As the blood flow begins to back up and cause increasing pressures in the pulmonary vasculature, the patient may experience **dyspnea**. In some cases, the bronchial vein will rupture into the lung parenchyma resulting in **hemoptysis**. Over time, chronic pulmonary

## Table 3-6 • Changes in the Intensity of Murmurs from Bedside Maneuvers

| Maneuver | Mitral Stenosis | Mitral Regurgitation | Mitral Valve Prolapse | Aortic Stenosis | Aortic Regurgitation | HCM | VSD |
|---|---|---|---|---|---|---|---|
| Standing (↓ preload) | ↓ | ↓ | Early click, longer murmur | ↓ | ↓ | ↑ | ↓ |
| Valsalva (↓ preload) | ↓ | ↓ | Early click, longer murmur | ↓ | ↓ | ↑ | |
| Squat (↑preload, ↑ afterload) | ↓ | ↑ | Delayed click, shorten murmur | ↑↓ | ↑ | ↓ | ↑ |
| Handgrip (↑ afterload) | ↑ | ↑ | Delayed click, shorten murmur | ↓ | ↑ | ↓ | ↑ |
| Inspiration (↑ blood to RV, ↓ blood to LV) | ↓ | ↓ | | | ↓ | ↓ | |
| Expiration (↓ blood to RV, ↑ blood to LV) | ↑ | ↑ | | | ↑ | ↑ | |

HCM—hypertrophic cardiomyopathy, LV—left ventricle, RV—right ventricle, VSD—ventral septal defect
Note: Left-sided murmurs (ie, mitral, aortic) and left-sided gallops (ie, $S_3$, $S_4$) are typically louder during expiration. Right-sided murmurs (ie, tricuspid, pulmonic) and right-sided gallops (ie, $S_3$, $S_4$) are usually louder during inspiration.

hypertension will lead to right-sided heart failure resulting in ↑ **JVP**, **hepatomegaly**, and **lower extremity edema**.

**Severity:** Normal mitral valve area is between 4 and 6 cm² with a mean gradient between the 2 chambers of 0 mm Hg and a pulmonary artery systolic pressure (PASP) less than 30 mm Hg. The severity of the stenosis is classified as **mild stenosis** (valve area >1.5 cm², mean gradient <5 mm Hg, PASP <30 mm Hg), **moderate stenosis** (valve area 1.0-1.5 cm², mean gradient 5-10 mm Hg, PASP 30-50 mm Hg), and **severe stenosis** (valve area <1 cm², mean gradient >10 mm Hg, PASP >50 mm Hg).

### Next Step:

**Step 1)** The best initial test is with a **transthoracic echocardiography (TTE)** with color flow Doppler imaging that can assess the severity of the stenosis, valve area, valve morphology, associated valve lesions, mean gradients, estimated PASP, and suitability for percutaneous mitral balloon valvotomy (PMBV). Other adjunctive testing may include the following:

  **EKG**—In the presence of left atrial enlargement, a large P wave that is broad and notched (M shaped) can be seen in lead II, also referred to as "P-mitrale." A biphasic P wave with a prominent negative component in the terminal portion of the P wave in lead $V_1$ is also consistent with left atrial enlargement. In the presence of pulmonary hypertension with subsequent right ventricular hypertrophy (RVH), a tall R wave can be seen in lead $V_1$ usually with a right axis deviation.

  **Chest x-ray**—Enlargement of the left atrium may produce a double shadowing of the cardiac silhouette ("double density"), upward displacement of the left mainstem bronchi,

and straightening of the left heart border. Kerley A, B, and C lines can sometimes be appreciated with increasing pulmonary congestion.

  **Transesophageal echocardiography (TEE)**—TEE is more invasive compared to the TTE, but it provides superior visualization of the posterior cardiac structures. The main indications for a TEE are equivocal information based on the TTE or to detect the presence of left atrial thrombi before DC cardioversion or percutaneous mitral balloon valvotomy (PMBV).

  **Cardiac catheterization**—Cardiac catheterization is an invasive test that can be used when the severity of the stenosis is still in question after echocardiography. Catheterization can provide information on the hemodynamics within the valve area.

**Step 2)** The clinical management for mitral stenosis can be best summarized into patients that are asymptomatic or symptomatic.

**Asymptomatic:** Patients with moderate to severe mitral stenosis (valve area ≤1.5 cm²) plus evidence of pulmonary hypertension (PASP >50 mm Hg at rest or >60 mm Hg with exercise) can undergo percutaneous mitral balloon valvotomy (PMBV).

**Symptomatic:** Patients with moderate to severe mitral stenosis (valve area ≤1.5 cm²) can undergo PMBV, but pharmacologic therapy may be appropriate to stabilize the patient or optimize loading conditions prior to intervention. The following conditions may require medical attention before intervention:

  **Pulmonary congestion**—Diuretics (usually loop diuretics) and sodium restriction.

  **Systolic heart failure**—Digoxin can be used as an inotropic agent in patients with decreased ventricular contractility.

**Atrial fibrillation**—Hemodynamically unstable patients require immediate electrical cardioversion. Hemodynamically stable patients may require rate control with beta-blockers (eg, metoprolol), calcium channel blockers (eg, verapamil, diltiazem), or less preferably with digoxin. In addition, long-term anticoagulation is recommended in patients with a left atrial thrombus, prior embolic event, or atrial fibrillation that is persistent, paroxysmal, or permanent. Warfarin can be used with a target INR of 2.5 with a range of 2.0 to 3.0.

**Step 3)** Patients with rheumatic mitral stenosis should receive **prophylactic antibiotics** for secondary prevention of rheumatic fever. It should be noted that if patients have acute rheumatic fever, a full course of therapeutic antibiotics should be given prior to initiating prophylactic antibiotics. Acceptable prophylactic antibiotics include benzathine penicillin G (intramuscular), penicillin V (oral), or sulfadiazine (oral).

**Follow-Up:**

A TTE should be performed anytime there is a change in clinical status. Patients that are stable and asymptomatic but have mild stenosis should have an echo every 3 to 5 years, with moderate stenosis every 1 to 2 years, and with severe stenosis every year.

**Pearls:**

- Routine infective endocarditis prophylaxis is no longer recommended in patients with common valvular disease (eg, aortic or mitral valve disease, mitral valve prolapse with regurgitation) except in patients with a **previous episode of infective endocarditis** or **prosthetic materials** used in heart repair. Amoxicillin or ampicillin can be used in these high-risk patients that require prophylaxis for dental, oral, or upper respiratory tract procedures. Routine infective endocarditis prophylaxis is not indicated in patients undergoing GI (eg, colonoscopy) or GU (eg, cystoscopy) procedures unless the patient has an ongoing GI or GU infection. If a patient has an ongoing infection, then amoxicillin or ampicillin are acceptable antibiotics prior to the procedure.

- A percutaneous mitral balloon valvotomy (PMBV) involves threading a catheter from the femoral vein into the right atrium and into the left atrium through a transseptal puncture and then across the mitral valve. A balloon is inflated and deflated to open the fused commissures.

- When PMBV is indicated, it is generally performed on patients with rheumatic mitral stenosis.

- Surgical intervention is preferred over PMBV in the setting of persistent left atrial thrombus despite anticoagulation, moderate to severe mitral regurgitation, unfavorable mitral valve morphology, mitral annular calcification, or congenital mitral stenosis.

- An open surgical commissurotomy allows direct visualization of the mitral valve and is often indicated when a valve is not amenable to PMBV.

- Mitral valve replacement (MVR) is considered the last alternative for treating mitral stenosis and is often indicated when a valve is not amenable to PMBV or open commissurotomy.

- The effects of pregnancy, especially an increase in heart rate and cardiac output, can cause mitral stenosis to manifest in previously asymptomatic patients or exacerbate existing symptoms. In most pregnant patients, mitral stenosis is due to rheumatic fever. Patients with mild to moderate mitral stenosis can be medically managed and PMBV reserved for severe symptoms that are refractory to medical management. It should be noted that warfarin is contraindicated, especially in the first trimester, because of teratogenicity; instead, heparin should be used for hospitalized patients.

- A prominent "a" wave can be seen in the right atrial pressure waveform in patients with pulmonary hypertension with right ventricular hypertrophy.

- **Connecting point** (pg. 58)—Know right axis deviation and right ventricular hypertrophy (RVH).

- **Connecting point** (pg. 223)—Know how to treat pharyngitis due to group A streptococcus (GAS).

- **On the CCS,** a "TTE" and a "TEE" are both available in the practice CCS.

- **On the CCS,** a "percutaneous mitral balloon valvotomy (PMBV)" is not available in the practice CCS, but if you type in "mitral" in the order menu, a list of mitral valve procedures are available including "mitral valve balloon valvuloplasty."

- **On the CCS,** once you demonstrate your skills sufficiently and have met the exam objectives, the CCS case will most likely end early.

# ■ CHRONIC MITRAL REGURGITATION

Mitral regurgitation (MR) is characterized by the failure of the mitral valve to close during systole resulting in a portion of the stroke volume being ejected back into the left atrium. **Primary causes** of MR that involve the valve apparatus are trauma, rheumatic heart disease, infective endocarditis, mitral annular calcification, congenital malformation, or mitral valve prolapse. **Secondary (functional) causes** of MR include ischemic heart disease (left ventricular remodeling), hypertrophic cardiomyopathy, or dilated cardiomyopathy.

**Clinical Features:**

**Murmur Type:** Systolic murmur (between $S_1$ and $S_2$)

**Heart Sounds:**

$S_1$—Soft $S_1$ reflecting the failure of the mitral valve to close.

$S_2$—Wide split $S_2$ can be due to early $A_2$ (shortened ejection time) and/or late $P_2$ (presence of pulmonary hypertension).

$S_3$—$S_3$ gallop is usually seen in chronic MR, which reflects the increase in blood return to the left ventricle in early diastole ($S_3$ is a normal finding in young adults and children).

**Murmur sound**—A **high-frequency pansystolic/holosystolic murmur** (ie, "blowing" quality) can be best heard over the apex with the patient in the left lateral decubitus position using the diaphragm of the stethoscope. The murmur will classically radiate to the left axilla or subscapular region. The intensity of the murmur will change upon different maneuvers (see Table 3-6).

**Clinical Progression:** As blood flows in a retrograde fashion from the left ventricle to the left atrium during systole, the left atrium enlarges and becomes more compliant in the gradual development of chronic mitral regurgitation (MR). Because of the atrial enlargement, the left atrial pressures are reduced and pulmonary congestion becomes less common. However, left atrial enlargement can predispose the patient to the development of **atrial fibrillation** with subsequent **thromboembolism**. In addition to left atrial enlargement, the left ventricle also undergoes compensatory dilatation (ie, **compensated phase**). Over time, the chronic volume overload results in **eccentric hypertrophy**. As a result of an increase in end-diastolic volume, the stroke volume increases, which translates into a preserved cardiac output (Frank-Starling mechanism). At some point, the myocardium begins to weaken and can no longer compensate for the regurgitation (the **transitional phase**). Eventually, the forward output deteriorates and signs and symptoms of heart failure develop (the **decompensated phase**).

**Severity:** For board purposes, the following is a general guideline for classifying the severity of MR seen in adults: **mild** (LA and LV size normal, regurgitant fraction <30%, regurgitant orifice area <0.2 cm²), **moderate** (LA and LV size normal to dilated, regurgitant fraction 30%-49%, regurgitant orifice area 0.2-0.39 cm²), and **severe** (LA and LV dilated, regurgitant fraction ≥50%, regurgitant orifice area ≥0.4 cm²).

**Next Step:**

**Step 1)** The best initial test is with a **transthoracic echocardiography (TTE)**. If the information provided by the TTE is suboptimal, the next best step is with a **transesophageal echocardiography (TEE)**. A **cardiac catheterization** can be considered if the information on TTE or TEE is equivocal or mechanical intervention is being considered in patients at risk of coronary artery disease. Other adjunctive testing may include the following:

**EKG**—EKG may demonstrate "P-mitrale" (ie, left atrial enlargement), tall R wave in lead $V_1$ with right axis deviation (ie, RVH), or a tall R wave in lead $V_5$ or $V_6$ with a deep S wave in lead $V_1$ (ie, LVH).

**Chest x-ray**—Enlargement of the left atrium (ie, double density, left bronchi upward displacement, left heart border straightened), enlargement of the left ventricle (ie, cardiac silhouette displaced to the left), or concomitant enlargement of both the atrium and ventricle (ie, cardiomegaly) can be seen.

**Step 2)** The clinical management for mitral regurgitation can be best summarized into patients that are asymptomatic or symptomatic. The recommendations for mitral valve surgery are based on the American College of Cardiology/American Heart Association (ACC/AHA) guidelines.

**Asymptomatic:**

1) Severe chronic MR + Dysfunctional LV (EF ≤60% and/or end-systolic dimension ≥40 mm) → Mitral valve surgery

2) Severe chronic MR + Preserved LV function (EF >60% and end-systolic dimension <40 mm) + Good chance of successful repair → Mitral valve surgery

3) Severe chronic MR + Preserved LV function + New-onset atrial fibrillation → Mitral valve surgery + Maze procedure (several cuts in the left atrium to disrupt electrical pathways)

4) Severe chronic MR + Preserved LV function + Pulmonary HTN (PASP >50 mm Hg at rest or >60 mm Hg during exercise) → Mitral valve surgery

**Symptomatic:**

**1) Medical Therapy**

- Vasodilators are not typically recommended in patients with asymptomatic chronic MR.
- Short-term vasodilator therapy (eg, IV nitroprusside) may be beneficial in patients with severe symptomatic chronic MR.
- Long-term vasodilator therapy (eg, oral hydralazine) is typically reserved for symptomatic patients who are not candidates for surgery.
- Patients with secondary (functional) MR with systolic heart failure should receive an ACE inhibitor (or ARB), diuretic, beta-blocker, and an aldosterone antagonist. It is important to optimize medical therapy since the long-term benefit of mitral valve surgery for severe secondary MR is still inconclusive.

**2) Surgery**

- Severe chronic MR + NYHA Class II-IV (see Pearls) + LV dysfunction that is not severe (EF ≥30% and/or end-systolic dimension ≤ 55 mm) → Mitral valve surgery
- Severe primary chronic MR (ie, not secondary MR) + NYHA Class III-IV (see Pearls) + Severe LV dysfunction (EF <30% and/or end-systolic dimension >55 mm) + Good chance of successful repair → Mitral valve surgery

**Step 3)** Patients with rheumatic mitral regurgitation should receive **prophylactic antibiotics** for secondary prevention of rheumatic fever.

**Follow-Up:**

A TTE should be performed anytime there is a change in clinical status. Patients that are asymptomatic but have moderate MR should have an echo every year, and those with severe MR should have an echo every 6 to 12 months. Patients that have mild MR should be seen every year, but an echo is not necessary unless there is a change in clinical status.

**Pearls:**

- Routine infective endocarditis prophylaxis is no longer recommended in patients with common valvular disease, including mitral regurgitation, unless the patient had a **previous episode of infective endocarditis** or **prior prosthetic repair**.
- New York Heart Association (NYHA) functional classification summarized:

Class I—Cardiac disease without physical limitation.

Class II—Slight limitation of physical activity, but comfortable at rest.

Class III—Marked limitation of physical activity, but comfortable at rest.

Class IV—Discomfort with any physical activity, and symptoms may be present at rest.

- Consider three types of holosystolic murmurs:

    1) VSD

    2) Tricuspid regurgitation—Typically associated with pulmonary HTN

    3) Mitral regurgitation—Characteristically seen in chronic MR

- Consider three types of early systolic murmurs:

    1) VSD—Associated with large VSDs with pulmonary HTN or small muscular VSDs

    2) Tricuspid regurgitation—Typically without pulmonary HTN

    3) Mitral regurgitation—Characteristically seen in acute MR

- If atrial fibrillation is encountered, rate control and anticoagulation may be warranted.

- The pulmonary capillary wedge pressure (PCWP) is an indirect measurement of the left atrial pressures.

- **Concentric hypertrophy** is seen in conditions with chronic pressure overload such as aortic stenosis or hypertension.

- In general, mitral valve repair is preferred over mitral valve replacement.

- Two types of mitral valve replacement can be performed, either with a mechanical valve (requires lifelong warfarin) or a bioprosthetic valve (limited "shelf" life due to degeneration).

- The bell of the stethoscope is used to detect low-frequency sounds, and the diaphragm is used to detect high-frequency sounds.

- Although there are a lot of details in this topic, it should be noted that once you understand the details you will have a better global (broader) understanding of mitral regurgitation and your overall clinical judgment will be sharper.

- **Foundational point**—Sarcomeres that are arranged in series (resulting in elongation of the heart) instead of in parallel are seen in eccentric hypertrophy.

- **Foundational point**—The Frank-Starling principle explains that the greater the end-diastolic volume (ie, ↑ muscle fiber stretch), the greater the stroke volume or cardiac output. At the same token, a reduced end-diastolic volume (eg, dehydration) would result in a reduced stroke volume.

- **CJ:** A 51-year-old man presents with sudden severe dyspnea, tachycardia, hypotension, pallor, and diaphoresis. Heart exam reveals an early systolic murmur ending before S$_2$ that can be heard along the left sternal border. EKG shows no significant abnormalities, CXR shows pulmonary edema, and a TTE shows a flail mitral leaflet. What are your next steps?
**Answer:** The patient has acute mitral regurgitation (MR). Causes of acute MR include trauma, infective endocarditis,

or MI, which can cause a papillary muscle rupture, chordae tendineae rupture, or a flail leaflet. In cases when the left atrium has not compensated, the regurgitant blood flow will cause high pressures that will eventually be transmitted to the pulmonary circulation resulting in rapid pulmonary edema. In cases when acute MR is superimposed on chronic MR, the presentation may not be so dramatic. In either case, the left atrial pressure waveform will have a prominent "v" wave, which is often referred to as a "cv" wave because the v wave merges with the preceding c wave. The corresponding "cv" wave reflects the increasing left atrial filling during systole. Surgical intervention is the definitive treatment, however, prior to surgery, the patient may need to be medically managed. If the patient is normotensive, then IV nitroprusside can be used to reduce the afterload and improve forward output. However if the patient is hypotensive, then administration of an inotropic agent (eg, dobutamine) or intraaortic balloon pump (IABP) should be inserted in conjunction with the nitroprusside.

- **On the CCS,** if your CCS case ends early, any remaining real time will not be added to other CCS cases.

## MITRAL VALVE PROLAPSE

Mitral valve prolapse (MVP) is a common valvular disorder that affects approximately 0.6% to 2.4% of the population in the United States. MVP can be characterized by the billowing of the mitral leaflets into the left atrium during systole. **Primary causes** of MVP include familial or sporadic cases. **Secondary causes** of MVP can be associated with connective tissue disorders (eg, Ehlers-Danlos syndrome, osteogenesis imperfecta, Marfan syndrome) or a sequel to acute rheumatic fever, endocarditis, trauma, or myocardial infarction (ie, chordae tendineae or papillary muscle rupture). MVP is a common cause of mitral regurgitation (MR) and typically a common cause of MR seen in pregnant women.

**Clinical Features:**

**Murmur Type:** Systolic murmur (between S$_1$ and S$_2$).

**Heart Sounds:** The classic auscultatory finding is a **midsystolic "click"** (single or multiple), which is thought to represent the sudden tensing of the chordae tendineae with billowing of the mitral leaflet into the left atrium. In some patients, the click is followed by a **late systolic murmur** (early in the disease) that crescendos into S$_2$. If there is a flail leaflet or severe prolapse, a holosystolic murmur will be heard instead. The click and murmur can be best heard over the cardiac apex using the diaphragm of the stethoscope with bedside maneuvers altering the sound pattern (see Table 3-6).

**Clinical Presentation:** MVP occurs more frequently in women than in men. Most patients with MVP are asymptomatic. However, another group of patients have MVP syndrome, which includes MVP plus nonspecific symptoms such as palpitations, chest pain, anxiety, dizziness, dyspnea, fatigue, or exercise intolerance. Although the validity of MVP syndrome is still in question, it is important to be aware of the condition for board purposes. On physical exam, common associated conditions include scoliosis, pectus excavatum, and low BMI.

## Next Step:

**Step 1)** The **clinical examination** is the best initial test. Upon auscultatory findings on exam, MVP can be confirmed with **2D-echocardiography** that demonstrates the valve prolapse of ≥2 mm above the mitral annulus in long axis views (parasternal and apical 3-chamber). The EKG and CXR are usually normal unless the patient has developed chronic mitral regurgitation.

**Step 2)** Consider the clinical management of MVP:

**Asymptomatic**—Provide reassurance. Patients that have mild to moderate MR with normal LV function can participate in all competitive sports. However, patients with severe MR or LV dysfunction should be restricted to less competitive sports.

**Autonomic dysfunction**—Patients that have palpitations, chest pain, or anxiety may respond to beta-blockers. In addition, they should be counseled to avoid alcohol, caffeine, and tobacco. A 24-hour Holter monitor may be beneficial to detect supraventricular or ventricular arrhythmias.

**Mitral regurgitation**—Indications for mitral valve surgery in patients with MVP are the same as those for other primary causes of MR (see step 2 in Chronic Mitral Regurgitation section).

**Infective endocarditis prophylaxis**—Routine infective endocarditis prophylaxis is no longer recommended in patients with common valvular disorders, including MVP even with mitral regurgitation, unless the patient had a **previous episode of infective endocarditis** or **prior prosthetic repair**.

**Step 3)** Patients with MVP due to rheumatic disease should receive **prophylactic antibiotics** for secondary prevention of rheumatic fever.

## Follow-Up:

Patients with MVP that are asymptomatic and without mitral regurgitation should be seen for a clinical exam every 3 to 5 years, but should be seen earlier anytime there is a change in clinical status.

## Pearls:

- The association between sudden cardiac death (SCD) and MVP is still unclear. However, patients that do survive a sudden cardiac arrest (SCA) through appropriate intervention may require an implantable cardioverter-defibrillator (ICD).
- The association between cerebral vascular events and MVP continues to be controversial. Different societies have differing recommendations on antithrombotic therapy, but the common agreement is (1) aspirin is recommended in patients with unexplained TIAs, and (2) anticoagulation (warfarin) is recommended if aspirin is ineffective (ie, recurrent TIAs) or there is established systemic embolism.
- The prevalence of panic disorder in patients with MVP is no different than in patients without MVP.
- **On the CCS**, the final diagnosis and reasons for your consult are not used in evaluating your performance.

# ❙ AORTIC STENOSIS

Aortic stenosis (AS) can be characterized by the obstruction of blood flow across the aortic valve. Three main causes of valvular AS are **congenital** (unicuspid or bicuspid valve), **calcific** (due to age-related degenerative changes), and **rheumatic disease** (usually coexisting with mitral valve disease).

**Clinical Features:**

**Murmur Type:** Systolic murmur (between $S_1$ and $S_2$).

**Heart Sounds:**

$S_1$—Usually normal.

$S_2$—Soft $A_2$ (reflecting the immobile aortic valve) followed by a $P_2$. With increasing severity of the AS, a delayed aortic valve closure can cause the $P_2$ to precede the $A_2$ resulting in a paradoxical split $S_2$. As the aortic valve becomes more stenotic, the $A_2$ may disappear, resulting in a single $S_2$ (ie, just a $P_2$).

$S_4$—$S_4$ can be heard, which reflects atrial contraction into a stiffened ventricle (ie, LV hypertrophy).

**Murmur sound**—A systolic **crescendo-decrescendo "ejection" murmur** (ie, "harsh" quality) can be best heard over the right second intercostal space with radiation that is transmitted equally over both carotid arteries. In elderly patients, the murmur may radiate to the apex instead of the carotids, which may be misinterpreted as mitral regurgitation (Gallavardin phenomenon). On palpation of the carotid artery, a diminished and delayed (parvus et tardus) carotid upstroke is a classic finding in severe aortic stenosis, but may be masked in elderly patients who have stiffened carotid vessels. The intensity of the murmur will change upon different maneuvers (see Table 3-6).

**Clinical Progression:** As the aortic orifice area becomes smaller and a pressure gradient begins to develop, the outflow obstruction leads to an increase in left ventricular systolic pressures. The left ventricle is able to compensate by increasing the wall thickness (ie, **concentric hypertrophy**). The wall thickness can now reduce the wall stress (Laplace's law) and ventricular function can be preserved with the patient being **asymptomatic** for a prolonged period. At some point, the left ventricular function becomes maladaptive and LV function begins to decline. Patients with advanced aortic stenosis can present with the classic symptoms, which can be easily remembered by the mnemonic "**SAD**" or **S**yncope, **A**ngina, and **D**yspnea (ie, heart failure).

**Severity:** In adults, the normal aortic valve area is between 3 and 4 cm² with a mean gradient <5 mm Hg and an aortic jet velocity of ≤2 m/sec. The severity of the stenosis can be classified as **mild stenosis** (valve area >1.5 cm², mean gradient <25 mm Hg, aortic jet velocity <3 m/sec), **moderate stenosis** (valve area 1.0-1.5 cm², mean gradient 25-40 mm Hg, aortic jet velocity 3-4 m/sec), **severe stenosis** (valve area <1 cm², mean gradient >40 mm Hg, aortic jet velocity >4 m/sec), and **critical aortic stenosis** (valve area <0.75 cm² and/or aortic jet velocity >5 m/sec). It should be noted that there is variability between symptoms and the severity of the stenosis (eg, patients classified with severe stenosis may have little to no symptoms and vice versa).

## Next Step:

**Step 1)** The best initial test is with a **transthoracic echocardiography (TTE)**. The TTE may also detect concurrent mitral valve disease and aortic regurgitation that can be seen with AS. The **transesophageal echocardiography (TEE)** is not routinely used, but would be the next best step if TTE does not provide adequate information. A **cardiac catheterization** can be considered if there is a discrepancy between the clinical and echocardiographic findings. In addition, coronary angiography becomes fairly important in patients with aortic stenosis since there is a higher prevalence of coronary artery disease (CAD). Patients who have signs and symptoms of coronary artery disease who are about to undergo valve surgery should have a coronary angiography. Also, patients that are ≥35 years old with risk factors for CAD should undergo a coronary angiography prior to valve surgery. Other adjunctive testing may include the following:

> **EKG**—EKG may be completely normal or may reveal left ventricular hypertrophy (LVH) and sometimes left atrial hypertrophy.
>
> **Chest x-ray**—CXR may be completely normal early in the disease, but later show rounding of the LV apex suggesting LVH. Another key finding is dilatation of the aortic root and/or ascending aorta, which may suggest that the patient has bicuspid aortic valves. It is important to be aware of such findings since dilatation of the aorta can lead to dissection or aneurysm formation. Therefore, a CT or MRI may be necessary to better visualize the aorta since echocardiography may be limited in its assessment. However, it should be noted that a TTE is the best initial test in patients with known bicuspid aortic valves to evaluate the aortic root and ascending aorta.

**Step 2)** The clinical management for aortic stenosis can be best summarized into patients that are asymptomatic or symptomatic.

**Asymptomatic:** It is generally recommended that asymptomatic patients with isolated severe aortic stenosis should not undergo routine prophylactic valve replacement. However, the ACC/AHA guidelines do support surgery if the patient has severe AS with a LVEF of <50%, or a patient with moderate to severe AS who will undergo a concurrent CABG, aortic surgery, or other valve surgery at the same time.

**Symptomatic:** Aortic valve replacement (AVR) is indicated when patients become symptomatic since the survival time is limited after the onset of symptoms and there is an increased risk of sudden cardiac death (especially in symptomatic severe AS). Pharmacologic therapy should be limited prior to surgery since it can potentially destabilize the patient.

**Step 3)** Patients with rheumatic aortic stenosis should receive **prophylactic antibiotics** for secondary prevention of rheumatic fever.

## Follow-Up:

A TTE should be performed anytime there is a change in clinical status. Patients with mild AS should receive an echo every 3 to 5 years, those with moderate AS every 1 to 2 years, and those with severe AS every year. In addition, the ACC/AHA recommends monitoring dilatation of the aortic root or ascending aorta (diameter >40 mm) every year with echocardiography, cardiac MRI, or CT.

## Pearls:

- Routine infective endocarditis prophylaxis is no longer recommended in patients with common valvular disease, including AS, unless the patient had a **previous episode of infective endocarditis** or **prior prosthetic repair**.

- Exercise testing is not recommended in patients with symptomatic AS.

- Atrial fibrillation is not a common event in isolated aortic stenosis. If atrial fibrillation is present, it is usually associated with heart failure.

- If atrial fibrillation is encountered, the management is similar to patients without AS.

- Percutaneous aortic balloon valvotomy is not considered an alternative to aortic valve replacement (AVR), but it can be used as a bridge to AVR or as a palliative measure in critically ill patients.

- If a patient has a contraindication to warfarin or does not want to take anticoagulation, consider a bioprosthetic valve over a mechanical valve.

- Both aortic and pulmonic valves are normally tricuspid.

- Patients with congenitally deformed aortic valves can have normal functioning valves at birth, but over time the aortic valve can develop fibrocalcific changes that can lead to progressive stenosis.

- Aortic stenosis due to a congenital cause is typically seen in younger patients.

- Aortic stenosis due to rheumatic disease is not as common in the United States, but is common worldwide.

- Aortic stenosis due to age-related degenerative calcific changes (also known as "senile" or sclerocalcific AS) is now considered the most common cause of adult aortic stenosis in the United States.

- Aortic valve sclerosis can be defined as thickening of one or more leaflets without impairment of the leaflet motion. On echo, the leaflets may show thickening and calcification, but the flow velocities are essentially normal. Aortic valve sclerosis can progress to aortic stenosis (not in all individuals), which is an important marker for an increased risk of atherosclerotic disease. Therefore, it is important to identify any cardiovascular risks in these patients (ie, age, sex, smoking, hyperlipidemia, HTN, DM).

- Aortic valve sclerosis is commonly found in the elderly and may present without a murmur or may have a midsystolic ejection murmur.

- **Caveat 1**—Diuretics should be used with caution (ie, avoid overdiuresis) since a decrease in preload may affect the cardiac output.

- **Caveat 2**—Vasodilators (eg, hydralazine, nitroglycerin) should be used with caution since they can cause hypotension.

- **Caveat 3**—Positive inotropic agents (eg, dobutamine) should be used with caution since they can cause stress on the heart (ie, myocardial ischemia).

- **Caveat 4**—Beta-blockers should be avoided in heart failure or symptomatic AS since a decrease in contractility can cause more stress on the already overloaded left ventricle.

- Patients that present with signs and symptoms of heart failure are the most worrisome since the approximate median survival time after the onset of symptoms is the following (in decreasing order of survival time): angina (5-year survival time) >syncope (3-year survival time) >heart failure (2-year survival time).

- Patients with aortic stenosis have an increased risk of bleeding from the skin, mucosa, and GI (ie, bleeding from the angiodysplasia).

- The increase risk of bleeding is now thought to be due to an acquired von Willebrand syndrome that results in the mechanical disruption of the von Willebrand multimers as they pass through the stenotic valve.

- **Foundational point**—Laplace's law explains that the wall stress is proportional to the intraventricular pressure and radius of the ventricle, but inversely related to the wall thickness.

- **Connecting point** (pg. 132)—Acquired von Willebrand disease can be seen in other conditions.

- **On the CCS**, type in "aortic" in the order menu and notice the options available to you.

- **On the CCS**, you will be given a 2-minute warning toward the end of your case to finalize care for your patient. If you use all 2 minutes to add or delete orders, you may not be able to type in your final diagnosis. You should still attempt to enter a diagnosis even though it is not part of your evaluation performance.

# CHRONIC AORTIC REGURGITATION

Aortic regurgitation (AR), also known as aortic insufficiency, can be characterized by the retrograde diastolic blood flow from the aorta into the left ventricle. Causes of AR can be due to valvular abnormalities or dilatation of the aortic root. Consider the following causes:

**Valvular:** Congenital (bicuspid), endocarditis, rheumatic fever, RA, fenfluramine-phentermine.

**Aorta:** HTN, syphilis (aortitis), Marfan syndrome, ankylosing spondylitis, reactive arthritis

## Clinical Features:

**Murmur Type:** Diastolic murmur (between $S_2$ and $S_1$).

**Heart Sounds:**

$S_2$—Soft $A_2$, but with severe AR; $A_2$ is usually absent.

$S_3$—$S_3$ gallop is usually seen in the presence of LV dysfunction.

**Murmur sound**—A **high-frequency decrescendo murmur** (ie, "blowing" quality) can be best heard along the left sternal border (usually due to valvular disease), at the third and fourth intercostal space using the diaphragm of the stethoscope. If the murmur is barely audible, it can be appreciated by having the patient sit up, lean forward, and hold his or her breath on expiration. If the murmur is heard best along the right sternal border, it suggests that the AR is due to an aortic root abnormality.

If a murmur is heard at the apex (using the bell of the stethoscope), consider an **Austin Flint murmur**, which is a low-frequency rumbling mid-diastolic murmur that is thought to represent turbulent flow as a result of mitral leaflet displacement from the aortic regurgitant jet flow. The intensity of the murmur will change upon different maneuvers (see Table 3-6).

**Clinical Progression:** Since the LV must pump the normal blood volume from the left atrium plus the regurgitant volume, the LV compensates gradually through dilatation and **eccentric hypertrophy**. The left atrium can also accommodate the increase in LV diastolic pressure by enlarging its chamber and reducing the likelihood of pulmonary congestion. Therefore, patients will remain **asymptomatic** for a prolonged period. As a result of LV dilatation, a higher stroke volume will be pumped out during systole (ie, higher systolic pressure), but at the same time a larger amount of regurgitant blood flow will occur during diastole (ie, lower diastolic pressure), which ultimately leads to a **widened pulse pressure**. At some point, the LV function deteriorates and symptoms of **heart failure** develop.

**Clinical Presentation:** The widened pulse pressure, which is manifested as marked distention and quick collapse on palpation of the peripheral arteries (eg, carotid or radial artery), is known as the "water-hammer" or Corrigan's pulse. Most of the widened pulse pressure accounts for other physical findings, which include (from head to toe):

**Head**—Head bobbing (de Musset's sign).

**Eyes**—Retinal artery pulsations (Becker's sign).

**Lips**—Pulsations can be seen on the lips or fingernails with light pressure applied to the nail tip (Quincke's sign).

**Liver**—Pulsation of the liver (Rosenbach's sign).

**Spleen**—Pulsation of the spleen (Gerhard's sign).

**Femoral artery**—"Pistol-shot" sound over the femoral artery (Traube's sign) and a to-and-fro murmur over the femoral artery with light compression (Duroziez's sign).

**Uvula**—Pulsation of the uvula (Müller's sign).

**Popliteal artery**—Popliteal systolic pressure 60 mm Hg higher than brachial systolic pressure (Hill's sign).

**Severity:** For board purposes, the following is a general guideline for classifying the severity of the AR seen in adults: **mild** (LV size normal, regurgitant fraction <30%, regurgitant orifice area <0.1 cm$^2$), **moderate** (LV size normal to dilated, regurgitant fraction 30%-49%, regurgitant orifice area 0.1-0.29 cm$^2$), and **severe** (LV size dilated, regurgitant fraction ≥50%, regurgitant orifice area ≥0.3 cm$^2$).

### Next Step:

**Step 1)** The best initial test is with a **transthoracic echocardiography (TTE)**. If the information provided by the TTE is suboptimal, the next best step is with a **transesophageal echocardiography (TEE)**. A **cardiac catheterization** can be considered when there is a discrepancy between clinical and echocardiographic findings, or when the patient is about to undergo valve surgery but has risk factors for coronary artery disease. Other adjunctive testing may include the following:

**EKG**—EKG may show signs of LVH and sometimes left atrial hypertrophy.

**Chest x-ray**—On frontal view, the apex may be displaced inferiorly and to the left (advanced AR). Other possible findings include a dilated aortic root and/or ascending aorta (consider AR due to bicuspid aortic valve) and evidence of heart failure.

**Exercise stress testing**—Exercise stress testing may be performed in patients to assess functional status prior to athletic activity or in patients with equivocal symptoms.

**Step 2**) The clinical management for aortic regurgitation can be best summarized into patients that are asymptomatic or symptomatic. The following recommendations are based on the American College of Cardiology/American Heart Association (ACC/AHA) guidelines.

**Asymptomatic:**

1) Severe AR + Not candidates for surgery + LV dysfunction → Chronic vasodilator therapy

2) Severe AR + Concurrent CABG, aortic or valve surgery at the same time → AVR

3) Severe AR + LV dysfunction at rest (EF ≤ 50%) → AVR

4) Severe AR + Normal LV function (EF >50%) + LV dilatation (end-systolic dimension >55 mm or end-diastolic dimension >75 mm) → AVR

**Symptomatic:**

1) Severe AR + Not candidates for surgery → Chronic vasodilator therapy

2) Severe heart failure symptoms + Severe LV dysfunction + Before proceeding with AVR → Short-term vasodilator therapy

3) Severe AR (irrespective of EF) → AVR

**Step 3**) Patients with rheumatic aortic regurgitation should receive **prophylactic antibiotics** for secondary prevention of rheumatic fever.

**Follow-Up:**

A TTE should be performed anytime there is a change in clinical status. As a general guideline, patients with mild AR (without LV dysfunction and dilatation) should have yearly clinical exams with routine echo every 2 to 3 years. Patients with moderate AR (without LV dysfunction and dilatation) should have yearly clinical exams with routine echo every 1 to 2 years. Those with severe AR (without LV dysfunction but with LV dilatation) require more frequent assessments such as clinical exams every

6 months and echo every 6 to 12 months. In addition, the ACC/AHA recommends monitoring dilatation of the aortic root or ascending aorta (diameter >40 mm) every year with echocardiography, cardiac MRI, or CT.

**Pearls:**

- Routine infective endocarditis prophylaxis is no longer recommended in patients with common valvular disease, including chronic AR, unless the patient had a **previous episode of infective endocarditis** or **prior prosthetic repair**.

- The prognosis in patients with AR is mainly determined by the presence of symptoms, LV function, and LV size.

- On EKG, right atrial hypertrophy is characterized by a biphasic P wave with a prominent positive deflection in the initial portion of the P wave in lead $V_1$.

- **CJ:** A 42-year-old man presents to the ED with blunt trauma to the chest. The patient presents with dyspnea, tachycardia, and hypotension. On cardiac exam, a low-pitched early diastolic murmur can be heard along the left sternal border in the third intercostal space. A soft $A_2$ with an accentuated $P_2$ (ie, presence of pulmonary hypertension) as well as an $S_3$ can also be appreciated. A bedside TTE suggests an acute aortic regurgitation. What are your next steps? **Answer:** Patients with acute AR require emergent aortic valve replacement or repair. In the interim, treat pulmonary edema with oxygen and respiratory failure with intubation (ie, high diastolic LV pressure transmitted to left atrium and lungs since the LV is relatively noncompliant). The patient may need to be temporarily stabilized in the ICU with IV vasodilators (eg, nitroprusside) and positive inotropic agents (eg, dobutamine or dopamine) to facilitate forward flow. Intraaortic balloon pump (IABP) is contraindicated in patients with acute AR since the balloon will worsen the regurgitant flow. Causes of acute AR include trauma, aortic dissection, and endocarditis. Clues to endocarditis would be the presence of fevers, chills, and a murmur heard along the left sternal border. Clues to an aortic dissection would include a "ripping" pain in the back or chest, greater than 20 mm Hg blood pressure difference between the left and right arm, and murmur heard along the right sternal border. Patients suspected of having an aortic dissection should have either a TEE or CT to make the diagnosis. In general, patients with an acute AR will not have a widened pulse pressure seen in chronic AR.

- **On the CCS**, once you receive the 2-minute warning toward the end of the case, you will not be able to relocate the patient, perform physical exams, make follow-up appointments, or view pending results.

# MYOCARDIUM DISORDER

## ▌ HYPERTROPHIC CARDIOMYOPATHY

Hypertrophic cardiomyopathy (HCM) is frequently referred to as hypertrophic obstructive cardiomyopathy (HOCM) or idiopathic hypertrophic subaortic stenosis (IHSS). HCM is distinct from

secondary hypertrophy (due to HTN or aortic stenosis) in that (1) Myocytes have a disorganized arrangement (unlike the orderly and enlarged myocytes seen in secondary hypertrophy) and (2) HCM can occur as a familial disease with autosomal dominant inheritance, or sporadically. HCM can have different morphologies (eg, septal, apical, or biventricular hypertrophy) with the end result of having diastolic dysfunction (ie, impaired filling).

**Clinical Features:**

**Murmur Type:** Systolic murmur (between $S_1$ and $S_2$).

**Heart Sounds:**

$S_2$—Normally a physiologic split, but with severe outflow obstruction, a paradoxical split can be heard.

$S_4$—$S_4$ is a common finding.

**Murmur sound**—A **harsh systolic crescendo-decrescendo murmur** can be best heard along the left lower sternal border, and sometimes it can radiate to the apex or base of the heart (usually not into the carotids). Unlike aortic stenosis, palpation of the carotid artery will reveal a brisk upstroke in the carotid pulse during early systole but then quickly decline in midsystole as a result of the outflow obstruction. In addition, the pulse is frequently biphasic or bifid (pulsus bisferiens). If a **holosystolic blowing murmur** is heard at the apex, then mitral regurgitation has developed from the outflow obstruction. The intensity of the murmur will change upon different maneuvers (see Table 3-6).

**Clinical Progression:** Some patients will develop HCM without an outflow tract obstruction. However, these patients will still develop increasing LV diastolic pressures (due to a stiff ventricle), which can eventually be transmitted back to the pulmonary vasculature and manifest as dyspnea. In other patients, outflow tract obstruction can accompany HCM with the systolic anterior motion (SAM) of the mitral leaflet against a hypertrophied septum. As a result of an improperly closed mitral valve during systole, mitral regurgitation can develop with subsequent development of dyspnea and atrial fibrillation. In a minority of patients, heart failure can develop in the late stages of the disease.

**Clinical Presentation:** HCM can occur at any age, and clinical manifestations can vary. However, features of HCM (similar to aortic stenosis) can be easily remembered by the mnemonic **"SAAAD"**:

**S**yncope—Syncope can be due to the outflow tract obstruction or arrhythmias.

**A**rrhythmias—Supraventricular (eg, atrial fibrillation, atrial flutter) and ventricular arrhythmias (eg, ventricular fibrillation, which can cause sudden cardiac death) can result in palpitations.

**A**symptomatic—Some patients may have minor to no symptoms. There is no strong correlation between the severity of the obstruction and symptoms.

**A**ngina—Even in the absence of CAD, angina may be due to an increase in myocardial $O_2$ demand and/or a decrease in myocardial $O_2$ supply.

**D**yspnea—Dyspnea is a common finding that can be due to diastolic dysfunction (ie, impaired diastolic relaxation), outflow obstruction with mitral regurgitation, or less commonly from heart failure, which may present as paroxysmal nocturnal dyspnea and orthopnea.

**Next Step:**

**Step 1)** The best initial tests are with a **transthoracic echocardiography (TTE)** and **EKG**. If information on the TTE is inconclusive, then a **transesophageal echocardiography (TEE)** would be the next best step to help guide management decisions. **Cardiac**

**catheterization** is usually unnecessary, but in the uncommon circumstances where there is a discrepancy between clinical findings and echocardiography, cardiac catheterization may be beneficial. The following are possible findings on the TTE and EKG:

**TTE**—Diastolic dysfunction, LVH with an increase in septal wall thickness, systolic anterior motion of the mitral valve, mitral regurgitation, increase in the LV outflow tract gradient, small LV cavity, or a "ground-glass" appearance of the hypertrophied myocardium.

**EKG**—EKG findings may include any of the following: LVH, left atrial enlargement, left axis deviation, prominent Q waves mimicking an MI in the inferior (II, III, aVF) and lateral leads (I, aVL, $V_4$-$V_6$), diffuse T-wave inversion in the precordial leads, or arrhythmias during ambulatory (Holter) monitoring.

Other adjunctive testing may include the following:

**Chest x-ray**—Chest x-ray is usually normal or may show mild to moderate enlargement of the cardiac silhouette.

**Exercise stress testing**—Exercise stress testing may be reasonable to assess functional capacity, SCD risk stratification (EKG monitoring), or to assess an inducible LV outflow obstruction (echocardiography monitoring) in patients without LV outflow obstruction at rest.

**Step 2)** The clinical management for HCM can be best summarized into patients that are asymptomatic or symptomatic.

**Asymptomatic:** Routine pharmacologic therapy (eg, beta-blockers, calcium channel blockers) and septal reduction therapy is not recommended in asymptomatic patients.

**Symptomatic:** Symptomatic patients can undergo pharmacologic therapy and/or surgery. Consider the following conditions:

**Syncope**—The next best step to manage patients with syncope is (1) order an echocardiography to evaluate for an obstruction, and/or (2) Holter monitor to evaluate for arrhythmias. Patients that continue to have syncope despite optimal medical therapy and known outflow tract obstruction are candidates for septal reduction therapy. However, if syncope cannot be explained by a specific cause, it is considered a risk factor for sudden cardiac death (SCD). Therefore, the next best step is to consider an implantable cardioverter defibrillator (ICD).

**Sudden cardiac death (SCD)**—Patients that survive an SCD through appropriate intervention should have a thorough evaluation for the possible cause (eg, EKG, Holter monitor, echo) and should be treated appropriately. Since patients that survive an SCD are at risk of another SCD event, patients should receive prophylactic ICD placement. In addition, patients are advised to avoid competitive sports and strenuous exercise.

**Acute hypotension**—HCM patients with an outflow tract obstruction can sometimes present with acute hypotension. In these patients, the first step is to elevate their legs. The next step is to administer IV fluids. Patients who do not respond to fluids should then receive **IV phenylephrine** (alpha-1 agonist).

**Atrial fibrillation**—If atrial fibrillation is encountered, patients can be managed with either rate control (eg, beta-blockers or calcium channel blockers) or rhythm control (eg, amiodarone or disopyramide with ventricular rate-controlling agent). If patients continue to have persistent or recurrent atrial fibrillation, then radiofrequency ablation or surgical maze procedure (only if the patient is undergoing concurrent cardiac surgery) can be performed. Anticoagulation is recommended in patients with persistent, paroxysmal, or chronic atrial fibrillation with HCM.

**Angina or dyspnea**—The following is the next step treatment approach for angina or dyspnea:

Step 1) The best initial therapy is with a negative inotropic agent such as low-dose **beta-blocker** or **verapamil**.

Step 2) If no response, titrate to a higher dose.

Step 3) If no response, switch to the other drug (ie, beta-blocker or verapamil).

Step 4) If no response, add **disopyramide** (class Ia anti-arrhythmic agent) to either beta-blocker or verapamil.

Step 5) If symptoms are refractory despite medical therapy and the patient has known outflow tract obstruction (ie, provokable or at rest), then consider a **septal myectomy**, **septal (alcohol) ablation**, or **dual-chamber pacing**.

**Step 3**) Since SCD has been associated with strenuous exercise, patients with HCM should be counseled to avoid competitive or high-intensity sports.

**Step 4**) First-degree relatives of an affected HCM patient should be screened for possible genetic inheritance with a thorough history, physical, echo, and EKG.

### Disposition/Follow-Up:

A TTE should be performed anytime there is a change in clinical status. First-degree relatives of an affected individual should continue to have periodic surveillance since delayed-onset HCM can occur and first-degree family members are still at risk of SCD. Patients who present with syncope in the emergency department with suspected HCM should be admitted to the hospital for further workup (eg, Holter monitor, echo, stress test).

### Pearls:

- Routine infective endocarditis prophylaxis is no longer recommended in patients with HCM, unless the patient had a **previous episode of infective endocarditis** or **prior prosthetic heart repair**.

- **Caveat 1**—Avoid diuretics, digoxin, and vasodilators (eg, nitroglycerin, ACE inhibitors, ARBs) in patients with HCM and significant LV outflow tract obstruction (remember patients can still have HCM without obstruction).

- **Caveat 2**—The calcium channel blockers (eg, nifedipine, verapamil, diltiazem) have vasodilatory properties that can cause hypotension. Therefore, calcium channel blockers should be avoided or used with caution in HCM patients with outflow tract obstruction.

- **Caveat 3**—Beta-blockers and verapamil should be used with caution in patients with sinus bradycardia.

- **Caveat 4**—Digoxin should be avoided in the management of atrial fibrillation since it has a positive inotropic effect that could worsen the outflow tract obstruction.

- **Caveat 5**—Be aware of volume status in patients with HCM since volume depletion can exacerbate the outflow tract obstruction, which may lead to worsening of symptoms.

- The Valsalva maneuver decreases preload, which makes the LV cavity smaller and allows the anterior mitral leaflet to come closer to the hypertrophied septum creating greater obstruction and increasing the intensity of the murmur.

- Competitive athletes that train with high intensity can develop "athlete's heart," which may resemble HCM. However, several distinctions should be made: (1) There is no impairment in diastolic filling (remember, they are athletes), (2) left atrium is usually normal, (3) LV wall thickness is usually symmetric, and (4) EKG findings usually reveal only LVH.

- The "**SAD**" (syncope, angina, dyspnea/heart failure) seen in aortic stenosis reflects end-stage disease. Patients can remain asymptomatic for a period of time before they encounter the classic symptoms of aortic stenosis. The "**SAAAD**" seen in HCM reflects a varied presentation that can occur at any one time.

- SCD is a major cause of mortality in patients with HCM. The incidence of SCD in children with HCM is as high as 6% per year, and it is 2% to 4% per year in adults.

- A prominent "a wave" may be seen on inspection of the neck veins.

- A double or triple apical impulse can be appreciated over the cardiac apex.

- **Connecting point** (pg. 163)—Know the inheritance pattern of autosomal dominant genes.

- **On the CCS**, be aware that in some CCS cases you will have to recognize when to refrain from further evaluation or treatment since the examination is assessing your clinical judgment.

# CONGENITAL DISORDERS

## ATRIAL SEPTAL DEFECT

Atrial septal defect (ASD) is a common congenital heart anomaly that is characterized by an interatrial septal defect that results in a left-to-right shunt (ie, acyanotic lesion). Septal tissue is absent in ASDs, which distinguishes this condition from a patent foramen ovale (PFO). ASDs can be an isolated disease or associated with other congenital lesions such as transposition of the great arteries, tricuspid atresia, tricuspid regurgitation, mitral regurgitation, or a VSD. There are four types of ASDs to consider, and it may be helpful to consider them in their relative anatomic location from a superior to inferior direction within the interatrial septum:

1) **Sinus venosus defect**—These are uncommon defects, and there are two types. The superior sinus venosus defect is located below the orifice of the SVC, and the inferior sinus venosus defect is located above the orifice of the IVC. Both types of sinus venosus defects can have anomalous pulmonary venous connections (eg, pulmonary veins connecting into the right atrium, SVC, or IVC).

2) **Ostium secundum defect**—This type is the most common defect and is located in the midseptum. This defect is more common in females than in males and is associated with mitral valve prolapse. Ostium secundum defects should not be confused with a PFO.

3) **Ostium primum defect**—This type of defect is located near the base of the interatrial septum or adjacent to the AV valves. This defect is associated with AV valve anomalies and is commonly seen in Down syndrome.

4) **Coronary sinus defect**—This is an uncommon defect that can be characterized by the absence of the wall between the coronary sinus and the left atrium. Many patients will also have a persistent left SVC that drains into the left atrium.

## Clinical Features:

### Heart Sounds:

$S_1$—$S_1$ can be normal or split with accentuation of the second component (tricuspid closure).

$S_2$—Wide, fixed splitting is usually seen with larger left-to-right shunts with normal pulmonary arterial pressures, which is thought to reduce the respiratory variation.

$S_4$—A right-sided $S_4$ can be heard if right ventricular hypertrophy (RVH) develops.

**Murmur sound**—There is **no murmur at the site of the ASD** because of an insufficient pressure gradient between the two atria. However, murmur sounds can be heard with larger left-to-right shunts that create more blood flow across the tricuspid valve (mid-diastolic murmur heard over the lower left sternal border) and across the pulmonary valve (systolic crescendo-decrescendo ejection murmur heard over the second intercostal space at the upper left sternal border). If an ostium primum defect or an ostium secundum defect is present, then a murmur sound of a mitral regurgitation or mitral valve prolapse may be heard respectively.

**Clinical Progression:** Patients with **small ASDs** (<8 mm in diameter) will typically have spontaneous closure while they are infants. It is uncommon to have spontaneous closure while they are children or adults. Patients with **moderate to large ASDs** will tend to have an increase in their left-to-right shunting as they age, and therefore, they will usually be symptomatic before the age of 40. In some cases, if significant pulmonary vascular disease develops over time, the direction of the shunt may reverse, causing a right-to-left shunt and manifesting as **Eisenmenger syndrome**, which is generally an irreversible condition. In this condition, blood bypasses the lungs and results in delivery of deoxygenated blood to the rest of the body, which will usually manifest as cyanosis and clubbing.

**Clinical Presentation**—The presentation usually depends on the size of the defect. Consider the following sizes:

**Small ASDs**—Small ASDs may be undetected during the first two years of life because the patient may be asymptomatic and have unimpressive auscultatory findings.

**Moderate to large ASDs**—Common manifestations include dyspnea, fatigue, and exercise intolerance. In childhood, patients may also present with recurrent respiratory infections. In adults, symptoms of heart failure are more prevalent by the fourth or fifth decades of life. Patients may also have palpitations associated with the heart failure, which may be due to atrial arrhythmias (eg, atrial fibrillation, atrial flutter) caused by right atrial enlargement.

## Next Step:

**Step 1)** A **transthoracic echocardiography (TTE)** is used to confirm the diagnosis of an ASD. If the image quality is suboptimal on TTE, the next best step is with a **transesophageal echocardiography (TEE)**. The TEE may be particularly useful in the diagnosis of a sinus venosus defect because it may potentially identify an anomalous pulmonary venous connection. A **cardiac catheterization** is not routinely performed to make the diagnosis. However, it may be useful if there are equivocal clinical findings, measure pulmonary vascular resistance (PVR), or to perform a transcatheter closure for small to moderate secundum ASDs. Other adjunctive testing may include the following:

**EKG**—EKG findings may include any of the following: left axis deviation, right axis deviation, RVH, first degree AV block, prolonged PR interval, atrial arrhythmias, or an rsR' pattern (RBBB) in lead $V_1$, which is thought to be related to RVH rather than a circuitry conduction problem.

**Chest x-ray**—With significant amount of left-to-right shunting, the right atrium and ventricle are usually enlarged. In addition, there is usually an increase in pulmonary vascular markings with a prominent pulmonary artery.

**Step 2)** Consider the clinical management of ASD:

**"Wait and See Approach":** A wait and see approach can be attempted in infants with an ostium secundum defect that is less than 8 mm since most defects will spontaneously close by 2 years of age. A wait and see approach can also be attempted in infants with larger secundum defects who are asymptomatic since there is still a possibility of spontaneous closure by 2 years of age.

**ASD Closure:** ASD closure can be accomplished through surgery or by percutaneous transcatheter closure. Transcatheter closure has the advantage of avoiding cardiopulmonary bypass, but the procedure is only amenable to ostium secundum defects. Sinus venosus, ostium primum, and coronary sinus defects should be surgically repaired. The following are indications and contraindications for ASD closure:

**Indications**—ASD closure is recommended in patients with either (1) evidence of right atrial and right ventricular enlargement with or without symptoms, or (2) significant left-to-right shunting that correlates to a pulmonary-to-systemic flow ratio (Qp/Qs) >2:1.

**Contraindications**—ASD closure is not recommended in patients with severe irreversible pulmonary hypertension and in patients with insignificant left-to-right shunts.

### Follow-Up:

A TTE should be performed anytime there is a change in clinical status. Patients that do not meet the indications for an ASD closure should be seen for a clinical exam and echocardiography at least every 2 to 3 years.

### Pearls:

- Routine infective endocarditis prophylaxis is no longer recommended in patients with an ASD unless the ASD is repaired with prosthetic materials. If prosthetic materials are used, then for the first 6 months after the repair, prophylactic antibiotics are recommended for dental, oral, or respiratory procedures.

- Infective endocarditis prophylaxis is also recommended in patients undergoing dental, oral, or respiratory procedures who have a repaired ASD with a residual defect adjacent to or at the site of prosthetic materials.

- Patients with an ASD will have an increase in oxygen saturation in the right atrium compared to the SVC or IVC.

- Paradoxical embolization occurs when an embolus originates from the venous system and crosses a PFO or ASD that eventually enters the arterial system, which could potentially cause a stroke. The embolus usually crosses the PFO or ASD when there is a transient right-to-left shunt gradient (eg, Valsalva maneuver, repetitive coughing) and does not necessarily have to occur with a chronic right-to-left shunt gradient (eg, Eisenmenger syndrome). An ASD closure is usually considered in the presence of a paradoxical embolism.

- Patients with an intracardiac shunt (eg, ASD, VSD, PFO, PDA) should avoid scuba diving because of the risk of paradoxical embolism and decompression illness.

- Pregnant women with uncomplicated ASDs typically do well during their pregnancy; however, complications to consider are arrhythmias, paradoxical embolization, and an increase in the left-to-right shunting in the presence of acute blood loss.

- Pregnancy is contraindicated in women who have developed Eisenmenger syndrome.

- **On the CCS**, "Atrial septal defect repair" is available in the practice CCS, but be sure to order a cardiac surgery consult prior to the repair.

- **On the CCS**, prior to a surgical procedure, preoperative care may include a CBC, BMP, type and crossmatch, and coagulation studies (PT, PTT).

## ▌VENTRICULAR SEPTAL DEFECT

Ventricular septal defect (VSD) is the most common congenital heart anomaly. VSD is characterized by a left-to-right shunt (ie, acyanotic lesion) with oxygenated blood still reaching the rest of the body. VSD can be an isolated disease or associated with other congenital heart defects such as tetralogy of Fallot, transposition of the great arteries, PDA, ASD, or atrioventricular canal defects. Consider four types of VSDs:

1) **Membranous defect**—This is the most common type of defect. When the defect extends into the muscular septum, it is referred to as perimembranous VSD. Aortic regurgitation with aortic valve prolapse is associated with this defect.

2) **Muscular defect**—This type of defect can close spontaneously. When there are multiple defects, the septum is often referred to as "Swiss cheese."

3) **Subpulmonic defect**—This type of defect is usually associated with aortic regurgitation caused by prolapse of the right aortic cusp of the aortic valve.

4) **Inlet defect**—This type of defect is associated with ASDs and Down syndrome. Inlet defects generally do not close spontaneously.

### Clinical Features:

**Murmur Type:** Systolic murmur with or without diastolic murmur.

### Heart Sounds:

$S_2$—A normal physiologic split is usually heard with small VSDs. In larger VSDs, the pulmonary arterial pressures can increase, which may result in a narrow split $S_2$ with a louder $P_2$ component. If there is pulmonic stenosis or concomitant RBBB (eg, complication from corrective surgery), then there may be a delayed $P_2$, which can result in a wide split $S_2$.

**Murmur sound**—A **harsh holosystolic murmur** can be best heard along the left lower sternal border and is sometimes accompanied by an **apical mid-diastolic flow rumble** which is thought to represent increasing blood flow across the mitral valve. If there is a large VSD with pulmonary hypertension, the shunting effect (ie, blood flow across the defect) may end before systole, and thus, it may be referred to as an **early systolic murmur**. An early systolic murmur can also occur in small muscular VSDs in the absence of pulmonary hypertension since the defect can close soon after the start of systole. The intensity of the murmur will change upon different maneuvers (see Table 3-6).

**Clinical Progression:** Patients with **small VSDs** will typically have spontaneous closure within the first two years of life. Small VSDs can persist into adulthood but are usually benign, although they can develop aortic regurgitation and endocarditis. **Moderate VSDs** may diminish in size over time and can spontaneously close, but less often than small VSDs. Patients with moderate VSDs can be asymptomatic or they can develop heart failure in childhood. **Large VSDs** usually do not close spontaneously, and parents seek medical attention early in life. The left-to-right shunt becomes prominent, which can result in volume overload in the right ventricle, pulmonary vasculature, left atrium, and left ventricle with subsequent development of heart failure by 3 to 4 weeks of age. If significant pulmonary vascular resistance increases over time, the shunt can reverse to a right-to-left shunt and manifest as **Eisenmenger syndrome**.

**Clinical Presentation**—The presentation usually depends on the size of the defect. Consider the following sizes:

**Small VSDs**—Patients are usually asymptomatic with normal feeding and weight gain.

**Moderate to large VSDs**—Patients may show signs of heart failure such as tachypnea, tachycardia, and hepatomegaly. Poor feeding with poor weight gain and growth may also be apparent. Diaphoresis (↑ sympathetic tone) and fatigue usually accompanies the feeds.

### Next Step:

**Step 1**) A **transthoracic echocardiography (TTE)** is used to confirm the diagnosis of a VSD. If the image quality is suboptimal on TTE, the next best step is with a **transesophageal echocardiography (TEE)**. The TEE may be particularly useful in visualizing aortic valve prolapse compared to the TTE. The TEE is also used intraoperatively to assess the surgical closure. A **cardiac catheterization** is infrequently performed, but it may beneficial to guide perioperative management, accurately assess hemodynamic status, measure pulmonary vascular resistance (PVR), or unravel equivocal clinical findings. Other adjunctive testing may include the following:

**EKG**—With small VSDs, the EKG is usually normal. In moderate to large VSDs with a significant amount of left-to-right shunting, left atrial enlargement and LVH can be seen with increasing blood return to the left part of the heart. If pulmonary vascular disease develops, RVH may also be apparent.

**Chest x-ray**—With small VSDs, the CXR is usually normal. In moderate to large VSDs with a significant amount of left-to-right shunting, there is usually an increase in pulmonary vascular markings with a prominent pulmonary artery.

**Step 2**) The clinical management of VSD depends on several factors such as the size of the VSD, presence of pulmonary hypertension, likelihood of spontaneous closure, and likelihood of a successful surgical repair. Consider the clinical management of VSD:

**Small VSD:** Asymptomatic patients do not require medical or surgical intervention. During the first year of life, the patient should have regularly scheduled follow-ups, and some physicians will elect to repeat an echocardiogram after the first year.

**Moderate to large VSDs:** Medical or surgical intervention is usually indicated when there is significant amount of left-to-right shunting causing symptoms. Consider the following:

**Heart failure**—The best initial pharmacologic therapy is with a **diuretic** (eg, furosemide) to relieve pulmonary congestion. An **ACE inhibitor** (eg, captopril, enalapril) can be used to reduce systemic vascular resistance and thus, ultimately reduce the left-to-right shunt. **Digoxin** is sometimes used to enhance contractility when diuresis or afterload reduction fails to relieve symptoms.

**Poor weight gain**—Infants have a high metabolic demand and require a certain amount of calories per day. Infants with a VSD may be tired with each feeding and therefore unable to meet their caloric requirements. Increasing the caloric density of the formula with each feeding may be successful. Infants should be monitored for their growth at least every 2 weeks. If infants cannot meet their nutritional requirements and growth is subpar, surgical repair is most likely to occur.

**VSD Closure:** VSD closure can be accomplished through surgery or by percutaneous transcatheter closure. Transcatheter closure can be performed on muscular VSDs and certain membranous VSDs. The following are indications and contraindications for VSD closure:

**Indications**—VSD closure is recommended in infants when patients continue to have symptoms despite optimal medical therapy, pulmonary-to-systemic flow ratio (Qp/Qs) >2:1 with elevated pulmonary arterial pressures, or in the presence of aortic regurgitation, which is seen in membranous and subpulmonic defects. VSD closure is recommended in adults when patients have a history of infective endocarditis, or pulmonary-to-systemic flow ratio (Qp/Qs) >2:1 with evidence of LV volume overload.

**Contraindications**—VSD closure is not recommended in patients with severe irreversible pulmonary hypertension.

### Follow-Up:

Patients with small VSDs and those who underwent cardiac surgical repair for a VSD require long-term follow-up.

### Pearls:

- Routine infective endocarditis prophylaxis is no longer recommended in patients with a VSD unless the VSD is repaired with prosthetic material. If prosthetic material is used, then for the first 6 months after the repair, prophylactic antibiotics are recommended for dental, oral, or respiratory procedures.

- Infective endocarditis prophylaxis is also recommended in patients undergoing dental, oral, or respiratory procedures who have a repaired VSD with a residual defect adjacent to or at the site of prosthetic materials.

- Increasing the afterload (ie, handgrip or squat) will increase the effect of the left-to-right shunt, thereby increasing the intensity of the murmur.

- Remember to keep a watchful eye on patients with a VSD and a narrow split $S_2$ with marked accentuation of the $P_2$ component because they are indications of increasing pulmonary arterial pressures, which may limit the patients' ability to undergo corrective surgical repair.

- In patients that developed right ventricular hypertrophy (RVH), a prominent "a" wave may be seen on jugular venous inspection.

- Pregnant women with small VSDs usually complete their pregnancy without complications.

- Pregnant women with moderate to large VSDs are at higher risk of developing complications.
- Pregnancy is contraindicated in women who have developed Eisenmenger syndrome.
- Patients with a VSD will have an increase in oxygen saturation in the right ventricle compared to the right atrium.
- **On the CCS**, patients that present to the office or ED with heart failure symptoms should initially be admitted to the hospital and managed on the inpatient unit.

- **On the CCS**, it is appropriate to consult a pediatric cardiologist in a patient with a VSD. Although the consultant may not say anything useful on the CCS exam, you are expected to implement a course of action (eg, echo, EKG, CXR).
- **On the CCS**, "VSD repair" is available in the practice CCS, but be sure to order a cardiac surgery consult prior to the repair.
- **On the CCS**, if the patient is not feeding well, be sure to order a "calorie count" or "dietary intake."

# CCS: ACUTE PERICARDITIS CASE INTRODUCTION

Day 1 @ 10:00
Emergency Room

A 42-year-old man from India comes to the emergency room because of chest pain.

**Initial Vital Signs:**
Temperature: 38.3°C (101°F)
Pulse: 85 beats/min
Respiratory: 16/min
Blood pressure: 128/85 mm Hg
Height: 185.4 cm (73.0 inches)
Weight: 79.3 kg (175 lb)
BMI: 23.1 kg/m²

**Initial History:**
Reason(s) for visit: Chest pain

**HPI:**
A 42-year-old man, who recently immigrated from India, is complaining of sudden chest pain for the past two days. The chest pain is a sharp retrosternal pain that radiates to the trapezius ridges. Coughing, inspiration, or lying supine aggravates the pain, but it is alleviated when sitting up and leaning forward. He rates his pain as a 5 on a 10-point scale. The patient states that he had a cough, runny nose, and a sore throat 1 week ago that has since resolved. He denies chills, shortness of breath, nausea, vomiting, abdominal pain, or any recent trauma.

| | |
|---|---|
| **Past Medical History:** | History of peptic ulcer disease |
| **Past Surgical History:** | None |
| **Medications:** | None |
| **Allergies:** | None |
| **Vaccinations:** | BCG vaccination |

| | |
|---|---|
| **Family History:** | Father, age 65, had a heart attack at age 60. Mother, age 63, is healthy. |
| **Social History:** | Smokes one pack per day × 20 years; denies drinking or drugs, married with two children, computer engineer, enjoys playing cricket |

**Review of Systems:**
| | |
|---|---|
| General: | See HPI |
| Skin: | Negative |
| HEENT: | See HPI |
| Musculoskeletal: | See HPI |
| Cardiorespiratory: | See HPI |
| Gastrointestinal: | Negative |
| Genitourinary: | Negative |
| Neuropsychiatric: | Negative |

Day 1 @ 10:00

**First Order Sheet:**
1) IV access
2) Pulse oximetry, stat — **Result:** 94%
3) Continuous cardiac monitor, stat — **Result:** Regular sinus
4) Continuous blood pressure cuff, stat — **Result:** 128/85 mm Hg
5) 12-lead EKG, stat — **Result:** Diffuse ST-segment elevations with upward concavity. Reciprocal ST-segment depressions in aVR and V₁. PR segment elevation in aVR, but PR segment depressions in other leads. Q waves absent.

**Second Order Sheet:**
1) Morphine, IV, one time
2) Oxygen, inhalation, continuous
3) Nitroglycerin, sublingual, one time
4) Aspirin, oral, one time

**Follow-Up History:**

Patient feels only partial relief and rates his pain as 4/10.

**Physical Examination:**

| | |
|---|---|
| General appearance: | Well nourished, well developed; in no acute distress. |
| HEENT/Neck: | Normocephalic. EOMI, PERRLA. Hearing normal. Ear, nose, mouth normal. Pharynx normal. Neck supple; trachea midline; no masses or bruits; thyroid normal. |
| Chest/Lungs: | Chest wall normal. Diaphragm and chest moving equally and symmetrically with respiration, but chest pain is elicited upon inspiration. Auscultation and percussion normal. |
| Heart/Cardiovascular: | Pericardial friction rub heard along the left sternal border. The intensity of the rub can be better appreciated with the patient leaning forward or resting his elbows on his knees. No reproducible chest pain on palpation of the anterior chest. No JVD. |
| Abdomen: | Normal bowel sounds; no bruits. No tenderness or masses. No abnormality on percussion. No rebound. No guarding. No hepatosplenomegaly. |
| Extremities/Spine: | No joint deformity or warmth. No cyanosis or clubbing. No edema. Peripheral pulses normal. Spine exam normal. No paraspinal tenderness. |

**Third Order Sheet:**
1) CBC with differential, stat — **Result:** WBC 12,500, H/H15/45%, Plt 250,000, Differential normal
2) BMP, stat — **Result:** Glu100, Urea 15, Na 140, K 4.0, Cl 100, HCO3 23, Cr 1,Ca 9.1
3) Troponin I, serum, stat — **Result:** 0.1 ng/mL (nl: 0-0.6)
4) ESR, stat — **Result:** 45 mm/hour (nl: 0-15)
5) PT/INR, stat — **Result:** PT-9.2 seconds (nl: <12), INR-1.0 (nl: 1.0-1.3)
6) PTT, stat — **Result:** 25 seconds (nl: <28)
7) Blood culture, stat — **Result:** No growth
8) Interferon gamma release assay — **Result:** Latent TB not detected
9) Chest x-ray, portable, stat — **Result:** Lungs clear, normal cardiac silhouette
10) Echocardiography, stat — **Result:** 5 mm of echo-free space. LVEF 60%

**Fourth Order Sheet:**
1) Indomethacin, oral, continuous
2) Colchicine, oral, continuous
3) Omeprazole, oral, continuous

**Actions:**
1) Change location to inpatient unit — **Note:** Vitals are automatically ordered for you in the practice CCS.

**Follow-Up History:**

Patient feels better and rates his pain as 2/10.

**Fifth Order Sheet:**
1) Check blood pressure — **Result:** 128/85 mm Hg
2) Check cardiac monitor — **Result:** Regular sinus

**This case will end in the next few minutes of "real time."**
You may **add** or **delete** orders at this time,
then enter a diagnosis on the following screen.

**Sixth Order Sheet:**
1) Cancel supplemental oxygen
2) ESR, routine
   Future date: In 14 days — **Result:** 8 mm/hour (nl: 0-15)
3) Counsel family/patient
4) Advise patient, no smoking
5) Advise patient, side effects of medication

**Please enter your diagnosis:**

Acute Pericarditis

**DISCUSSION:**

Acute pericarditis refers to inflammation of the pericardium, which consists of the visceral and parietal pericardium. Most cases of acute pericarditis are idiopathic in nature, but most likely of viral origin. Other causes of acute pericarditis includes bacterial infections, fungal infections, TB, inflammatory conditions (eg, RA, SLE, IBD, scleroderma, rheumatic fever), metabolic conditions (eg, uremia, hypothyroidism), cardiac conditions (eg, Dressler's syndrome, aortic dissection), radiation-induced, neoplastic disease, drug-induced (eg, hydralazine, procainamide, isoniazid, minoxidil, doxorubicin), iatrogenic, or trauma.

## Clinical Features:

Patients with acute pericarditis may present in different ways depending on the etiology. For example, malignancy (eg, weight loss, lymphadenopathy), infections (eg, fever, leukocytosis), SLE (eg, arthritis, photosensitivity), Crohn's disease (eg, abdominal pain, nonbloody diarrhea), or TB (eg, night sweats, cough). In addition to the specific manifestations of the underlying cause, the vast majority of patients will also present with chest pain. The pain is typically an acute onset, but it can be gradual. The pain is precordial or retrosternal that radiates to the back, neck, shoulder, arm, or to the trapezius ridge. The pain is usually characterized as sharp and pleuritic. Lying flat often aggravates the pain, but sitting up and leaning forward relieves the pain by reducing the pressure on the parietal pericardium. Sometimes patients may complain of dysphagia due to an irritation of the esophagus from the posterior pericardium. An associated condition that is usually seen with viral etiologies is a "flulike" illness prior to the onset of acute pericarditis. On physical exam, the presence of a pericardial friction rub is pathognomonic for acute pericarditis. The rub is best heard with the diaphragm of the stethoscope applied between the left lower sternal border and the cardiac apex with the patient leaning forward in suspended respiration. Cardiac tamponade can sometimes develop in patients with a neoplastic etiology, trauma, or from an iatrogenic cardiac perforation. Clues to look for in cardiac tamponade include Beck's triad (ie, hypotension, JVD, muffled heart sounds) and pulsus paradoxus (ie, systolic blood pressure decreases more than 10 mm Hg on inspiration).

## Next Step Summary:

**Step 1)** In this patient that presented with chest pain, the initial clinical management focused on ruling out a myocardial infarction or ischemia. However, consider your differential diagnosis in this patient, which should include a pulmonary embolism, aortic dissection, costochondritis, peptic ulcer disease, or esophageal spasm.

**Step 2)** The diagnosis of acute pericarditis is usually based on the clinical history (ie, pleuritic chest pain with improvement by sitting up and leaning forward), physical exam (ie, pericardial friction rub), and EKG changes. Consider all the following possible options in evaluating a patient with suspected acute pericarditis, but use your clinical judgment on what tests are appropriate for that given patient.

CBC—Leukocytosis may be present with an infectious or inflammatory etiology.

BMP—Keep a watchful eye on an elevated BUN as a cause for uremic pericarditis.

Troponins—Elevated troponins can be seen with inflammation that has reached the myocardium, and the patient is then considered to have myopericarditis rather than pericarditis only.

ESR or CRP—These are markers of inflammation, but not specific for acute pericarditis.

Coags—PT and PTT will give you an idea if there is a risk for hemorrhagic pericarditis or tamponade.

Blood cultures—Recommended in patients with fever >38°C (100.4°F) or suspected bacterial etiology.

Interferon gamma release assay (IGRA)—Unlike a PPD, a false positive test will not occur when using an IGRA in a BCG-vaccinated patient. If a patient did not receive a BCG vaccination and comes from an endemic area where TB is high (eg, India), a PPD is acceptable to use on the CCS. In this case, the patient immigrated from an area where TB is endemic and therefore a potential cause for TB pericarditis.

ANA or rheumatoid factor—Consider these tests in patients with suspected rheumatologic diseases.

Viral culture—Not recommended since it is low-yield and does not alter management.

HIV serology—Order if clinically indicated.

CXR—Typically normal in acute pericarditis, but an enlarged cardiac silhouette suggests a pericardial effusion (ie, 200 mL needed before silhouette enlarges).

Echocardiography—Recommended in all patients suspected of having pericardial disease as it can detect a cardiac tamponade or large pericardial effusions (ie, echo-free space >20 mm). Although a pericardial effusion supports the diagnosis of pericarditis (ie, inflammation-induced effusion), the absence of an effusion does not exclude the diagnosis.

Pericardiocentesis—Not routinely performed in acute pericarditis with small or moderate sized effusions, unless there is a cardiac tamponade, large effusions despite medical therapy, or suspected bacterial or neoplastic pericarditis.

EKG—There are four stages in the EKG changes of acute pericarditis that include: Stage 1) diffuse ST elevation with reciprocal ST depression; PR elevation and depressions (see first order sheet); Stage 2) return to isoelectric; Stage 3) diffuse T-wave inversions; and then Stage 4) return to isoelectric or continue with T-wave inversions indefinitely.

**Step 3)** Treatment of acute pericarditis is focused on treating the underlying cause (eg, TB pericarditis requires antituberculous therapy). Most patients with idiopathic or presumed viral pericarditis (such as in our CCS patient) will respond to medical management, which includes the following:

NSAIDs—Ibuprofen or indomethacin can be used for the duration of the patient's symptoms, which is typically 1 to 2 weeks, but be aware that NSAIDs do not alter the course of the disease. NSAIDs and glucocorticoids should be avoided in patients following an acute MI since they can interfere with healing and remodeling.

**Aspirin**—Aspirin is the preferred agent following an acute MI.

**Glucocorticoids**—Glucocorticoids (eg, prednisone) can be considered in patients that have a contraindication to NSAIDs or are refractory to a regimen of NSAIDs + colchicine. Glucocorticoids should be avoided in patients following an acute MI and in patients with purulent bacterial pericarditis (these patients require drainage and antibiotics, not steroids).

**Colchicine**—Colchicine can be added to any of the above three regimens as it is considered an adjunctive therapy to NSAIDs, aspirin, or glucocorticoids. Colchicine is thought to prevent recurrences, and it is fairly well tolerated in patients. Duration of therapy is typically 3 months or longer.

**Proton pump inhibitors (PPIs)**—PPIs (eg, omeprazole, lansoprazole) offer GI protection, and it is reasonable to give PPIs in patients with a history of peptic ulcer disease, age >65 years, high-dose NSAIDs, or concurrent use with aspirin, anticoagulants, or glucocorticoids. In this particular case, a PPI was given to the patient since he had a history of peptic ulcer disease.

### Disposition:

Most patients who present with acute pericarditis in the emergency department do not require admission to the hospital. However, patients should be admitted if they have any of the following:

- Cardiac tamponade
- Large pericardial effusion (ie, echo-free space >20 mm)
- Temperature >38°C (100.4°F)
- Elevated troponins (ie, suggesting myopericarditis)
- Immunosuppressed
- Concurrently taking anticoagulants
- NSAID drug failure
- Recent trauma
- Subacute onset

### Pearls:

- The EKG changes seen in acute pericarditis differs from acute MI in that (1) Q waves are generally absent in acute pericarditis (unless the inflammation has reached the myocardium), (2) ST elevations have a concave shape (convex shape in STEMI), (3) widespread ST elevations in pericarditis (remember the pericardium surrounds the entire heart),

and (4) reciprocal ST depressions are limited to aVR and $V_1$ in acute pericarditis.

- Early repolarization (normal variant) can also have widespread ST-segment elevations, but differ from acute pericarditis in that (1) the evolution of ST-T wave changes is absent in early repolarization, and (2) the ratio of ST amplitude to T-wave amplitude seen in lead $V_6$ is <0.25 in early repolarization, but a ST/T ratio >0.25 suggests acute pericarditis.

- Electrical alternans can be seen in pericardial effusions or cardiac tamponade, which can be characterized by the beat-to-beat alternations of the QRS complex (ie, alternating between a reduced QRS amplitude and an increased QRS amplitude complex). The alternating pattern is thought to be due to shifting of the heart, back and forth, within the pericardial fluid.

- When a pericardial effusion is present, the echocardiography can identify echo-free fluid in the pericardial space.

- The normal thickness of the pericardial layers is less than 2 mm on echocardiography.

- Patients with uremic pericarditis respond well to dialysis.

- Post-infarct pericarditis can occur in the **first few days after an MI**. Consistent with the diagnosis is the presence of pleuritic chest pain and pericardial friction rub, and the EKG may show an atypical ST-T wave evolution because of changes seen in the MI. Anticoagulation is typically held if a pericardial effusion develops or effusion size increases. Routine NSAID treatment is avoided, but when symptomatic, aspirin is the preferred agent.

- Postcardiac injury (Dressler's syndrome) occurs **weeks to months after an acute MI** and is thought to be immune mediated. Consistent with the diagnosis is the presence of pleuritic chest pain, pericardial friction rub, fever, leukocytosis, and pulmonary infiltrates. Patients generally respond to NSAIDs.

- **Connecting point** (pgs. 252, 253)—Familiarize yourself with IGRA and know the treatment for TB.

- **On the CCS**, "interferon gamma release assay (IGRA)" is not recognized in the practice CCS.

- **On the CCS**, if you want to taper a medication (eg, prednisone), just discontinue the medication (ie, the CCS has done it for you without any patient problems on the actual CCS exam).

- **On the CCS**, do not assume that any orders will be written for you (eg, vitals) during the CCS cases.

- **On the CCS**, remember to order things that are pertinent and appropriate for the patient since unnecessary testing or treatments would be considered suboptimal management.

# Color Plate 1

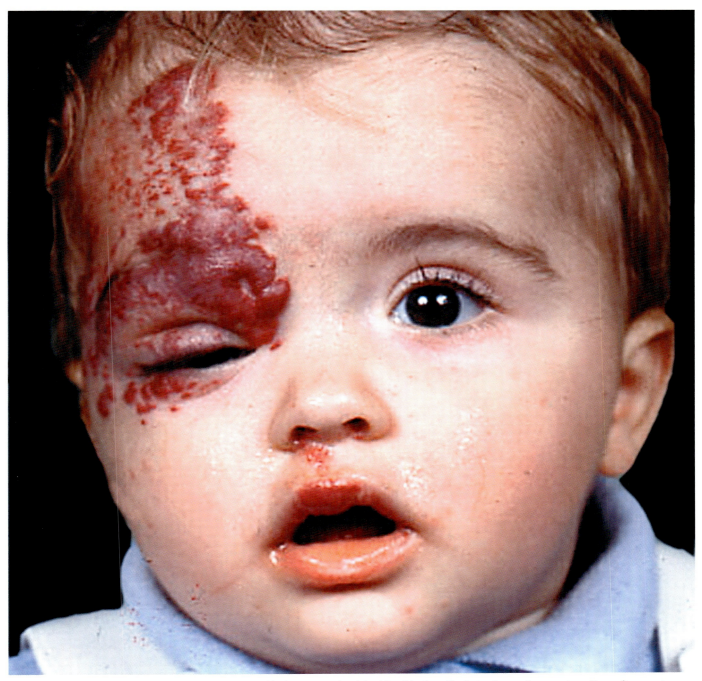

**FIGURE 4-1 • Infantile hemangioma.** A segmental plaquelike lesion over the right side of the face. The lesion has a crimson color with a soft appearing texture. Involution is apparent over the forehead. The lesion on the upper eyelid and the medial canthus is impairing proper function of the lid, and this indicates that vision might be impaired in the future. In this patient, treatment was indicated. (Reproduced with permission from Wolff K, Johnson RA. *Fitzpatrick's Color Atlas of Synopsis of Clinical Dermatology*. 6th ed. New York: McGraw-Hill; 2009:196.)

# Color Plate 2

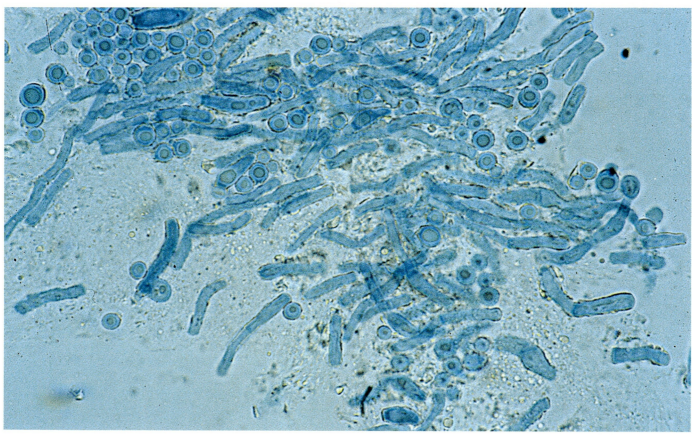

**FIGURE 4-2 • *Malassezia furfur* on KOH preparation.** Examination of both round yeast and elongated pseudohyphae reveals the characteristic "spaghetti and meatballs" pattern. (Reproduced with permission from Wolff K, Johnson RA. *Fitzpatrick's Color Atlas of Synopsis of Clinical Dermatology*. 6th ed. New York: McGraw-Hill; 2009:735.)

# Color Plate 3

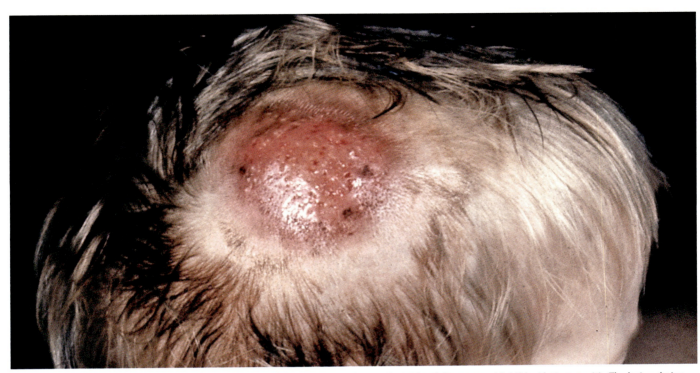

**FIGURE 4-3 • Kerion.** An extremely painful, boggy, purulent inflammatory nodule on the scalp of this 4-year-old child with tinea capitis. The lesion drains pus from multiple openings, and there is a retroauricular, tender lymphadenopathy. Infection was due to a zoophilic dermatophyte, *Trichophyton verrucosum*, that was contracted from an infected rabbit. (Reproduced with permission from Wolff K, Johnson RA. *Fitzpatrick's Color Atlas of Synopsis of Clinical Dermatology*. 6th ed. New York: McGraw-Hill; 2009:713.)

## Color Plate 4

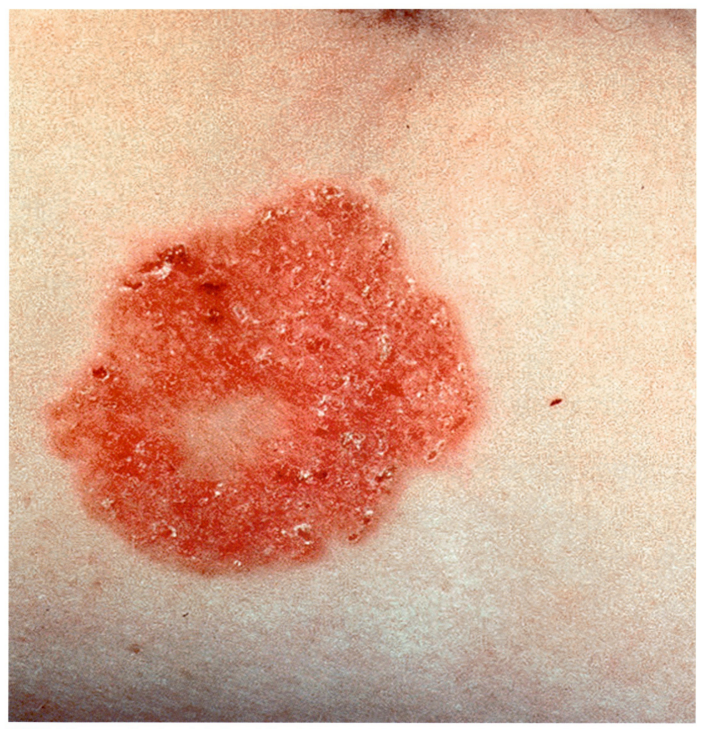

**FIGURE 4-4 • Squamous cell carcinoma in situ (bowen's disease).** A large, sharply demarcated, scaly, erythematous plaque simulating a psoriatic lesion. (Reproduced with permission from Wolff K, Johnson RA. *Fitzpatrick's Color Atlas of Synopsis of Clinical Dermatology*. 6th ed. New York: McGraw-Hill; 2009:279.)

# Color Plate 5

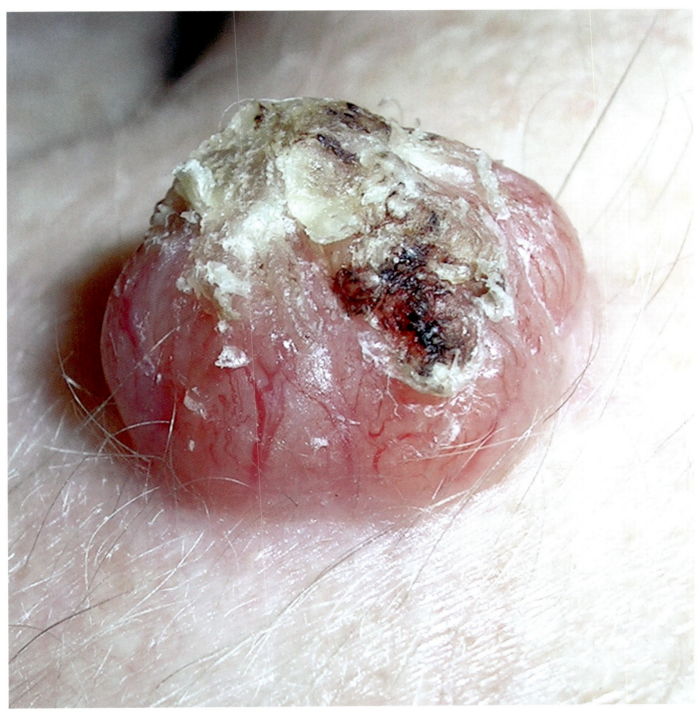

**FIGURE 4-5 • Keratoacanthoma.** A keratoacanthoma is seen on the face of a woman. Note the telangiectasias and central keratin core. (Reproduced with permission from Usatine RP, et al. *The Color Atlas of Family Medicine.* 2nd ed. New York: McGraw-Hill; 2013:977.)

# Color Plate 6

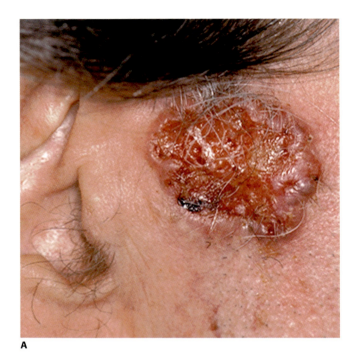

A

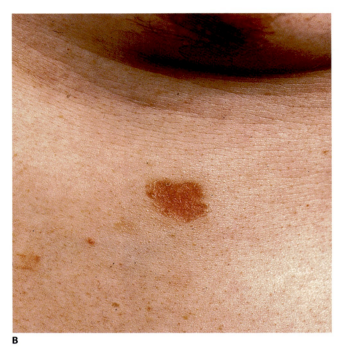

B

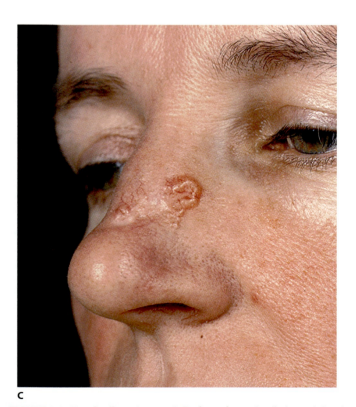

C

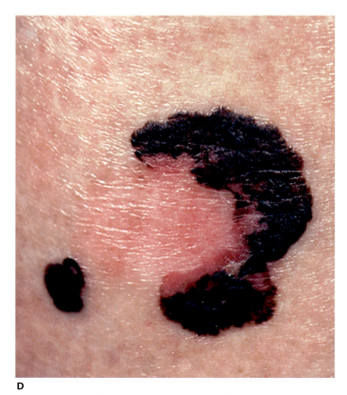

D

**FIGURE 4-6 • Basal cell carcinoma. A. Rodent ulcer**—A rolled, pearly border surrounds an ulcer with yellow necroses and a tiny black crust. **B. Superficial BCC**—A solitary, flat, bright red lesion with a slightly elevated rolled border that can be detected with "side lighting." **C. Sclerosing BCC**—A scarlike lesion on the nose with ill-defined margins. **D. Pigmented BCC**—An irregular pitch-black plaque with a central area of regression. This pigmented BCC is clinically indistinguishable from superficial spreading melanoma. (Reproduced with permission from Wolff K, Johnson RA. *Fitzpatrick's Color Atlas of Synopsis of Clinical Dermatology*. 6th ed. New York: McGraw-Hill; 2009: 290, 291, 292, 295.)

# Color Plate 7

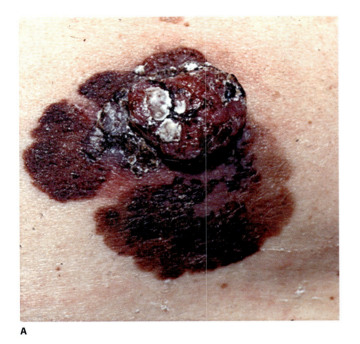

A

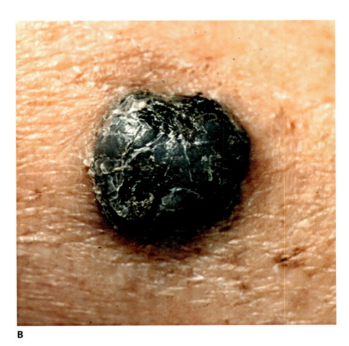

B

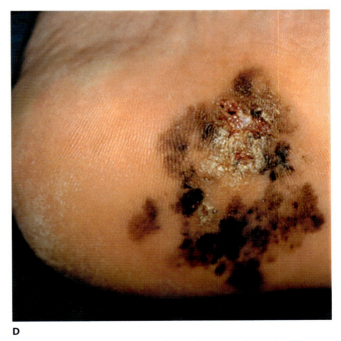

C

D

**FIGURE 4-7 • Melanoma. A. Superficial spreading**—Depicted is a flat plaque that demonstrates asymmetry, irregular borders, and color variegation (tan, brown, black, and red). Note the partially crusted nodule, which indicates a transition into the vertical growth phase. **B. Nodular**—A discrete darkly pigmented papule. This lesion has been present for less than 1 year. **C. Lentigo maligna**—An irregularly shaped, flat macular lesion with color variegation (tan, brown, black) that represents an in situ melanoma. **D. Acral lentiginous**—A lesion on the heel that reveals color variegation (brown, gray, black) and a nodular component that is hyperkeratotic, reddish, and ulcerated. (Reproduced with permission from Wolff K, Johnson RA. *Fitzpatrick's Color Atlas of Synopsis of Clinical Dermatology*. 6th ed. New York: McGraw-Hill; 2009: 313, 319, 322, 325.)

## Color Plate 8

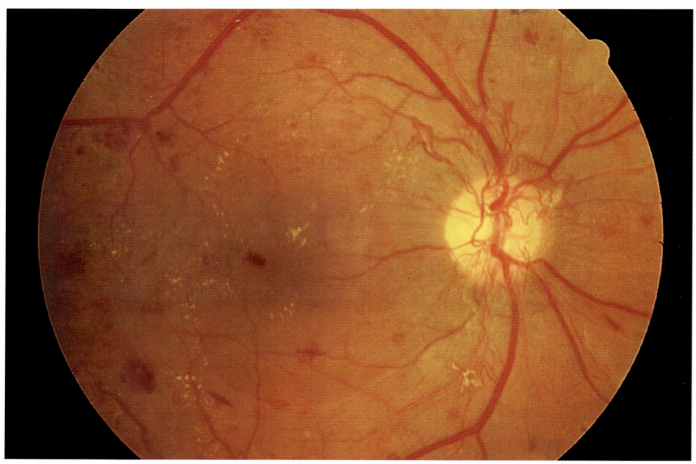

**FIGURE 6-2 • Proliferative diabetic retinopathy.** Proliferative retinopathy displaying yellow exudates, scattered hemorrhages, and neovascular vessels proliferating from the optic disc, requiring urgent panretinal laser photocoagulation. (Reproduced with permission from Lango DL, Fauci AS, Kasper DL, et al. *Harrison's Principles of Internal Medicine*. 18th ed. New York: McGraw-Hill, www.accessmedicine.com.)

**Color Plate 9**

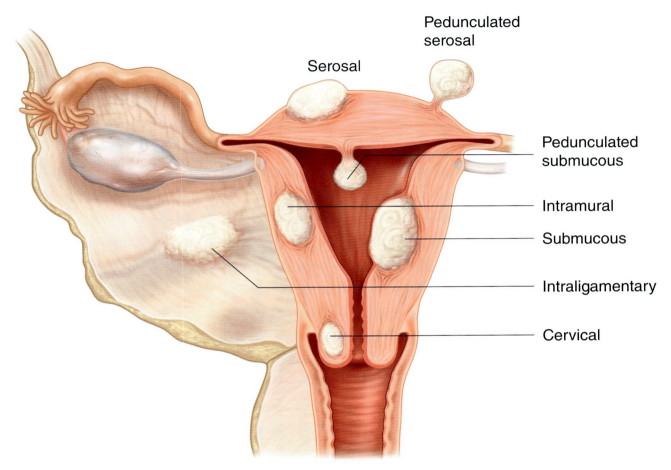

Pedunculated
serosal

Serosal

Pedunculated
submucous

Intramural

Submucous

Intraligamentary

Cervical

**FIGURE 9-1 • Leiomyomas.** Uterine fibroids can be classified by their location. Subserosal myomas grow near the uterine serosa. Submucous myomas are adjacent to the endometrium. Intramural myomas are within the uterine walls. Cervical myomas are located in the cervix. Pedunculated myomas have an attached stalk. Infrequently, myomas can be found in the broad ligament, ovary, fallopian tube, vagina, and vulva. (Reproduced with permission from Hoffman BL, Schorge JO, Schaffer JI, et al. *Williams Gynecology*. 2nd ed. New York: McGraw-Hill, www.accessmedicine.com.)

# Color Plate 10

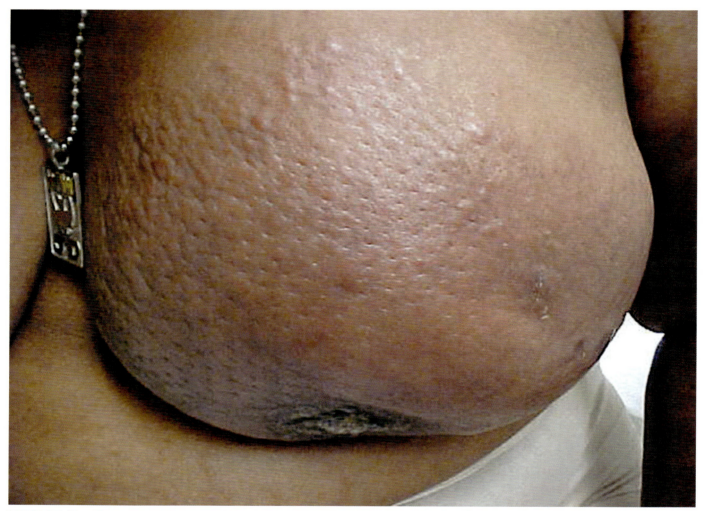

**FIGURE 9-2 • Peau d' orange.** Note the texture of the skin, which appears as an "orange peel." The skin is thickened with enlarged pores secondary to lymphedema. (Reproduced with permission from Usatine RP, Smith MA, Mayeaux EJ Jr, et al. *The Color Atlas of Family Medicine*. 2nd ed. New York: McGraw-Hill; 2013:553.)

## Color Plate 11

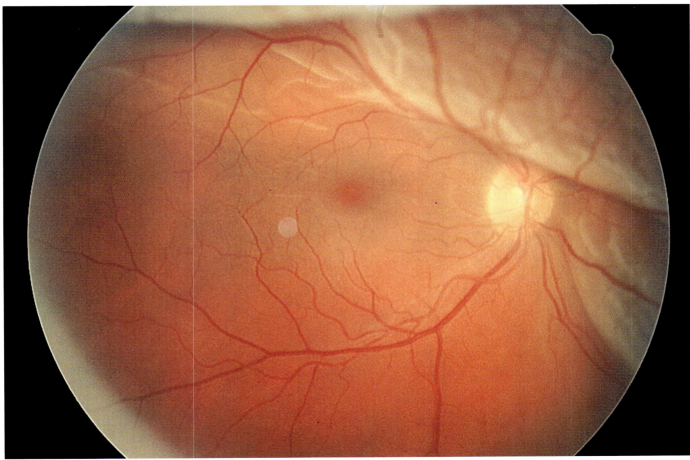

**FIGURE 13-1 • Retinal detachment.** Depicted is a superior retinal detachment with billowing or elevation of the retina with folds that can produce an inferior scotoma. Also, note that the fovea was spared, which led to normal visual acuity in this patient. (Reproduced with permission from Hauser SL, Josephson SA, et al. *Harrison's Neurology in Clinical Medicine*. 2nd ed. New York: McGraw-Hill; 2010:183.)

## Color Plate 12

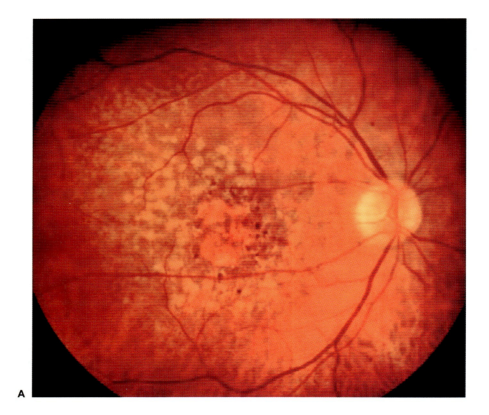

A

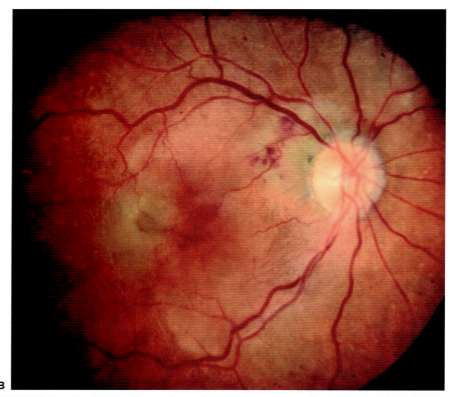

B

FIGURE 13-2 • Macular degeneration. A. Dry ARMD—Depicted are soft yellow drusen that are beginning to coalesce. B. Wet ARMD—A clearly evident subretinal hemorrhage over the macula may not always be present as in this case. However, further investigation with a fluorescein angiogram revealed leakage of fluorescein dye (hyperfluorescence) into the subretinal space of the macula in this patient. (Reproduced with permission from Gerstenblith AT, Rabinowitz MP, et al. *The Wills Eye Manual: Office and Emergency Room Diagnosis and Treatment of Eye Disease*. 6th ed. Philadelphia, LWW; 2012:323-324.)

# Color Plate 13

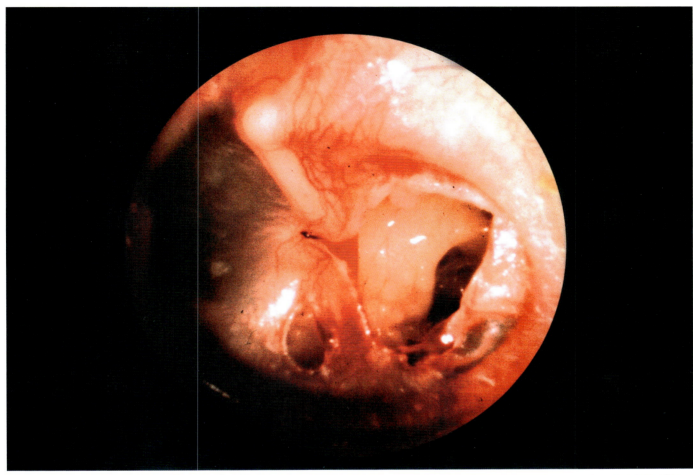

**FIGURE 15-1 • Acute tympanic membrane perforation.** Note the clean-cut margins of the perforation, which is commonly seen in traumatic cases. Also examine the hyperemic tympanic membrane, which suggests an acute process. (Photo Contributor: Richard A. Chole, MD, PhD. Reproduced with permission from Knoop KJ, et al. *The Atlas of Emergency Medicine.* 3rd ed. McGraw-Hill, www.accessmedicine.com.)

# Color Plate 14

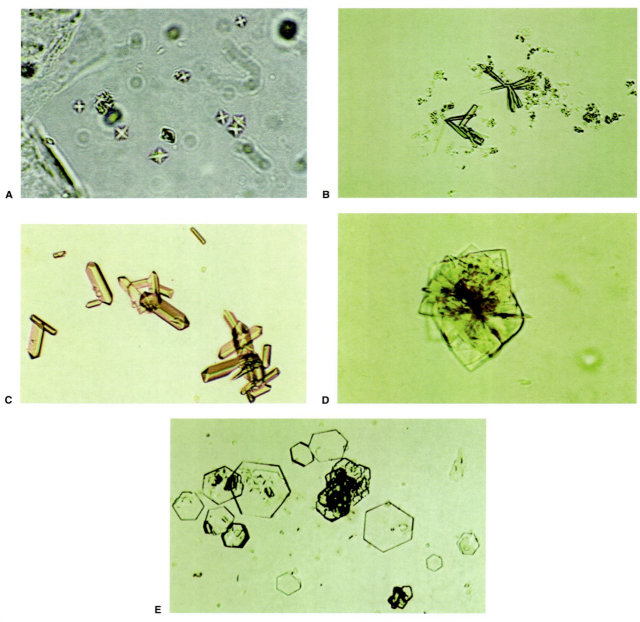

**FIGURE 18-1 • Urinary crystals. A. Calcium oxalate**—Envelope-shaped crystals with a prominent "X" crossing at the center. **B. Calcium phosphate**—Needle-shaped crystals. **C. Triple phosphate**—"Coffin lid" appearance. **D. Uric acid**—Rosette formation. **E. Cystine**—Hexagonal plates. (Reproduced with permission from Mundt LA, Shanahan K. Graff. *Textbook of Urinalysis and Body Fluids*. 2nd ed. Philadelphia, LWW; 2011: 66, 67, 76, 123, 133.)

## Color Plate 15

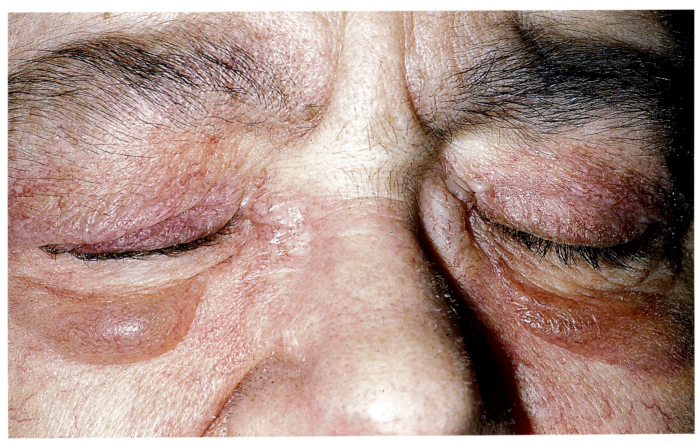

**FIGURE 19-1 • Heliotrope rash.** Note the reddish-purple rash over the upper eyelid with edema over the lower lids. The purplish hue is likened to the flower *Heliotropium peruvianum*. This patient developed severe muscle weakness of the shoulder girdle and presented with a lump in the breast that proved to be carcinoma. (Reproduced with permission from Wolff K, Johnson RA. *Fitzpatrick's Color Atlas of Synopsis of Clinical Dermatology*. 6th ed. New York: McGraw-Hill; 2009:371.)

**Color Plate 16**

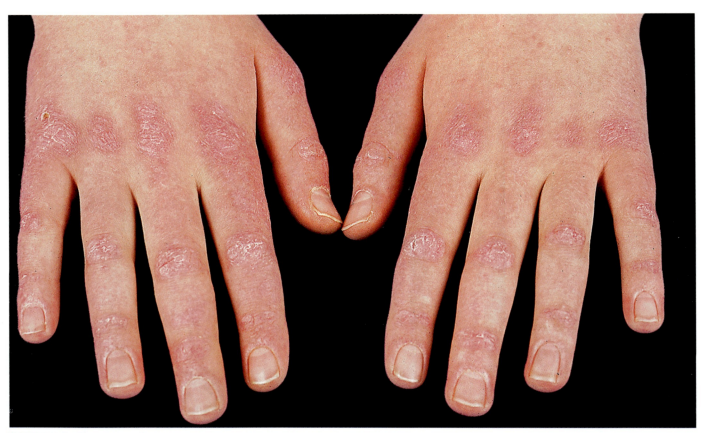

**FIGURE 19-2 • Gottron papules.** A raised, erythematous, scaly eruption can be seen over the dorsa of the hands and fingers, especially over the metacarpophalangeal and interphalangeal joints. (Reproduced with permission from Wolff K, Johnson RA. *Fitzpatrick's Color Atlas of Synopsis of Clinical Dermatology*. 6th ed. New York: McGraw-Hill; 2009:372.)

# 4

# Dermatology

## KEYWORDS REVIEW

**Macule**—A flat spot without skin elevation or depression.

**Patch**—A flat spot without skin elevation or depression, but larger than a macule.

**Papule**—A solid elevation of the skin.

**Nodule**—A solid elevation of the skin that is deeper and larger than a papule.

**Plaque**—A well-defined plateaulike elevation of the skin.

**Wheal**—A transient pinkish plaque with varying sizes and shapes.

**Vesicle**—A circumscribed elevation of the skin filled with fluid.

**Bulla**—A circumscribed elevation of the skin filled with fluid, but larger than a vesicle.

**Pustule**—A circumscribed elevation of the skin filled with pus.

**Paronychia**—Inflammation of the nail fold.

# INFLAMMATORY CONDITIONS

## ▌ ACNE VULGARIS

The pathogenesis of acne vulgaris is not fully understood, but it is thought that follicular keratinization obstructs sebum secretion resulting in keratin plugs or comedones. Androgens have been implicated in increasing sebum production, which provides a medium for the bacterium *Propionibacterium acnes* to grow within the follicle. Subsequently, *P. acnes* triggers an inflammatory response to the pilosebaceous units.

## Clinical Features:

Lesions can occur on the face, neck, chest, back, or upper arms. Comedones are usually the earliest manifestation of acne. The comedones can be open (blackheads) or closed (whiteheads). Although there is no universal classification system for describing acne, the following has been provided as a guideline for board purposes. Mild acne can generally be characterized by comedones, papules, and pustules. Moderate acne can be characterized by comedones, inflammatory papules and pustules, ± nodules. Severe acne is generally characterized by comedones, numerous inflammatory papules, pustules, nodules, and scarring. Nodules and pseudocysts can coalesce to form linear mounds (ie, sinus tracts) resulting in nodulocystic acne, which is considered severe acne.

## Next Step:

**Step 1)** Acne vulgaris is a clinical diagnosis. However, you have to consider hyperandrogenism if the patient presents with a combination of acne, acanthosis nigricans, menstrual irregularity, or virilization. In these types of cases, the next best step is to order total testosterone, free testosterone, and DHEA-S levels. It is also imperative to ask the patient what type of medications he or she is taking since some drugs can cause acne. Some of the more notable agents that can cause acne include lithium, phenytoin, glucocorticoids, isoniazid, azathioprine, and vitamins $B_2$, $B_6$, and $B_{12}$.

**Step 2)** Treatment for acne vulgaris can be managed by the following:

### Mild Acne

**Option 1:** For comedonal acne, patients can be treated with topical retinoids (eg, tretinoin, adapalene, tazarotene) since these meds aim to normalize follicular keratinization.

**Option 2:** In the presence of papules and pustules, treat the patient with a topical retinoid + topical benzoyl peroxide + topical antibiotic (eg, clindamycin, erythromycin, sulfacetamide, dapsone).

### Moderate Acne

**Option 1:** Topical retinoid + topical benzoyl peroxide + oral antibiotic (eg, tetracycline, doxycycline, minocycline, erythromycin, azithromycin, clindamycin, TMP-SMX).

### Severe Acne

**Option 1:** Oral isotretinoin is used in patients with cystic or nodulocystic acne. It can also be used in patients who have acne that is resistant to other therapies, including systemic antibiotics.

Prior to using isotretinoin, patients should have a pregnancy test since the drug is a teratogenic (category X). The patient should also be on birth control while taking the medication.

**Step 3)** Patients that improve with therapy can use topical retinoids for long-term maintenance therapy.

## Follow-Up:

Oral antibiotics should be used for a limited time (ie, <4 months). Oral isotretinoin can be given over a 4- to 6-month course.

## Pearls:

- It is still unclear if diet and stress contribute to the development of acne.
- Side effects of isotretinoin include hypertriglyceridemia, hepatotoxicity, idiopathic intracranial hypertension (pseudotumor cerebri), myalgias, visual changes, cheilitis, and dry skin.
- **Caveat 1**—Avoid using a tetracycline derivative (eg, doxycycline, tetracycline, minocycline) in conjunction with isotretinoin since isotretinoin and the tetracycline derivatives can both cause pseudotumor cerebri.
- **Caveat 2**—Tazarotene is contraindicated in pregnant women since it is also a category X drug, however, adapalene is a category C drug.
- **Caveat 3**—Minocycline, doxycycline, and tetracycline can cause photosensitivity, and patients should be advised about sun protection.
- **Caveat 4**—Avoid using minocycline, doxycycline, or tetracycline during pregnancy or in children since it can cause discoloration of the teeth and reduced bone growth.
- Benzoyl peroxide is an antimicrobial agent and is comedolytic. It is often used in conjunction with a topical or oral antibiotic to reduce the emergence of antibiotic resistance.
- Antibiotics are used to treat against *Propionibacterium acnes* with the aim of reducing the inflammatory response that comes along with the bacteria.
- **Foundational point**—*Propionibacterium acnes* is a gram-positive, catalase-positive rod that can produce propionic acid, acetic acid, and lactic acid.
- **Connecting point** (pg. 121)—Know the clinical features and management of PCOS.
- **Connecting point** (pg. 165)—Take a look at the pregnancy drug ratings.

# VASCULAR DISORDERS

## ▌ INFANTILE HEMANGIOMA

Infantile hemangiomas are the most common vascular tumors of infancy. Infantile hemangiomas are benign, and they can be characterized by a proliferation and an involution phase.

## Clinical Features:

Infantile hemangiomas are usually not present at birth but occur within the first few days to months after birth. The earliest sign will be an area of blanching with telangiectasias that will progress to a reddish macule. The lesion will enter the **proliferating phase**, which occurs during the first year. Rapid growth can be seen during the first 6 months of life and will slow down by the end of the first year. The color of the lesion can be bright red, crimson, deep purple, or a halo of white speckles (vascular blanching). The lesion can be soft, rubbery, firm, compressible, or ulcerated. The lesion can be superficial and take the appearance of a nodule, papule, or plaque. The lesion can also be subcutaneous with a normal appearing overlying skin, or it can take on a bluish hue appearance ± telangiectatic patch. More commonly, the lesion can appear with both superficial and subcutaneous components. The lesion can be solitary, multiple, or segmental (see Figure 4-1 and Color Plate 1). Hemangiomas tend to appear on the head and neck, but they can occur on the trunk, legs, lumbosacral area, mucous membranes, and even in internal organs. Following the proliferating phase is the **involution phase**, which can be characterized by a color change of the skin lesion, the lesion shrinks, and the consistency of the lesion becomes softer. Unfortunately, most of the skin lesions do not return to "normal skin" but will have residual effects such as discoloration, scarring, atrophy, redundant skin, or telangiectasias. Approximately 50% of patients will have complete involution by 5 years, 70% by 7 years, and 90% by 9 years.

## Next Step:

**Step 1)** Diagnosis of infantile hemangiomas is made clinically. If the diagnosis is still in question after a thorough history and physical, then a biopsy can be performed for definitive diagnosis.

**Step 2)** Imaging is sometimes performed under special circumstances. **Ultrasound** is usually performed in infants <6 months with ≥5 small multiple cutaneous lesions to look for

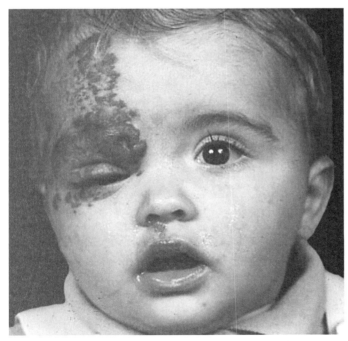

**FIGURE 4-1 • Infantile hemangioma.** A segmental plaquelike lesion over the right side of the face. The lesion has a crimson color with a soft appearing texture. Involution is apparent over the forehead. The lesion on the upper eyelid and the medial canthus is impairing proper function of the lid, and this indicates that vision might be impaired in the future. In this patient, treatment was indicated. (Reproduced with permission from Wolff K, Johnson RA. *Fitzpatrick's Color Atlas of Synopsis of Clinical Dermatology.* 6th ed. New York: McGraw-Hill; 2009:196.)

hemangiomas in the internal organs (ie, gastrointestinal, liver, and brain). **MRI** is usually performed in patients that have hemangiomas in the lumbosacral area to look for spinal dysraphism or genitourinary anomalies.

**Step 3)** In the majority of uncomplicated infantile hemangiomas, there is **no need for intervention** unless vital structures are compromised. Under special circumstances a consultation should be requested:

**Pediatric ophthalmologist**—If a hemangioma affects the periorbital area, especially when it involves the upper eyelid, then the vision might be compromised and a consultation would be prudent.

**Pediatric otolaryngologist**—If a hemangioma affects the "beard" distribution (ie, preauricular skin, mandible, lower lip, chin, and anterior neck), the patient may have hoarseness, stridor, and cough. These are symptoms that an airway hemangioma may be present, and early consultation is warranted.

**Plastic surgeon**—When there is a risk of disfigurement or scarring at such locations as the nose, lip, and ear, an excision can be considered, but the outcome of the surgery must be weighed into consideration. In most cases, surgery should only be considered on involuted lesions and not proliferating lesions since they have the potential to bleed.

## Follow-Up:

Educating parents about the clinical course of infantile hemangiomas is important. Although there may be residual skin changes, it is important to discuss the realistic outcome with any type of intervention.

## Pearls:

- Medical and surgical intervention for infantile hemangioma may include pulsed dye laser, excisional surgery, intralesional steroids, systemic steroids, interferon-alpha, vincristine, and propranolol.

- Congenital hemangiomas are benign vascular tumors that grow in utero and are fully developed by birth.

- Complications of hemangiomas include airway obstruction, visual impairment, ulceration, bleeding, and high-output cardiac failure (secondary from hepatic or large cutaneous hemangiomas).

- Patients that have a segmental facial hemangioma should be aware of the PHACES syndrome because the segmental lesion is one of the hallmarks of the syndrome. If the syndrome is present, then a cardiac, dermatologic, neurologic, and ophthalmologic workup is necessary. PHACES stands for:

  **P**—Posterior fossa malformations

  **H**—Hemangiomas (usually a segmental lesion on the face)

  **A**—Arterial anomalies

  **C**—Cardiac anomalies

  **E**—Eye and endocrine abnormalities

  **S**—Sternal cleft and/or supraumbilical raphe

# INFECTIONS

## ▌TINEA VERSICOLOR

Tinea versicolor, also known as pityriasis versicolor, is a noncontagious, superficial fungal infection caused by a saprophyte in the genus *Malassezia*. Although there are other *Malassezia* (formerly known as *Pityrosporum*) species that can cause tinea versicolor, *Malassezia furfur* has been synonymous with this disease. *Malassezia furfur* was previously known as *Pityrosporum ovale* and *Pityrosporum orbiculare*.

### Clinical Features:

The affected skin may have several (*versi-*) shades of color. The skin may be hypopigmented, hyperpigmented, or have a salmon-color appearance. In light-skinned individuals, lesions may appear hypopigmented on tanned skin. In darker-skinned individuals, lesions may appear as dark brown macules. The lesions may appear as well-marginated, oval-to-round macules. Sometimes the macules can coalesce forming irregularly shaped patches. Most often, the infection has a tendency to affect sebum-rich areas or oily skin. However, lesions can be seen on the face, neck, upper arms, axilla, upper trunk, abdomen, groin, or thighs. Sometimes a fine scale can be appreciated over the skin lesion. In most cases, patients will be asymptomatic, but some will complain of mild pruritus.

### Next Step:

**Step 1)** Tinea versicolor is a clinical diagnosis. However, a confirmatory test with KOH scraping of the scale will demonstrate clusters of oval budding yeasts cells and branching hyphae in the classic "spaghetti and meatballs" appearance (see Figure 4-2 and Color Plate 2).

**Step 2)** Treatment involves topical or systemic therapy. Initially, topical therapy should be attempted first unless there is treatment failure with topicals or recurrent or widespread infection, in which case systemic therapy would be more appropriate.

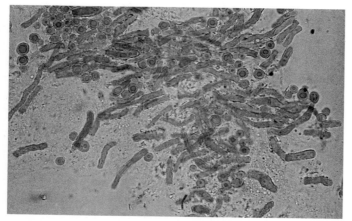

**FIGURE 4-2 • *Malassezia furfur* on KOH preparation.** Examination of both round yeast and elongated pseudohyphae reveals the characteristic "spaghetti and meatballs" pattern. (Reproduced with permission from Wolff K, Johnson RA. *Fitzpatrick's Color Atlas of Synopsis of Clinical Dermatology.* 6th ed. New York: McGraw-Hill; 2009:735.)

**Topical therapy**—Selenium sulfide, "azole" antifungals (eg, ketoconazole, clotrimazole, econazole) or terbinafine can be applied for 2 weeks.

**Systemic therapy**—Oral "azole" antifungals such as keto-conazole, fluconazole, or itraconazole can be used. Oral terbinafine and griseofulvin should be avoided since they are both ineffective in this condition.

### Follow-Up:

Patients should be aware that discoloration of the skin may persist for 1 to 2 months even after successful therapy. Although recurrence is not uncommon, physicians should think about immunosuppression in the individual.

### Pearls:

- Tinea versicolor is not a dermatophyte infection.
- Tinea versicolor is a very superficial fungal infection localized to the stratum corneum, unlike the dermatophytes, which can go deeper into the epidermis.
- A Wood's lamp will reveal a yellow-green fluorescence of the lesion in the dark.
- Hepatotoxicity has been associated with systemic "azole" antifungals.
- Tinea versicolor has a predisposition for warm tropical climates.

## ▌DERMATOPHYTE INFECTIONS

Dermatophyte infections are fungal infections that can break down keratin and therefore affect the skin, nails, and hair. Three common dermatophytes include *Trichophyton*, *Microsporum*, and *Epidermophyton*.

### Clinical Features:

**Tinea capitis**—Tinea capitis is commonly seen in children. Clinical presentation can vary, but common symptoms include pruritus, scaling, and bald spots. Sometimes a sharply defined area of alopecia can be seen that appears as a **"gray patch."** Tinea capitis can also present as diffuse, poorly circumscribed patches of alopecia that on close inspection appear as **"black dots"** because of broken hair shafts. Scalp lesions can also appear as **cup-shaped yellow crusts.** In some cases, an immune response to the fungal infection will result in a **kerion**, which is manifested as a raised, boggy, red, painful, purulent lesion ± posterior cervical lymphadenopathy (see Figure 4-3 and Color Plate 3).

**Tinea corporis**—Tinea corporis usually presents as a pruritic, erythematous, scaly lesion that expands peripherally with raised advancing borders while clearing centrally, resulting in a ring-shaped lesion. Tinea corporis can be contracted from contaminated soil, animals, skin-to-skin contact such as wrestlers (ie, tinea corporis gladiatorum), or from autoinoculation (eg, tinea capitis to tinea corporis).

**Tinea cruris**—Also known as jock itch. Similar presentation to tinea corporis, but will affect the inner thighs, groin, and sometimes the buttocks and perineum area. The infection will usually spare the scrotum and penis. Consider candidal intertrigo when it affects the scrotum and penis along with satellite papules or

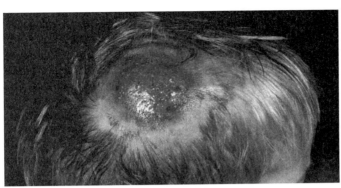

**FIGURE 4-3 · Kerion.** An extremely painful, boggy, purulent inflammatory nodule on the scalp of this 4-year-old child with tinea capitis. The lesion drains pus from multiple openings, and there is a retroauricular, tender lymphadenopathy. Infection was due to a zoophilic dermatophyte, *Trichophyton verrucosum*, that was contracted from an infected rabbit. (Reproduced with permission from Wolff K, Johnson RA. *Fitzpatrick's Color Atlas of Synopsis of Clinical Dermatology.* 6th ed. New York: McGraw-Hill; 2009:713.)

pustules. Tinea cruris can be contracted by autoinoculation or by fomites (eg, towels, bedsheets).

**Tinea pedis**—Also known as athlete's foot. Clinical presentation can vary, but most commonly, patients will complain of pruritus. The lesion can affect the interdigital area, which can be wet (ie, macerated ± ulceration) or dry (ie, scaling). Sometimes painful bullae or vesicles can be found on the plantar surface or toes. Another presentation includes diffuse scaling to hyperkeratosis with distinct areas of erythema on the plantar surface and lateral borders of the feet, which is notably referred to as the moccasin type.

**Tinea unguium**—Also known as dermatophytic onychomycosis. However, onychomycosis can also be caused by molds and yeast with *Candida albicans* as a common cause of fingernail onychomycosis with paronychia. Clinical presentation for dermatophytic onychomycosis can vary, but look for a discoloration of the nail plate, which can be brown, yellow, or a chalky white appearance.

### Next Step:

**Step 1)** Diagnosis of the tinea infections is by KOH preparation with hyphae and/or spores visible under microscope. If the diagnosis is still in question, a culture can be performed for definitive diagnosis.

**Step 2)** Treatment involves topical or systemic therapy. Initially, topical therapy should be attempted first in tinea corporis,

cruris, and pedis unless there is treatment failure with topicals or extensive disease, in which case systemic therapy would be more appropriate.

**Topical therapy**—Tinea corporis, cruris, and pedis can be treated with topical ketoconazole, clotrimazole, econazole, miconazole, oxiconazole, sertaconazole, sulconazole, terbinafine, naftifine, butenafine, ciclopirox, or tolnaftate. Do not use topical nystatin for dermatophytic infections, but it is okay to use for candidal infections.

**Systemic therapy**—Tinea capitis should be treated with oral griseofulvin, terbinafine, itraconazole, or fluconazole. Tinea unguium should be treated with either oral terbinafine or itraconazole with a duration of 6 weeks for fingernails or 12 weeks for toenails.

### Follow-Up:

Patients who develop a kerion and are appropriately treated with an antifungal medication should see improvement of the kerion (ie, treat the underlying infection).

### Pearls:

- Avoid using topical steroids for tinea corporis, cruris, and pedis because it can alter the clinical presentation such as decreased erythema with poorly defined borders; this condition is then referred to as tinea incognito.

- Erythrasma can present similarly to tinea cruris and tinea pedis; however, a Wood's lamp will demonstrate the characteristic coral red fluorescence in erythrasma.

- Hepatotoxicity has been associated with oral "azoles," griseofulvin, and terbinafine.

- When dermatophytes infect beyond the epidermis into the dermis, a deep folliculitis can occur that is referred to as Majocchi's granuloma. Papules, pustules, or nodules can be present. It is most commonly seen in women who frequently shave their legs, immunocompromised individuals, or those who apply topical steroids on the skin.

- ID reactions (ie, dermatophytid reactions) are an immune response to dermatophytic infections. They can be characterized by pruritic, papulovesicular eruptions occurring at distant sites from the original fungal infection. The lesions are devoid of any organisms at the distant site, and patients usually improve when the original fungal infection is treated appropriately.

# NEOPLASMS

## SQUAMOUS CELL CARCINOMA

Squamous cell carcinoma (SCC) is the second most common skin cancer after basal cell carcinoma.

### Clinical Features:

Squamous cell carcinoma has a predilection for the scalp, face (forehead, nose, cheeks, ears, outside border of the lower lip), upper chest, upper back, dorsal aspects of the hands and forearms, genital area, and shins. Clinical presentation can vary but can be best characterized when the lesion is in situ or invasive:

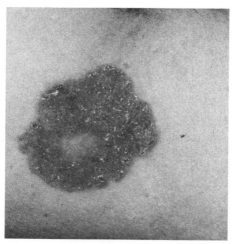

**FIGURE 4-4 • Squamous cell carcinoma in situ (Bowen's Disease).** A large, sharply demarcated, scaly, erythematous plaque simulating a psoriatic lesion. (Reproduced with permission from Wolff K, Johnson RA. *Fitzpatrick's Color Atlas of Synopsis of Clinical Dermatology.* 6th ed. New York: McGraw-Hill; 2009:279.)

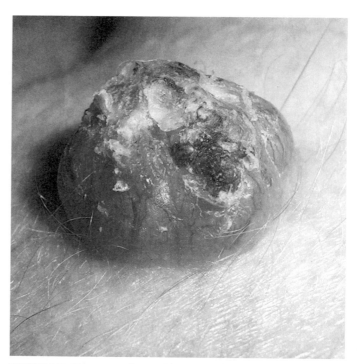

**FIGURE 4-5 • Keratoacanthoma.** A keratoacanthoma is seen on the face of a woman. Note the telangiectasias and central keratin core. (Reproduced with permission from Usatine RP, et al. *The Color Atlas of Family Medicine.* 2nd ed. New York: McGraw-Hill; 2013:977.)

**SCC in situ (Bowen's disease)**—Lesions are confined to the epidermis without invasion into the dermis layer. Lesions are typically presented as a sharply defined, scaly patch or plaque ± hyperkeratosis. The color can range from pink to red (see Figure 4-4 and Color Plate 4). Lesions tend to grow slowly, and once it becomes invasive, a nodular lesion usually appears within the plaque. When in situ lesions affect the penis, the lesion is referred to as erythroplasia of Queyrat. Patients are usually asymptomatic with in situ lesions.

**SCC invasive**—Invasive lesions can be a papule, nodule, or plaque that can be scaly, crusted, or ulcerated with heaped-up edges. Lesions can be further characterized by their differentiation. Well-differentiated lesions are usually harder and have hyperkeratosis. Poorly differentiated lesions are usually softer, fleshy, and friable without hyperkeratosis. Patients are also asymptomatic but rapidly evolving lesions can be painful.

### Next Step:

**Step 1)** Confirm the diagnosis with a biopsy (ie, "tissue is the issue").

**Step 2)** Surgical excision is the most common form of treatment. Prevention is also an important part of skin cancer management, which should include sunscreens and protective clothing.

### Follow-Up:

The overall 5-year cure rate is >90% for primary cutaneous squamous cell carcinoma.

### Pearls:

- Risk factors for SCC include sun exposure, ionizing radiation, immunosuppression, arsenic exposure, industrial carcinogens, and actinic keratosis.

- Actinic keratosis typically presents as yellowish-brown hyperkeratotic scales on a red-tinged background of macules on sun-exposed skin. Removing the scales can be quite painful for the patient. Although the progression from actinic keratosis to SCC is fairly low, for lesions that grow rapidly, ulcerate, or for which the diagnosis is uncertain, a biopsy should be performed. Avoid prolonged sun exposure and wear sunscreens. Treatment includes cryotherapy, photodynamic therapy, topical 5-FU, or topical imiquimod.

- A keratoacanthoma is most likely a variant of SCC and presents as a **rapidly growing** nodule that appears domed-shaped with central hyperkeratosis (see Figure 4-5 and Color Plate 5). Shedding or removal of the central keratotic plug results in a craterlike appearance. Regression of the lesion begins within a few months and can take as long as 1 year. Since keratoacanthomas can be indistinguishable from SCC, a biopsy is often recommended. Treatment is by excision.

- Hyperkeratosis can result in a hornlike projection of the skin. Hyperkeratosis can be seen in actinic keratosis, keratoacanthoma, SCC in situ, and invasive SCC. A biopsy should be taken because of the possibility of invasive SCC at the base of the horn.

- Verrucous carcinoma is a subtype of SCC and is characteristically presented as "cauliflower-like" lesions.

- SCC rarely metastasizes; approximately 5% to 10% of patients with SCC will develop regional to distant metastasis.

- **Foundational point**—Histologically, invasive squamous cell carcinoma may demonstrate keratin production ("keratin

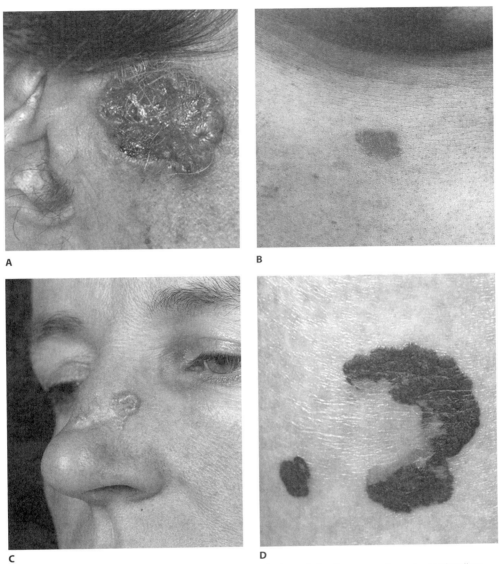

**FIGURE 4-6 • Basal cell carcinoma. A. Rodent ulcer**—A rolled, pearly border surrounds an ulcer with yellow necroses and a tiny black crust. **B. Superficial BCC**—A solitary, flat, bright red lesion with a slightly elevated rolled border that can be detected with "side lighting." **C. Sclerosing BCC**—A scarlike lesion on the nose with ill-defined margins. **D. Pigmented BCC**—An irregular pitch-black plaque with a central area of regression. This pigmented BCC is clinically indistinguishable from superficial spreading melanoma. (Reproduced with permission from Wolff K, Johnson RA. *Fitzpatrick's Color Atlas of Synopsis of Clinical Dermatology*. 6th ed. New York: McGraw-Hill; 2009: 290, 291, 292, 295.)

pearls") and intercellular attachment sites (desmosomes or "intercellular bridges").

- **Connecting point** (pg. 260)—Know the other histologic features from different neoplasias.

## BASAL CELL CARCINOMA

Basal cell carcinoma (BCC) is the most common skin cancer. BCC develops from the **basal** layer of the epidermis.

### Clinical Features:

Basal cell carcinoma has a predilection for the scalp, face (medial and lateral canthi, nasolabial fold, ears), and trunk. BCC typically grows slowly, and patients are often asymptomatic. Consider four different types of BCC (see Figure 4-6 and Color Plate 6):

**Nodular**—Most common type of BCC, which typically presents as a smooth, "**pearly**" nodule or papule with telangiectasias. If untreated, nodular BCC can ulcerate into a "rodent ulcer," called this because the appearance of the lesion is like something that has been gnawed on by a rodent.

**Superficial**—These lesions tend to occur on the trunk as solitary or multiple lesions. They typically present as a red, scaly, patch or plaque with threadlike borders.

**Sclerosing (morpheaform)**—These lesions can present as a scarlike, flesh-colored, lesion with ill-defined borders.

**Pigmented**—These lesions are often confused with melanoma since they may appear as a brown-black plaque or nodule.

**Next Step:**

**Step 1)** Confirm the diagnosis with a biopsy (ie, "tissue is the issue").

**Step 2)** Surgical excision is the most common form of treatment. Prevention is also an important part of skin cancer management, which should include sunscreens and protective clothing.

**Follow-Up:**

The prognosis for patients with BCC is excellent; however, significant morbidity can occur if the lesion is left untreated.

**Pearls:**

- Risk factors for BCC include sun exposure, ionizing radiation, immunosuppression, arsenic exposure, and basal cell nevus syndrome.

- Basal cell nevus syndrome is an autosomal dominant disorder that results in multiple BCCs along with other numerous anomalies such as frontal bossing, palmar and plantar pitting, intracranial calcification, rib anomalies, and odontogenic (bone) keratocysts.

- Xeroderma pigmentosum is an autosomal recessive disease that results in the inability to repair damaged DNA caused by ultraviolet light. Consequently, patients can develop basal cell carcinoma, squamous cell carcinoma, melanoma, or neurologic and ocular conditions.

- Treatment options for BCC can also include cryotherapy, electrodesiccation and curettage, topical 5-FU, imiquimod, photodynamic therapy, radiation, or Mohs surgery.

- Mohs surgery is the best approach when there is concern for recurrence or for cosmetic reasons (eg, tissue sparing). In the Mohs surgery, tissue is resected at oblique angles and evaluated under the microscope, providing excellent evaluation of the peripheral margins while minimizing the amount of tissue needed to be resected.

- There are no known "in situ" lesions in BCC compared to SCC.

- There is no hyperkeratosis in BCC compared to SCC.

- BCC very rarely metastasizes; approximately <0.5% of patients with BCC will develop regional or distant metastasis.

- **Foundational point**—Histologically, the tumor cells of nodular BCC are arranged in a characteristic palisading pattern at the periphery. The stroma tends to shrink away from the tumor nests creating a cleft (ie, retraction artifact).

- **Foundational point**—Mutations in the tumor suppressor gene, patched 1 (PTCH1), has been identified as one of the cause for the development of BCC.

# ▌MELANOMA

Melanoma is the fifth most common cancer in men and seventh most common cancer in women in the United States. Most melanomas have a characteristic horizontal (ie, radial) growth before transitioning to a vertical growth pattern with further invasion into the dermis.

**Risk Factors:**

UVA and UVB radiation exposure (especially intense intermittent exposure), family history, personal history of melanoma, tanning beds, psoralen + UVA radiation therapy (PUVA), typical nevi (>50), dysplastic nevi (>5), congenital nevi, eye color (blue, green, hazel), hair color (red, blond), ↑ freckles, sunburns in childhood or adolescence.

**Clinical Features:**

There are four major subtypes of invasive melanomas. In descending order of frequency, these melanomas include (see Figure 4-7 and Color Plate 7):

**Superficial spreading**—This type of lesion is the most common. It can occur anywhere on the body but has a predilection for the back in both men and women and on the legs of women. Radial growth is fairly slow with up to a period of 2 years before switching to vertical growth. The lesion can take on a variety of colors, along with irregular borders and asymmetry. The presence of a nodule usually indicates progression into the vertical growth phase.

**Nodular**—These lesions do not have a radial growth phase but begin their growth in the vertical direction, making the prognosis very concerning. These lesions grow fairly rapidly within a period of 1 to 2 years. Lesions appear as dome-shaped nodules with minimal variation in color and have more of a uniform blue-black appearance. For unknown reasons, there is a high frequency of this type in Japanese people.

**Lentigo maligna**—This lesion typically occurs on sun-exposed areas such as the head, neck, and dorsa of the hands. These lesions begin as in situ lesions. Lentigo malignas are very-slow-growing lesions that can take up to 20 years before transforming into an invasive lesion. Initially, the lesions start out as a brown-tan macule that develops into a larger, darker, asymmetric lesion. The presence of a nodule or papule often indicates the transition into the vertical growth phase, and then the term lentigo maligna melanoma is used.

**Acral lentiginous**—These lesions are the least common of the melanomas, but commonly occur in Asians and dark-skinned individuals. They can occur on the palms of the hands, soles of the feet, under the nails, and on mucosal surfaces. The lesions begin with radial growth that may go unnoticed for several years before transitioning to vertical growth where nodules usually appear.

**Next Step:**

**Step 1)** The **ABCDE** mnemonic (**A**symmetry, **B**order irregularities, **C**olor variegation, **D**iameter ≥6 mm, **E**volving) can assist with the initial clinical diagnosis.

**Step 2)** A full-thickness, narrow-margin excisional biopsy should be performed on any suspicious lesion to confirm the diagnosis.

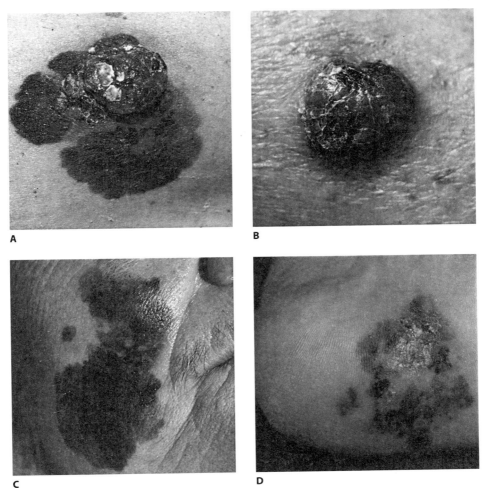

**FIGURE 4-7 • Melanoma. A. Superficial spreading**—Depicted is a flat plaque that demonstrates asymmetry, irregular borders, and color variegation (tan, brown, black, and red). Note the partially crusted nodule, which indicates a transition into the vertical growth phase. **B. Nodular**—A discrete darkly pigmented papule. This lesion has been present for less than 1 year. **C. Lentigo maligna**—An irregularly shaped, flat macular lesion with color variegation (tan, brown, black) that represents an in situ melanoma. **D. Acral lentiginous**—A lesion on the heel that reveals color variegation (brown, gray, black) and a nodular component that is hyperkeratotic, reddish, and ulcerated. (Reproduced with permission from Wolff K, Johnson RA. *Fitzpatrick's Color Atlas of Synopsis of Clinical Dermatology*. 6th ed. New York: McGraw-Hill; 2009: 313, 319, 322, 325.)

It is not recommended to perform a shave biopsy because the **Breslow depth** is the most important prognostic parameter in the evaluation of a melanoma.

**Step 3)** Surgical therapy with a wide local excision is the primary form of treatment for cutaneous malignant melanomas. Prevention with sunscreens and protective clothing is an important part of skin cancer management since patients that develop melanomas are at risk of developing another melanoma in the future.

**Follow-Up:**

The prognosis depends on the thickness of the lesion. For example, a thickness >3.6 mm correlates to an 8-year survival rate of 33.3%. When there is lymph node involvement, the 5-year survival rate is approximately 30% to 45%. With distant metastases, the 5-year survival rate diminishes to <10%.

**Pearls:**

- Melanomas can arise from in situ lesions from the subtypes of superficial spreading, lentigo maligna, and acral lentiginous but not from nodular.

- Melanomas metastasize more frequently compared to SCC or BCC.

- **Foundational point**—Serum S-100 is a tumor marker for melanoma. Serum levels of this protein are correlated with the stage of the disease. S-100 is not specific for melanoma since it can also be found in schwannomas, neurofibromas, and different cell types (eg, macrophages, adipocytes).

# 5

# EKG

# EKG REVIEW

## ▍ RATE

Step 1) Find an R wave that lands on a heavy black line.

Step 2) From there, count the sequence "300-150-100-75-60-50" for each of the large boxes (ie, 5 small squares) until the next R wave is seen. Note that the next R wave may not fall exactly on another heavy black line, and therefore, you have to approximate the heart rate from the last two numbers that were counted from your sequence.

**Pearl:**

- Bradycardia (<60 bpm), tachycardia (>100 bpm), paroxysmal tachycardia (150-250 bpm), flutter (250-350 bpm), fibrillation (350-450 bpm).

## ▍ RHYTHM

Sinus rhythm should have the following components:

1) P wave before QRS.
2) The presence of a QRS after every P wave.
3) Upright P wave in leads I, II, aVF, $V_4$-$V_6$.
4) Negative P wave in aVR.
5) Heart rate between 60 and 100 bpm.

## ▍ INTERVALS AND COMPLEXES

P wave: <3 small boxes (<0.12 seconds), and amplitude <2.5 small boxes (<0.25 mV)

PR interval: 3 to 5 small boxes (0.12-0.20 seconds)

QRS complex: ≤2.5 small boxes (≤0.10 seconds)

QT interval: QT interval depends on the heart rate (ie, corrected QT or QTc). For example, a faster heart rate can result in a shorter QT. The QTc in men is ≤0.44 seconds, and the QTc in women is ≤0.45 to 0.46 seconds. A simple method to detect a normal QT interval when the heart rate is within normal range (60-100 bpm) is to visually compare the **R-R** interval length to the **QT** interval length. If the QT interval appears less than half of the R-R interval, then you have a normal QT.

**Pearl:**

- One small box (1 mm) going horizontally represents 0.04 seconds, and one large box (5 small squares) represents 0.2 seconds. One small box (1 mm) going vertically represents 0.1 millivolt (mV), and one large box (5 small squares) represents 0.5 millivolts (mV).

# AXIS DEVIATION

Axis deviation represents the net direction of the electrical currents generated during ventricular depolarization. Consider the following:

Normal axis (−30° to 90°): Net positive (ie, upright) QRS deflection in both leads I and II.

Left axis (−30° to −90°): QRS in lead I is net positive, but QRS in lead II is net negative.

Right axis (90° to 180°): QRS in lead I is net negative, but QRS in aVF is net positive.

Extreme axis (180° to −90°): Net negative (ie, downward) QRS deflection in both leads I and II.

**Pearl:**

- For causes of left axis deviation, think of LVH, left bundle branch block, inferior MI, pregnancy, and hyperkalemia. For causes of right axis deviation, think of RVH, right bundle branch block, and lateral wall MI. It should be noted that the word "net" refers to the overall direction of the QRS complex (eg, upward deflection > downward deflection).

# ATRIAL ENLARGEMENT

Left atrial enlargement (LAE): A broad notched P wave in lead II and/or a diphasic P wave in lead $V_1$ with a prominent negative component in the end portion of the diphasic wave.

Right atrial enlargement (RAE): Increased P wave amplitude in lead II (P ≥2.5 mm) and/or in lead $V_1$ (P ≥1.5 mm).

# VENTRICULAR HYPERTROPHY

Left ventricular hypertrophy (LVH): A pattern recognition of a left axis deviation, left atrial abnormalities (eg, biphasic P wave, P wave >3 small boxes), widened QRS (>2.5 small boxes), increased voltage of the QRS complex (ie, tall R waves in lead $V_5$ or $V_6$, deep S wave in $V_1$ or $V_2$), or ST-T wave changes (eg, T wave inversions, ST depressions).

Right ventricular hypertrophy (RVH): A pattern recognition of a right axis deviation, right atrial enlargement, prominent R wave in lead $V_1$ (R > S wave), or ST-T wave changes (eg, T wave inversions, ST depressions).

**Pearl:**

- For causes of LVH, think of aortic stenosis, aortic regurgitation, mitral regurgitation, hypertrophic cardiomyopathy, and dilated cardiomyopathies. For causes of RVH, think of pulmonary stenosis, pulmonary HTN, cor pulmonale, and lung diseases.

# INFARCTS

Injury to the myocardial tissue secondary to an occluded artery can be identified on specific EKG leads that are associated with the anatomic regions of the heart (see Table 3-5).

**Pearls:**

**Hyperkalemia**—Peaked T waves, P wave flattens, and QRS widens.

**Hypokalemia**—U waves occur after the T wave, which is best seen in leads $V_4$-$V_6$, T wave flattens or inverted.

**Hypercalcemia**—Shortened QT interval secondary to shortened ST segment.

**Hypocalcemia**—Prolonged QT interval.

**Hypothermia**—Osborne wave, which is an elevation of the J point (ie, sits between the QRS and ST segment).

**Digoxin toxicity**—Digoxin toxicity can cause almost any arrhythmia (eg, asystole, PVCs, AV blocks, ventricular fibrillation).

# ATRIA

## MULTIFOCAL ATRIAL TACHYCARDIA

Multifocal atrial tachycardia (MAT) is the result of multiple ectopic foci generating impulses. These areas of automaticity can lead to an elevated heart rate that exceeds 100 beats per minute (bpm). The cause of MAT is related to the underlying illness. Common underlying illnesses associated with MAT include COPD, acute respiratory failure, pulmonary embolism, pneumonia, sepsis, coronary artery disease, heart failure, valvular heart disease, hypertension, right atrial enlargement, hypokalemia, hypomagnesemia, hypoxia, and medications (eg, theophylline, aminophylline, isoproterenol).

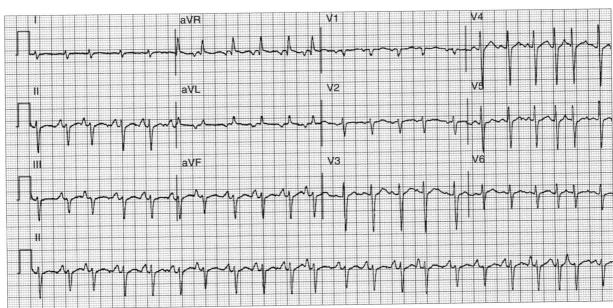

**FIGURE 5-1 • Multifocal atrial tachycardia.** Reproduced with permission from Loscalzo J, et al. *Harrison's Cardiovascular Medicine.* New York: McGraw-Hill; 2010:508.

## EKG Features:

(1) P waves have at least 3 different morphologies (eg, inverted, biphasic, upright), (2) Atrial rate >100 bpm, (3) P-P, P-R, and R-R intervals vary, and (4) A flat isoelectric baseline between the P waves distinguishes MAT from atrial fibrillation (AF). See Figure 5-1.

## Next Step Treatment:

**Step 1)** Treat the underlying illness.

**Step 2)** Pharmacologic therapy can be considered for acute heart rate control. Rate control therapy with either a calcium channel blocker (IV verapamil) or with a beta-blocker (IV metoprolol) has been used. Verapamil is the preferred agent over metoprolol in patients with bronchospasms or COPD since there are concerns of bronchoconstriction if a beta-blocker is used. However, neither agent should be used in the presence of a second- or third-degree AV block or sinus node dysfunction unless a pacemaker has been implanted.

## Disposition:

Admit patients to the hospital for further cardiac monitoring if acute heart rate control was attempted in the ED.

## Pearls:

- DC cardioversion is ineffective.
- The use of antiarrhythmic drugs is questionable.
- The clinical manifestations of MAT typically correlate with the underlying illness.
- **On the CCS**, if you're going to give the patient intravenous rate control, be sure to have the appropriate monitoring (eg, cardiac monitor, blood pressure monitor, pulse oximetry).

# AV NODE

## ▌FIRST-DEGREE AV BLOCK

First-degree AV block is a delay in the impulse between the atria and ventricles. The site of conduction delay usually occurs in the AV node if the QRS duration is normal.

## EKG Features:

PR interval >5 small boxes (>0.20 seconds) that does not vary. See Figure 5-2.

## Next Step Treatment:

**Step 1)** No pacemaker is required in most patients.

## Follow-Up:

Patients with an isolated first-degree AV block have a good prognosis, but patients with coexistent coronary artery disease should be closely observed since they are at higher risk of morbidity and mortality.

## Pearls:

- Atrioventricular blocks can be the result of reversible causes (eg, ↑ vagal tone, beta-blockers, calcium channel blockers, digoxin) or structural causes (eg, MI, myocarditis, catheter ablation).
- **On the CCS**, when placing an order for an EKG test, there are different types to choose from (eg, 12-lead, ambulatory, monitor, rhythm strip, and EKG stress test). The EKG 12-lead

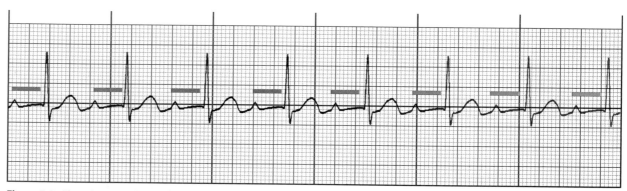

**Figure 5-2 • First-degree AV block.** Reproduced with permission from Jones SA. *ECG Success: Exercises in ECG Interpretation*. Philadelphia: F.A. Davis Company; 2008:56.

will give you the most useful information in terms of rhythm, axis, intervals, and interpretation.

# SECOND-DEGREE AV BLOCK—TYPE I

Second-degree AV block is a result of intermittent failure of atrial impulses reaching the ventricles. Second-degree AV block type I (Mobitz type I or Wenckebach block) typically occurs within the AV node and is associated with a normal QRS interval. Rarely, does type I progress to a complete heart block.

## EKG Features:

Progressive prolongation of the PR interval preceding a non-conducted P wave (ie, no QRS complex). See Figure 5-3.

## Next Step Treatment:

**Step 1)** The clinical management for Mobitz type I can be summarized into patients that are asymptomatic or symptomatic.

**Asymptomatic:** No specific therapy.

**Symptomatic:**

1) Identify any reversible causes (eg, meds, MI, ↑ vagal tone), if none found, then …

2) IV atropine, q5 minutes, not to exceed 3.0 mg.

3) If atropine is unsuccessful, consider transcutaneous pacing (ie, temporary pacing).

## Disposition:

Admit patient to the hospital for further cardiac monitoring and consultation with a cardiologist for a permanent pacemaker

in patients with symptomatic bradycardia without a reversible etiology.

## Pearls:

- In approximately 90% of patients, the right coronary artery (RCA) supplies the AV node. Therefore, an obstruction in the RCA can result in an inferior MI and a Mobitz type I block.

- There is a higher risk in mortality in patients with an inferior MI and an associated Mobitz type I block.

- **Connecting point** (pg. 26)—Know the associated leads for an inferior MI.

- **On the CCS**, "transcutaneous pacemaker, temporary," and "pacemaker, permanent" are both available in the practice CCS.

# SECOND-DEGREE AV BLOCK—TYPE II

Second-degree AV block type II (Mobitz type II) typically occurs below the AV node (infranodal) and frequently progresses to a complete heart block.

## EKG Features:

A fixed PR interval prior to and after a nonconducted P wave (ie, no QRS complex). Patients with type II blocks typically do not have a normal QRS duration, but rather a wide QRS interval which is indicative of a block in the infranodal system (eg, bundle of His, bundle branches). See Figure 5-4.

## Next Step Treatment:

**Step 1)** Identify any reversible causes (eg, meds, MI, ↑ vagal tone).

**Step 2)** Similar to Mobitz type I, symptomatic bradycardia with signs of hypoperfusion may require atropine and transcutaneous pacing.

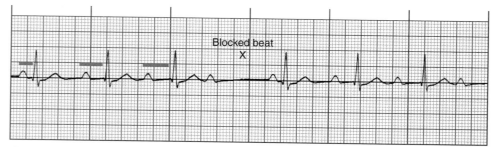

**Figure 5-3 • Second-degree AV block—Type I.** Reproduced with permission from Jones SA. *ECG Success: Exercises in ECG Interpretation*. Philadelphia: F.A. Davis Company; 2008:57.

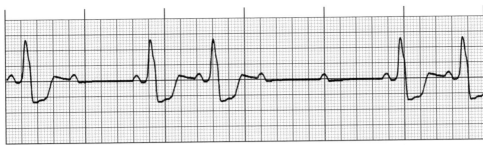

**Figure 5-4 • Second-degree AV block—Type II.** Reproduced with permission from Jones SA. *ECG Success: Exercises in ECG Interpretation.* Philadelphia: F.A. Davis Company; 2008:57.

**Step 3)** If no reversible causes are found, then the next best step is to implant a permanent pacemaker in almost all patients with a Mobitz type II block.

**Disposition:**

Admit symptomatic patients to the hospital for further monitoring since patients with Mobitz type II blocks can have syncopal attacks (Stokes-Adams attacks).

**Pearls:**

• Mobitz type I and Mobitz type II cannot be differentiated on EKG in the presence of a 2:1 block. In a 2:1 block, every other P wave is not conducted.

• **On the CCS**, when you order a consult, remember that you are functioning as a primary care physician and not the specialist.

## THIRD-DEGREE AV BLOCK

Third-degree AV block (complete heart block) results in no AV conduction. The escape rhythm that controls the ventricles can occur at any level below the region of the conduction block.

**EKG Features:**

There is complete dissociation between the P waves and QRS complexes. If a third-degree AV block occurs within the AV node or bundle of His, the escape rhythm will usually have a narrow QRS complex. If the escape rhythm originates distal to the block (eg, ventricles), the QRS complex will usually be wider and rates will be slower (eg, <40 bpm). See Figure 5-5.

**Next Step Treatment:**

**Step 1)** Identify any reversible causes (eg, meds, MI, ↑ vagal tone) and remove the offending agent.

**Step 2) Short-term management:** Unstable patients (symptomatic bradycardia) should be managed with (1) **A**irway, **B**reathing, **C**irculation, (2) monitoring equipment (eg, blood pressure, cardiac monitor, pulse oximetry), (3) oxygen (if hypoxemic), (4) IV access, and 5) 12-lead EKG. Unstable patients should initially be treated with IV atropine (q5 minutes, 3 mg maximum). If atropine is ineffective, prepare for transcutaneous pacing. Acceptable alternatives to temporary pacing are IV infusions of either dopamine or epinephrine. If transcutaneous pacing or the above medications are ineffective, consider transvenous pacing.

**Step 3) Long-term management:** If no reversible causes are found, then the next best step is to implant a permanent pacemaker in almost all patients with a third-degree AV block.

**Disposition:**

Hemodynamically unstable patients may require the ICU. Hemodynamically stable patients can be sent to the telemetry floor.

**Pearls:**

• Some patients may respond favorably to atropine, which is indicative of an abnormal conduction in the AV node. The more distal the conduction block is from the AV node (ie, less vagal activity), the less the response with atropine.

• As a result of the slow rate in third-degree AV blocks, patients can experience lightheadedness or syncope.

• **On the CCS**, telemetry is also known as cardiac monitor in the practice CCS. If you want future results from the cardiac monitor, you have to type in "check cardiac monitor" in the order form.

• **On the CCS**, "pacemaker, temporary, transvenous" is available in the practice CCS.

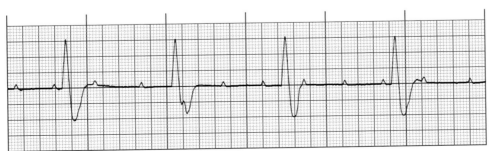

**Figure 5-5 • Third-degree AV block.** Reproduced with permission from Jones SA. *ECG Success: Exercises in ECG Interpretation.* Philadelphia: F.A. Davis Company; 2008:58.

- **On the CCS**, suboptimal management includes delaying transcutaneous pacing in patients with symptomatic bradycardia and signs of poor perfusion.

- **On the CCS**, remember to "bridge" your therapy by treating any acute issues (symptomatic bradycardia) with the long-term management of a third-degree AV block (permanent pacemaker).

# ACCESSORY PATHWAY

## WOLFF-PARKINSON-WHITE

Wolff-Parkinson-White (WPW) is characterized by a ventricular preexcitation via an accessory pathway. Patients can have a symptomatic arrhythmia (WPW syndrome), or they can be asymptomatic but have the classic EKG pattern (WPW pattern). WPW syndrome can be associated with other conditions such as atrial fibrillation, atrial flutter, sudden cardiac death (SCD), and AVRT, also known as atrioventricular reentrant tachycardia (orthodromic or antidromic).

### EKG Features:

A shortened PR interval that is usually <3 small boxes (<0.12 seconds) secondary to a rapid conduction through the accessory pathway. A slurred upstroke of the QRS, also known as the **delta wave,** secondary to a slowed ventricular activation, which can result in a widened QRS complex. See Figure 5-6.

### Next Step Treatment:

**Step 1)** The clinical management for patients who are asymptomatic but have the WPW pattern on EKG is usually observation. The management approach for WPW syndrome can be summarized into short-term or long-term management.

### Short-term Management:

**Hemodynamically unstable**—Electrical cardioversion.

**Atrial fibrillation**—IV procainamide, amiodarone, or ibutilide.

**AVRT (Orthodromic)**—Attempt vagal maneuvers first; if no success, then IV adenosine, verapamil, or esmolol (short-acting beta-blocker).

**AVRT (Antidromic)**—IV procainamide.

### Long-term Management:

Catheter ablation is considered a first-line therapy for patients with WPW syndrome and associated conditions (eg, AVRT, atrial fibrillation, atrial flutter).

### Disposition:

Patients treated in the ED for symptomatic arrhythmias should be admitted to the hospital for further monitoring and consultation with a cardiologist.

### Pearls:

- Orthodromic AVRT is characterized by an antegrade conduction through the AV node to the ventricles, but a retrograde conduction (back to the atria) via an accessory pathway. This results in a narrow QRS complex with tachycardia.

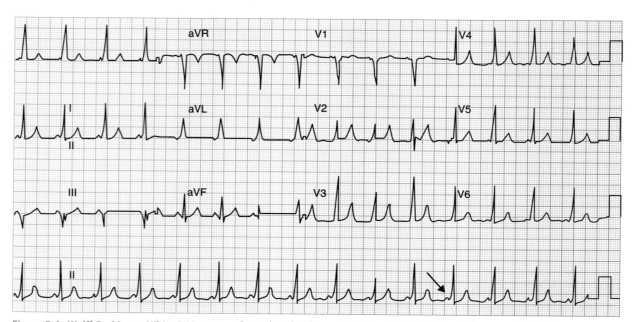

**Figure 5-6 • Wolff-Parkinson-White EKG pattern.** Reproduced with permission from Tintinalli JE, et al. *Emergency Medicine: A Comprehensive Study Guide.* 7th ed. New York: McGraw-Hill; 2011:986.

- Antidromic AVRT is characterized by an antegrade conduction through the accessory pathway, but a retrograde conduction via the AV node. This results in a wide QRS complex with tachycardia.

- Avoid using AV nodal blocking drugs (eg, beta-blockers, calcium channel blockers, adenosine, digoxin) in atrial fibrillation or atrial flutter since using these drugs can promote conduction through the accessory pathway.

- Patients with the WPW syndrome may develop palpitations, chest pain, dizziness, lightheadedness, or syncope.

- Patients with sudden cardiac death usually die from ventricular fibrillation (VF), which is usually generated from an episode of atrial fibrillation (AF → VF → SCD).

- WPW syndrome is associated with Ebstein's anomaly of the tricuspid valve.

- Patients with only the WPW pattern on EKG may have the abnormality disappear over time.

- Electrophysiologic study (EPS) is not required to make the diagnosis of WPW, but can be used in equivocal cases.

- **On the CCS**, the vagal maneuver, "massage carotid" is available in the practice CCS.

- **On the CCS**, "electrophysiologic testing" is available in the practice CCS.

- **On the CCS**, "synchronous cardioversion" is available in the practice CCS.

- **On the CCS**, remember to "bridge" your therapy by treating any acute issues (eg, termination of the tachycardia) with the long-term management of WPW syndrome (eg, prevention).

# VENTRICLES

## TORSADES DE POINTES

Torsades de pointes is a distinct form of polymorphic ventricular tachycardia that is associated with a prolonged QT interval. The presence of a prolonged QT increases the risk of developing torsades de pointes because it is often triggered by a ventricular premature complex (VPC) during the prolonged repolarization period. QT prolongation may be congenital (eg, Romano-Ward syndrome) or acquired. Consider the following acquired causes:

> **Acquired long QT**—Hypokalemia, hypomagnesemia, hypocalcemia, hypothyroidism, tricyclic antidepressants, antipsychotics (eg, haloperidol, thioridazine, phenothiazines), antibiotics (eg, erythromycin, clarithromycin, azithromycin, levofloxacin, moxifloxacin, gatifloxacin), antifungals (eg, pentamidine, voriconazole), antiarrhythmics (eg, quinidine, procainamide, amiodarone, ibutilide, sotalol), AV blocks, MI, cocaine, ondansetron, organophosphate insecticides, intracranial disease, liquid protein diets, anorexia nervosa.

### EKG Features:

Torsades de pointes literally has a "twisting of the points" appearance. The ventricular rate is usually >150 complexes per minute. In the following figure, the tachycardia is preceded by a short R-R interval followed by a long R-R interval with a ventricular premature complex (VPC) falling during repolarization. The arrow denotes the R on T phenomenon (ie, ventricular depolarization occurring at the end of repolarization). See Figure 5-7.

### Next Step Treatment:

**Step 1)** Withdraw any offending agents and correct electrolyte abnormalities.

**Step 2)** The clinical management for torsades de pointes can be summarized into short-term or long-term management.

### Short-term Management:

**Hemodynamically unstable**—Electrical cardioversion

**Acquired long QT**

- IV magnesium sulfate is a first-line therapy to treat and prevent recurrence.

- Temporary pacemaker can shorten the QT interval and is usually tried after an unsuccessful attempt with magnesium sulfate.

- IV isoproterenol (given as a continuous infusion) can also shorten the QT interval and can be given as an interim agent until pacing is available.

**Congenital long QT**

- Beta-blockers (eg, propranolol) are the cornerstone for treatment in symptomatic patients.

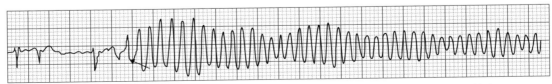

**Figure 5-7 • Torsades de pointes.** Reproduced with permission from Fuster V, et al. *Hurst's The Heart.* New York: McGraw-Hill; 2011:2109.

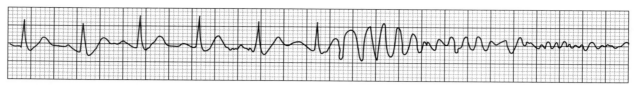

**Figure 5-8 • Ventricular fibrillation.** Reproduced with permission from Stone KC, Humphries RL. *Current Diagnosis and Treatment: Emergency Medicine.* 6th ed. New York: McGraw-Hill; 2008: Figure 33-19.

**Long-term Management:**

**Acquired long QT**—Identify the precipitating factor. Patients with AV blocks or symptomatic bradycardia may benefit from a permanent pacemaker.

**Congenital long QT**—Beta-blockers, avoid strenuous activity, and consider an implantable cardioverter defibrillator (ICD) in patients who are remain symptomatic despite beta-blocker therapy.

## Disposition:

Patients treated for acute management of torsades de pointes should be admitted to the hospital for further monitoring.

## Pearls:

- Torsades de pointes can be sustained, nonsustained, or it can degenerate into ventricular fibrillation.

- Consider torsades de pointes as the "sitting duck" of arrhythmias since a prolonged QT is vulnerable to the firing of a depolarization from a PVC onto a T wave (repolarization) that can trigger the "twisting of the points."

- **On the CCS**, "ICD" is available in the practice CCS.

- **On the CCS**, remember to "bridge" your therapy by treating any acute issues (eg, tachycardia) and addressing any chronic issues (eg, prolonged QT).

# ■ VENTRICULAR FIBRILLATION

Ventricular fibrillation (VF) results in disorganized electrical activity that leads to irregular ventricular contraction and, subsequently, into cardiac arrest (absent pulse). A common cause for VF is due to coronary artery disease with resultant MI. Other causes of VF include long QT syndrome, short QT syndrome, myocarditis, valvular heart disease, dilated cardiomyopathies, hypertrophic cardiomyopathy, congenital heart disease, WPW syndrome (AF → VF → SCD), antiarrhythmics, electrolyte abnormalities, and acid-base abnormalities.

## EKG Features:

The rhythm appears to have a chaotic irregular appearance without recognizable P waves, QRS complexes, or T waves. At the onset of VF, high amplitude fibrillatory waves may be seen and are referred to as coarse VF (type I VF). Later, the fibrillatory waves may be of low amplitude (small undulations) and are referred to as fine VF (type II VF). Fine VF may be very difficult to distinguish from asystole. In the following figure,

after 6 beats, the sinus rhythm degenerates into ventricular fibrillation. See Figure 5-8.

**Next Step Treatment:**
(The following steps are based on the ACLS guidelines.)

**Step 1)** CPR until defibrillator arrives.

**Step 2)** Asynchronous cardioversion (monophasic 360 Joules or diphasic 200 Joules).

**Step 3)** Resume CPR and obtain IV/IO access.

**Step 4)** If a shockable rhythm is present, then defibrillate.

**Step 5)** Resume CPR, deliver IV epinephrine q3-5 minutes or IV vasopressin x 1 can replace the first or second dose of epinephrine. During this step, consider intubation.

**Step 6)** If a shockable rhythm is present, then defibrillate.

**Step 7)** Resume CPR, deliver IV amiodarone in patients that are unresponsive to defibrillation, CPR, and epinephrine. If amiodarone is unavailable, you can use IV lidocaine. During this step, treat any reversible causes (eg, hypovolemia, hypoxia, hydrogen ions, hypo-/hyperkalemia, hypothermia, tension pneumothorax, tamponade, toxins, thrombosis coronary or pulmonary).

**Disposition/Follow-Up:**

Patients with a successful reversion should be transferred to the ICU. The long-term follow-up plan for patients with corrected reversible causes of VF should be considered for an implantable cardioverter defibrillator (ICD).

**Pearls:**

- Vigilance should be taken within the next several hours (<5 hours) in patients with an acute MI since VF usually strikes during that window.

- Early defibrillation is key to patient survival.

- In VF, you want to use unsynchronized cardioversion because you do not want to delay the machine from sensing a QRS complex, which is seen in synchronous cardioversion.

- **On the CCS**, "defibrillation" is available in the practice CCS, which is synonymous with unsynchronized cardioversion.

- **On the CCS**, in patients with VF, look for the patient with no pulse, unresponsiveness, and agonal gasps.

- **On the CCS**, this case is an emergency, move the simulated time judiciously.

- **On the CCS**, this is a type of case in which you'll be judged on your timing, sequence of actions, and appropriateness of your actions.

# Endocrinology

## KEYWORDS REVIEW

**Acroparesthesia**—Paresthesia in the extremity.

**Calciphylaxis**—Systemic calcification of the arteries that can lead to tissue ischemia and necrosis.

**Hyperhidrosis**—Excessive sweating.

**Hyperprolactinemia**—Elevated levels of prolactin in the blood.

**Pretibial myxedema**—An infiltrative dermopathy seen in Grave's disease that will present as a nonpitting induration of the skin, also described as an "orange-peel" appearance, over the lower legs.

**Renal osteodystrophy**—Renal bone disease that is seen in patients with chronic kidney disease as a result of derangements in electrolytes and endocrine function (eg, PTH). Examples of renal osteodystrophy include osteitis fibrosa cystica, osteomalacia, and adynamic bone disease.

# PITUITARY DISORDERS

## ACROMEGALY

Acromegaly is a disease that results from hypersecretion of growth hormone (GH). Hypersecretion is most commonly due to an anterior pituitary somatotroph adenoma. The term *acromegaly* is used when hypersecretion of GH occurs after the epiphyseal plates have closed. The term *pituitary gigantism* is used when hypersecretion of GH occurs before the epiphyseal plates have closed (results in disproportionately long arms and legs).

**Clinical Features:**

Acromegaly is an insidious disease. The clinical presentation of acromegaly can be best understood by either "on-site" or "off-site" effects.

**On-Site Effects (Direct Tumor Effects)**

**Neurologic**—Headaches, cranial nerve palsies, visual defects (bitemporal hemianopsia), pituitary damage (ie, ↓ ACTH, ↓ LH, ↓ FSH, ↓ TSH, ↑ prolactin)

**Off-Site Effects (Distant Effects due to Excess GH/IGF-1)**

Consider the effects from a relative head to toe fashion:

**Head**—Frontal bossing, coarse facial features, prognathism, sleep apnea (central and obstructive), macroglossia, dental malocclusion, enlarged salivary glands

**Neck**—Thyroid enlargement (visceromegaly), diffuse or multinodular goiter, deepened voice

**Cardiac**—Cardiomyopathy, HTN, CHF, LVH, hypertriglyceridemia, arrhythmias, valvular heart disease

**Renal**—Enlarged kidneys, ↓ renin levels, ↑ aldosterone levels, hypercalciuria, hyperphosphatemia

**Hepatic**—Hepatosplenomegaly

**GI**—Colonic polyps, colonic diverticula, adenocarcinoma

**Pancreas**—Diabetes mellitus, insulin resistance, hyperinsulinemia

**Prostate**—Enlarged prostate

**Reproduction**—Menstrual irregularities, galactorrhea, ↓ libido, impotence

**Skin**—Oily texture, hyperhidrosis, body odor, skin tags, women can have hirsutism, acanthosis nigricans

**Musculoskeletal**—Large hands and feet, ↑ ring size, hypertrophic arthropathy (eg, spine, hips, knees, ankles), acroparesthesia secondary to nerve entrapment (eg, carpal tunnel syndrome), proximal muscle weakness

**Next Step:**

**Step 1)** The best initial test is obtaining **serum IGF-I**. A normal IGF-I concentration indicates that the patient does not have acromegaly.

**Step 2)** If serum IGF-I levels are high or equivocal, then the next best step is to obtain a serum GH level after administering oral glucose (ie, oral glucose tolerance test). In normal individuals, GH is suppressed to ≤1 ng/mL after a 75 gram oral glucose load, but in patients with acromegaly the GH levels are inadequately suppressed (ie, GH concentration usually cannot go below 2 ng/mL after a 75 gram glucose load).

**Step 3)** Identify the tumor with a brain MRI if the GH level is elevated after OGTT. In some cases, a pituitary adenoma may not be identified, and the next thing you have to consider is an ectopic secretion of GH or an ectopic secretion of GHRH. In such cases, consider further imaging (chest, abdomen) or biochemical testing for GHRH levels.

**Step 4)** The goal of therapy is to control the levels of GH and IGF-I. Consider the following treatment modalities:

**Surgical Intervention**

**Transsphenoidal surgery**—Surgical resection is the treatment of choice for most patients, especially in the presence of a mass effect (eg, bitemporal hemianopsia). The cure rate is approximately 70% for microadenomas and less than 50% for macroadenomas (size ≥10 mm).

**Medical Intervention**

**Somatostatin analogs** (eg, octreotide, lanreotide)—Inhibit GH secretion and are considered the best option if the adenoma does not look resectable or if the risks outweighs the benefit of surgery. Somatostatin analogs can cause nausea, abdominal discomfort, flatulence, fat malabsorption, and diarrhea. Octreotide and lanreotide can be both given as SubQ or IM (depot injection).

**Dopamine agonists** (eg, cabergoline, bromocriptine)—Inhibits GH secretion but not as well as the somatostatin analogs. However, these agents would be a good choice to consider for patients that cosecrete prolactin since dopamine reduces prolactin secretion. Dopamine agonists can also be added as a combination therapy with other somatostatin analogs. Administer orally.

**GH receptor antagonist** (eg, pegvisomant)—Pegvisomant blocks the binding of endogenous GH resulting in a decrease in IGF-I. The use of pegvisomant has been associated with an increase in serum GH concentration. Pegvisomant can be considered if somatostatin analogs and dopamine agonists are ineffective. Pegvisomant can also be added as a combination therapy with other somatostatin analogs. Side effects include elevated liver enzymes and lipohypertrophy. Administer SubQ.

**Radiation Intervention**

**Radiation therapy**—Used as an adjuvant therapy or contraindication to surgery. Radiation is mainly considered when surgery or medical treatments have been ineffective.

**Follow-Up:**

Patients are followed up and monitored periodically with the clinical assessment, serum IGF-I levels, MRI (if pituitary adenoma was seen on initial MRI), and colonoscopy (remember patients have a risk for colonic polyps). Patients with acromegaly have an increased risk in mortality, and most die from cardiovascular disease. Therefore, it is important to periodically assess and treat any cardiovascular issues.

## Pearls:

- IGF-I is GH dependent (ie, GH stimulates the secretion of IGF-I).

- IGF-I binding protein-3 (IGFBP-3) is also GH dependent and is a major IGF-I binding protein in serum. The levels of IGFBP-3 are also elevated in acromegaly, but there is considerable overlap with normal levels, which makes this measurement of limited value.

- Children with pituitary gigantism tend to have rapid weight gain along with an accelerated linear growth pattern since the epiphyseal plates have not closed.

- Adults with acromegaly do not become taller since the epiphyseal plates have closed. Instead, patients may experience hypertrophic arthropathy.

- Once treatment is initiated and serum IGF-I levels return to normal, patients may continue to have symptoms and bony abnormalities may persist.

- Complications of transsphenoidal surgery include central diabetes insipidus, CSF leak, and meningitis.

- One of the advantages of medical intervention (somatostatin analogs, dopamine agonists, GH receptor antagonist) is that it does not cause hypopituitarism, unlike surgery or radiation therapy.

- **Foundational point**—Approximately 40% of somatotroph adenomas have a mutation in the alpha subunit of the stimulatory GTP binding protein. The result is an increase in adenylyl cyclase activation ($\uparrow$ cAMP), which can increase GH secretion.

- **CJ:** In the office, you decide to obtain serum GH levels in addition to the serum IGF-I. Is that acceptable? **Answer:** Obtaining measurements of serum GH levels is not recommended because of the wide fluctuation in GH levels during a 24-hour period. IGF-I does not have as wide a variability in serum levels as GH.

- **On the CCS**, if a pituitary adenoma is found on MRI, remember to consult with a neurosurgeon.

- **On the CCS**, when you order labs during the CCS case, the normal reference values will be provided next to the actual values.

- **On the CCS**, in almost every case and probably in the real clinical world, you have to consider "bridging your therapy." Ask yourself, "Do I have to treat any acute issues and address any long-term (chronic) issues?" This style of thinking is comprehensive and will gain you points on the exam.

## PROLACTINOMA

Prolactinoma is a pituitary lactotroph adenoma that secretes excessive amounts of prolactin. The adenoma may be referred to as a microadenoma (<1 cm) or a macroadenoma (>1 cm).

### Clinical Features:

Both men and women may experience a local mass effect from the adenoma (eg, visual field defects, headaches). However, men and women may present with different signs and symptoms from the hyperprolactinemia. Consider the following:

**Women**—In a young adolescent, delayed puberty may occur (eg, late menarche). In a reproductive-aged female, patients may present with menstrual irregularities, infertility, galactorrhea, vaginal dryness, hot flashes, or decrease bone mineral density.

**Men**—In a prepubescent boy, hyperprolactinemia can result in small testicles. In an adult, patients may present with impotence, $\downarrow$ libido, infertility, or less commonly gynecomastia and galactorrhea.

### Next Step:

**Step 1**) The best initial step is to determine the **serum prolactin level**. If the value is elevated, this will support the suspicion of hyperprolactinemia. It should be noted that normal prolactin levels should be less than 20 ng/mL and values greater than 100 ng/mL are usually associated with a macroadenoma.

**Step 2**) Determine the etiology of the hyperprolactinemia (see Table 6-1). For example, order a qualitative β-HCG in a reproductive-aged female, TSH plus $T_4$ level for hypothyroidism, LFTs for liver disease, BUN/Cr for renal insufficiency, or determine if there is a medication-induced hyperprolactinemia.

**Step 3**) Once the secondary causes of hyperprolactinemia have been excluded, the next best step is to order a brain **MRI** to evaluate for a pituitary adenoma. Be aware that not all microadenomas will show up on imaging, and they may lead to a diagnosis of idiopathic hyperprolactinemia.

**Step 4**) First-line treatment for any size lactotroph adenoma are the dopamine agonists (eg, bromocriptine, cabergoline) since they will decrease the size of the adenoma and secretion of the prolactin. Transsphenoidal surgery is considered if dopamine agonists have been unsuccessful, the size of the adenoma persists despite medical therapy, or there is drug intolerance. Radiation therapy is regarded as a second-line treatment, but is considered in patients that do not respond to drugs or surgery.

### Follow-Up:

Once the patient is treated for a prolactinoma, the follow-up consists of clinical assessments, serum prolactin levels, and imaging of the pituitary.

### Pearls:

- Prolactin has an inhibitory effect on GnRH resulting in infertility. Therefore, treating the patient with a dopamine agonist (ie, inhibits prolactin) will help patients with hyperprolactinemic anovulation.

- Prolactinomas can potentially increase in their size during pregnancy because of the elevated estrogen levels during pregnancy.

- The mechanism of elevated prolactin levels secondary to hypothyroidism is unclear. However, thyrotropin-releasing hormone (TRH) has been implicated as a cause for elevated prolactin.

- If the cause of hyperprolactinemia is due to hypothyroidism, treat the hypothyroidism and the elevated prolactin levels should normalize.

- Hyperprolactinemia can recur after surgery or discontinuation of the dopamine agonists.

| Table 6-1 • Causes of Hyperprolactinemia | | | | |
|---|---|---|---|---|
| **Physiologic** | | | | |
| • Pregnancy (↑ estrogen causes ↑ prolactin) <br> • Nipple stimulation <br> • Stress <br> • Sleep <br> • Exercise | | | | |
| **Medical** | | | | |
| **Neurologic**—Prolactinoma, hypothalamic-pituitary stalk damage (e.g. trauma, tumor, surgery, sarcoidosis), seizures, acromegaly (GH can be cosecreted with prolactin) <br> **Thyroid**—Hypothyroidism <br> **Chest wall**—Chest wall injury (e.g. burns, herpetic infection, trauma, surgery) can cause an increase in prolactin <br> **Renal**—Chronic renal failure <br> **Hepatic**—Cirrhosis <br> **Idiopathic**—Unknown cause for some patients | | | | |
| **Medications—Antipsychotics** | **Antidepressants** | **Antihypertensives** | **GI Meds** | **Opiates** |
| • Haloperidol <br> • Chlorpromazine <br> • Prochlorperazine <br> • Thioridazine <br> • Fluphenazine <br> • Risperidone <br> • Olanzapine | • Amitriptyline <br> • Clomipramine | • Verapamil <br> • Methyldopa <br> • Reserpine | • Metoclopramide <br> • Cimetidine | • Morphine <br> • Codeine |

- **Foundational point**—Lactotroph adenomas are mainly composed of chromophobic or weakly acidophilic cells.
- **Connecting point** (pg. 108)—Elevated prolactin levels can cause primary and secondary amenorrhea.
- **CJ:** A 27-year-old woman is in her first trimester of pregnancy and is experiencing visual problems. An MRI was ordered and confirms the presence of a macroadenoma with a size of 12 mm. What is your next step? **Answer:** Macroadenomas have a higher propensity to enlarge during pregnancy compared to microadenomas. In this case, the patient should initially be treated with a dopamine agonist

(eg, bromocriptine). If the patient does not respond to medical therapy and vision is compromised, the next best step is to consider transsphenoidal surgery for surgical decompression.

- **On the CCS,** when rescheduling a patient to come back for an office visit, weekend schedule appointments will be defaulted to the following Monday.
- **On the CCS,** remember to "advise patient, side effects of medication" since dopamine agonists can cause nausea, constipation, nasal stuffiness, postural hypotension, Raynaud phenomenon, and dizziness.

# THYROID DISORDERS

## ▍THYROTOXICOSIS

Thyrotoxicosis is a condition of excess quantities of endogenous or exogenous thyroid hormones. Hyperthyroidism can lead to thyrotoxicosis, but should not be synonymous with thyrotoxicosis. Hyperthyroidism (ie, excessive thyroid function) is characterized by the excess synthesis and secretion of thyroid hormone and can be divided into primary hyperthyroidism (eg, Grave's disease, toxic multinodular goiter, toxic adenoma, metastatic follicular thyroid carcinoma) and secondary hyperthyroidism

(eg, TSH-secreting pituitary adenoma, hCG-secreting tumor). Other causes of thyrotoxicosis include exogenous causes (eg, excess ingestion of thyroid hormones) or thyroid inflammation damage leading to release of thyroid hormones (eg, subacute thyroiditis, silent thyroiditis).

### Clinical Features:

The signs and symptoms of thyrotoxicosis can vary (see Table 6-2). Consider the following clinical manifestations in a relative head to toe fashion:

**Psychiatric**—Anxiety, irritability, depression, psychosis, nervousness, insomnia, emotional lability

## Table 6-2 • Thyrotoxicosis Causes and Treatment

| Name | MOA | Clinical Features | Diagnostic Clues | RAIU | Next Step Treatment |
|---|---|---|---|---|---|
| Graves' disease (Hyperthyroid) | TSH receptor antibodies activate the receptor | • Diffusely nontender enlarged gland<br>• Exophthalmos<br>• Pretibial myxedema | ↓ TSH, $FT_3$ and $FT_4$ can be normal to ↑<br>TSI-positive<br>TBII-positive<br>(see Pearls section) | ↑<br>Diffuse uptake | Symptomatic → β-blocker + PTU or MMI<br>Definitive Tx → RAI or surgery<br>Large obstructive goiter → Consider surgery |
| Toxic adenoma (Hyperthyroid) | Autonomous production | • Discrete nodule<br>• Hot nodule or hyperfunctional nodule will produce symptoms | ↓ TSH, $FT_3$ and $FT_4$ can be normal to ↑ | ↑<br>Single nodule uptake but rest of gland is suppressed | Symptomatic → β-blocker + PTU or MMI<br>Definitive Tx → RAI or surgery |
| Toxic multinodular (Plummer's disease) | Autonomous production | • Multiple nodules | ↓ TSH, $FT_3$ and $FT_4$ can be normal to ↑ | ↑<br>Patchy uptake; both hot or cold nodule may be seen | Symptomatic → β-blocker + PTU or MMI<br>Definitive Tx → RAI or surgery |
| Subacute thyroiditis (de Quervain's) | ↑ preformed release of hormone 2° to inflammation due to a possible virus | • Enlarged thyroid<br>• **Painful** | **3 phases** (Thyrotoxic → Hypothyroid → Recovery)<br>In thyrotoxic phase:<br>↓ TSH, $FT_3$ and $FT_4$ can be normal to ↑ | ↓ | Step 1) Try NSAIDs<br>Step 2) Try glucocorticoids (eg, prednisone) if NSAIDs are ineffective. |
| Silent thyroiditis (Subacute lymphocytic thyroiditis) | ↑ preformed release of hormone 2° to inflammation<br>• Considered a variant of Hashimoto's thyroiditis | • Slightly enlarged gland<br>• **Painless** | Also has 3 phases. In thyrotoxic phase:<br>↓ TSH, $FT_3$ and $FT_4$ can be normal to ↑<br>• ↑ Anti-TPO<br>• ↑ Anti-TG | ↓ | Asymptomatic → Observe<br>Symptomatic → β-blocker |
| Iodine-induced (eg, contrast, amiodarone) | ↑ hormone release | • Look for nodular goiter | ↓ TSH, ↑ $FT_4$, and/or ↑$FT_3$, | ↓ | Remove the offending agent. |
| Struma ovarii (Teratoma made up of thyroid) | • Extrathyroidal | • Pelvic mass | ↓ TSH, ↑ $FT_4$, and/or ↑$FT_3$<br>U/S-ovarian mass | ↓ | Definitive Tx → Surgical resection of the ovarian tumor |
| Metastatic follicular thyroid carcinoma | • Extrathyroidal | • Bone and lung involvement | T3-toxicosis (↓ TSH, ↑ $FT_3$, normal $FT_4$) | ↓ | • Surgery + RAI + Thyroid hormone replacement |
| Thyrotoxicosis factitia | • Exogenous | • Symptomatic<br>• No goiter | ↓ TSH, $FT_3$ and $FT_4$ can be normal to ↑<br>• ↓ thyroglobulin | ↓ | • Reduce or discontinue thyroid hormones. |

*MMI—methimazole; MOA—mechanism of action; RAI—radioactive iodine; RAIU—radioactive iodine uptake; TBII—thyrotropin-binding inhibitory immunoglobulin; TG—thyroglobulin; TPO—thyroid peroxidase; TSI—thyroid-stimulating immunoglobulin; U/S—ultrasound*

**Neurologic**—Heat intolerance, tremor, cognitive dysfunction

**Ocular**—Staring gaze, lid lag, diplopia, proptosis (exophthalmos)

**Respiratory**—Dyspnea secondary to respiratory muscle weakness

**Cardiovascular**—Tachycardia, systolic HTN, widened pulse pressure, atrial fibrillation

**GI**—Weight loss despite an increase in appetite, frequent bowel movements, diarrhea

**Genitourinary**—Urinary frequency, amenorrhea, oligomenorrhea, erectile dysfunction, ↓ libido

**Musculoskeletal**—Osteoporosis, fatigue, weakness

**Dermatologic**—Warm and moist skin, sweating, fine hair, onycholysis, pretibial myxedema

**Hematologic**—Normochromic, normocytic anemia

**Metabolic**—Impaired glucose tolerance, low HDL levels

## Next Step:

**Step 1)** The best initial screening test is **serum TSH level**. If TSH level is low, order an unbound **free $T_4$ ($FT_4$)** and **free $T_3$ ($FT_3$)**. If TSH is low and both $FT_4$ and $FT_3$ are high, thyrotoxicosis is confirmed. In some cases, when TSH is low but $FT_4$ is elevated and $FT_3$ is normal, it is considered a $T_4$ toxicosis. When you have $T_4$ toxicosis, you should think of $T_4$ ingestion, nonthyroidal illness, excess iodine, and amiodarone therapy (ie, inhibits conversion from $T_4$ to $T_3$). On the contrary, with a low TSH, but $FT_3$ is elevated and $FT_4$ is normal, then it is considered a $T_3$ toxicosis. With $T_3$ toxicosis, you should think of Graves' disease, toxic adenoma, nodular goiter, and increased conversion from $T_4$ to $T_3$ (ie, $T_3$ is the more active thyroid hormone). Finally, if you have a low TSH but normal $FT_4$ and $FT_3$, then the patient has subclinical hyperthyroidism.

**Step 2)** If the etiology of thyrotoxicosis is unclear even after a clinical assessment and laboratory testing, the next best step is with scintigraphy, also referred to as radioactive iodine uptake (RAIU). RAIU uses either $^{123}$I or technetium-99m. It should be noted that measuring thyrotropin receptor antibodies is not routinely performed, but should be considered if RAIU is contraindicated. See Table 6-2 for the clinical clues for each type of thyrotoxicosis.

**Step 3)** The next step treatment involves medical therapy, radiation, or surgery. Consider the following:

## Medical Intervention

**Beta-blockers**—β-blockers (eg, propranolol, atenolol, metoprolol) are used to treat hyperadrenergic symptoms such as tachycardia, tremulousness, palpitations, anxiety, and heat intolerance. It should be noted that beta-blockers can be coadministered with thionamides.

**Thionamides**—Thionamides (eg, propylthiouracil [PTU], methimazole [MMI]) decrease the synthesis of thyroid hormones. Thionamides are considered the best initial therapy for children and adolescents.

**Iodine**—Iodine elixirs (eg, potassium iodide) and iodinated contrast agents (eg, iopanoic acid, sodium ipodate) can inhibit the peripheral conversion of $T_4$ to $T_3$. However, this type of medical therapy is considered second-line therapy and not available in the United States.

## Radiation Ablation

**Radioactive Iodine Therapy**—Radiation ablation involves administering the radioactive iodine orally in a dose of $^{131}$I to destroy the thyroid tissue within 6 to 20 weeks.

## Surgical Intervention

**Surgery**—Subtotal or total thyroidectomy is a definitive form of treatment, but it is not considered first-line treatment because of the success with medications and radioactive iodine therapy. However, surgery is considered when there is an obstructive goiter, intolerance to meds or radioactive therapy, or severe ophthalmopathy.

## Follow-Up:

Patients taking thionamides should have a thyroid function test every 4 to 6 weeks until levels are stabilized. Patients who underwent radioactive iodine therapy will have destruction of their thyroid tissue within 2 to 5 months, and it is important to check thyroid function every 4 to 6 weeks because at some point they can be hypothyroid and may need thyroid hormone replacement. Thyroid function test should be obtained in 4 to 8 weeks postoperatively in patients who underwent a thyroidectomy.

## Pearls:

- Antibodies against thyroid peroxidase (TPO) and thyroglobulin (TG) are fairly nonspecific.

- Thyrotropin-binding inhibitory immunoglobulin (TBII) and thyroid-stimulating immunoglobulin (TSI) are assays that are used to detect TSH receptor antibodies (TSHR-Ab) that can be seen in Graves' disease.

- Conditions that can increase the levels of hCG include hydatidiform mole, hyperemesis gravidarum, and choriocarcinoma. Elevated hCG levels can stimulate TSH receptors and thereby cause thyrotoxicosis.

- Graves' disease is characterized by hyperthyroidism, Graves' ophthalmopathy, goiter, and dermopathy.

- Clinical manifestations in elderly patients may appear more atypical. For example, they may appear apathetic, absence of tremor and tachycardia, constipation, and toxic multinodular goiter appears to be more common.

- **Caveat 1**—Pregnancy and breastfeeding is a contraindication to RAIU.

- **Caveat 2**—Methimazole and propylthiouracil can both cause agranulocytosis and hepatitis, therefore order baseline labs before initiating thionamides.

- **Caveat 3**—Thionamides can cross the placenta during pregnancy, but they have been given during pregnancy. Remember they are a category D drug.

- **Caveat 4**—Radiation therapy and surgery can both lead to hypothyroidism.
- **Caveat 5**—Patients that have a relative contraindication to beta-blockers can be given a selective beta 1-blocker (eg, metoprolol, atenolol).
- **Caveat 6**—Radioactive iodine therapy can actually make Graves' ophthalmopathy worse.
- **Caveat 7**—After radioactive iodine therapy, patients should wait at least 6 months prior to conception.
- **Caveat 8**—Always check an hCG in a reproductive female before administering radioactive iodine.
- **Foundational point**—$T_4$ is converted to the more active form $T_3$ by the enzyme deiodinase.
- **Foundational point**—$T_4$ (thyroxine) is produced solely by the thyroid. $T_3$ (triiodothyronine) can be produced by the thyroid, but also by other tissues (ie, peripheral conversion).
- **Foundational point**—Thyroglobulin (Tg) is a thyroid protein that is produced in the thyroid follicular cell and is predominantly found in the lumen of the thyroid follicles. Tg is involved in the biosynthesis of $T_4$ and $T_3$ in the thyroid gland.
- **Foundational point**—Thyroxine-binding globulin (TBG) is one of three carrier proteins that carry $T_4$ and $T_3$ in the bloodstream.
- **Foundational point**—$T_3$ resin uptake (T3RU) is used to estimate free $T_4$ by measuring unbound TBG. T3RU is sometimes ordered with the total $T_4$ to take into account abnormalities in protein binding such as an increase or decrease in thyroxine-binding globulin (TBG) levels.
- **Foundational point**—TBG levels are lowered in chronic liver failure, chronic renal failure, and glucocorticoid use, which may result in low total $T_4$ and high T3RU.
- **Foundational point**—Estrogen, pregnancy, and OCPs can increase TBG levels and may show high total $T_4$ and low T3RU.
- **Foundational point**—A high T3RU and high total $T_4$ is suggestive of hyperthyroidism, while a low T3RU and low total $T_4$ is suggestive of hypothyroidism.
- **Foundational point**—Methimazole blocks the oxidation of iodine in the thyroid gland, which inhibits the ability of iodine to combine with tyrosine and thereby form $T_4$ and $T_3$.
- **Foundational point**—Propylthiouracil blocks the oxidation of iodine, but also the conversion of $T_4$ to $T_3$.
- **CJ:** A 45-year-old man is undergoing $^{131}$I radiation. He has two small children at home. Is it okay for him to play with them? **Answer:** Avoid contact with children and pregnant women for one week and avoid using utensils and other dishes while on treatment. Also, no sex!
- **On the CCS**, ordering "antibody thyroid, serum" will give you antibody results of both thyroid peroxidase and thyroglobulin in the practice CCS software.
- **On the CCS**, ordering "I 123 uptake, thyroid" and "I 131" are available in the practice CCS, but remember one is for imaging (I 123) and the other one is for treatment (I 131).
- **On the CCS**, remember to "advise patient, side effects of medication" which is available in the practice CCS.
- **On the CCS**, remember to "bridge" your therapy. For example, if a hyperthyroid patient presents with hyperadrenergic symptoms (eg, tremors, palpitations), treat the acute issues with a beta-blocker and the long-term management (eg, hyperthyroidism) with thionamides, radioactive ablation, or surgery.

# HYPOTHYROIDISM

Hypothyroidism can be characterized by the inadequate production of thyroid hormone. Iodine deficiency remains the most common cause of hypothyroidism worldwide. In iodine-sufficient areas, chronic autoimmune (Hashimoto's) thyroiditis remains the most common cause of hypothyroidism. The cause of hypothyroidism can be understood at the level of the thyroid gland (primary), pituitary (secondary), or hypothalamus (tertiary). Consider the following etiologies:

**Primary**

**Autoimmune**—Hashimoto's thyroiditis

**Drugs**—Lithium, amiodarone, thionamides, interferon alpha

**Iodine**—Iodine excess and deficiency can both cause hypothyroidism

**Iatrogenic**—Neck radiation, thyroidectomy, radioactive iodine

**Transient**—Subacute thyroiditis, silent thyroiditis, postpartum thyroiditis

**Secondary**

Sheehan's syndrome, panhypopituitarism, pituitary adenoma, drugs that ↓ TSH (eg, dopamine, octreotide, glucocorticoids), infiltrative diseases (eg, hemochromatosis), trauma, tumor, radiation

**Tertiary**

Infiltrative diseases (eg, sarcoidosis), trauma, tumor, radiation

## Clinical Features:

The clinical manifestations of hypothyroidism can vary. It may be helpful to think from a relative head to toe fashion:

**Psychiatric**—Depression, ↓ concentration, forgetfulness, emotional lability

**Neurologic**—Cold intolerance, cognitive dysfunction, ↓ DTRs, nerve entrapment syndromes

**ENT**—Decreased hearing, macroglossia, hoarseness, periorbital edema, goiter, fullness in throat

**Respiratory**—Dyspnea on exertion, respiratory muscle weakness

**Cardiovascular**—Bradycardia, diastolic HTN, pericardial effusions

**GI**—Weight gain, constipation

**Reproduction**—Menorrhagia, impaired fertility

**Musculoskeletal**—Myalgia, arthralgia, paresthesia, muscle weakness, fatigue

**Dermatologic**—Dry skin, coarse hair, hair loss, brittle nails, myxedema (nonpitting edema)

**Hematologic**—Normochromic, normocytic anemia, pernicious anemia

**Metabolic**—Hyperlipidemia, hyperhomocysteinemia, hyperprolactinemia, hyponatremia

## Next Step:

**Step 1)** The best initial test is a **serum TSH level**. If TSH level is elevated, order an unbound free $T_4$ ($FT_4$). Since approximately 25% of patients with hypothyroidism will have a normal free $T_3$ ($FT_3$), a routine $FT_3$ is generally not indicated. An elevated TSH and a low $FT_4$ confirms the diagnosis of hypothyroidism. In some cases, the TSH level can be low, normal, or slightly high, and now you have to consider a central cause (ie, 2° or 3° hypothyroidism). The next best step is to order a $FT_4$ (see Table 6-3). Finally, if there is an elevated TSH but a normal $FT_4$, the patient has subclinical hypothyroidism. It should be noted that since most cases of hypothyroidism are due to Hashimoto's thyroiditis in iodine-sufficient areas, ordering a thyroid peroxidase antibodies (TPO-Ab) is generally not indicated since most will be positive for the antibodies. However, a TPO-Ab can be ordered in a patient with lab values that are not suggestive of hypothyroidism but the patient has a goiter, or in a patient with subclinical hypothyroidism.

**Step 2)** The treatment of choice for hypothyroidism is with synthetic thyroxine ($T_4$), also known as **levothyroxine**. Other formulations that exist include liothyronine ($T_3$) and liotrix (mixture of $T_4$ and $T_3$ in a 4:1 ratio).

## Follow-Up:

Once thyroid replacement is initiated, the patient should be seen every 6 to 8 weeks until TSH levels normalize. Thereafter, patients can be seen every 6 to 12 months for a TSH checkup.

### Table 6-3 • Hypothyroidism Patterns

| Hypothyroidism | TSH | Free $T_4$ |
|---|---|---|
| Primary | ↑ | ↓ |
| Secondary-"Central" (TSH deficiency) | Low, normal, or slightly ↑ | Low to low-normal |
| Tertiary-"Central" (TRH deficiency) | Low, normal, or slightly ↑ | Low to low-normal |
| Subclinical | ↑ | Normal |

$FT_4$—free thyroxine; TRH—thyrotropin releasing hormone; TSH—thyroid-stimulating hormone

## Pearls:

- Hashimoto's thyroiditis is characterized by the destruction of thyroid cells from an autoimmune process. There are two forms to consider. First, goitrous thyroiditis (presence of a goiter), and second, atrophic thyroiditis (decrease in thyroid tissue), which can be seen in the later stages of the disease.

- Although antibodies against thyroid peroxidase and thyroglobulin are nonspecific, the presence of both antibodies suggests Hashimoto's.

- Hashimoto's thyroiditis may be associated with other autoimmune diseases such as SLE, Sjögren's syndrome, RA, DM type 1, vitiligo, pernicious anemia (may present as $B_{12}$ deficiency), celiac disease, and Addison's disease.

- Hypothyroidism during pregnancy may have several important consequences such as spontaneous abortions, preeclampsia, placental abruption, low birth weight, and cognitive impairment.

- Levothyroxine is a category A drug that is safe to use during pregnancy but may require an increase in dosage during pregnancy.

- **Foundational point**—Iodine deficiency can not only cause hypothyroidism, but excess iodine can do it as well. Excess iodine inhibits organification (ie, oxidation) of iodide, and thereby, synthesis of $T_4$ and $T_3$ (Wolff-Chaikoff effect).

- **Connecting point** (pg. 68)—Hypothyroidism can result in hyperprolactinemia.

- **CJ:** In the ED, a patient with a history of long-standing **untreated hypothyroidism** and **recurrent infections** presents with **hypotension, bradycardia, hypothermia, and altered mental status**. Labs were drawn and revealed **hyponatremia, hypoglycemia**, normal TSH level, and low $FT_4$ levels. Myxedema coma is suspected. What is your next step? **Answer:** Once you suspect myxedema coma on presentation, you should consider (1) intubation if breathing is compromised, (2) fluids to support the pressure (remember not to give a diluted solution since they can be hyponatremic), (3) consider empiric antibiotics, (4) IV levothyroxine ($T_4$) plus IV liothyronine ($T_3$), and (5) stress-dose glucocorticoids (eg, IV hydrocortisone) since you do not know if a hypopituitarism is causing both secondary hypothyroidism and concurrent adrenal insufficiency. Give the stress-dose steroids until adrenal insufficiency has been ruled out (eg, cortisol level, ACTH stimulation test).

- **On the CCS**, once hypothyroidism is confirmed on initial serum levels, consider ordering a "lipid profile" to look for ↑ LDL and ↓ HDL levels. In most cases, it is the routine cholesterol screening that suggests hypothyroidism.

- **On the CCS**, "levothyroxine," "liothyronine," and "liotrix" are available in the practice CCS.

- **On the CCS**, you are expected to advance the clock to "make things happen" such as changes to the patient's condition, test results, procedures, or an effect on treatment that you ordered.

# PARATHYROID DISORDERS

## PRIMARY HYPERPARATHYROIDISM

Primary hyperparathyroidism is characterized by excessive PTH secretion resulting in **hypercalcemia** (see Table 6-4). The etiology can be due to a single adenoma (approximately 85% of cases), multiple gland hyperplasia (15% of cases), or parathyroid carcinoma (1% of cases). Several other causes are neck irradiation, MEN 1 (ie, "**Triple Ps**"—**P**arathyroid tumor, **P**ituitary tumor, **P**ancreatic tumor), and MEN 2A (ie, parathyroid tumor, pheochromocytoma, medullary thyroid cancer).

### Clinical Features:

Patients may be asymptomatic, but the clinical manifestations vary. Remember the mnemonic for hypercalcemia is "bones, stones, abdominal groans, and psychic moans." Consider the following clinical manifestation in a relative head to toe fashion:

**Psychiatric**—Depressed mood, lethargy

**Neurologic**—Confusion, cognition dysfunction

**Cardiovascular**—HTN, bradycardia, short QT interval

**Renal**—Nephrolithiasis, polyuria, polydipsia, ↓ GFR, hypercalciuria, hypophosphatemia, hypomagnesemia, nephrocalcinosis

**GI**—Abdominal pain, nausea, vomiting, peptic ulcer, pancreatitis, constipation, anorexia

**Musculoskeletal**—Bone pain, muscle weakness, osteoporosis, osteopenia, osteitis fibrosa cystica

### Next Step:

**Step 1)** The best initial step is to order a **serum calcium level** to determine if hypercalcemia exists.

**Step 2)** If calcium levels are elevated, the next best step is to order an **intact PTH** level because if it's elevated, then you know it must be due to a PTH-mediated phenomenon (eg, parathyroid adenoma, MEN 1, 2A). If the PTH level is low, then the hypercalcemia is most likely due to a PTH-independent phenomenon (eg, malignancy, ↑ vitamin D, ↑ vitamin A, lithium, thiazides, granulomatous diseases).

**Step 3)** If the calcium levels are elevated with an elevated intact PTH, the next thing you have to consider is familial hypocalciuric hypercalcemia (FHH), which presents similarly to primary hyperparathyroidism. The next best step is to order a **24-hour calcium urine excretion** because the key difference between primary hyperparathyroidism and FHH is the amount of calcium in the urine. Remember FHH has the word "hypocalciuric" in the disorder, therefore a urine calcium level <100 mg/24 hr is most likely FHH, while a urine calcium level >250 mg/24 hr is most likely primary hyperparathyroidism (see Table 6-4).

**Step 4)** Treatment for primary hyperparathyroidism may include observation, surgery (parathyroidectomy), and medications. Consider the following:

**Parathyroidectomy**

- Surgery should be considered in patients that are symptomatic.
- Surgery should be considered in patients with severe hypercalcemia (eg, >15 mg/dL).
- Surgery can be considered in patients that are asymptomatic and who meet the guidelines from the Third International Workshop on Asymptomatic Primary Hyperparathyroidism:

  Age <50 years

  Serum calcium 1 mg/dL above the upper limit of normal

  Cr clearance reduced to <60 mL/min

  T-score <−2.5 at the lumbar spine, hip, femoral neck, radius

**Observation**

- Observation can be considered in patients who want to avoid surgery.
- Observation can be considered in patients who do not meet the above guidelines.

**Medications**

- **Bisphosphonates**—Bisphosphonates (eg, alendronate) inhibit bone resorption and can be given to patients with osteopenia or osteoporosis who are unable to have surgery.
- **Calcimimetics**—Calcimimetics (eg, cinacalcet) increases the sensitivity of the calcium-sensing receptor and thereby lowers PTH secretion. Cinacalcet is an option for patients with severe hypercalcemia who are not candidates for surgery.

### Table 6-4 • Calcium Disorders

| Disorder | Intact PTH | Serum Ca | Serum PO$_4$ | Key Findings |
|---|---|---|---|---|
| Primary hyperparathyroidism | ↑ | ↑ | ↓ | Urine Ca >250 mg/24 hr |
| Familial hypocalciuric hypercalcemia (FHH) | Normal to ↑ | ↑ | Normal to ↓ | Urine Ca <100 mg/24 hr |
| Vitamin D deficiency | ↑ | Normal to ↓ | Normal to ↓ | ↓ 25-OHD |
| Renal failure | ↑ | ↓ | ↑ | ↓ 1,25-OHD |
| Tertiary hyperparathyroidism | ↑ | ↑ | Normal to ↑ | History of secondary hyperparathyroidism |
| Hypoparathyroidism | ↓ | ↓ | ↑ | 1,25-OHD can be low to normal |
| Pseudohypoparathyroidism | ↑ | ↓ | ↑ | Shortened fourth and fifth metacarpals |

**Follow-Up:**

Asymptomatic patients who do not undergo surgery are typically followed up with serum calcium levels, creatinine levels, and bone density. Patients with MEN 1 or MEN 2A should have genetic counseling since both conditions are inherited in an autosomal dominant pattern.

**Pearls:**

- Almost all patients with hypercalcemia will have an elevated free (ionized) calcium level. However, abnormal albumin levels can influence the total calcium level since calcium binds to albumin. In such cases of hypoalbuminemia (eg, liver disease, malnutrition) or hyperalbuminemia (eg, severe dehydration), a corrected total calcium should be performed. In the majority of cases, the initial diagnostic approach for determining primary hyperparathyroidism is with a serum total calcium in the presence of a normal albumin level. A free (ionized) calcium can be added as an adjunct in patients with abnormal albumin levels.

- Patients with primary hyperparathyroidism can have lower levels of 25-OHD and slightly higher levels of 1,25-OHD.

- **Foundational point**—Familial hypocalciuric hypercalcemia (FHH) is due to an inactivating mutation for a gene that codes for the calcium-sensing receptor that is expressed in many tissues (eg, parathyroid, kidney, intestine).

- **Foundational point**—PTH increases serum calcium levels by (1) bone resorption, (2) reabsorption of calcium in the distal tubule, (3) increasing the synthesis of calcitriol in the proximal tubules by stimulating the enzyme 1-alpha hydroxylase to convert calcidiol (25-OHD) to calcitriol (1,25-OHD), which is the more active form of vitamin D, and (4) increase intestinal calcium absorption that is mediated by 1,25-OHD.

- **CJ:** In the ED, a 52-year-old man presents with confusion, severe abdominal pain, HR 55 bpm, BP 160/92, and serum total calcium level of 15 mg/dL. What is your next step? **Answer: Unstable** symptomatic patients with severe hypercalcemia (ie, >14 mg/dL) should be treated accordingly:

  **Step 1**) Administer isotonic fluids such as normal saline (0.9% NaCl) to expand intravascular volume.

  **Step 2**) Administration of salmon calcitonin (IM or SubQ), which is effective within 2 hours.

  **Step 3**) Administration of a bisphosphonate such as IV zoledronic acid or IV pamidronate. The maximal effect of a bisphosphonate can take several days after administration. Step 2 and step 3 are "bridging" the therapeutic effects since one medication works faster than the other.

- **Connecting point** (pg. 282)—Know the bone mineral density scores.

- **On the CCS,** "Calcitonin-Salmon therapy" is available in the practice CCS.

- **On the CCS,** "genetics counseling" is available in the practice CCS.

- **On the CCS,** "ionized calcium, serum" is available in the practice CCS.

- **On the CCS,** a "24-hour urine calcium" is available in the practice CCS.

- **On the CCS,** remember to "bridge" your therapy by treating any acute issues of hypercalcemia with the long-term management of hypercalcemia.

- **On the CCS,** remember to order medications by generic or trade names, not by the class of medications (eg, "beta-blockers").

# SECONDARY HYPERPARATHYROIDISM

Secondary hyperparathyroidism is characterized by an excess secretion of PTH in response to **hypocalcemia.** Secondary hyperparathyroidism is seen in patients with renal failure, vitamin D deficiency, or with inadequate calcium intake.

**Clinical Features:**

Since the PTH levels are elevated, one of the functions of PTH is bone resorption. Naturally, patients are prone to develop renal bone disease, also referred to as renal osteodystrophy. Patients can develop osteomalacia, osteitis fibrosa cystica, mixed osteodystrophy, or adynamic bone disease. Therefore, patients will complain of musculoskeletal problems such as bone pain, muscle pain, or weakness.

**Next Step:**

**Step 1**) Initial laboratory testing should include an intact PTH, serum calcium, serum phosphate, and 25-hydroxyvitamin D levels. See Table 6-4 for expected findings.

**Step 2**) X-rays may be warranted in patients who complain of bone pain to rule out fractures or other pathological diseases secondary to renal osteodystrophy.

**Step 3**) Medical therapy is the cornerstone for treating secondary hyperparathyroidism, but surgery (parathyroidectomy) is considered in cases of fractures, bone pain, or calciphylaxis. Consider the following treatment approach:

**For Hyperphosphatemia**

- Dietary phosphate restriction
- Phosphate binders (eg, calcium carbonate, calcium acetate, sevelamer)

**For Hypocalcemia**

- Provide calcium supplementation, but keep in mind in prolonged disease, patients can develop hypercalcemia.

**For Elevated PTH**

- Calcimimetics (eg, cinacalcet) to reduce the secretion of PTH.

**Vitamin Deficiency**

- Vitamin D replacement, but treat the hyperphosphatemia first because raising the calcium levels before treating the hyperphosphatemia can result in calciphylaxis.

**Follow-Up:**

Once medical therapy is initiated, patients are followed up with the clinical assessment, PTH, calcium, phosphate, and 25-OHD.

**Pearls:**

- 25-hydroxyvitamin D (25-OHD) is the "inactive" form of vitamin D produced in the liver before it becomes hydroxylated to the "active" form of 1,25-OHD in the kidney, with subsequent actions to ↑ Ca absorption in the intestines and to ↓ Ca and phosphate excretion in the kidneys.

- **CJ:** Why are serum phosphate levels higher in renal failure than in vitamin D deficiency? **Answer:** Serum phosphate levels will tend to be higher in renal failure than in vitamin D deficiency because of poor renal clearance of phosphate.

- **On the CCS**, if you want to order vitamin $D_2$ therapy, it will be recognized as either "vitamin D, therapy" or "ergocalciferol."

- **On the CCS**, if you want to order vitamin $D_3$ therapy, it will be recognized as either "vitamin $D_3$" or "cholecalciferol."

- **On the CCS**, if you want to know the 25-hydroxyvitamin D level, it will be recognized as "vitamin D 25-OH, serum, total" on the practice CCS.

# TERTIARY HYPERPARATHYROIDISM

Tertiary hyperparathyroidism is characterized by excessive PTH secretion that is no longer responsive to medical therapy.

**Clinical Features:**

Patients will have signs and symptoms of hypercalcemia. Patients may also have renal bone disease and calciphylaxis.

**Next Step:**

**Step 1)** Initial laboratory testing should include an intact PTH, serum calcium, serum phosphate, and 25-hydroxyvitamin D levels. See Table 6-4 for expected findings.

**Step 2)** X-rays may be warranted in patients who complain of bone pain to rule out fractures or other pathological diseases secondary to renal osteodystrophy.

**Step 3)** Treatment is based on a subtotal or total parathyroidectomy with autotransplantation of the parathyroid tissue into the forearm.

**Follow-Up:**

Obtain serum calcium, phosphate, and PTH levels postoperatively.

**Pearls:**

- **CJ:** Two days postoperatively from a parathyroidectomy, the patient develops tetany and complains of tingling of the fingers. What syndrome is associated with this scenario? **Answer:** Hungry bone syndrome is a complication after a parathyroidectomy. Hungry bone syndrome is a result of a precipitous fall in the calcium, phosphate, and magnesium levels. Literally, the bone is hungry to uptake calcium, phosphate, and magnesium secondary to an abrupt decrease in PTH. Correct the electrolyte abnormalities.

- **On the CCS**, "parathyroidectomy" is recognized in the practice CCS.

- **On the CCS**, if you require a consult during the case, a reason for the consultation in 10 words or less is required.

# HYPOPARATHYROIDISM

Hypoparathyroidism is characterized by low levels of circulating PTH resulting in a state of **hypocalcemia**. Consider the following etiologies of hypoparathyroidism:

**Acquired**—Parathyroid surgery, neck radiation, hyper/hypomagnesemia, Wilson's disease, hemochromatosis, sarcoidosis, carcinoma.

**Autoimmune**—Polyglandular autoimmune syndrome type 1 (ie, hypoparathyroidism, candidiasis, adrenal insufficiency).

**Genetics**—Di George syndrome (ie, **CATCH** → **C**ardiac abnormality (TOF), **A**bnormal facies, **T**hymic aplasia, **C**left palate, **H**ypocalcemia from failure of the parathyroid glands to develop).

**Clinical Features:**

Patients will have signs and symptoms of hypocalcemia. The classic Trousseau's sign (ie, carpopedal spasm elicited by inflating a blood pressure cuff) and Chvostek's sign (ie, tapping on the zygoma or the area of the facial nerve to elicit facial spasms) may be present. Consider the following clinical manifestations in a relative head to toe fashion:

**Psychiatric**—Anxiety, depression, emotional lability

**Neurologic**—Tetany, paresthesias (eg, fingers, toes, perioral), seizures, muscular twitching, ectopic calcifications (basal ganglia), ↑ deep tendon reflexes, parkinsonism

**ENT**—Papilledema, dental hypoplasia

**Respiratory**—Laryngospasm, bronchospasm, hyperventilation (respiratory alkalosis)

**Cardiovascular**—Prolonged QT, arrhythmia

**Dermatologic**—Dry skin, brittle nails

**Next Step:**

**Step 1)** Initial laboratory testing should include an intact PTH, serum calcium, serum phosphate, serum magnesium, and 25-hydroxyvitamin D levels. See Table 6-4 for expected findings.

**Step 2)** **Short-term management:** Acute symptomatic hypocalcemic patients should be treated with IV calcium gluconate. Care must be taken in patients receiving digitalis since hypercalcemia may precipitate an arrhythmia or digitalis toxicity.

**Step 3)** **Long-term management:** The goal of long-term therapy is to address any symptoms and to maintain calcium levels within normal range. Patients can be given calcium supplements (eg, calcium carbonate, calcium citrate) and vitamin D. It should be noted that vitamin D supplements (cholecalciferol or ergocalciferol) are acceptable choices, but the preferred vitamin D is the active vitamin D (1,25-OHD), calcitriol. Remember, in the absence of PTH, patients cannot convert 25-OHD to 1,25-OHD, therefore, giving calcitriol will bypass that requirement.

### Follow-Up:

Monitor electrolytes to maintain a near-normal calcium level and to prevent hypercalciuria (ie, risk for stone formation).

### Pearls:

- Pseudohypoparathyroidism is characterized by a resistance or insensitivity to circulating PTH (see Table 6-4).
- Patients with hypoparathyroidism can have concurrent hypomagnesemia. In the presence of hypomagnesemia, hypocalcemia can be difficult to treat, therefore treat the hypomagnesemia before or in conjunction with the hypocalcemia.

- In the presence of alkalosis, calcium has a higher affinity to bind with albumin, thereby lowering ionized calcium and precipitating symptoms of hypocalcemia.
- **On the CCS,** sometimes you will be given preexisting medications at the beginning of the case. You have to determine whether to discontinue them or allow them to be active throughout the case. Think about whether or not the medication is affecting the patient's current condition, and if there will be a potential for a drug-drug interaction with future medications you order during the case.
- **On the CCS,** for any patient presenting with an arrhythmia, be sure to monitor the patient (ie, telemetry, cardiac monitor) when correcting the calcium levels.
- **On the CCS,** remember to "bridge" your therapy by treating any acute issues of hypocalcemia with the long-term management of hypocalcemia.

# ADRENAL DISORDERS

## ▌CUSHING'S SYNDROME

Cushing's syndrome is a constellation of various clinical findings from prolonged exposure to elevated glucocorticoids. Cushing's syndrome can be due to an ACTH-secreting pituitary tumor (Cushing's disease), ACTH-secreting ectopic tumor (nonpituitary), cortisol-secreting adrenal adenoma or carcinoma, or exogenous glucocorticoids.

### Clinical Features:

The characteristic features are central obesity, buffalo hump, moon facies, peripheral muscle wasting, and proximal weakness. However, the presentation can vary, and it may be helpful to consider the clinical manifestations in a relative head to toe fashion:

**Psychiatric**—Emotionally labile, depression, ↓ cognition

**Neurologic**—Headaches, visual disturbances from pituitary tumors

**Cardiovascular**—HTN

**GI**—Weight gain

**Genitourinary**—Oligomenorrhea, amenorrhea, impotence, polyuria, polydipsia, kidney stones

**Musculoskeletal**—Osteoporosis, avascular necrosis

**Dermatologic**—Abdominal striae, ecchymoses, hyperpigmentation, supraclavicular fat pads, hirsutism, poor wound healing, acne

**Metabolic**—Glucose intolerance

### Next Step:

**Step 1)** The initial tests to order are the 24-hour urine cortisol level to determine if there is truly an excess cortisol secretion and an overnight low-dose dexamethasone suppression test to assess the function of the hypothalamic-pituitary-adrenal axis

(see Figure 6-1). It should be noted that if two tests are abnormal, then it rules in the diagnosis of Cushing's syndrome, but not the etiology.

**Step 2)** If there are two abnormal tests, the next thing you have to consider is the level of the ACTH. Determining the ACTH level will help delineate the cause into an ACTH-independent or ACTH-dependent condition. Remember that an ACTH-dependent cause would be a condition where ACTH is needed to drive the elevated cortisol level. An ACTH-independent condition does not need ACTH to elevate the cortisol level; the lesion itself is producing the cortisol.

**Step 3)** Further testing with imaging to localize the etiology and high-dose dexamethasone suppression test (8 mg) to differentiate between pituitary and ectopic causes of Cushing's syndrome are usually pursued (see Figure 6-1).

**Step 4)** Treatment of Cushing's syndrome depends on the etiology. Consider the following:

### Cushing's Disease

- Transsphenoidal surgery is considered the treatment of choice.
- Pituitary irradiation is considered in patients who refuse surgery or when surgery is not successful.
- Bilateral adrenalectomy is considered second-line treatment.

### Ectopic ACTH Tumor

- Surgical removal of the tumor.
- If the mass is not identified, then control the hypercortisolism with adrenal enzyme inhibitors (eg, ketoconazole, fluconazole, etomidate, metyrapone) until the culprit is found.

### Adrenal Tumor

- Adrenalectomy is the treatment of choice.

### Exogenous Glucocorticoids

- Gradual withdrawal of glucocorticoids.

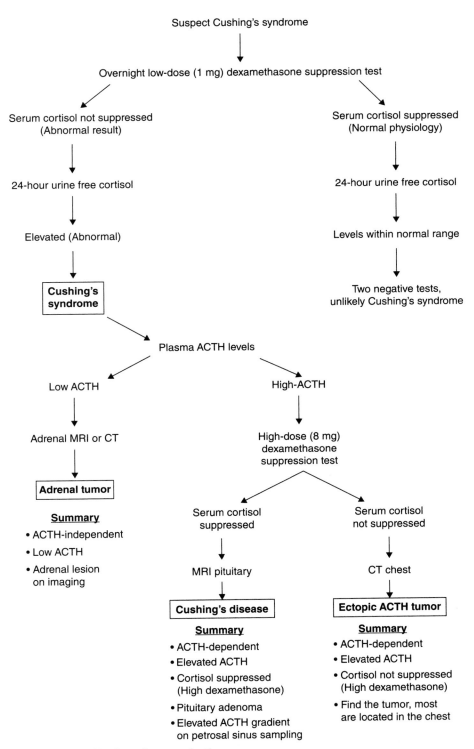

**FIGURE 6-1 • Cushing's syndrome evaluation.**

**Follow-Up:**

Finding the cause of Cushing's syndrome is important since hypercortisolism can lead to significant morbidity.

**Pearls:**

- Exogenous administration of glucocorticoids is the most common cause of Cushing's syndrome.

- Patients who undergo surgery should have stress doses of glucocorticoids intraoperatively and immediately postoperatively.

- Patients who undergo transsphenoidal surgery for Cushing's disease require lifelong glucocorticoid therapy.

- Patients who undergo bilateral adrenalectomy require lifelong glucocorticoid and mineralocorticoid therapy.

- Petrosal sinus sampling with corticotropin-releasing hormone (CRH) stimulation can be performed in patients that do not have a clear pituitary lesion on MRI. This test can help differentiate an ectopic ACTH tumor from Cushing's disease. An elevated plasma ACTH gradient (central to peripheral) is diagnostic for Cushing's disease.

- **CJ:** A 20-year-old woman with Cushing's disease refuses transsphenoidal surgery and pituitary irradiation because of fear of brain complications. She instead consents for a bilateral adrenalectomy. Over the course of the year, she notices visual disturbances, headaches, and hyperpigmentation of the skin. What syndrome is associated with a bilateral adrenalectomy? **Answer:** Patients who undergo bilateral adrenalectomy can develop **Nelson's syndrome**, which is characterized by an enlargement of a pituitary adenoma causing a local mass effect and the development of hyperpigmentation of the skin secondary to an increase in ACTH levels from a suppressed negative feedback because of inadequate cortisol levels. Transsphenoidal surgery or irradiation are the treatments of choice.

- **On the CCS,** "dexamethasone suppression test" is recognized in the order menu, but the results will only provide you with the low-dose dexamethasone in the practice CCS.

- **On the CCS,** when you have a patient with multiple problems, try to select the most appropriate physical exam that will potentially give you relevant results. Remember that unnecessary parts of the physical exam can cost you time and potentially deduct from your score.

# PHEOCHROMOCYTOMA

Pheochromocytoma is a catecholamine-secreting tumor. The tumor is composed of chromaffin cells and arises from the adrenal medulla. A chromaffin cell tumor outside of the adrenal medulla such as the sympathetic ganglion is more appropriately called a paraganglioma, although it may still be referred to as an extra-adrenal pheochromocytoma.

## Clinical Features:

The classic presentation is **diaphoresis, headaches, palpitations,** and **hypertension (episodic or sustained)**. However, patients can still be asymptomatic with only an incidental finding of the tumor. The presentation for pheochromocytoma is variable, and it is important to consider the other clinical findings in a relative head to toe fashion:

**Neurologic**—Tremor, anxiety ("impending doom"), visual disturbances

**Cardiovascular**—Chest pain, arrhythmias, myocarditis, postural hypotension

**GI**—Nausea, epigastric pain, weight loss, constipation

**Dermatologic**—Pallor, flushing spells

## Next Step:

**Step 1)** Biochemical testing with a 24-hour urine collection for fractionated catecholamines and metanephrines. Alternatively, plasma fractionated metanephrine can also be measured since it has a high sensitivity but rather poor specificity. It should be noted that there is no consensus as to the "best diagnostic test" for pheochromocytoma.

**Step 2)** If biochemical testing is elevated, further investigation to locate the tumor with either an adrenal/abdominal CT or MRI should be performed.

**Step 3)** If CT or MRI are negative but clinical suspicion is still high (ie, clinical symptoms, positive biochemical tests), then the next best step is to order a 123-I-meta-iodobenzylguanidine (MIBG) scintigraphy (ie, a test that uses a radioactive tracer that is picked up by adrenergic tissue).

**Step 4)** Once pheochromocytoma is confirmed, a preoperative preparation with medication is important. Start with an **alpha-blocker first** with the preferred agent, phenoxybenzamine, to control the blood pressure. Other alpha-1 blockers that can be used are prazosin, doxazosin, or terazosin. Typically, an alpha-blocker is used for 10 to 14 days preoperatively. Once adequate alpha blockade is achieved, then a **beta-blocker** (eg, propranolol) should be initiated.

**Step 5)** Surgical resection by a laparoscopic approach is the preferred procedure.

## Follow-Up:

Patients with MEN 2A, MEN 2B, and Von Hippel–Lindau disease should have genetic counseling.

## Pearls:

- Patients may have elevated glucose levels because of an increase in catecholamine release.

- Rules of 10 for pheochromocytoma: 10% malignant, 10% bilateral, 10% extra-adrenal, 10% familial, 10% found in children.

- Pheochromocytoma can occur sporadically or they can be associated with familial syndromes.

- Familial syndromes:

  **MEN 2A**—Pheochromocytoma, medullary thyroid CA, Hirschsprung's, hyperparathyroidism (look for ↑ calcium levels). Associated with mutations in the *ret* proto-oncogene.

  **MEN 2B**—Pheochromocytoma, medullary thyroid CA, Hirschsprung's, intestinal ganglioneuromas, marfanoid habitus. Associated with mutations in the *ret* proto-oncogene.

  **Von Hippel–Lindau disease**—Pheochromocytoma, hemangioblastomas, clear cell renal cell carcinoma

- Concurrent illnesses and medications (eg, TCAs, psychoactive meds, decongestants, acetaminophen, amphetamines, benzodiazepines, alcohol, labetalol, clonidine, levodopa) can alter the interpretation of the biochemical lab measurements.

- Metabolites of catecholamine include metanephrine, normetanephrine, and vanillylmandelic acid (VMA).

- **Foundational point**—The adrenal gland is composed of the adrenal cortex or **GFR**, which stands for the outermost layer, zona **G**lomerulosa (secretes aldosterone), then zona **F**asciculata (secretes glucocorticoids), and then the innermost layer zona **R**eticularis (secretes androgens). After the cortex is the inner portion of the adrenal gland, the adrenal medulla, which secretes catecholamines.

- **CJ:** In the office, you have been taking the necessary steps in preparing your patient for a laparoscopic adrenalectomy secondary to a pheochromocytoma. However, you've been treating your patient with a beta-blocker first instead of an alpha-blocker. Is that acceptable? **Answer:** Beta blockade should not be administered before alpha blockade because there can be a paradoxical increase in blood pressure in the presence of an unopposed alpha-adrenergic stimulation from the catecholamine-secreting tumor.

- **On the CCS,** if you order a 24-hour urine catecholamine in the practice CCS, you will get results of all the catecholamines (eg, epinephrine, norepinephrine, dopamine).
- **On the CCS,** a "24-hour urine metanephrine, total" is available in the practice CCS.
- **On the CCS,** "MIBG scan, pheochromocytoma" is recognized in the practice CCS.
- **On the CCS,** in acute cases, remember to do targeted physical exams.

# GLUCOSE HOMEOSTASIS DISORDERS

## DIABETES MELLITUS TYPE 1

Type 1 diabetes mellitus (T1DM) is characterized by a deficiency in insulin production secondary to destruction of the beta cells in the islets of Langerhans of the pancreas through an autoimmune (type 1A) or nonautoimmune/idiopathic process (type 1B).

Clinical Features:

Type 1 diabetes typically presents in childhood. Consider the following clinical manifestations of T1DM:

- Polyuria
- Polydipsia (secondary from ↑ serum osmolality and fluid loss)
- Polyphagia
- Weight loss (mainly from fluid loss and increased catabolism)
- Abdominal pain
- Fatigue
- Blurred vision (secondary from the hyperosmolar state of the lens and refractive index changes from the vitreous and aqueous humor)
- Children can initially present with DKA in some cases

Next Step:

**Step 1)** Diagnosis of diabetes mellitus requires at least **one** of the following criteria:

- Fasting glucose ≥126 mg/dL (fasting for at least 8 hours)
- Random glucose ≥200 mg/dL with symptoms (eg, polyuria, polydipsia, or weight loss)
- 2-hour plasma glucose ≥200 mg/dL after a 75 gm glucose load (test known as oral glucose tolerance test, OGTT)
- Glycated hemoglobin A1C ≥6.5%

**Step 2)** Repeat any one of the criteria above on a different day to confirm diabetes mellitus, unless there is no doubt that hyperglycemia is present on testing.

**Step 3) Insulin therapy** is the treatment of choice for T1DM (see Table 6-5). Multiple insulin regimens exist, but one common example is the basal/bolus insulin therapy, which includes a premeal injection of a rapid- or short-acting insulin to cover spikes in glucose from the meals along with a once-a-day injection of a long-acting insulin to cover basal requirements. An alternative to frequent injections is a continuous subcutaneous insulin infusion using a rapid- or short-acting insulin by an external pump, which offers a more flexible lifestyle.

**Step 4)** The following are the glycemic recommendations for diabetic adults from the American Diabetes Association (ADA):

### Table 6-5 • Insulin Agents

| Insulin | Onset | Peak | Duration | Note |
|---|---|---|---|---|
| **Rapid-acting** | | | | • Rapid-acting can be given 15 minutes before mealtime. |
| Lispro | ~15 min | ~1 hr | ≤5 hrs | • Short-acting can be given 30 minutes before mealtime. |
| Aspart | ~15 min | ~1 hr | ≤5 hrs | • Both rapid- and short-acting insulins are useful for postprandial |
| Glulisine | ~15 min | ~1 hr | ≤5 hrs | glycemic control. |
| **Short-acting** | | | | • Both intermediate and long-acting are useful for basal glycemic control. |
| Regular | ~30 min | 2-4 hrs | Up to 8 hrs | • Route of administration for all insulins should be given subcutaneously (SubQ). |
| **Intermediate-acting** | | | | |
| NPH | 1-2 hrs | 4-12 hrs | Up to 24 hrs | |
| **Long-acting** | | | | |
| Glargine | ~2 hrs | No peak | ≥24 hrs | |
| Detemir | ~2 hrs | 3-9 hrs | Up to 24 hrs | |

*NPH—neutral protamine of Hagedorn*
*Note: The insulin agents are noted in generic names.*

## Table 6-6 • Diabetic Health Maintenance

### Microvascular Prevention

| | |
|---|---|
| Retinopathy | Patients with T1DM should have an eye exam within 5 years after the onset of diabetes and then annually. |
| | Patients with T2DM should have an eye exam at initial diagnosis and then annually. |
| Nephropathy | Patients with T1DM should have a urine microalbumin test within 5 years after the onset of diabetes and then annually. |
| | Patients with T2DM should have urine microalbumin test at initial diagnosis and then annually. |
| | Patients with T1DM and T2DM should have annual serum creatinine levels. |
| Neuropathy | Patients with T1DM and T2DM should have distal symmetric polyneuropathy (DPN) screen at diagnosis and then annually. T1DM patients should be screened for autonomic neuropathy 5 years after the diagnosis, but T2DM should be screened at diagnosis. |

### Macrovascular Risk Reduction

| | |
|---|---|
| Blood pressure | Check at every office visit with goal of <130/80. |
| Lipids | Check annually with goal of LDL <100 mg/dL, Trigs <150 mg/dL, HDL >40 mg/dL. |
| Aspirin | Aspirin is a key component in mitigating the inflamed and hypercoaguable vascular system (endothelial dysfunction) as a result of diabetes. Start aspirin 75-162 mg/dy in patients who have diabetes in men >50 years old or women >60 years old who have one additional risk factor such as HTN, dyslipidemia, family history of CHD, or smoking. Those who have aspirin allergy may use clopidogrel. In patients with known cardiovascular disease start aspirin, statin, and ACE I if no contraindication exists. |
| Smoking | Advise smoking cessation at every visit. |

### Vaccinations

| | |
|---|---|
| Influenza | Annually in patients ≥6 months of age. |
| Pneumococcal | Diabetic patients ≥2 years old, and one-time revaccination >64 years old if they were immunized when they were less than 65 years old and the vaccine was given more than 5 years ago. |

### Miscellaneous

| | |
|---|---|
| Foot care | Visual inspection at every office visit and annual comprehensive foot exam to identify risk factors predictive of ulcers and amputations. |
| A1C | Check every 3 months after initial diagnosis and when changing medication therapy, and then every 6 months once controlled, with goal of <7%. |

- Keep A1C <7.0
- Preprandial plasma glucose between 70 and 130 mg/dL
- Postprandial plasma glucose of <180 mg/dL (1-2 hours after the beginning of a meal).

### Follow-Up:

Routine diabetic care as recommended by the ADA is an essential component to the patient's health (see Table 6-6).

### Pearls:

- A few weeks after initiating insulin therapy, patients may require less exogenous insulin because of the **"honeymoon phase,"** which can last up to several months. During this phase, any remaining functional beta cells are still able to secrete endogenous insulin. It is important to monitor blood glucose during this phase to prevent a hypoglycemic episode. As exogenous insulin requirements increase, the honeymoon phase is coming to its end.

- Associated autoimmune disorders with T1DM include autoimmune thyroiditis, celiac disease, Addison's disease, and polyglandular autoimmune syndrome type 2.

- Improving glycemic control improves the risk of **microvascular** complications, which include retinopathy, nephropathy, and neuropathy in both type 1 and type 2 diabetes.

- Diabetic retinopathy is a chronic complication of diabetes that is classified as proliferative or nonproliferative diabetic retinopathy. The hallmark of proliferative retinopathy is the formation of new blood vessels (neovascularization) arising from the disc and/or retinal vessels (see Figure 6-2 and Color Plate 8).

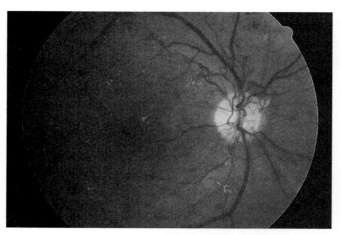

**FIGURE 6-2 • Proliferative diabetic retinopathy.** Proliferative retinopathy displaying yellow exudates, scattered hemorrhages, and neovascular vessels proliferating from the optic disc, requiring urgent panretinal laser photocoagulation. (Reproduced with permission from Lango DL, Fauci AS, Kasper DL, et al. *Harrison's Principles of Internal Medicine.* 18th ed. New York: McGraw-Hill, www.accessmedicine.com.)

Nonproliferative diabetic retinopathy is characterized by the absence of neovascularization but the presence of any of the following: microaneurysm, exudates (eg, yellow lipid), cotton wool spots (ie, nerve fiber layer infarcts, which have a dull white appearance), hemorrhages, dilated or tortuous vessels.

- Not all patients with nonproliferative retinopathy will go on to develop proliferative retinopathy.
- Insulin injections may be given in the abdomen, outer thigh, back of arm, and buttock region.
- Insulin injection at the site of the abdomen has the quickest absorption compared to the thigh, arm, or buttocks and would be an ideal site prior to meals.
- Lipohypertrophy is tissue scar formation from repeated injections in the same area. This can lead to poor insulin absorption and possible depot formation that can then randomly release insulin.
- Urine dipstick is not sensitive enough to detect moderately increased albuminuria (formerly called microalbuminuria), which is in the range of 30 to 300 mg/dy. Instead, a 24-hour urine collection (which is more cumbersome) or a urine albumin-to-creatinine ratio (also referred to as spot urine) can be used.
- **Somogyi phenomenon** is the notion that nocturnal hypoglycemia due to an increased dose of insulin at bedtime would lead to morning hyperglycemia secondary to release of stress or counterregulatory hormones from the hypoglycemic state.
- **Dawn phenomenon** is the notion that morning hyperglycemia is not due to nocturnal hypoglycemia, but rather from natural overnight release of hormones (eg, growth hormone, cortisol, glucagon, epinephrine).
- **On the CCS**, "spot urine, microalbumin" and "microalbumin, 24-hour urine" are available in the practice CCS. The two

orders are different, and the results will give you values with their normal reference ranges.

- **On the CCS**, if you ever get stuck in a case, let the order menu help you. For example, if your case is diabetes, type in "diabetes" in the order sheet and a drop-down menu will help you order other important diabetic care such as diabetic teaching, diabetic foot care counseling, or diabetic diet.
- **On the CCS**, remember to always counsel your diabetic, hypertensive, asthmatic, and hyperlipidemic patients.

## ▮ DIABETES MELLITUS TYPE 2

Type 2 diabetes mellitus (T2DM) is characterized by insulin resistance in the peripheral tissue and insufficient amounts of insulin production from the beta cells of the pancreas (see Table 6-7).

### Clinical Features:

Clinical manifestations of T2DM typically present well after the onset of the disease, and many patients will even have established cardiovascular complications at the time of diagnosis. The classic presentation seen in T1DM may also be present (eg, polyuria, polydipsia, polyphagia), but they may appear to be less acute. Patients with type 2 diabetes who are in chronic hyperglycemia may also be predisposed to poor wound healing and recurrent infections (particularly yeast). Several risk factors for T2DM will help differentiate from T1DM, including:

- Age ≥45 years
- Family history of diabetes
- History of gestational diabetes
- History of impaired glucose tolerance

| Table 6-7 • Comparison Between Type 1 and Type 2 Diabetes Mellitus | | |
|---|---|---|
| Features | Type 1 | Type 2 |
| Age of onset | Typically <30 years old, particularly in childhood or adolescence | Typically >40 years old |
| Body habitus | Thin | Obese |
| Etiology | Destruction of beta cells | Insulin resistance and insufficient amounts of insulin production from beta cells |
| Endogenous insulin levels/C-peptide levels | Low to absent once all beta cells destroyed | Present, but can become relatively deficient once insulin production slows down |
| Genetic predisposition | Moderate | Strong |
| HLA association | Yes | No |
| Autoimmune association | Yes (eg, hypothyroid, celiac disease, Addison's, polyglandular autoimmune type 2) | None known |
| Onset of symptoms | Rapid | Insidious |
| Acute complications | DKA | HHNS, but sometimes DKA |
| Chronic complications | Retinopathy, nephropathy, neuropathy | Retinopathy, nephropathy, neuropathy |
| Medical therapy | Insulin agents | Oral agents and sometimes insulin |

DKA—diabetic ketoacidosis; HHNS—hyperosmolar hyperglycemic nonketotic state; HLA—human leukocyte antigen

- History of cardiovascular disease (CVD)
- Obesity
- Sedentary lifestyle
- Conditions associated with insulin resistance (acanthosis nigricans, polycystic ovary syndrome, HTN (≥140/90), dyslipidemia (↑ trigs, ↓ HDL)
- Ethnicity (African American, Hispanic, Native American, Asian)

Next Step:

**Step 1)** Diagnosis for T2DM is the same as for T1DM (refer to T1DM section).

**Step 2)** The best initial therapy is **lifestyle modification**, which includes diet, exercise, and smoking cessation. If lifestyle measures fail to achieve the targeted blood glucose goal within 2 to 3 months, medical therapy with **metformin** should be initiated if there are no contraindications (eg, hypersensitivity to metformin, Cr >1.5 mg/dL in males, Cr >1.4 mg/dL in females). Key features of metformin are that it does not cause weight gain, rarely causes hypoglycemia, but can cause lactic acidosis (see Table 6-8).

**Step 3)** If glycemic control is not achieved with metformin even at the recommended maximum dosage, add a different class of an antidiabetic oral agent. One common combination is to add

### Table 6-8 • Oral Antidiabetic Agents

| Agents | MOA | Advantages | Disadvantages |
|---|---|---|---|
| **Sulfonylureas** | | | |
| Glyburide Glipizide Glimepiride | ↑ insulin release | • Considered first-line agents when there is a contraindication to metformin. | • Weight gain<br>• Hypoglycemia |
| **Meglitinides** | | | |
| Repaglinide Nateglinide | ↑ insulin release | • Targets postprandial glucose since they are rapid-acting agents that mimic physiological insulin secretion.<br>• Useful in patients with irregular or erratic eating habits. | • Weight gain<br>• Hypoglycemia |
| **α-Glucosidase Inhibitors** | | | |
| Acarbose Miglitol | Delays carbohydrate absorption in the gut. | • Targets postprandial glucose.<br>• Weight neutral. | • Flatulence<br>• Diarrhea<br>• Abdominal pain<br>• Can cause elevated serum transaminases (AST, ALT). |
| **Thiazolidinediones** | | | |
| Rosiglitazone Pioglitazone | ↓ hepatic glucose production<br>↑ peripheral glucose uptake (insulin sensitivity) | ↓ Trigs, ↑ HDL | • ↑ LDL<br>• Weight gain<br>• Edema<br>• Bone fractures<br>• Contraindicated in patients with NYHA Class III and IV CHF.<br>• Do not use in patients with liver disease.<br>• Can cause elevated serum transaminases (AST, ALT). |
| **Biguanide** | | | |
| Metformin | ↓ hepatic glucose production<br>↑ peripheral glucose uptake (insulin sensitivity)<br>↓ intestinal glucose absorption | • Does not induce weight gain and may actually cause weight loss, preferred agent for obese patients.<br>• Minimal risk of hypoglycemia. | • Lactic acidosis<br>• Do not use when Cr >1.5 mg/dL in males, or Cr >1.4 mg/dL in females.<br>• Do not use immediately after radiocontrast procedures.<br>• Do not use in patients with hepatic insufficiency.<br>• Do not use in patients with decompensated CHF.<br>• Can cause ↓ vitamin $B_{12}$ levels.<br>• May cause GI discomfort. |

*CHF—congestive heart failure; Cr—creatinine; MOA—mechanism of action; NYHA—New York Heart Association*

a **sulfonylurea** to metformin. However, it is important to know the drug profile of each antidiabetic agent to assist in your clinical judgment on the board exam (see Table 6-8).

**Step 4)** If glycemic control is still not achieved with dual oral agents, some clinicians may add a third agent if the patient is close to the targeted blood glucose, or they may add **insulin** to the regimen.

### Follow-Up:

Patients should initially be seen every 3 months until Hb A1C is <7% and then at least every 6 months thereafter. As with T1DM, routine diabetic care is important (see Table 6-6).

### Pearls:

- ACE inhibitors and ARB have renal protective effects in patients with diabetes.
- Patients with the metabolic syndrome have a higher risk of developing T2DM.
- **CJ:** A 45-year-old man with T2DM has elevated blood glucose despite being on metformin and glipizide. His primary care physician decided to add insulin to his regimen, and in the following week, the patient became unconscious at his home. His wife immediately took a blood glucose reading of 19 mg/dL. What is the best treatment to reverse his hypoglycemia? **Answer:** Glucagon intramuscularly or subcutaneously in an **unconscious** patient. Conscious patients who are able to take oral intake can consume juices, glucose tablets, or a snack.

- **Connecting point** (pg. 24)—Know the components of the metabolic syndrome.
- **On the CCS,** when ordering an oral antidiabetic agent, be sure to give the specific name of the medication.
- **On the CCS,** "counsel patient/family."
- **On the CCS,** "advice patient, no smoking."
- **On the CCS,** "advise patient, side effects of medication."
- **On the CCS,** a sample checklist of items for the physical examination in a diabetic patient should include the following:

**Neuro/Psych**—Assesss for peripheral sensation, or signs of neuropathy.

**HEENT/Neck**—Assess the fundus of the eye, also assess for the thyroid.

**Chest/Lungs**—Assess for coexisting respiratory conditions.

**Heart/Cardiovascular**—Assess for signs of cardiovascular disease.

**Abdomen**—Assess for hepatomegaly (usually due to fatty liver).

**Skin**—Look at the injections sites and look for signs of acanthosis nigricans.

**Extremities/Spine**—Check for peripheral pulses and foot examination.

# CCS: DKA CASE INTRODUCTION

Day 1 @ 16:00
Emergency Room

A 22-year-old Hispanic man presents to the emergency department because of severe abdominal pain, nausea, and vomiting.

**Initial Vital Signs:**
Temperature: 37.0°C (98.6°F)
Pulse: 102 beats/min
Respiratory: 30/min
Blood pressure: 107/70 mm Hg
Height: 175.3 cm (69 inches)
Weight: 75 kg (165 lb)
BMI: 24.4 kg/m$^2$

**Initial History:**
Reason(s) for visit: abdominal pain, nausea, vomiting.

**HPI:**
A 22-year-old college student has been experiencing diffuse abdominal pain for the past several hours. He states the abdominal pain is 7/10 in severity, with no aggravating or alleviating factors. He has nausea with five episodes of nonbloody, nonbilious emesis over the past 6 hours. In addition, he has been drinking more water than usual and has been urinating more frequently. The patient states that he was diagnosed with type 1 diabetes 12 years ago and admits that he has not been compliant with his insulin medication. He has visited the emergency department twice this year for the same condition.

**Past Medical History:** Type 1 diabetes diagnosed at age 10.
**Past Surgical History:** Tonsillectomy at age 9.

**Medications:** Lispro, Glargine
**Allergies:** None

**Vaccinations:** Up to date

**Family History:** Father, age 50, and mother, age 48, are healthy. No siblings. Uncle has history of type I diabetes.

**Social History:** Smokes half pack per day × 3 years; drinks on the weekends with room-mates; admits to occasional cocaine use with fraternity friends and recent use within the last two days; single; no children; full-time college student; enjoys playing baseball and going to movies.

**Review of Systems:**

General: See HPI
HEENT: Negative
Musculoskeletal: Negative
Cardiorespiratory: Negative
Gastrointestinal: See HPI
Genitourinary: See HPI
Neuropsychiatric: Negative

Day 1 @ 16:07

**Physical Examination:**

General appearance: Patient is in pain and uncomfortable.
HEENT/Neck: Normocephalic. EOMI, PERRLA. "Fruity" breath smell. Dry oral mucosa and nasal mucosa; septum midline. Trachea midline; no masses or bruits; thyroid normal.
Chest/Lungs: Tachypneic, deep labored respirations (Kussmaul respirations).
Heart/Cardiovascular: Tachycardia. No murmurs, rubs, gallops, or extra sounds. No JVD.
Abdomen: Normal bowel sounds; diffuse tenderness on palpation. No rebound or guarding. No hepatosplenomegaly.
Neuro/Psych: Awake, but inattentive. Normal motor, sensory, and cranial nerve exams. No focal deficits.

**First Order Sheet:**
1) IV access
2) Continuous cardiac monitor, stat — **Result:** Sinus tachycardia
3) Continuous blood pressure cuff, stat — **Result:** 107/70 mm Hg
4) Pulse oximetry, stat — **Result:** 98%
5) Finger-stick glucose, stat — **Result:** 650 mg/dL
6) Urinalysis, stat — **Result:** Glucose-positive, Ketones-positive, Nitrite-negative, Leukocyte esterase-negative, Microscopic exam-unremarkable

**Second Order Sheet:**
1) NS, 0.9% NaCl, IV, continuous
2) Ondansetron, IV, one time

**Note:** Patient is tachycardic, hypotensive, and signs of dehydration → Start fluids.

**Third Order Sheet:**
1) BMP, stat — **Result:** Glu-650, Urea-17, Na-132, K-3.0, Cl-100, $HCO_3$-12, Cr-1, Ca-9
2) CBC with differential, stat — **Result:** WBC-10,000, H/H-14/42%, Plt-300,000, Differential-normal
3) ABG, stat — **Result:** pH-7.25, $pCO_2$-25 mm Hg, $pO_2$-85 mm Hg, $HCO_3$-12, $O_2$ sat.-97%
4) 12-Lead EKG, stat — **Result:** Rhythm- sinus tachycardia, Axis- +30 degrees, P-waves- wnl, QRS complexes- wnl, ST-T waves- wnl, Other findings-wnl, Interpretation- sinus tachycardia
5) Urine culture, routine — **Result:** No growth
6) Blood culture, routine — **Result:** No growth

**Fourth Order Sheet:**
1) KCL, IV, continuous

**Note:** Patient's potassium level is low, and the only real indication to delay insulin therapy is if the potassium is below 3.3 mEq/L since insulin can drive the potassium into the cell and thereby exacerbate the hypokalemia.

**Actions:**
1) Change location to ICU

**Note:** Vitals are automatically ordered for you in the practice CCS.

**Fifth Order Sheet:**
1) NPO
2) Bed rest
3) Urine output, q8 hrs, stat
4) BMP, routine, q2 hr, stat — **Result:** Glu-650, Urea-17, Na-132, K-3.4, Cl-100, $HCO_3$-12, Cr-1, Ca-9

**Sixth Order Sheet:**
1) Insulin, Regular, IV, continuous

**Seventh Order Sheet:**
1) Vital signs, stat — **Result:** 37.0°C, HR-95, RR-25, BP-120/78

2) Check cardiac monitor, stat — **Result:** Regular sinus

3) Venous pH — **Result:** 7.33
**Note:** Obtaining a venous pH is less painful than the ABG, and still provides the acid-base status. The venous pH is approximately 0.03 lower than the arterial pH.

**Follow-Up History:**
Patient is feeling a little bit better.

**BMP result is now available**
**Result:** Glu-450, Urea-17, Na-135, K-3.5, Cl-100, $HCO_3$-19, Cr-1, Ca-9
**Note:** Anion gap is beginning to close from 20 to 16

**Eighth Order Sheet:**
1) D/C, Normal saline, 0.9%, IV — **Note:** Click the item on the order sheet to cancel the order.

2) 1/2 NS, 0.45%, IV, continuous — **Note:** One-half normal saline can be used if the corrected serum sodium is normal or elevated. However, if the corrected serum sodium is still low, continue with normal saline. To correct for the sodium value, add 1.6 mEq to the sodium for every 100 mg/dL of glucose over 100 mg/dL.

**BMP result is now available**
**Result:** Glu-210, Urea-17, Na-135, K-3.6, Cl-100, $HCO_3$-24, Cr-1, Ca-9

**Ninth Order Sheet:**
1) D/C, 1/2 NS, 0.45%, IV, continuous

2) Dextrose 5% in 0.45% saline, IV, continuous

3) Insulin, Regular, Sub Q, one time — **Note:** The metabolic acidosis has improved with anion gap of 11.

**This case will end in the next few minutes of "real time."**
You may **add** or **delete** orders at this time, then enter a diagnosis on the following screen.

**Tenth Order Sheet:**
1) Counsel patient/family
2) Diabetic teaching
3) Diabetic diet
4) Advise patient, no smoking
5) Advise patient, no illegal drug use

**Please enter your diagnosis:**

DKA

**DISCUSSION:**
DKA is characterized by the triad of **hyperglycemia** (>200 mg/dL), **ketosis** (presence of ketone bodies), and **metabolic acidosis** (pH ≤7.3, plasma bicarbonate <15 mEq/L). Precipitating factors include acute illness, noncompliance with meds, illicit drugs (eg, cocaine), medications (eg, lithium, thiazides, steroids, antipsychotics), infection, surgery, or new-onset diabetes. In this case, both noncompliance and probably drugs such as cocaine might have precipitated the event. One simple way to manage DKA patients is to first correct intravascular volume, then potassium levels, and finally sugar levels in this particular order because hydration is important in the early stages of management, and administering insulin depends on the potassium level. You can remember this simple format by the word DKA or "D" for dehydration, "K" for potassium, and "A" for azucar (sugar in Spanish).

**"D"**—Fluid replacement is important early in the management of DKA patients. DKA patients can lose up to 6 liters of fluid, while patients who are in hyperosmolar hyperglycemic nonketotic state (HHNS) can lose up to 9 liters of total water. It is recommended to initially treat with an isotonic solution such as normal saline to establish intravascular repletion. However, it is important not to replace the water deficit too quickly as it can cause cerebral edema. Once the patient is stabilized and corrected sodium levels are either normal or elevated, switch to a less isotonic solution such as one-half normal saline. If the corrected sodium is still hyponatremic, continue with the isotonic solution. Once glucose levels are between 200 and 250 mg/dL, switch intravenous fluids to dextrose 5% in one-half normal saline to prevent hypoglycemia. Keep in mind that the CCS will not require you to know the rate or the amount of fluids to give.

**"K"**—Patients may initially present with hypokalemia or hyperkalemia. In either case, there is a total body deficit of potassium. Hyperkalemia can be explained by a deficiency in insulin (ie, insulin promotes potassium cell uptake). Acidosis or the $H^+$/$K^+$ shift plays a minor role in hyperkalemia, probably since hyperkalemia can still be seen in HHNS where there is no acidosis. Hypokalemia can be explained by urinary excretion due to osmotic diuresis and the need to balance electroneutrality since negative ketoacid anions are being excreted along with the positive K$^+$. If the potassium level is <3.3 mEq/L, continue to hydrate the patient and replace the potassium (eg, KCl). Once the potassium is ≥3.3 mEq/L, insulin can be administered.

**"A"**—Treatment of elevated "azucar" levels is with insulin. Regular insulin is the preferred agent. Again, dosage is not required on the CCS. If the initial potassium level is less than 3.3 mEq/L, it is not recommended to initiate insulin therapy since the insulin will drive the potassium into the cell. At a potassium level of 3.3 and above, an insulin drip can be started and should be done in a monitored setting such as the ICU. When the anion gap (ie, serum Na$^+$ − [Cl$^-$ + HCO$_3^-$]) is less than 15, the transition from intravenous insulin to subcutaneous insulin should begin. Once the subcutaneous insulin is given, the overlap of the insulin drip should continue for at least 1 to 2 hours.

**Pearls:**

- Monitor glucose levels every hour and electrolyte levels every 2 hours until stable.

- The use of bicarbonate is controversial, and therefore, it is not routinely used in DKA management, however, bicarbonate is sometimes given when the pH is <6.9.

- The metabolic acidosis caused by the ketoacids results in a compensatory hyperventilation (Kussmaul's respiration) to blow off the CO$_2$, which results in a fall in the pCO$_2$.

- DKA patients often have elevated amylase and lipase levels even though they do not have pancreatitis.

- The management of DKA and HHNS is essentially the same, which is to give fluids, insulin, and electrolyte correction. However, the clinical features are slightly different (see Table 6-9).

- In this particular CCS case, the clinical judgment was not to give empiric antibiotics because the precipitating factor for DKA was the recent drug use and noncompliance with medication. In addition, the patient did not have a fever, the leukocyte esterase and nitrites were negative, the white count was within normal range, and there were no elevated bands ("left shift").

- **Foundational point**—There is a total of 3 ketone bodies produced during DKA. The major circulating ketoacid is the **beta-hydroxybutyric acid**. The other ketoacid is **acetoacetic acid** and a neutral ketone called **acetone**.

- **Foundational point**—Nitroprusside tablets can only detect acetoacetic acid and acetone but not the beta-hydroxybutyric acid.

- **On the CCS**, perform a focused physical examination. In any acute cases that require immediate attention, a complete physical examination would be considered suboptimal management.

- **On the CCS**, become comfortable relocating patients to different settings (practice with the CCS software).

- **On the CCS**, the diagnosis is sometimes clearly evident in the HPI. It is your workup, the sequence of your actions, appropriateness of your medical decisions, and efficiency that will score you points on the examination.

- **On the CCS**, ordering "continuous blood pressure cuff" and "continuous cardiac monitoring" will keep the cuff and leads on the patient throughout the case. When you want future results, you have to type in "check blood pressure" or "check cardiac monitor" in the order sheet.

- **On the CCS**, continuous cardiac monitoring is the same as telemetry or EKG monitor. Remember, it is important to monitor the patient in this type of case.

- **On the CCS**, if your advancing the time to fast during the case, sometimes a "PATIENT UPDATE" screen may appear which is usually indicative of a "warning sign" (ie, slow down and reevaluate what you're doing).

- **On the CCS**, when you transfer a patient to the ICU or inpatient unit, the vitals will be ordered for you. However, you should not assume any orders will be written for you during the CCS cases.

## Table 6-9 • Comparison Between DKA and HHNS

| Features | DKA | HHNS |
|---|---|---|
| Age | Typically <30 years old | Typically >30 years old |
| Onset of symptoms | Rapid | Insidious |
| Abdominal pain | Common | Uncommon |
| Neurologic symptoms | Yes, occurs with increasing plasma osmolality. | Yes, occurs with increasing plasma osmolality. |
| Plasma osmolality | Typically <320 mOsm/kg | Typically >320 mOsm/kg |
| Plasma glucose | Typically <600 mg/dL but as high as 800 mg/dL | Typically >600 mg/dL and can exceed 1,000 mg/dL |
| Total body deficit of potassium (K$^+$) | Yes | Yes |
| Plasma bicarbonate | <15 mEq/L | >15 mEq/L |
| Ketone bodies | Yes | No |
| pH | <7.35 | >7.30 |
| Total water lost | 6 liters | 9 liters |

*DKA—diabetic ketoacidosis, HHNS—hyperosmolar hyperglycemic nonketotic state*

# 7

# Ethics

## PRINCIPLES OF MEDICAL ETHICS

**Autonomy**—The patient has the right to refuse or accept medical treatment.

**Beneficence**—Acting in the best interest of or benefit to the patient.

**Nonmaleficence**—Do no harm to the patient.

**Justice**—The decision to be fair and equal with the distribution of health-care resources to patients (eg, who gets an organ transplantation).

**Truthfulness**—Full disclosure and honesty to patients.

## INFORMED CONSENT

Informed consent is an agreement or authorization to perform a specific intervention. The patient must understand the following even if it requires translation into another language:

- Diagnosis, if known
- Proposed intervention
- Risk and benefits of the intervention
- Consequence of not receiving the intervention
- Alternatives
- Risk and benefits of the alternatives

**Clinical Judgment:**

- Patient speaks and understands a different language → Get a translator to explain everything and document it in the chart.
- A procedure was performed on a patient, but afterward the patient found out there could have been an alternative option → The physician is liable for not explaining other alternatives prior to the procedure.

- A patient who was fully alert and conscious discussed and documented with his or her physician about not performing a specific intervention two days ago in the office. The following day the patient becomes unconscious and the health-care proxy wants the specific intervention performed → Honor the request of the patient.

- A pregnant woman is informed about the risk and benefit about a particular medical treatment. The benefit outweighs the risk of the proposed treatment and without the treatment the fetus would be in jeopardy. The patient initially refuses the medical treatment → Continue to educate and counsel the patient about the intervention without coercion.

- An unconscious patient needs a specific intervention but the health-care proxy is in another state → Telephone consent is acceptable as long as a second witness speaks with the health-care proxy and is documented in the chart.

- An unconscious patient arrives in the ER and requires blood → Give blood in life-threatening cases in which the patient is unknown to you and no health-care proxy is available.

- A child comes into the ER and requires urgent treatment but the parents refuse → Treat → Then seek a court order.

- A child needs a specific intervention in a nonurgent case and the parents refuse → Inquire about the parents' concerns → If parents are still refusing → Get a court order before treatment.

- A 14-year-old girl is in her first trimester of pregnancy and requests an abortion → Some states require parental consent, while other states do not. In some cases, a minor can ask a judge to excuse her from getting permission in those states that require parental consent, which is referred to as "judicial bypass." → For board purposes, the key element is to have a nonjudgmental discussion with the minor of all the options regarding pregnancy. It is also important to explore if she is willing to inform her parents, since some adolescents will disclose the information to their parents on their own. For those who are hesitant, you can schedule another follow-up visit to continue the discussions, or you can offer your assistance by being present during the discussion with her parents. It should be noted that there is no legal requirement to notify the father of the baby prior to the abortion.

# COMPETENCY

*Competency* is a legal term based on a court's decision to determine if a patient can comprehend and make rational decisions. *Capacity* is a clinical evaluation made by a physician that is based on the patient's ability to understand and make reasonable decisions. In most cases, patients that are minors (ie, <18 years old) do not have the capacity to understand their medical condition and therefore require parental consent. However, the following are exceptions to parental consent:

- Emancipated minor (ie, married, raising children, self-supporting, or serving in the military)
- Contraception
- Prenatal care
- Treatment for STDs
- Treatment for drug and alcohol abuse
- Treatment for psychiatric illness

**Clinical Judgment:**

- An 80-year-old man has dementia and does not have the capacity to make decisions. The patient is in need of a specific medical intervention → Look for advance directives → If no advance directives → Contact the health care proxy.

- A schizophrenic patient is compliant with his medications and appears to have no impairment in reasoning or making decisions → Patient can accept or refuse treatment.

- A suicidal patient is refusing medical treatment → The patient does not have the capacity to make sound decisions.

- A patient consented to a written DNR order but recently changed her decision by verbalizing it to her physician → Make sure that the patient has the mental capacity to understand her decision, and after a full discussion change the DNR status. Also document the discussion in the chart.

- A 30-year-old patient who has the capacity to understand and make decisions refuses blood for religious reasons (eg, Jehovah's witness) → Honor the request of the patient.

# CONFIDENTIALITY

Physicians are expected to maintain and respect patient privacy. The exceptions to break confidentiality include:

- Patient waiver
- Court orders
- Threat to self-harm (eg, suicide)
- Threat to others in violence (eg, child abuse, elder abuse, or homicidal potential)
- Threat to the public (eg, impaired airplane pilot)
- Threat to others by transmitting infectious diseases

**Clinical Judgment:**

- Family members want to know the result of a biopsy test before the patient → Disclose only to the patient unless the patient waived his rights to privacy.

- The patient's urologist wants to have medical records from the patient's primary care physician → Patient must sign a release form.

- Law enforcement comes to your office without a court order and is requesting information about a patient → Without a court order, no information should be given.
- A newly diagnosed HIV patient does not want to tell his or her partner → Encourage the patient to tell the partner. Ultimately, the partner will have to be told even if it means breaking confidentiality.

- A teenage girl comes to your office and is accompanied by her parent → Politely ask the parent to step outside the room so that a private interview can occur. Most teenagers do not feel comfortable discussing sexual matters in front of their parents. Maintaining a good rapport with the teenager is important in developing trust. Assure her that these discussions are confidential unless violence, infectious disease, or self-harm are involved.

# MALPRACTICE

Lawsuits are generally successful if all **four Ds** have been committed. The four Ds of malpractice are **duty, deviation, damage**, and **direct causation**. In other words, did the physician have a duty to the patient in which there was negligence or deviation from the standard of care that resulted in damage to the patient directly caused by deviating from the standard of care?

**Clinical Judgment:**

- Your wife's best friend called you to obtain medical advice over the phone. The next few weeks she took your advice, and she became extremely ill and had to go to the hospital because of your advice. She now wants to sue you → Unlikely she'll win because there was never a doctor-patient relationship and therefore no duty to your wife's best friend.
- A patient has been prescribed Drug A for a cardiovascular problem. Drug A has been around for many years and is considered the standard of care for the specific cardiovascular problem. The patient has also been prescribed Drug B for a GI problem. Drug B has been around for many years and is considered the standard of care for the GI problem. New clinical findings now show that there are adverse interactions in the concomitant use of Drug A and Drug B. The patient is experiencing the adverse side effects and wants to sue → Unlikely the patient will win since the physician never deviated from the standard of care at the time of prescribing either medication.

# REPORTABLE DISEASES

Reporting certain infectious diseases to the state health departments or national agencies (eg, CDC) are important for the greater public health. They permit surveillance on disease occurrence and assist with disrupting the spread of transmissible diseases to the public. The following is a list of reportable diseases:

AIDS
Anthrax
Botulism
Brucellosis
Chancroid
Chickenpox
Chlamydia trachomatis
Cholera
Cryptosporidiosis
Dengue
Diphtheria
Encephalitis (Eastern virus, St. Louis virus)
Encephalitis (Western virus, West Nile virus)
Encephalitis (California virus)
Giardiasis
Gonorrhea
Haemophilus influenza, invasive
Hansen's disease (leprosy)
Hemolytic uremic syndrome
Hepatitis A, B, C
HIV infection
Legionellosis
Listeriosis
Lyme disease
Malaria
Measles
Meningococcal disease
Mumps
Pertussis
Plague
Poliomyelitis
Poliovirus infection, nonparalytic
Psittacosis
Q fever
Rabies
Rocky Mountain spotted fever
Rubella
Salmonellosis
Shigellosis
Smallpox
Streptococcus pneumoniae, invasive
Syphilis
Tetanus
Tuberculosis
Tularemia
Typhoid fever
Varicella
Vibriosis
Yellow fever

**Clinical Judgment:**

- A 35-year-old man has genital herpes → Not a reportable disease.
- A newly diagnosed HIV patient does not want to tell his or her partner → Encourage the patient to tell the partner. Ultimately the Department of Health will contact the patient's partner, but they may not disclose the patient's name to the partner.

# PHYSICIAN'S RESPONSIBILITIES

### Child Abuse

- Any child abuse that is suspected should be reported to the Department of Children and Family Services. Do not let the child go back home until a full evaluation is conducted by the agency.

### Elder Abuse

- Any person over the age of 60 who has been subjected to abuse, neglect, or financial exploitation should be reported to the Department of Aging.

### Domestic Violence

- Ask the patient if there is domestic abuse in the relationship in a nonthreatening approach. Reporting to law enforcement or protection agencies is not the role of a physician, unless there is potential for homicide. In addition, ask if there is any child abuse in the home as well. Otherwise, offer supportive counseling and referral to support services.

### Impairment

- Impaired medical student → Report to Dean.
- Impaired resident → Report to residency director.
- Impaired licensed physician → Report to state licensing board.

### Sexual Relations

- Refrain from any sexual or romantic relationships with a patient even after the medical relationship between the doctor and patient ends.

### Truth Telling

- Tactful honesty is very important.
- If a physician made a mistake, it is important to be forthright about the error.
- If a patient wants to know about his or her medical illness, it is important to inform the patient and not withhold information. However, you can ask the patient how much he or she wants to know since some patients do not want to know all the facts of their illness.

### Physician Rights

- Physicians have the right not to accept a new patient into their office. However, if a physician decides that he or she no longer wants to provide medical treatment to a current patient, then the treating physician should continue the care until the patient finds another physician. It is important not to suddenly abandon the patient, but to help and guide the patient until he or she finds the best physician for him or her.

# END-OF-LIFE CONCERNS

### Brain Death

- The irreversible cessation of cerebral and brainstem functions. When considering the diagnosis of brain death, at least 4 important elements should be assessed: (1) **Absence of cerebral function**. There is no spontaneous movement, no purposeful movement, no response to painful stimuli, deeply comatose, absence of seizures, and the absence of decorticate or decerebrate posturing. However, spinal cord reflexes may still be present in some cases; (2) **Absence of brainstem function**. Absent corneal, pupillary, oculocephalic (doll's eyes), oculovestibular (caloric response), cough, sucking, and gag reflexes. There is no facial movements, loss of eye movements, and the pupils are dilated or midposition; (3) **Destruction of the medulla**. The presence of apnea as demonstrated by the apnea test. Apnea is confirmed if there is no spontaneous respiration in the presence of elevated $PaCO_2$ ($\geq$60 mm Hg) that serves as a stimulus for respiratory activity in the medullary centers; (4) **Exclusion of reversible medical conditions that may confound the clinical assessment** (eg, hypothermia, hypotension, electrolyte abnormalities, acid-base abnormalities, shock, drug intoxication, neuromuscular blockade).

### Organ Donation

- Organ donation may be **refused** if the family objects to donation even if the patient has an organ donor card.

### Euthanasia

- Euthanasia is the deliberate act of ending a person's life, which is ethically unacceptable. Euthanasia can take several forms:

  **Voluntary active euthanasia**—The physician intentionally and directly causes death of a patient at the patient's request (eg, administering a lethal dose of a drug), which is not legal in the United States.

  **Involuntary active euthanasia**—The physician intentionally and directly causes death of a patient without the patient's request, which is not legal in the United States.

  **Passive euthanasia**—The physician withholds life-sustaining medical treatment (eg, nutrition, ventilation) with the proxy's or patients' consent, which is legal and ethical in the United States.

### Physician-assisted Suicide

- The physician provides the means or imparts information to enable a patient to end his or her life. Only Oregon and Washington State have legalized physician-assisted suicide.

**Advance Directives**

- In the event that a patient cannot make decisions for himself or herself, an advance directive is a way to communicate the patient's wishes. Advance directives can take several forms:

  **Living will**—A document that states the patient's specific instructions on medical intervention in the event that the patient loses his or her capacity to make decisions.

  **Health-care proxy**—Also known as durable power of attorney, a health-care proxy is appointed and documented by the patient to make decisions for the patient in the event that the patient loses his or her capacity to make decisions. The health-care proxy should make decisions based on what the patient would want and not what the health-care proxy would want.

  **Do not resuscitate (DNR)**—Do not perform cardiopulmonary resuscitation in the event that the patient experiences cardiac arrest. However, in the event that the validity of the DNR order is in doubt or the patient's best interest is in question without a DNR order, then the next best step is to initiate resuscitative measures.

  **Do not intubate (DNI)**—Neither an endotracheal tube nor an esophageal obturator airway can be placed to secure the airway or to assist in ventilation.

**Palliative Care**

- The means of providing relief from pain and suffering and encouraging dignity and autonomy to the dying patient. Caution must be taken from providing active euthanasia or physician-assisted suicide. Not uncommonly, palliative care medicine will encounter the "principle of double effect" in which an intended action (eg, pain relief) may cause an unintended effect (eg, death). For example, a terminal patient may require a significant amount of pain medication to relieve pain, but at the potential consequence of respiratory depression, which would hasten the patient's death. The most important element in the double effect is that the intention of the action (ie, giving pain meds to relieve pain, not to cause death) is for good, even if the bad effect (death) is expected.

**Hospice Care**

- In hospice care, patients have 6 or less months to live as certified by a physician, and palliative care is instituted instead of curative treatments. Hospice care can be given in a hospital, nursing home, private home, or any other hospice care facility.

# 8

# Gastroenterology

## KEYWORDS REVIEW

**Endoscopic ultrasound (EUS)**—EUS is a technique that combines endoscopy with ultrasound to evaluate a variety of lesions within the gastrointestinal tract. EUS can serve as a diagnostic and therapeutic procedure (eg, draining procedure).

**ERCP**—Endoscopic retrograde cholangiopancreatography is a technique that combines endoscopy with fluoroscopic imaging to evaluate the biliary and pancreatic ductal system. Contrast material is injected into the ductal system followed by fluoroscopic imaging to produce either a cholangiogram or a pancreatogram. ERCP can serve as a diagnostic and therapeutic procedure (eg, stent placement).

**MRCP**—Magnetic resonance cholangiopancreatography is a noninvasive technique that is used to assess the intrahepatic duct, extrahepatic bile duct, and pancreatic duct. No contrast material or intervention (eg, stone extraction) is used with this technique.

**Phlegmon**—A walled-off inflammatory mass without bacterial infection.

**Pyrosis**—Heartburn.

**Sinus tract**—An abnormal channel that allows the escape of fluid. Sinus tracts can give rise to fistulas, but not all fistulas are derived from sinus tracts.

# ESOPHAGUS

## BARRETT'S ESOPHAGUS

Barrett's esophagus is a condition in which there is a metaplastic change from stratified squamous epithelium to columnar epithelium in the distal esophagus. GERD is the most common cause of Barrett's esophagus, and it is thought that the metaplastic columnar epithelium is more resistant to the acid damage compared to squamous epithelium. The overall risk of esophageal adenocarcinoma in Barrett's esophagus is approximately 0.5% per year, or in other words, 1 in 200 patients per year.

**Risk Factors:**

Older age (>50 years old), male, white race, high BMI, smokers, chronic GERD, hiatal hernia.

**Clinical Features:**

There are no symptoms or physical findings that are characteristic of Barrett's esophagus other than those that would be found in patients with GERD such as heartburn, dysphagia, or regurgitation.

**Next Step:**

**Step 1)** Patients suspected of having Barrett's esophagus based on multiple risk factors require an **upper endoscopy with biopsy** of the distal esophagus to confirm the diagnosis. Mucosal biopsies should show the presence of **specialized intestinal metaplasia** (also known as specialized columnar epithelium) from the columnar-lined distal esophagus.

**Step 2)** Precancerous changes seen on biopsy that are graded as "low-grade dysplasia" or "high-grade dysplasia" should be confirmed by a second pathologist who is, ideally, an expert in esophageal histopathology.

**Step 3)** Treatment of Barrett's esophagus is the following:

**GERD**—GERD therapy should continue as it is for patients without Barrett's esophagus.

**Eradication therapy**—Patients with confirmed high-grade dysplasia may undergo various types of eradication therapy such as endoscopic mucosal resection, radiofrequency ablation, photodynamic therapy, or alternatively an esophagectomy (higher morbidity). The choice of treatment usually depends on the patient's comorbidities, local expertise, and the patient's functional fitness.

**Follow-Up:**

The following endoscopic surveillance intervals are recommended by the American Gastroenterological Association (AGA):

No dysplasia: 3 to 5 years

Low-grade dysplasia: 6 to 12 months

High-grade dysplasia in the absence of eradication therapy: 3 months

**Pearls:**

- There is no association between *H pylori* infection and GERD since the organism does not infect the esophagus.

- There are 3 types of columnar epithelium to consider, they include cardia-type epithelium, gastric-fundic-type epithelium, and specialized intestinal metaplasia. Only specialized intestinal metaplasia has a clear association with carcinoma.

- The specialized intestinal metaplasia comprise a collection of columnar cell types such as goblet cells, intestinal-like cells, and gastric-type cells.

- The AGA notes that the use of proton pump inhibitors (PPIs) in patients with Barrett's esophagus solely to reduce the risk of progression to dysplasia or cancer is indirect and has not been proven in a long-term controlled trial.

- The AGA recommends against attempts to eliminate esophageal acid exposure for the prevention of esophageal adenocarcinoma. Examples of such attempts include antireflux surgery, PPI doses greater than once daily, or esophageal pH monitoring to titrate PPI dosing.

- **On the CCS,** if you order "Endoscopy, upper gastrointestinal" in the practice CCS, the evaluation will not provide biopsy results. Therefore, you will need to order "Biopsy, esophagus" to confirm the diagnosis of Barrett's esophagus.

# STOMACH

## PYLORIC STENOSIS

Pyloric stenosis, also known as infantile hypertrophic pyloric stenosis (IHPS), is characterized by hypertrophy of the muscular layers of the pylorus, which can lead to gastric outlet obstruction. The etiology of pyloric stenosis is unknown, but it is thought to be multifactorial.

**Clinical Features:**

Pyloric stenosis classically presents between 3 to 6 weeks of life. The condition is characterized by nonbilious, projectile vomiting soon after a feeding. On physical examination, a firm, nontender, mobile "olive" can be felt immediately after emesis at the lateral edge of the rectus abdominis muscle in the right upper quadrant. Prior to emesis, peristaltic waves may be seen moving from the patients left to right as the peristalsis is trying to overcome the obstruction. As a result of improper feeding, patients may have various degrees of dehydration. The following are signs to look for:

**Mild dehydration**—Heart rate normal, respirations normal, palpable pulses present, fontanel normal, skin turgor normal, mucous membrane moist.

**Moderate to severe dehydration**—Tachycardia, respirations deep and rapid, palpable pulses decreased, fontanel depressed, skin turgor reduced, mucous membranes dry.

**Next Step:**

**Step 1)** Definitive diagnosis is commonly made with an **ultrasound**, although an upper gastrointestinal (UGI) contrast study can also make the diagnosis.

**Step 2)** Prior to any type of surgical correction, the patient's fluid status and electrolytes should first be corrected. The classic electrolyte finding in pyloric stenosis is a **hypochloremic, hypokalemic, metabolic alkalosis** (↑ HCO3).

**Treatment for Mild Dehydration with Normal Electrolytes**
- Treat with maintenance fluids (eg, D5 0.25% NaCl + KCl).

**Treatment for Moderate to Severe Dehydration**
- Treat with higher concentrations of NaCl (ie, one-half normal saline to normal saline)
- Consider a bolus of fluids initially.
- Make sure the kidneys are functioning properly before administrating KCl.

**Step 3)** Definitive treatment for pyloric stenosis is with a surgical pyloromyotomy.

**Follow-Up:**

Up to 80% of patients will regurgitate after surgery; however, this issue should not delay feedings.

**Pearls:**
- Up to 30% of patients with pyloric stenosis will be firstborn males.

- Become familiar with the equivalent fractions and percentages: one-quarter normal saline (0.22% NaCl), one-third normal saline (0.3% NaCl), one-half normal saline (0.45% NaCl), and normal saline (0.9% NaCl).
- Most patients with pyloric stenosis are "chloride responsive" and can be treated by replacing the chloride through saline solution and KCl, which in turn will enhance renal bicarbonate excretion.
- Failure to correct the alkalosis prior to surgery can lead to postoperative apnea.
- Administering oral erythromycin, especially in the first 2 weeks of life, has been associated with pyloric stenosis.
- Hypokalemia is typically seen in patients who have been vomiting for a period of time (ie, >3 weeks).
- No single sign is pathognomonic in the upper GI contrast study, but possible findings include the "beak" sign (tapered pyloric canal), "shoulder" sign (dilated prepyloric antrum), "string" sign (narrowed pyloric lumen), or "double-track" sign (2 tracks of barium as a result of a compressed pyloric mucosa).
- **On the CCS,** prior to the exam day, type in "fluids" in the order menu, and become familiar with the different types of fluids and when you would want to use them.
- **On the CCS,** informed consent is assumed for any procedure that you order. In addition, consent is also given for any child or infant in the cases.

# INTESTINES—INFLAMMATORY BOWEL DISEASE

## CROHN'S DISEASE

Crohn's disease (CD) is a chronic, **transmural** inflammatory process that can lead to progressive fibrosis, stricturing, or perforating disease. Crohn's disease can affect any part of the gastrointestinal tract from the mouth to the anus. In descending order of frequency, the following are locations of gastrointestinal tract involvement: **ileocecal region (ileocolitis) > terminal ileum only (ileitis) > colon only > mouth or gastroduodenal area > esophagus**. The etiology of Crohn's disease is still unknown.

### Clinical Features:

The onset of symptoms in Crohn's disease is typically insidious. Most patients will have recurring episodes of abdominal pain, nonbloody diarrhea, weight loss, fever, and fatigue interspersed with periods of remission. As with ulcerative colitis, extraintestinal manifestations are frequently encountered with Crohn's disease (see Table 8-1). However, consider the clinical manifestations of Crohn's disease based on the following affected gastrointestinal location in a superior to inferior direction:

**Esophagus**—Dysphagia, odynophagia

**Stomach**—Upper abdominal pain, symptoms of gastric outlet obstruction due to fibrotic strictures

**Intestines**—Small bowel or colonic obstruction, periumbilical pain, RLQ pain, steatorrhea, phlegmon, malabsorption, "bile salt" diarrhea, constipation secondary from an obstruction, abscess, sinus tracts, fistulas (ie, bowel to bowel, bowel to bladder, bowel to vagina, or bowel to skin)

**Perianal**—Perianal fistulas, fissures, perirectal abscess, anal stenosis, hemorrhoids

### Next Step:

**Step 1)** The diagnosis of Crohn's disease is based on a compatible clinical picture along with supportive endoscopic or imaging studies.

### Endoscopy

**Colonoscopy**—Colonoscopy with biopsy can increase the diagnostic accuracy. To establish a diagnosis in the ileocecal region, a colonoscopy with a terminal ileum intubation (ie, ileoscopy) should be performed. Endoscopic findings may reveal a "cobblestone" appearance, focal ulcerations, linear

## Table 8-1 • Extraintestinal Manifestations Seen in Crohn's Disease and Ulcerative Colitis

| System | Manifestations |
|---|---|
| **Neurologic** | Peripheral neuropathy, myelopathy, myasthenia gravis, pseudotumor cerebri |
| **Ocular** | Episcleritis, anterior uveitis |
| **Oral** | Aphthous ulcers |
| **Cardiac** | Pericarditis, myocarditis, endocarditis |
| **Respiratory** | Pulmonary fibrosis, vasculitis, bronchitis, bronchiectasis, interstitial lung disease, BOOP |
| **Hepatobiliary** | Cholelithiasis, cholangiocarcinoma, primary sclerosing cholangitis (PSC), pericholangitis, autoimmune hepatitis, fatty liver |
| **Renal** | Calcium oxalate and uric acid kidney stones, hydronephrosis, amyloidosis |
| **Musculoskeletal** | Arthritis (eg, sacroiliitis, ankylosing spondylitis, peripheral arthritis), osteoporosis |
| **Dermatologic** | Erythema nodosum, pyoderma gangrenosum |
| **Hematologic** | Vitamin $B_{12}$ deficiency, folate deficiency, iron deficiency, anemia of chronic disease, autoimmune hemolytic anemia, thromboembolism |

ulcers, stellate ulcers, serpiginous ulcers, aphthous ulcers (not just the mouth), normal rectum, normal vascular pattern adjacent to affected tissue, discontinuous lesions ("skip lesions"), edema, strictures, or pseudopolyps. Histological findings may reveal crypt abscesses, crypt atrophy, mixed acute and chronic inflammation, **noncaseating granulomas**, or deep fissures.

**Esophagogastroduodenoscopy (EGD)**—EGD is effective when there is gastroduodenal involvement. EGD is also helpful in differentiating Crohn's disease from other gastrointestinal diseases (eg, peptic ulcer disease).

**Capsule ("pill") endoscopy**—The indications for capsule endoscopy are still evolving, however it is being used more frequently in patients with Crohn's disease with suspected small bowel involvement. Capsule endoscopy should not be used in patients with suspected strictures since it can lead to an obstruction.

### Imaging Studies

**Upper GI series**—An upper GI series with small bowel follow-through (SBFT) is typically the initial test to evaluate the small intestines. Possible findings may include ulcerations, abscess formation, "string" sign (luminal narrowing), fistulas, bowel wall thickening, segmental stricturing, nodularity, or cobblestone appearance.

**Barium enema**—Barium enema can be performed to evaluate the lower bowel, but it should be considered as an alternative when colonoscopy cannot be performed.

### Adjunctive Studies

**CBC**—Leukocytosis may be detected due to an abscess, chronic inflammation, or steroid treatment. Anemia may also be detected due to iron deficiency, vitamin $B_{12}$ deficiency, or folate deficiency.

**CMP**—Hypoalbuminemia is common in Crohn's patients. Liver function tests may be elevated due to PSC or pericholangitis.

**ESR or CRP**—Typically elevated in patients with Crohn's disease.

**ASCA**—Usually positive in Crohn's disease.

**p-ANCA**—Usually negative in Crohn's disease.

**Stool for occult blood**—Frequently test positive, but typically no gross blood is seen.

**Stool culture, bacterial**—Normal flora.

**Stool for white cells**—Leukocytes may be seen, indicative of gut inflammation.

**Stool for ova and parasites**—Negative.

**Stool for *C difficile* toxin assay**—Negative.

**Stool fat, 72-hour**—Usually elevated in patients with bacterial overgrowth or bile acid malabsorption.

**Step 2)** The goal of therapy is to achieve remission and maintain remission. Consider the different stages of treatment:

### Active Disease

**Glucocorticoids**—**Prednisone** may be used for a short course of therapy for active disease. **Budesonide** is another glucocorticoid that appears to be less effective than conventional glucocorticoids, but has the advantage of inducing less systemic side effects because of a high first-pass hepatic metabolism.

**5-Aminosalicylic acid (ASA)**—The use of 5-ASA derivatives for Crohn's disease is controversial. Although some authorities continue to use 5-ASA in the management of Crohn's, it should be noted that there is a clearer therapeutic benefit for patients with ulcerative colitis.

**Antibiotics**—Similar to 5-ASA agents, the utility of antibiotics is not well established. Aside from treating an abscess or a wound infection related to Crohn's disease, the use of metronidazole or the combination of metronidazole and ciprofloxacin are still used to treat active Crohn's disease.

### Refractory Disease

**Immunomodulators**—**Azathioprine (AZA)** or **6-mercaptopurine (6-MP)** are used in patients that are refractory to steroid therapy or as a steroid-sparing agent in attempt to withdraw steroids from steroid-dependent patients. **Methotrexate**

**(MTX)** is an alternative drug for patients that have contraindications or do not respond to AZA or 6-MP therapy.

**Biologic therapies**—Anti-TNF therapies such as **infliximab**, **adalimumab**, and **certolizumab pegol** are typically used in Crohn's patients that are refractory to conventional treatment.

**Surgery**—Surgery is considered in patients that have symptoms refractory to optimal medical therapy or development of a complication related to Crohn's disease.

### Severe Disease

**Hospitalize**—Patients with severe disease will typically have persistent symptoms despite optimal medical therapy as an outpatient. Patients should be admitted to the hospital for bowel rest, intravenous glucocorticoids (eg, prednisolone), and parenteral nutrition. Broad-spectrum antibiotics (IV metronidazole + IV ciprofloxacin) should be added in patients with fevers, elevated white count, fulminant features (ie, abruptly occurring symptoms), or any indication of toxicity.

### Maintenance Therapy

**Immunomodulators**—AZA, 6-MP, and MTX are used for maintenance remission.

**Biologic therapies**—The anti-TNF agents are used for maintenance remission.

**Glucocorticoids**—Conventional glucocorticoids are not effective in maintaining remission; however, budesonide has been approved for maintenance remission for up to 3 months.

**Step 3)** The risk of colon cancer in Crohn's disease and ulcerative colitis appears to be equivalent for a similar extent and duration of disease. Therefore, in patients with Crohn's colitis, surveillance colonoscopy is typically started after 8 years of disease followed by annual examinations.

### Follow-Up:

Patients with mild to moderate active Crohn's disease can be managed as an outpatient with close follow-up with their physician.

### Pearls:

- Microscopic GI bleeding can occur, but there is usually no gross bleeding.
- Be aware that extraintestinal manifestations may be the initial complaint in patients with inflammatory bowel disease.
- Thiopurine methyltransferase (TPMT) genotype or phenotype testing is recommended before the initiation of AZA or 6-MP therapy to prevent unwanted toxicities and to make the appropriate empiric dose adjustments.
- On pathological examination of diseased bowel in Crohn's disease, sometimes mesenteric fat will wrap around the bowel surface ("creeping fat").
- Since transmural inflammation can reach the serosal level, the inflammation itself can promote adhesion of the bowel surface to the mesentery.
- Endoscopy is considered a primary tool in the diagnosis of inflammatory bowel disease because it allows for direct visualization and targeted biopsies, which usually leads to a definitive diagnosis. However, an endoscopy should not be performed if there is a toxic megacolon, severe acute colitis, or a patient cannot undergo adequate bowel preparation.
- The terminal ileum is the site for bile salt and vitamin $B_{12}$ absorption.
- "Bile salt" diarrhea occurs when bile salts are not absorbed at the terminal ileum because of disease or resection in that region, which results in bile salts entering the colon causing a secretory diarrhea.
- Patients with bile salt diarrhea may benefit from bile acid sequestrants (eg, cholestyramine, colestipol).
- Steatorrhea may be the result of bacterial overgrowth or bile acid malabsorption (hence elevated stool fat content in the 72-hour collection).
- Avoid antidiarrheal agents (eg, loperamide) in patients with active colitis since they can precipitate a toxic megacolon.
- Infliximab has been approved for fistulizing Crohn's disease.
- **Foundational point**—Azathioprine (AZA) is an immunosuppressant agent that is first converted to 6-mercaptopurine (6-MP) and eventually into a nucleotide, thioinosinic acid. The nucleotide analogs can inhibit enzymes involved in purine metabolism and have a cytotoxic effect on lymphoid cells.
- **Connecting point** (pg. 289)—Biologic agents are also used in patients with rheumatoid arthritis. Prior to treatment, remember to perform latent TB screening with a PPD.
- **Connecting point** (pg. 252)—Know the management for a positive PPD.
- **On the CCS**, "advise patient, medication compliance."
- **On the CCS**, "advise patient, side effects of medication."
- **On the CCS**, try to practice the CCS on a computer with each chapter you review so that you can become familiar with the possible options in that particular field.

## ULCERATIVE COLITIS

Ulcerative colitis (UC) is a chronic inflammatory condition that involves the **mucosal layer** of the colon that can lead to diffuse friability and erosions with bleeding. The rectum is virtually always involved and extends proximally in a **continuous retrograde fashion**. Approximately 50% of patients will have disease confined to the rectosigmoid region (proctosigmoiditis), 30% extend to the splenic flexure (left-sided colitis), and 20% extend beyond the splenic flexure and even up to the cecum (pancolitis). Similar to Crohn's disease, the etiology of ulcerative colitis is unknown (see Table 8-2).

### Clinical Features:

The clinical course of ulcerative colitis is of a chronic intermittent exacerbation interspersed with periods of remission. In some patients, the first attack is followed by a prolonged period of inactivity. Possible clinical findings may include abdominal pain, bloody diarrhea, weight loss, fever, tenesmus, passage of

**Table 8-2 • Distinctive Features of Inflammatory Bowel Disease (IBD)**

| Features | Crohn's Disease (CD) | Ulcerative Colitis (UC) |
|---|---|---|
| Etiology | Unknown | Unknown |
| Age of onset | Bimodal (15-40 and 50-80) | Bimodal (15-40 and 50-80) |
| Ethnicity | Jewish > Non-Jewish | Jewish > Non-Jewish |
| Genetics | First-degree relative may have either CD or UC | First-degree relative may have either CD or UC |
| Smoking | Increases risk | Decreases risk |
| Appendectomy | Appears to increase the risk of developing CD | Appears to be protective against the development of UC |
| Perianal involvement | Yes, approximately 30% of patients | No |
| Rectal involvement | Spared | Almost always |
| Colon involvement | Usually | Always |
| Terminal ileum involvement | Common | Sometimes ("Backwash ileitis") |
| Distribution | Skip lesions | Continuous |
| Segmental colitis | Yes | No |
| Depth of inflammation | Transmural | Mucosal, sometimes submucosal |
| Granulomas | Noncaseating granulomas | No |
| Ulcers | Yes | Yes |
| Pseudopolyps | Yes | Yes |
| "Cobblestone" appearance | Yes | No |
| Mesenteric encased bowel ("Creeping fat") | Yes | No |
| Crypt abscess | Yes | Yes |
| Crypt atrophy | Yes | Yes |
| Fistulas | Yes | No |
| Strictures | Common | Sometimes |
| Gross blood | No | Yes |
| Mucus | Sometimes | Yes |
| Bloody diarrhea | No | Yes |
| Bile salt diarrhea | If there is diseased or resected terminal ileum | Rare, unless there is diseased terminal ileum from "backwash ileitis" |
| Severe abdominal pain | Common | Sometimes |
| Extraintestinal manifestations | Yes | Yes |
| Risk of colon cancer | Yes | Yes |
| ASCA | Positive | Negative |
| p-ANCA | Negative | Positive |
| Fecal leukocytes | Yes | Yes |
| Recurrence after surgery | Yes | No |
| 5-ASA agents | Used, but controversial | Clear therapeutic benefit |
| Methotrexate | Used | Not supported |

mucus, anemia, tachycardia, or red blood on rectal examination. As with Crohn's disease, extraintestinal manifestations are encountered in ulcerative colitis (see Table 8-1). However, consider the severity of the disease in ulcerative colitis:

**Mild disease**—Clinical findings may include: <4 bowel movements per day, small amounts of blood in the stool, no fevers, no weight loss, no tachycardia.

**Moderate disease**—Clinical findings may include: 4 to 6 bowel movements per day, moderate amounts of blood in the stool, low-grade fevers, some weight loss, heart rate in the upper limit of normal, mild anemia.

**Severe disease**—Clinical findings may include: >6 bowel movements per day, large amounts of blood in the stool, fevers, weight loss, tachycardia, hypovolemia, anemia.

**Next Step:**

**Step 1)** The diagnosis of ulcerative colitis is based on a compatible clinical picture along with endoscopy.

**Endoscopy**

**Flexible sigmoidoscopy**—In patients with an acute flare, flexible sigmoidoscopy can provide an adequate diagnosis since it can assess the disease activity (see endoscopic findings in Colonoscopy section) and exclude other diagnosis (eg, infectious or ischemic colitis).

**Colonoscopy**—Colonoscopy with biopsy can make the definitive diagnosis in equivocal cases, but it should not be performed during an acute flare or in severe disease since it may precipitate a toxic megacolon or cause a perforation. Endoscopic findings may reveal an erythematous mucosa, granular surface, friability, spontaneous bleeding, erosions, pseudopolyps, purulent exudates, edema, loss of normal vascular pattern, continuous and circumferential involvement, or ulcerations extending into the submucosa in more severe disease. Histologic findings may reveal crypt abscesses, crypt atrophy, or diffuse mixed inflammation.

**Adjunctive Studies**

**Plain abdominal x-ray**—Colonic dilatation may be seen in patients with severe colitis.

**CT abdomen**—Bowel wall thickening may be seen but is nonspecific.

**Barium enema**—Not commonly used since the advent of flexible sigmoidoscopy and colonoscopy. Findings may reveal pseudopolyps, collar button ulcers (ie, penetration through the mucosa), or loss of haustra (lead-pipe appearance). Barium enema should be avoided in patients with severe disease since it may precipitate a toxic megacolon.

**CBC**—Leukocytosis, anemia, and thrombocytosis may be present.

**CMP**—Hypoalbuminemia is often found in extensive disease. LFTs may be elevated due to PSC or pericholangitis.

**ESR or CRP**—Elevated, which usually correlates with disease activity.

**ASCA**—Usually negative in ulcerative colitis.

**p-ANCA**—Usually positive in ulcerative colitis.

**Stool for occult blood**—Positive, and on examination, gross blood with mucus is usually seen.

**Stool culture, bacterial**—Normal flora.

**Stool for white cells**—Fecal leukocytes are usually present.

**Stool for ova and parasites**—Negative.

**Stool for *C difficile* toxin assay**—Negative.

**Step 2)** Therapy is based on the severity and extent of the disease. Consider the different stages of treatment:

**A—Active Disease**

*Proctitis (rectum)*
Mild to moderate disease:
  Option 1: 5-ASA suppository
  Option 2: Hydrocortisone foam (rectal)
  Option 3: Hydrocortisone suppository
Severe disease → Hospitalize
Fulminant disease → Hospitalize

*Proctosigmoiditis (rectum + sigmoid)*
Mild to moderate disease:
  Option 1: 5-ASA enema
  Option 2: Hydrocortisone enema
Severe disease → Hospitalize
Fulminant disease → Hospitalize

*Left-sided colitis or pancolitis*
Mild to moderate disease:
  Oral 5-ASA + Suppository (5-ASA or steroid) + Enema (5-ASA or steroid)
Severe disease → Hospitalize
Fulminant disease → Hospitalize

**B—Refractory Disease**

**Glucocorticoids**—Oral steroids (eg, prednisone) are usually considered when there is an inadequate response to maximal tolerated dosage of 5-ASA agents. Once remission is achieved, a gradual taper can begin.

**Azathioprine (AZA) or 6-mercaptopurine (6-MP)**—AZA or 6-MP is usually considered in patients who are steroid dependent and/or steroid refractory. The onset of full activity for both AZA and 6-MP can take up to 3 to 6 months. TPMT testing should be performed before therapy.

**Infliximab**—Infliximab is an available option for patients who are not responding to corticosteroids, AZA, or 6-MP, but have reservations about undergoing surgery or want to avoid the side effects of cyclosporine (eg, neurotoxic, nephrotoxic, hypertension, ↑ risk of skin cancer).

**Cyclosporine**—Cyclosporine (calcineurin inhibitor) has a rapid onset of action and is considered a last-ditch effort for medical intervention. It is an option for patients who have failed intravenous steroids, but do not want to have surgery. Cyclosporine is usually given as an intravenous infusion, and then can be switched to PO for outpatient use for a few months, but not for long-term maintenance.

**Surgery**—Surgery is an option for patients that have failed cyclosporine, infliximab, or intravenous steroids. Unlike Crohn's disease, a colectomy can lead to a cure in ulcerative colitis.

### C—Severe Disease

**Severe disease**: Patients with severe disease have the potential to progress to toxic megacolon or fulminant colitis. The following actions should take place:

1) Hospitalize the patient
2) NPO, IV fluids, electrolyte correction
3) Intravenous glucocorticoids (eg, prednisolone)
4) Consider surgery or IV cyclosporine in patients who do respond to IV steroids after 7 to 10 days.

**Acute severe (fulminant) disease**: Patients with fulminant disease will have a rapid progression of severe toxic symptoms (eg, rapid weight loss, fever, severe bloody diarrhea, peritoneal signs), which can progress to toxic megacolon or bowel perforation. The following actions should take place:

1) Hospitalize the patient.
2) NPO, IV fluids, electrolyte correction.
3) Nasogastric suction if obstruction or toxic megacolon is suspected.
4) Abdominal x-rays.
5) Intravenous glucocorticoids (eg, prednisolone).
6) Broad-spectrum antibiotics are usually given in patients with fever, leukocytosis, elevated bands, peritoneal signs, or suspicion for toxic megacolon. Recommended antibiotics include:

   IV metronidazole (covers anaerobes) + IV ciprofloxacin (covers gram-negatives).

7) Consider surgery in patients who fail to improve in 48 to 72 hours to prevent a perforation.

### D—Maintenance Therapy

**Proctitis**: 5-ASA suppository; avoid IV and PO steroids to prevent systemic side effects

**Proctosigmoiditis**: 5-ASA enema; avoid IV or PO steroids to prevent systemic side effects

**Left-sided colitis and pancolitis**: Oral 5-ASA ± 5-ASA enema; avoid IV or PO steroids to prevent systemic side effects

**Steroid-dependent colitis**: 6-MP, AZA, or infliximab (for those who responded to induction therapy)

**Step 3)** Since patients are at risk of colon cancer, a colonoscopic surveillance should start after 8 years of disease and then annually.

**Follow-Up:**

Patients that are receiving AZA or 6-MP require weekly blood monitoring for the first month to minimize the dose-dependent toxicities.

**Pearls:**

- "Backwash ileitis" refers to the presence of inflammation at the terminal ileum in patients with ulcerative colitis that have pancolitis.
- "Backwash ileitis" can be differentiated from Crohn's ileocolitis by obtaining a colonoscopy with ileoscopy and biopsy (ie, granulomatous inflammation should be seen in Crohn's disease).
- The 5-ASA agents include sulfasalazine, mesalamine, balsalazide, and olsalazine.
- Sulfasalazine is the original drug in the 5-ASA class, but it has unfavorable side effects such as nausea, vomiting, headache, dyspepsia, pruritus, fever, rash, male infertility, and agranulocytosis.
- Mesalamine is better tolerated and has fewer adverse effects than sulfasalazine.
- All the 5-ASA agents can be given orally, but mesalamine can also be given as an enema or as a suppository.
- Suppositories are generally effective in the rectum, but enemas can reach the sigmoid colon and potentially up to the splenic flexure.
- Hydrocortisone is available in PO, IV, IM, enemas, suppositories, and foams.
- Patients with toxic megacolon (ie, colonic dilatation ≥6 cm) are managed the same as fulminant disease. In addition, nasogastric suction should be initiated and patients should roll side to side intermittently to help redistribute the gas.
- Antidiarrheals should not be used during acute flares or severely ill patients.
- Patients with ulcerative colitis are at risk of colon cancer, but it also appears that having concomitant primary sclerosing cholangitis (PSC) increases the risk of colon cancer.
- Pseudopolyps are commonly seen in patients with long-standing disease and are the result of epithelial regeneration.
- Pseudopolyps are commonly seen in ulcerative colitis, but they are not specific for the disorder.
- Periappendiceal inflammation ("cecal patch") can sometimes be seen in patients with ulcerative colitis but may not be contiguous with the disease.
- Most of the studies on serologic markers have revolved around antibodies to the yeast *Saccharomyces cerevisiae* (ASCA) and perinuclear antineutrophil cytoplasmic antibodies (p-ANCA).
- A colonoscopy can assess the disease activity as well as the extent of the disease in ulcerative colitis.
- **Foundational point**—Sulfasalazine is a sulfa drug that is poorly absorbed in the small intestine, but when it reaches the colon the intestinal bacteria splits the drug into sulfapyridine (antibacterial) and 5-aminosalicylic acid (anti-inflammatory). The 5-ASA (ie, mesalamine) is the active component of sulfasalazine. It should be noted that balsalazide and olsalazine are prodrugs that are also converted to the active form of 5-ASA (ie, mesalamine) by colonic bacteria.

- **On the CCS**, if you want to order mesalamine as an enema or suppository, it will only be recognized as "rectal" under the route of administration.

- **On the CCS**, if you need a consult during the case, type in "consult" in the order menu and a robust list of consults are available for you to choose.

# PANCREAS

## ▌ PANCREATIC PSEUDOCYST

Pancreatic pseudocysts are localized fluid collections of pancreatic enzymes that are encased by fibrous and granulation tissue (ie, no epithelial lining, hence "pseudo" cyst). Pancreatic pseudocysts are seen following acute pancreatitis, chronic pancreatitis, or blunt trauma (frequently associated with children).

### Clinical Features:

There are no signs or symptoms that are pathognomic for pancreatic pseudocysts. Pseudocysts should be considered in patients with a history of pancreatitis or trauma that present with persistent abdominal pain, abdominal mass, or anorexia. The clinical progression of the pseudocyst can be affected by many factors. Consider the following:

**Infection**—An infected pseudocyst can lead to fever, leukocytosis, or a tender epigastric mass.

**Expansion**—Abdominal pain, abdominal mass, abdominal fullness.

**Obstruction**—Biliary or duodenal obstruction can lead to jaundice, scleral icterus, nausea, or vomiting.

**Fistulization**—Fistulization into the abdomen (ie, ascites) or chest (ie, pleural effusions).

**Rupture**—Rupture of the pseudocyst can result in peritoneal signs.

**Erosion**—Erosion into an adjacent vessel can result in a "pseudoaneurysm." If there is a communication between the pseudocyst and the pancreatic duct, blood may now flow through the ampulla of Vater and into the GI tract (ie, hemosuccus pancreaticus), which may be the cause of unexplained anemia. If there is no communication between the pseudocyst and the pancreatic duct, the pseudocyst will simply enlarge and cause abdominal pain.

### Next Step:

**Step 1)** After a careful **clinical assessment**, especially in a patient with a history of pancreatitis or trauma with persistent abdominal pain, the first-line imaging modality is an **abdominal CT scan**. However, consider the features of the following imaging modalities:

### Ultrasound

- Ultrasound has a sensitivity of 75% to 90%.
- Overlying bowel gas can decrease the sensitivity.
- Useful in distinguishing solid from cystic masses.
- Visualization is limited by patient's habitus.
- Technique is highly operator dependent.

### CT Scan

- CT scan has a sensitivity of 90% to 100%.
- CT scan can provide information of the surrounding anatomy such as pancreatic duct dilatation, common bile duct dilatation, calcifications, pseudoaneurysm, and extension of the pseudocyst.
- CT scans cannot differentiate pseudocysts from pancreatic cystic neoplasms.

### MRCP

- MRCP is not routinely performed as the initial diagnostic test because CT scans provides most of the diagnostic information.

### ERCP

- ERCP is not necessary to establish a diagnosis of a pancreatic pseudocyst, but it may be useful in planning a strategy for drainage.

### Endoscopic Ultrasound (EUS)

- EUS is often performed when there is diagnostic uncertainty because it provides high-quality images due to the close proximity of the ultrasound transducer to the area of interest, and the lesion can be sampled through fine needle aspiration (EUS-FNA), which can then be analyzed for cytology, molecular markers, or tumor markers (eg, CEA level).
- EUS is helpful in planning pseudocyst drainage sites since it can detect small portal collaterals (eg, gastric varices) that would otherwise not be detected by other means, which would potentially reduce the risk of bleeding.

**Step 2)** Management of pancreatic pseudocysts involves observation or intervening with some type of draining procedure.

### No Intervention

- Most pseudocysts will resolve with supportive care.
- Medical supportive care may include analgesics, antiemetics, IV fluids, and TPN or nasoenteral feeding if the patient cannot tolerate oral intake.

### Intervention

- Indications to intervene are the presence of symptoms or complications of the pseudocyst such as infection, bleeding, or gastric outlet or biliary obstruction.
- Drainage of the pseudocyst can be accomplished by surgery, endoscopy, or percutaneous catheter drainage using CT or US guidance.

**Follow-Up:**

Patients that have stents in place for drainage or are being observed are usually monitored by simple palpation on daily exam and serial CT scans to observe for resolution of the pseudocyst.

**Pearls:**

- Pancreatic pseudocysts can be single or multiple.
- Pancreatic pseudocysts may have communication or no communication with the pancreatic ductal system.
- Pancreatic cysts may be associated with von Hippel–Lindau disease or polycystic kidney disease.
- Although larger-sized pseudocysts are prone to cause more symptoms and complications, the size or duration of the pseudocyst (ie, greater than 6 cm or longer than 6 weeks) is not an indication to intervene.
- To date, there are no randomized comparative studies between endoscopic, surgical, and percutaneous drainage. Therefore, the type of drainage procedure is often based on local expertise.
- Pancreatic abscess is a liquid collection of pus that can be formed secondary to an infected pseudocyst.
- Pancreatic abscesses should be drained, usually by surgery or percutaneous techniques.
- Amylase levels are usually high within the pseudocyst, but low in pancreatic cystic neoplasms.
- There are 4 main subtypes of pancreatic cystic neoplasms, which include serous cystic tumors, mucinous cystic neoplasms, intraductal papillary mucinous neoplasms, and solid pseudopapillary neoplasms. Of the four subtypes, serous cystadenomas have little to no malignant potential.

- History and imaging features of pancreatic cystic neoplasms that might be worrisome include no history of pancreatitis or trauma, dilated pancreatic duct or branches, solid component, mural nodularity, septated cyst, macroseptation, multiloculated microcystic appearance, grape-like clusters, honeycomb pattern, external lobulation, or central scar.
- **CJ:** A 50-year-old man with known pancreatic pseudocyst has sudden abdominal pain, presence of abdominal bruit, a slight drop in blood pressure, and is stool hemoccult positive with an unexplained GI bleed. How do you manage this patient? **Answer:** The first step in this patient, who has a pseudoaneurysm, is to stabilize him (eg, fluids). Ultimately, the patient needs to have a mesenteric angiography, which can confirm the diagnosis, and at the same time, perform an embolization of the bleeding vessel. It should be noted that any patient with suspected pseudoaneurysm should not undergo endoscopic drainage unless arterial embolization is performed first.
- **On the CCS,** "angiography, mesenteric" is available in the practice CCS.
- **On the CCS,** remember to monitor your patients (eg, physical exam) after any kind of treatment.
- **On the CCS,** suboptimal management would be to make an incorrect diagnosis, since erroneously treating a pancreatic cystic neoplasm as a pseudocyst can lead to serious problems.

# CCS: EARLY GASTRIC CANCER CASE INTRODUCTION

Day 1 @ 14:00
Office

A 50-year-old Asian man comes to the office because of mild epigastric pain.

**Initial Vital Signs:**
Temperature: 37.0°C (98.6°F)
Pulse: 68 beats/min, regular rhythm
Respiratory: 18/min
Blood pressure: 120/75 mm Hg
Height: 162.6 cm (64.0 inches)
Weight: 81.8 kg (180 lb)
BMI: 30.9 kg/m²

**Initial History:**
Reason(s) for visit: Epigastric pain

**HPI:**

The patient, a 50-year-old grocery store manager, has been experiencing mild epigastric pain without radiation for the past 4 months. The pain is described as a "gnawing pain" that occurs shortly after meals. He rates his pain as a 5 on a 10-point scale. He has not taken any over-the-counter medications to alleviate his pain. He has tried drinking warm milk and hot tea without success. Lying down on the couch or bending over does not exacerbate the pain. He continues to have a normal appetite without early satiety. He denies having fevers, chills, dysphagia, regurgitation, bloody stools, passage of mucus, or unintended weight loss. He denies any trauma or recent travel.

**Past Medical History:**    None
**Past Surgical History:**    None
**Medications:**    None

**Allergies:** None

**Vaccinations:** Up to date

**Family History:** Father died of gastric cancer at age 58. Mother, age 75, has hypertension. One sister, age 48, is healthy.

**Social History:** Smokes one pack per day × 30 years; drinks 5 to 6 beers after work and drinks whiskey and vodka on the weekends; denies use of illegal drugs; eats a high-salt diet with low vegetables; eats a sufficient amount of cured meats; married; three children; works as a full-time grocery store manager; enjoys hosting dinner parties for friends and family.

**Review of Systems:**

| | |
|---|---|
| General: | See HPI |
| Skin: | Negative |
| HEENT: | Negative |
| Musculoskeletal: | Negative |
| Cardiorespiratory: | Negative |
| Gastrointestinal: | See HPI |
| Genitourinary: | Negative |
| Neuropsychiatric: | Negative |

Day 1 @ 14:10

**Physical Examination:**

**General appearance:** Well nourished, well developed; in no apparent distress.

**Skin:** Normal turgor. No lesions. Hair and nails normal.

**Lymph nodes:** No lymphadenopathy.

**HEENT/Neck:** Normocephalic. EOMI, PERRLA. Hearing normal. Ear, nose, mouth normal. Pharynx normal. Neck supple; trachea midline; no masses or bruits; thyroid normal.

**Chest/Lungs:** Chest wall normal. Diaphragm and chest moving equally and symmetrically with respiration. Auscultation and percussion normal.

**Heart/Cardiovascular:** S1 and S2 normal. No murmurs, rubs, gallops, or extra sounds. No JVD.

**Abdomen:** Normal bowel sounds; no bruits. Tenderness in the epigastric area. No masses. No abnormality on percussion. No rebound. No guarding. No rigidity. No hernias. No hepatosplenomegaly.

**Rectal:** Normal sphincter tone. No masses. No occult blood; stool brown.

**First Order Sheet:**
1) CBC with differential, routine — **Result:** WBC-9,000, H/H-14/45%, Plt-150,000, Differential-WNL

2) BMP, routine — **Result:** Glu-90, Urea-10, Na-141, K-3.9, Cl-101, HCO3-23, Cr-1.0, Ca-9.2

3) Lipase, serum, routine — **Result:** 0.50 U/mL (nl: 0.10-1.00)

4) Amylase, serum, routine — **Result:** 100 U/L (nl: 25-125)

5) H. pylori antibody, serum, routine — **Result:** IgG antibody-Positive, IgA antibody-Positive

6) Stool for occult blood, routine — **Result:** Negative

**Second Order Sheet:**
1) Consult, gastroenterology, routine

2) EGD with biopsy, routine — **Reason:** EGD with biopsy to rule out cancer and H. pylori

**Result:** Endoscopic examination shows an ulcerated circumferential mass measuring 30 mm in the antrum of the stomach without active bleeding. Esophageal and duodenal mucosa normal. Pathology results will be reported in approximately 24 hours.

3) H. pylori stain gastric biopsy, routine — **Result:** H. pylori detected

**Third Order Sheet:**
1) Lansoprazole, oral, continuous
2) Amoxicillin, therapy, oral, continuous
3) Clarithromycin, oral, continuous
4) Advise patient, side effects of medication

**Actions:**
1) Change location to home

**Gastric mucosa biopsy result is now available (24 hours later):**
Presence of intestinal-type gastric adenocarcinoma at the level of the submucosa without invasion into the muscularis propria.

**Actions:**
1) Change location to office

**Fourth Order Sheet:**
1) Advise patient, cancer diagnosis
2) CT, abdomen/pelvis, with contrast, routine — **Result:** No focal defect seen in the liver, spleen, kidneys, and pancreas. Gallbladder appears normal. No para-aortic adenopathy

3) Chest x-ray, PA/lateral, routine

**Result:** Normal findings

4) PET scan, routine

**Result:** No abnormal metabolic activity

5) LFT, routine

**Result:** AST-35, ALT-15, Albumin-4.0, T Bil-0.9, Direct Bil-0.2, Total protein-7.2, Alk Phos-72

6) PT/INR, routine

**Result:** PT-7 seconds (nl: <12), INR-1.0 (nl: 1.0-1.3)

7) PTT, routine

**Result:** 22 seconds (nl: <28)

**Fifth Order Sheet:**
1) Consult, general surgery, routine

**Reason:** Biopsy confirms gastric adenocarcinoma, T1 lesion, in the lower two-thirds of the stomach.

**General surgery consult recommendations:** After discussion with the patient regarding alternative treatments, risks and benefits with surgery, the patient agrees with surgery. A subtotal gastrectomy is scheduled for tomorrow morning. Thank you for the consult.

**This case will end in the next few minutes of "real time."**
You may **add** or **delete** orders at this time,
then enter a diagnosis on the following screen.

**Sixth Order Sheet:**
1) Urea breath test, routine

Future date: In 60 days

**Result:** No radiolabeled carbon dioxide detected.

2) Counsel family/patient
3) Advise patient, no smoking
4) Advise patient, no alcohol
5) Low sodium diet

**Please enter your diagnosis:**

Early Gastric Cancer (EGC)

## DISCUSSION:

Gastric cancer is a very common cancer worldwide. Rates are highest in Asia, South America, and Eastern Europe, but lowest in North America. Approximately 85% of gastric cancers are adenocarcinomas, and 15% are due to leiomyosarcomas, gastrointestinal stromal tumors (GIST), and lymphomas (eg, MALT lymphomas). Adenocarcinomas can be subdivided into diffuse type and intestinal type. Intestinal type is the more common type of adenocarcinoma, and is typically seen in older people and males. Diffuse type (infiltrative type) is not as common, but typically seen in younger people and affects both sexes equally. Early gastric cancer refers to invasion of the lesion no deeper than the submucosa, irrespective of the lymph node status.

## Risk Factors:

H. pylori, high salt intake, low intake of fruits and vegetables, dietary nitrates, obesity, smoking, EBV infection, gastric surgery, gastric ulcers, blood group A, pernicious anemia, family history, hereditary diffuse gastric cancer (HDGC), heavy alcohol drinking (moderate alcohol drinking has no clear association with an increased risk for gastric cancer)

## Clinical Features:

Patients with early gastric cancer may be completely asymptomatic, and if they are symptomatic, the symptoms are usually nonspecific. Since gastric cancers and gastric ulcers share a common risk factor (H. pylori), some patients will have manifestations of a gastric ulcer. It should be noted that duodenal ulcers have not been shown to increase the risk of gastric cancers. Although the clinical history cannot accurately differentiate gastric from duodenal ulcers, the following findings may be suggestive of either gastric or duodenal ulcers. A "gnawing" or "burning" sensation may occur after meals in both gastric and duodenal ulcers. Gastric ulcer pain typically occurs shortly after meals, but 2 to 5 hours later in patients with duodenal ulcers. Approximately two-thirds of duodenal ulcers and one-third of gastric ulcers and nonulcer dyspepsia (NUD) will have nocturnal pain with awakenings during sleep. Duodenal ulcers are usually relieved with food or antacids, while in gastric ulcers, antacids usually provide minimal relief and food precipitates the pain.

In more advanced, invasive gastric cancers, patients may present with "alarm features" such as unexplained weight loss, recurrent vomiting, hematemesis, melena, anemia, dysphagia, odynophagia, abdominal mass, jaundice, early satiety, bloating, or family history of gastric cancer. In addition, physical exam may reveal hepatomegaly, left-sided supraclavicular lymph node (Virchow's nodes), periumbilical nodule (Sister Mary Joseph node), left axillary node (Irish node), a mass in the cul-de-sac on rectal exam (Blumer's shelf), or ovarian metastasis (Krukenberg's tumor). Paraneoplastic syndromes can also be seen in advanced disease such as acanthosis nigricans, seborrheic keratoses, dermatomyositis, Trousseau's syndrome, or microangiopathic hemolytic anemia.

## Next Step Summary:

**Step 1)** In a patient with multiple risk factors for gastric cancer but without "alarm" symptoms, there are two considerations for the workup: (1) determine if H. pylori is present so that you can appropriately treat it, and (2) determine if there is an ulcer that might be malignant. Consider the following strategies in this patient with epigastric pain not caused by NSAIDs.

**Option 1:** Empirically treat with antisecretory therapy (eg, PPIs, $H_2$ antagonists).

**Caveat 1:** This may delay the diagnosis of H. pylori, delay the diagnosis of gastric cancer, and have potentially false negative results with further diagnostic testing for H. pylori if antisecretory products are taken.

**Option 2**: Empirically treat for H. pylori.

**Caveat 2**: This may delay the diagnosis of gastric cancer.

**Option 3**: Test for H. pylori, and if:

Positive → Treat for H. pylori

Negative → Trial of PPI for 4 to 6 weeks

**Caveat 3**: This may delay the diagnosis of gastric cancer

**Option 4**: Go straight to endoscopy (EGD)

**Caveat 4**: This may be too invasive as the initial test in a patient with only "mild epigastric pain" without alarm symptoms.

**Option 5**: Noninvasive testing for H. pylori (eg, serologic testing) followed by endoscopy with biopsy if the test is positive.

**Caveat 5**: This may not be cost effective.

Keep in mind that not every option will be suitable for all patients. However, in this particular CCS case, the judgment was made to undergo an EGD after a positive result from serologic testing. In this approach, a biopsy can rule out cancer, but at the same time confirm the diagnosis of H. pylori. Remember, an endoscopy should not be used solely to establish the H. pylori status, but in this case, it was used for multiple reasons (eg, presence of ulcer, cancer, H. pylori).

**Step 2)** Treat the H. pylori infection with the following:

**First-line combination**: PPI (eg, omeprazole) + amoxicillin + clarithromycin × 10 to 14 days

**Penicillin allergic**: PPI (eg, pantoprazole) + metronidazole + clarithromycin × 10 to 14 days

**Failed treatment**: PPI (eg, rabeprazole) + metronidazole + tetracycline + bismuth × 10 to 14 days

**Step 3)** Stage the gastric cancer once it has been confirmed on biopsy. Staging can assess the extent of the disease and determine management options. Labs and imaging are typically used in the staging process. Consider a chest CT instead of a chest x-ray in patients with a proximal gastric cancer. Endoscopic ultrasound (EUS) can be used to assess the depth of invasion of the gastric cancer, but is usually performed in patients with early disease without evidence of distant metastasis. Similarly, a staging laparoscopy can be considered in patients without distant metastasis, but is usually performed in patients with more advanced disease.

**Step 4)** Treatment of early gastric cancers can be accomplished by either endoscopic resection or surgery.

**Endoscopic Resection**

- Typically reserved for patients with tumor confined to the mucosa, no lymph node involvement, size <2 cm without ulceration, and intestinal-type adenocarcinomas.

**Surgery**

- Typically reserved for patients with tumor extending into the submucosa, lymph node involvement, size >3 cm with ulcerations, or diffuse-type adenocarcinomas.

- A total gastrectomy is typically reserved for patients with lesions located in the upper one-third of the stomach.

- A subtotal gastrectomy is typically reserved for patients with lesions located in the lower two-thirds of the stomach.

**Follow-Up:**

Patients who had treatment for early gastric cancer have a good prognosis with a 5-year survival rate greater than 90%. Patients should continue to have follow-up visits every 3 to 6 months for the first year. Patients treated for H. pylori should have noninvasive testing (eg, urea breath test or stool antigen) to confirm eradication. Testing should be postponed for at least 4 weeks after treatment of the infection to prevent false-negative results.

**Pearls:**

- Dietary nitrates (cured meats, food additives, contaminated water) can be converted to nitrites and eventually into N-nitroso compounds (contains -NO group). It is the N-nitroso compounds that have been associated with gastric cancer risk.

- A penetrating posterior gastric ulcer can result in pancreatitis, which can cause pain that radiates to the back.

- Signs and symptoms suggestive of GERD include pyrosis, regurgitation, dysphagia, or discomfort after bending over or lying supine.

- Gastric metastasis can occur in the liver, lymph nodes, lung, ovaries, peritoneum, bone, CNS, or soft tissues.

- Although there is a clear association between H. pylori and gastric adenocarcinomas, only a small percentage of patients will actually develop gastric cancer.

- H. pylori can increases the risk of mucosa-associated lymphoid tissue (MALT) lymphomas.

- Serological testing for antibodies against H. pylori is a noninvasive and cost-effective initial test. However, it should not be used to confirm eradication because the antibodies can persist for several years. Another caveat is that a positive result cannot differentiate between active infection and past exposure. The overall sensitivity is high (90%-100%), but specificity is variable (75%-95%).

- Urea breath test and stool antigen assay for H. pylori are noninvasive tests that have fairly high sensitivity and specificity (>90%). Either test can be used for initial diagnosis or confirming eradication following therapy. In contrast to serological testing, neither test is affected from previous exposure.

- Urease testing is an invasive test for detecting H. pylori because it requires a gastric biopsy from the EGD. Urease testing has near equivalent sensitivity and specificity compared to histology (>90%).

- Histology is also an invasive test that permits additional information on biopsy other than the presence of H. pylori such as MALT lymphoma or intestinal metaplasia.

- Since the stool antigen test, urea breath test, biopsy urease test, and histology depends on the H. pylori load, prior treatment with antibiotics, bismuth, and antisecretory therapy can decrease the sensitivity of all the tests and lead to false negative results. Therefore, patients should be off antibiotics and bismuth for at least 4 weeks, and PPIs for at least 2 weeks to reduce the chance of false negative results.

- Avoid using the stool antigen test and biopsy urease test in patients with a GI bleed since results can be affected.

- In a patient with early gastric cancer with a positive serology (ie, IgG) for H. pylori, but a negative biopsy for H. pylori, the patient should still be treated for the infection because the onset of gastric cancer can actually decrease the H. pylori load and, hence, the sensitivity of the biopsy.

- Tumor markers such as CEA or CA-125 are not typically used in the staging, unless the patient will undergo neoadjuvant therapy.

- Diffuse type gastric cancers are highly metastatic and carry a poor prognosis. This type has a tendency to invade the gastric wall, which results in a very rigid-appearing stomach termed linitis plastica or "leather bottle."

- **Foundational point**—Histologically, diffuse-type gastric carcinomas can result in **signet ring cells** where abundant mucin formation within the tumor cells pushes the nucleus to the periphery creating an appearance of a finger hole with the nucleus mimicking the face of a ring.

- **On the CCS**, if you forget the name of a test, let the order menu assist you. For example, typing in "H. pylori" in the order menu will provide you a list of different tests.

- **On the CCS**, failure to obtain a biopsy in a patient with a nonbleeding gastric ulcer, especially in the presence of multiple risk factors for gastric cancer, would be considered suboptimal management.

- **On the CCS**, failure to detect H. pylori and appropriately treat the infection with a first-line medication would be considered suboptimal management.

- **On the CCS**, in most cases the consultants offer very little assistance. However, in some cases, if you have enough information (ie, thorough workup), the consultants may be helpful.

- **On the CCS**, as you read the HPI it may be helpful to jot down a couple of differential diagnoses on the dry-erase board provided to you in the exam. As you refer to your notes, it may be helpful to order tests based on the chief complaint and your differentials. Remember that a thorough methodical workup will probably not deduct from your score, but keep in mind that you want to order your tests as "appropriate" as possible.

# Gynecology

## KEYWORDS REVIEW

**Colposcopy**—A diagnostic procedure that uses a magnifying instrument (colposcope) to examine the cervix, vagina, and in some cases the vulva. Once acetic acid is applied to the cervix, the solution will highlight areas of tissue abnormality. The colposcope (ie, standing microscope), which does not touch the patient, will be able to magnify the tissue of interest and help guide directed biopsies.

**Dyschezia**—Painful or difficult defecation.

**Dyspareunia**—Painful or difficult sex.

**Hematochezia**—Passage of bloody stools.

**Hematocolpos**—Sequestration of menstrual blood in the vagina, which is usually due to an imperforate hymen or other obstruction.

**Hypomenorrhea**—Reduction in menstrual flow or duration occurring at regular cycle intervals.

**Loop electrosurgical excision procedure (LEEP)**—A thin wire loop that uses electric current to remove a cone-shaped segment of the cervix.

**Menometrorrhagia**—Excessive uterine bleeding at regular and irregular intervals.

**Menorrhagia**—Also referred to as hypermenorrhea. Heavy or prolonged menstrual flow occurring at regular cycle intervals.

**Metrorrhagia**—Intermenstrual bleeding (ie, irregular intervals).

**Oligomenorrhea**—Infrequent menses with intervals that vary from 35 days to 6 months.

**Polymenorrhea**—Abnormally frequent menstruation occurring at regular intervals of 21 days or less.

**Primary amenorrhea**—Absence of menses by age 15 in the presence of normal growth and secondary sexual characteristics. The cause is usually due to genetic or anatomic abnormalities.

**Primary dysmenorrhea**—Painful menstruation with no identifiable pelvic pathology. Instead, there is excessive endometrial prostaglandin $F_2$ alpha that can cause uterine contractions and GI symptoms (eg, nausea, vomiting, diarrhea). NSAIDs (prostaglandin synthetase inhibitors) can provide symptomatic relief.

**Secondary amenorrhea**—Absence of menses for more than 3 cycle intervals or 6 months in an individual who was previously menstruating. Pregnancy is the most common cause, but other causes can occur along the hypothalamic (eg, exercise, stress, trauma, tumor)–pituitary (eg, pituitary adenomas, infarcts)–ovarian (eg, PCOS, premature ovarian insufficiency) axis. Other endocrine disorders (eg, hypothyroidism, hyperthyroidism, diabetes mellitus) and anatomic abnormalities (eg, Asherman's syndrome) can result in secondary amenorrhea.

**Secondary dysmenorrhea**—Painful menstruation with an attributable pelvic pathology. It may be due to abnormalities in the ovaries (eg, ovarian cysts), uterus (eg, leiomyomas, adenomyosis, endometriosis, endometrial polyps, IUD, PID), or cervix (eg, cervical stenosis).

**Virilization**—Masculinization, particularly in a female or prepubertal boy.

# OVARIES

## ▌OVARIAN TORSION

Ovarian torsion refers to the rotation of the ovary around the supporting ligaments, most commonly the suspensory ligament of the ovary (ie, infundibulopelvic ligament) and the ovarian ligament. When the fallopian tube twists along with the ovary, it is referred to as adnexal torsion.

### Risk Factors:

Large ovarian cysts or tumors (especially size ≥5 cm), pregnancy, ovulation induction, congenitally elongated fallopian tubes, elongated utero-ovarian ligaments.

### Clinical Features:

The classic presentation of ovarian torsion is an acute, severe, unilateral, lower abdominal and pelvic pain. The pain can be characterized as sharp, stabbing, or crampy and may radiate to the back, pelvis, or thigh. Exertion such as exercise may be a precipitating factor. Associated features include nausea, vomiting, and fever. If fever is present, it suggests adnexal necrosis, which is a late finding. On examination, a tender adnexal mass may sometimes be felt that is a result of an edematous and cyanotic ovary secondary to an obstruction of the lymphatic and venous outflow. Atypical presentations do occur, and features may include a mild pain, bilateral involvement, no tenderness, no adnexal mass, or intermittent episodes of pain. It is thought that the previous episodes of pain are attributable to partial torsion with spontaneous reversal.

### Next Step:

**Step 1)** Ovarian torsion is a gynecologic emergency. Provide analgesics for pain control and antiemetics (eg, ondansetron) for nausea and vomiting.

**Step 2)** Obtain both transvaginal and transabdominal ultrasound with color Doppler flow to get good visualization of the pelvic structures. It should be noted that an abnormal color Doppler flow suggests an ovarian torsion, but a normal color Doppler flow study does not rule out an ovarian torsion. Initial testing should also include the following:

**β-hCG**—Rule out a pregnancy or ectopic pregnancy.

**CBC**—Check for anemia secondary to hemorrhage and leukocytosis secondary to an infection from the necrosis.

**BMP**—Check the electrolytes.

**Step 3)** The clinical management of suspected ovarian torsion is to proceed with surgery. At the time of surgical evaluation, the definitive diagnosis can be made by visualizing the rotated ovary. The surgeon may then untwist the vascular pedicle, perform a possible ovarian cystectomy if a benign mass is present, or perform a salpingo-oophorectomy in the presence of a necrotic ovary or suspected malignancy.

### Disposition:

After initial management in the ED, patients with suspected ovarian torsion should be sent to surgery for definitive diagnosis and therapeutic treatment.

### Pearls:

- Ovarian torsion is more common on the right side than the left side, which may confuse you with appendicitis.

- Differential diagnosis includes appendicitis, ectopic pregnancy, tubo-ovarian abscess, and small intestinal obstruction.

- Ovarian torsion can occur at any age (eg, fetus, neonates, prepubertal girls, reproductive years, postmenopausal).

- Ovarian torsion can recur.

- With early diagnosis and treatment, the prognosis of the affected ovary improves.

- **Foundational point**—Compression of the ovarian vessels initially affects the lymphatic and venous outflow because they have fairly thin walls. This results in ovarian congestion and cyanosis.

Further progression eventually interrupts the arterial vessel (ie, muscular walls), which can lead to ovarian hypoxia causing intense pelvic pain. Without intervention, the ovary can undergo necrosis, infarction, and possibly hemorrhage.

- **On the CCS**, "ovarian artery Doppler" is available in the practice CCS.
- **On the CCS**, if you suspect ovarian torsion, do not delay treatment, since that would be considered suboptimal management (eg, ordering an MRI).
- **On the CCS**, poor management would include the failure to order a pelvic ultrasound.

- **On the CCS**, if your ob-gyn consultant agrees with surgery, remember to order the pre-op work up (eg, blood type and crossmatch, PT/INR, PTT).
- **On the CCS**, your simulated timing will be important in this type of case.
- **On the CCS**, if you're not sure what type of surgical procedure the patient should have, type in the word "laparoscopic" and a menu of different procedures will be available to you.

# UTERUS

## LEIOMYOMA

Leiomyoma (fibroids or myomas) is a benign smooth muscle neoplasm that is the most common pelvic tumor in women. The etiology is unclear.

### Risk Factors:

**Increased risk**—Early menarche, blacks, elevated BMI, early pregnancy (first trimester), reproductive-aged female, increasing age (high prevalence in the fifth decade)

**Decreased risk**—Smoking, increased parity, postmenopausal

### Clinical Features:

Patients can be asymptomatic, especially if the myomas are small. Symptomatic patients typically complain of bleeding, pain, pressure sensation, or infertility. The severity of the symptoms is usually dictated by the number, size, and location of the myoma (see Figure 9-1 and Color Plate 9). Bleeding typically presents as

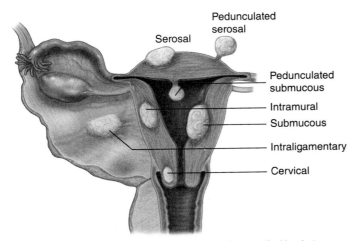

**FIGURE 9-1 • Leiomyomas.** Uterine fibroids can be classified by their location. Subserosal myomas grow near the uterine serosa. Submucous myomas are adjacent to the endometrium. Intramural myomas are within the uterine walls. Cervical myomas are located in the cervix. Pedunculated myomas have an attached stalk. Infrequently, myomas can be found in the broad ligament, ovary, fallopian tube, vagina, and vulva. (Reproduced with permission from Hoffman BL, Schorge JO, Schaffer JI, et al. *Williams Gynecology.* 2nd ed. New York: McGraw-Hill, www.accessmedicine.com.)

menorrhagia. Menorrhagia is often accompanied by pain (dysmenorrhea). Acute pelvic pain is uncommon, unless there is a degenerating myoma or torsion of a pedunculated tumor. Enlarged myomas can compress nearby pelvic organs such as the rectum (constipation), bladder (urinary frequency, incontinence), and infrequently, the ureter (hydronephrosis). Distortion of the uterine cavity, especially with submucous leiomyomas, can result in infertility. Upon bimanual pelvic examination, an enlarged, firm, asymmetrical, irregular contoured uterus may be felt. A single mass or multiple masses may also be appreciated on exam.

### Next Step:

**Step 1)** In a reproductive-aged woman with uterine enlargement, order a β-hCG level to rule out a pregnancy. In a postmenopausal woman with uterine bleeding and a rapidly growing enlarging uterine mass, a workup to rule out a uterine leiomyosarcoma (ie, aggressive uterine cancer) should be performed.

**Step 2)** Diagnosis of a leiomyoma is based on the clinical evaluation and most commonly with the transvaginal ultrasound. Leiomyomas can vary in their echogenicity from hypo- to hyperechoic on ultrasound findings. Submucosal leiomyomas may be diagnosed by saline infusion sonography or hysteroscopy which both provide better visualization of the mass within the endometrial cavity. MRI's are not routinely performed, but may be considered in patients with distorted anatomy or surgical planning. Hysterosalpingography (HSG) is a radiologic procedure that uses radio-opaque material to characterize the contour of the uterus. HSG is often used to determine tubal patency in an infertile woman.

**Step 3)** The clinical management of leiomyomas can vary. Consider the following approaches:

### Observation

There are two populations to consider for expectant management. First, in a reproductive-aged woman with small, asymptomatic myomas. Second, in a perimenopausal woman who is close to menopause since the condition usually improves with lower levels of estrogen.

### Pharmacologic Therapy

**NSAIDs**—NSAIDs can be useful for patients with painful menses, but not for reducing the bulk of the myoma.

**GnRH agonist**—GnRH agonist (ie, leuprolide) induces a hypogonadal state. It can reduce the uterine size within 3 months, and it can improve anemia. GnRH agonist should not be used as a form of long-term management, but rather as a preoperative medication for 3 to 6 months prior to surgery and in conjunction with iron supplements. Side effects include amenorrhea, hot flashes, bone loss, insomnia, and myalgias. Due to the side effects of GnRH agonist, add-back therapy with low-dose estrogen-progestin (eg, conjugated estrogen plus medroxyprogesterone acetate) is often administered to counter the side effects, especially bone loss and vasomotor symptoms. Leuprolide is administered as a onetime IM injection every month or every 3 months (ie, higher dosage).

### Interventional Procedures

**Hysterectomy**—Hysterectomy is considered definitive therapy. It is ideal in patients who have completed their childbearing and who are refractory to other forms of treatment.

**Myomectomy**—Myomectomy is ideal in patients who have not completed their childbearing and want to retain their uterus. The disadvantage of myomectomy is the formation of adhesions and leiomyoma recurrence. Additionally, there is a risk of uterine rupture with subsequent pregnancy, and therefore, patients are usually advised to undergo a C-section.

**Uterine artery embolization (UAE)**—UAE is an alternative to surgery in symptomatic patients that are refractory to medical management. UAE can alleviate leiomyoma-related symptoms and induce shrinkage of the myoma. Although UAE can preserve the uterus, it is not ideal for patients that have not completed their childbearing since pregnancy-related complications have been associated following UAE.

### Follow-Up:

Asymptomatic patients with small myomas can be followed-up every 6 months for a pelvic exam to reassess the rate of growth.

### Pearls:

- Following discontinuation of GnRH agonists, normal menses resume, leiomyomas regrow, and uterine volume returns to the original size.
- Most women, not all, that are in menopause typically have shrinkage of their leiomyomas.
- Low-dose oral contraceptives do not cause leiomyomas to grow.
- Parasitic myomas are considered a subserosal variant. In this type, a pedunculated subserosal myoma can attach itself into the peritoneal cavity and derive blood supply from another organ (eg, omentum). Subsequently, the parasitic myoma may or may not detach itself from the parent myometrium.
- **Foundational point**—Leiomyoma cells have a high density of estrogen receptors on the cell surface.
- **Foundational point**—On cut section of a leiomyoma, a characteristic "whorled" pattern of smooth muscle bundles can be seen.
- **Foundational point**—On histology, smooth muscle cells are elongated with an eosinophilic cytoplasm and an oval or

cigar-shaped nucleus. Mitotic activity is uncommon in leiomyoma, but it is frequently present in leiomyosarcoma.

- **Foundational point**—An outer connective tissue surrounds a leiomyoma, which serves as a cleavage plane for the surgeon to easily shell out the mass, unlike adenomyomas, which are not easily excised because they lack a good cleavage plane.
- **On the CCS**, "transvaginal ultrasound," "saline infused sonogram of uterus," "hysterosalpingography," and "hysteroscopy" are available in the practice CCS. If you decide to order a hysterosalpingography or hysteroscopy, an ob-gyn consult is required.
- **On the CCS**, if you order "OCP," you will be required to pick the strength (eg, low, medium, high) of the OCP.
- **On the CCS**, if a patient presents with menorrhagia, remember to order a CBC to check for anemia and a TSH to rule out hypothyroidism.
- **On the CCS**, even if you made the correct management decisions during the CCS case, you may still receive no credit for those decisions if you placed them in the wrong sequence of actions (eg, ordering a hysterectomy before a transvaginal ultrasound).

## ADENOMYOSIS

Adenomyosis is characterized by the presence of ectopic endometrial glands and stroma deep within the myometrium. The myometrium reacts to the ectopic tissue by hyperplasia and hypertrophy resulting in a diffusely enlarged uterus or in a focal circumscribed nodule, also referred to as an adenomyoma. The etiology is unknown.

### Risk Factors:

Parity (opposite of leiomyoma), increasing age (usually seen in the fourth or fifth decade), uterine trauma.

### Clinical Features:

Patients can be asymptomatic. Symptomatic patients typically complain of menorrhagia and secondary dysmenorrhea. Infrequently, patients may complain of dyspareunia or infertility. On pelvic examination, diffuse adenomyosis will present as a uniformly enlarged uterus or "globular" enlargement. The uterus will be symmetrical in shape and will generally not exceed a 12-week size gestation. A focal adenomyosis (adenomyoma) is typically confined to a discrete area and results in an asymmetrical uterus. The uterus is usually tender immediately before and during menstruation.

### Next Step:

**Step 1)** In a reproductive-aged woman with uterine enlargement, order a β-hCG level to rule out a pregnancy. In a postmenopausal woman with uterine bleeding, the initial evaluation may begin with an endometrial biopsy and/or transvaginal ultrasound to rule out a malignancy.

**Step 2)** Diagnosis of an adenomyosis is based on the clinical evaluation and transvaginal ultrasound (TVUS) or MRI.

However, MRI is more accurate and it can differentiate between focal and diffuse adenomyosis. MRI can also delineate between a leiomyoma and adenomyosis. The transvaginal ultrasound is operator dependent, but results will typically demonstrate heterogeneity in the myometrium and hypoechoic cysts (ie, endometrial cystic glands) or hypoechoic nodules (ie, adenomyoma).

**Step 3)** Hysterectomy is considered definitive treatment. It is ideal in patients who have completed their childbearing and who have significant symptoms. Unfortunately, there are no superior medical treatments for adenomyosis. NSAIDs, estrogen-progestin contraceptives, and progestin-only (eg, levonorgestrel-releasing IUD) therapies are used for menorrhagia and dysmenorrhea.

### Follow-Up:

Symptomatic patients may require ongoing follow-ups, unless they decide to undergo a hysterectomy.

### Pearls:

- Diffuse adenomyosis is more common than focal adenomyosis.
- The clinical presentation of focal adenomyosis can resemble leiomyomas.

- Adenomyosis can also occur in patients with leiomyomas and endometriosis.
- Definitive diagnosis is made from histologic exam of the uterus following a hysterectomy.
- Needle biopsy is not routinely performed in the evaluation of adenomyosis.
- *Adeno-* means gland in Greek. Therefore, it is easy to remember that the gland tissue is in reference to the endometrial glands.
- **Foundational point**—Adenomyosis is derived from the basalis layer of the endometrium.
- **Foundational point**—The endometrial glands and stroma found in the myometrium rarely undergo the same proliferative and secretory changes of a normal uterine endometrium during the menstrual cycle.
- **Foundational point**—On cut section of the uterus, there is a spongy appearance with focal areas of hemorrhage.
- **On the CCS**, if you order something that is truly not indicated and it poses a threat to your patient, you will lose points (eg, ordering a laparoscopic ovarian biopsy for an adenomyoma).

# CERVIX

## CERVICAL DYSPLASIA

Cervical dysplasia is a precancerous condition in which abnormal cell growth occurs within the cervix. The transformation zone (TZ) is an area of active cell division that poses a high risk for neoplasia. This area represents a transition of stratified squamous epithelium to columnar epithelium. The position of the TZ can change based on the woman's age, hormonal status (eg, pregnancy, menopause, hormonal contraception), vaginal pH, or prior cervical procedures. Cervical dysplasia usually causes no symptoms and is often discovered by routine screening.

### Risk Factors:

HPV 16 and 18, cigarette smoking, immunosuppression (eg, HIV, immunosuppressive therapy), sex at a young age, multiple sexual partners.

### Cytological and Histological Features:

The Pap smear allows for cytologic evaluation while colposcopy-directed biopsies are often used for histologic examination.

### Squamous Cell Abnormalities

**Low-grade squamous intraepithelial lesion (LSIL)**—The risk of invasive cervical cancer is low in this category and is consistent with mild dysplasia, HPV, and CIN 1.

**High-grade squamous intraepithelial lesion (HSIL)**—The risk of invasive cervical cancer is fairly high in this category and is consistent with moderate to severe dysplasia, carcinoma in situ (CIS), and CIN 2 or CIN 3.

**Atypical squamous cell—cannot exclude a high-grade lesion (ASC-H)**—Findings indicate a concern for a significant lesion, but not conclusively. There is still a potential risk for malignant disease in this category.

**Atypical squamous cell of undetermined significance (ASC-US)**—ASC-US is the most common type of cervical cytologic abnormality. Consider this type as a "gray zone" category because it has some features associated with squamous lesions, but it does not fit the criteria for squamous intraepithelial lesion (SIL).

### Histologic Abnormalities

**CIN 1**—A low-grade lesion that exhibits koilocytotic atypia (HPV viral cytopathic effect). There are mild cellular changes in the lower one-third of the epithelium.

**CIN 2**—A high-grade lesion with progressive atypia seen in the basal two-thirds of the epithelium.

**CIN 3**—A high-grade lesion with severe cellular changes of more than two-thirds of the epithelium and usually lacks squamous maturation throughout the thickness of the epithelium.

### Next Step:

**Step 1)** Cervical cancer screening guidelines are based on several organizations (eg, USPSTF, ACS, ASCCP, ASCP, ACOG) with slight differences in their screening parameters. It should be noted that the recognition of HPV in cervical cancer has led to the incorporation of HPV screening in women 30 to 65 years old. The following screening parameters are based on the above organizations and should be served as a basis for board examination:

**21 years old:** Initiate screening (no earlier), regardless of age of sexual initiation

**21-29 years:** Cytology every 3 years

**30-65 years:** Cytology + HPV testing every 5 years or cytology alone every 3 years

**>65 years:** Not indicated if high risk is absent and 3 consecutive negative cytology results or 2 consecutive negative co-tests in the past 10 years

**Step 2)** The cervical cytology results is an initial assessment to detect abnormal cervical cells. The Pap smear is not used to establish a diagnosis nor initiate treatment. Consider the following cervical cellular abnormalities and the associated clinical management:

## LSIL

**21-24 years old:** LSIL → Repeat Pap test in 1 year. If repeat shows HSIL or ASC-H perform colposcopy, but if repeat shows LSIL or ASC-US repeat Pap test in 1 year.

**25-29 years old:** LSIL → Colposcopy.

**≥30 years old:**

LSIL + HPV (+) → Colposcopy

LSIL + HPV (−) → Repeat Pap + HPV in 1 year or colposcopy

LSIL → Colposcopy

**Pregnant:** LSIL → Colposcopy without endocervical curettage (ECC). Only biopsy if you suspect a high-grade lesion.

## HSIL

**21-24 years old:** HSIL → Colposcopy (Do not do LEEP).

**≥25 years old:** HSIL→ Colposcopy or immediate LEEP.

**Pregnant:** HSIL → Colposcopy without ECC or LEEP. Only biopsy if you suspect a high-grade lesion.

## ASC-H

**21-24 years old:** ASC-H → Colposcopy.

**≥25 years old:** ASC-H → Colposcopy.

**Pregnant:** ASC-H → Colposcopy without ECC. Only biopsy if you suspect a high grade lesion.

## ASC-US

**21-24 years old:** ASC-US → HPV testing now or repeat Pap test in 1 year. If results show HSIL or ASC-H, perform colposcopy, but if results show HPV (+), LSIL, or ASC-US, repeat Pap in 1 year.

**≥25 years old:** ASC-US → HPV testing now or repeat Pap test in 1 year. If results show ASC-US, ASC-H, HSIL, LSIL, or HPV (+), perform colposcopy, but if results show HPV (−), retest in 3 years with Pap test + HPV.

**Pregnant:** ASC-US → Colposcopy without ECC. Only biopsy if you suspect a high-grade lesion.

**Step 3)** Upon confirmed CIN 1, CIN 2, or CIN 3 via colposcopy-directed biopsies, observation or treatment may be recommended. Consider the following CINs:

## CIN 1 with Prior Low-grade Lesions (LSIL or ASC-US)

**21-24 years old:** Repeat Pap test in 1 year. If results show HSIL or ASC-H, perform colposcopy, but if results show LSIL or ASC-US, repeat Pap in 1 year.

**≥25 years old:** Repeat Pap + HPV in 1 year. If results show HPV (+), ASC-US, ASC-H, or HSIL, perform colposcopy, but if results show HPV (−) and a normal Pap test, resume screening in 3 years.

**Persistent CIN 1 ≥2 years:** Observation or treatment (excision or ablation).

**Pregnant:** No excision or ablation, reevaluate 6 weeks postpartum.

## CIN 1 with Prior High-grade Lesions (HSIL or ASC-H)

**21-24 years old:** Pap test + colposcopy every 6 months for 2 years.

**≥25 years old:** Repeat Pap + HPV at 12 and 24 months or diagnostic excisional procedure.

**Persistent CIN 1 ≥2 years:** Observation or treatment (excision or ablation).

**Pregnant:** No excision or ablation, reevaluate 6 weeks postpartum.

## CIN 2 or CIN 3

**Treat:** Excision or ablation.

**Young women who have not finished childbearing:** Observation (Pap + colposcopy) or treatment.

**Pregnant:** Reevaluate 6 weeks postpartum or Pap test + colposcopy without ECC. Only biopsy if you suspect invasive cancer.

**Follow-Up:**

Patients with CIN 2 or CIN 3 who have been treated (excision or ablation) should have follow-up testing with a Pap smear plus HPV testing in 12 and 24 months.

**Pearls:**

- CIN 1 is typically caused by the low-risk HPV types and is not considered precancerous unless the lesion has been present for ≥2 years. CIN 1 is considered a transient HPV infection that usually regresses over several months.

- CIN 2 and 3 are true precancerous lesions.

- A higher "CIN" number reflects a high-grade lesion; this can easily be remembered in that the higher the "sin" the greater the risk of malignant disease.

- There are over 100 genotypes of HPV. The "high-risk" types that can cause cervical cancer include HPV 16 and 18, which are the major types. HPV 31, 33, 35, 45, 52, and 58 can also cause cervical cancer. The "low-risk" types that can cause benign condylomatous genital warts are HPV 6 and 11.

- Smoking and coexistent HPV infection have a synergistic effect on cervical cancer and CIN formation.

- Most of the screening recommendations incorporate HPV testing after 30 years of age because prior to 30 years old, most of the HPV infections are transient.

- Bivalent (types 16, 18) HPV vaccine is available under the trade name Cervarix and should be used for females only.

- Quadrivalent (types 6, 11, 16, 18) HPV vaccine is available under the trade name Gardasil and is used for females and males. In males, HPV vaccine can be effective in preventing genital warts and anal intraepithelial neoplasia in men who have sex with men (MSM).

- HPV vaccines do not remove preexisting HPV infections.

- HPV vaccines are most effective when females or males have not been infected with the HPV infection (ie, before their first sexual encounter). However, females and males can still be vaccinated even if they have been sexually active or are positive for HPV infection, presence of genital warts, abnormal Pap tests in females, or anal intraepithelial neoplasia in males.

- HPV vaccination is not recommended for pregnant women until more information is available on its safety even though the drug rating in pregnancy is a category B.

- HPV vaccination is recommended for patients who are immunocompromised.

- HPV vaccines can be given as early as 9 years of age, but the recommended age is 11 or 12 years old. Catch-up vaccinations may be given to patients 13 to 26 years of age who have not been vaccinated. It is a 3-dose series that can be given at 0, 2, and 6 months of follow-up visits.

- A Pap smear involves the direct transfer of cervical cells onto a microscope slide for evaluation. Liquid-based cytology involves the transfer of the cervical cells to a liquid vial. The cells are then place in a monolayer onto a glass slide for evaluation. Either procedure is acceptable, and there is no significant advantage of liquid-based testing compared to the conventional Pap smear.

- The cervical screening recommendations for patients that have undergone a hysterectomy for a benign disease vary from different organizations. In general, patients in this category are at lower risk of cervical cancer, especially if the cervix was removed. A collective summary and agreement of the recommendations from the various organizations propose that screening is not indicated if the patient had no history of CIN 2, CIN 3, or cervical cancer. Screening recommendations will vary based on evidence of adequate negative prior screening.

- Ablation modalities are used for treatment, but excisional modalities are used for treatment plus diagnostic information (eg, inadequate colposcopy, recurrent CIN 2, 3).

- Ablation therapies include cryotherapy, $CO_2$ laser, cold coagulation, and electrocoagulation diathermy.

- Excisional therapies can be performed using a scalpel (cold knife conization), laser, or electrosurgery (ie, LEEP). The procedure involves a cone-shaped biopsy (cervical conization) that includes the entire transformation zone. Unfortunately, excisional therapies frequently result in cervical stenosis compared to ablation therapies.

- Patients with a history of cervical conization are at risk of future second trimester pregnancy loss.

- Glandular cells on cytology usually derive from the endometrium or endocervix. Glandular cells can be categorized as atypical glandular cells (AGC)–endocervical, endometrial, or not otherwise specified (NOS). There is also a category of AGC favoring neoplastic–endocervical or not otherwise specified (NOS).

- **CJ:** A 35-year-old woman underwent a Pap smear that demonstrated AGC-endocervical cells on cytology. What is your next step? **Answer:** All AGC categories except endometrial cells should undergo a colposcopy with endocervical sampling. In addition, all women ≥35 years old or at risk for endometrial hyperplasia (eg, late menopause, early menarche, unopposed estrogen use, tamoxifen use, nulliparity, PCOS, postmenopausal with uterine bleeding) should undergo endometrial sampling. Patients with AGC-endometrial cells are managed differently. The initial workup requires endometrial sampling plus endocervical sampling. If the results are negative for any premalignant lesion, then the next best step is to perform a colposcopy.

- **Foundational point**—Most women are born with columnar epithelium on the face of the cervix. The columnar cells are replaced by squamous epithelium via squamous metaplasia during the time of menarche, when the vagina becomes fairly acidic. The squamous epithelium is more resistant to the acidic environment.

- **Foundational point**—During colposcopy, acetic acid is applied to the cervix. It is thought that the acetic solution causes dehydration of squamous cells but not columnar cells. This results in an increased nuclear density or nuclear-cytoplasm ratio in the squamous cells, which would be more prominent in actively dividing cells (eg, dysplastic cells, metaplastic cells). Essentially, the acetic solution causes an increased light reflectivity in the abnormal tissue and thus creates a visual contrast from the normal tissue.

- **Foundational point**—During colposcopy, if no lesion is seen with acetic acid, an iodine solution is applied to the cervix. Normal mature squamous cells contain a large amount of glycogen, and when iodine is applied, it will be taken up and stained a dark brown color. Rapidly dividing cells contain little glycogen, and when iodine is applied, it will not be taken up and these cells will stain a light yellow.

- **On the CCS,** "Gardasil" is available in the practice CCS, but not "Cervarix."

- **On the CCS,** if you're not sure on the type of diagnostic excisional procedure to perform (eg, laser, LEEP, cold knife conization), type in "cervical" in the order menu and select from the list.

# VAGINA/VULVA

## ▌ BACTERIAL VAGINOSIS

Bacterial vaginosis is characterized by a shift in normal vaginal flora from a hydrogen peroxide-producing lactobacilli to an increasing number of anaerobes, particularly *Gardnerella vaginalis*, *Prevotella species*, and *Mobiluncus* species. An inflammatory response is lacking in bacterial vaginosis, hence the term *vaginosis* rather than *vaginitis*.

**Risk Factors:**

Sexual activity, douching

**Clinical Features:**

Patients can be asymptomatic. Symptomatic patients typically complain of a "fishy" or "musty" vaginal odor, particularly after sex or during menses. It is thought that following intercourse, the alkaline semen releases aromatic amines. Patients usually do not complain of vaginal pruritus, dysuria, or dyspareunia. On examination, the vaginal discharge has a thin, gray-white appearance that adheres to the vaginal walls. Typically, there is little evidence of inflammation of the vaginal walls. In some cases, not all, patients may have a frothy discharge.

**Next Step:**

**Step 1)** The diagnosis of bacterial vaginosis is based on the Amsel criteria, which require at least 3 of the following 4 findings:

- Vaginal pH >4.5 (normal pH values are from 3.8 to 4.5)
- Presence of a thin, gray-white, homogenous discharge
- Fishy odor upon adding KOH to vaginal discharge (positive whiff test)
- Presence of clue cells (>20% seen on the wet smear)

**Step 2)** The goal of treatment is to shift the high concentration of anaerobes back to the dominant lactobacilli. Metronidazole and clindamycin are good agents against anaerobes, and over time, the hope is for the regeneration of normal vaginal flora. Consider the following regimens:

**Option 1:** Metronidazole (oral) × 7 days
**Option 2:** Metronidazole (intravaginal gel) × 5 days
**Option 3:** Clindamycin (intravaginal cream) × 7 days
**Option 4:** Clindamycin (vaginal suppository) × 3 days
**Option 5:** Clindamycin (oral) × 7 days

**Follow-Up:**

Patients do not require a follow-up if symptoms resolve with antibiotic therapy.

**Pearls:**

- *Gardnerella vaginalis* is actually part of the normal vaginal flora, but its concentrations increase in bacterial vaginosis.
- Male sexual partners of affected women do not have to be treated.
- Asymptomatic women do not have to be treated.
- Vaginal culture has no role in the evaluation and diagnosis of bacterial vaginosis since the organisms you culture will be part of the normal vaginal flora.
- Infected pregnant patients with bacterial vaginosis are at risk of premature rupture of membranes, preterm delivery, and endometritis.
- There is no effective treatment in replacing lactobacilli.
- In the absence of lactobacilli, the vaginal pH rises creating an environment for anaerobes to grow and *Gardnerella vaginalis* to adhere to vaginal epithelial cells (clue cells).
- **Foundational point**—Clue cells represent vaginal epithelial cells studded with coccobacilli.
- **On the CCS,** "vaginal pH" and "Whiff test" are available in the practice CCS.
- **On the CCS,** "metronidazole" and "clindamycin" are available in the practice CCS with both oral and vaginal routes of administration.

## ▌ TRICHOMONIASIS

Trichomoniasis is the most common nonviral, nonchlamydial STD in women. Trichomoniasis is caused by a flagellated protozoan, *Trichomonas vaginalis*, which is primarily transmitted through sexual intercourse.

**Risk Factors:**

Sexual activity with an infected partner, history of STDs, multiple partners.

**Clinical Features:**

The clinical presentations are different for women and men. Consider the following:

**Women**—Patients may complain of copious, malodorous vaginal discharge. Patients may also have vaginal pruritus, burning, dysuria, dyspareunia, and postcoital bleeding. On examination, the vaginal discharge may be green-yellow, white, or gray. In some cases, not all, patients may have a frothy discharge. Edema and erythema may be present in the vagina and vulva. Punctate hemorrhages ("strawberry cervix") may be seen on the vagina or cervix, but this finding is uncommon.

**Men**—Men can be asymptomatic (carrier state). However, untreated men can develop signs and symptoms of urethritis, which may include dysuria, pruritus, burning, or a discharge that is mucoid or mucopurulent. Patients may also have findings consistent with epididymitis, prostatitis, or balanoposthitis.

**Next Step:**

**Step 1)** The clinical features of trichomoniasis are not sufficient to make the diagnosis. The diagnosis can be confirmed by examining the motile trichomonads on saline wet mount. Consider the following adjunctive tests that can be used to support the diagnosis.

- Vaginal pH between 5.0 and 7.0.
- Increased numbers of PMNs on saline microscopy.
- Fishy odor upon adding KOH to vaginal discharge (positive whiff test).
- Cultures can be performed in the absence of a motile trichomonad on saline microscopy, but with a high clinical suspicion for trichomoniasis.
- Molecular testing for DNA, RNA, or antigen comes in rapid diagnostic kits that can be useful when cultures and saline microscopy are unavailable.

**Step 2)** Treatment involves both symptomatic and asymptomatic women and men. Both sexual partners should be treated simultaneously and should abstain from sexual intercourse until after treatment and until they are asymptomatic. Consider the following regimens with the 5-nitroimidazole drugs:

**Option 1:** Metronidazole (oral) × 1 day (ie, single dose with 2 grams)

**Option 2:** Metronidazole (oral) × 7 days (ie, 500 mg BID)

**Option 3:** Tinidazole (oral) × 1 day (ie, single dose with 2 grams)

#### Follow-Up:

No follow-up is necessary for both patient and partner if they are asymptomatic after therapy. Keep in mind that since trichomoniasis is associated with STDs, patients should have the appropriate testing to rule out other sexually transmitted infections.

#### Pearls:

- Neither a frothy discharge nor a positive whiff test (amine odor test) is pathognomonic for bacterial vaginosis or trichomoniasis.
- Wet mount microscopy is not effective in diagnosing trichomonas in men. Men should have either a culture or nucleic acid amplification test to make the diagnosis.
- Systemic therapy with the 5-nitroimidazole agents are the choice of therapy compared to topical therapy because the drug can reach the hidden reservoirs such as the Skene's gland and Bartholin's gland, which can be a cause of recurrence other than not treating the sexual partner.
- Infected pregnant women with trichomoniasis are at risk of premature rupture of membranes, preterm delivery, and intrauterine infections.
- **Foundational point**—The trophozoite, *Trichomonas vaginalis*, replicates by binary fission.
- **On the CCS,** "Trichomonas vaginal smear" and "wet mount, vaginal secretions" are both available in the practice CCS, and they are considered the same order.
- **On the CCS,** remember to "advise patient, sexual partner needs treatment."
- **On the CCS,** remember to "advise patient, no intercourse."
- **On the CCS,** remember to "advise patient, medication adherence."
- **On the CCS,** remember to "advise patient, side effects of medication" since metronidazole and tinidazole can cause

nausea, vomiting, metallic taste, and a disulfiram-like reaction if alcohol is consumed.
- **On the CCS,** remember to "advise patient, no alcohol."
- **On the CCS,** you do not have to know the drug doses on the exam, but you should know the duration of treatment.

## CANDIDA VULVOVAGINITIS

Candida vulvovaginitis is a fungal infection that is caused by *Candida albicans* in the majority of cases. Nonalbicans species such as *Candida glabrata* and *Candida parapsilosis* can also cause infection, but they generally produce milder symptoms. Candida vulvovaginitis is not considered an STD.

**Risk Factors:**

Broad-spectrum antibiotics, immunosuppression (eg, HIV, glucocorticoids, chemotherapy), diabetes mellitus, high dose estrogen, pregnancy.

**Clinical Features:**

The predominant symptom is pruritus. Patients may also have burning, dysuria, and dyspareunia. On examination, there may be vulvar erythema, edema, and excoriations. The vagina can appear erythematous. Patients may have no discharge, or they may have a thick, white, clumpy "cottage cheese" discharge that usually has no odor. The speculum exam usually reveals a normal cervix. Candida vulvovaginitis can be classified as a complicated or uncomplicated infection. Features of an uncomplicated infection include signs and symptoms that are mild to moderate, sporadic, nonrecurrent, and infection with *Candida albicans*. Features of a complicated infection include signs and symptoms that are severe, recurrent (≥4 infections per year), comorbid conditions (eg, diabetes), and infection that is nonalbicans (eg, *Candida glabrata*).

**Next Step:**

**Step 1)** The clinical diagnosis of Candida vulvovaginitis should be confirmed with further testing. The diagnosis can be confirmed with a wet mount of the discharge and adding 10% KOH to the prep, which will dissolve the epithelial cells leaving behind the hyphae, pseudohyphae, or buds. Consider the following adjunctive tests that can be used to support the diagnosis.

- Vaginal pH between 4.0 and 4.5 (ie, basically a normal pH).
- Negative whiff test (no odor).
- Cultures can be performed in recurrent infections or the absence of hyphae, pseudohyphae, or buds on KOH prep but with a high clinical suspicion for Candida vulvovaginitis.

**Step 2)** Treatment of Candida vulvovaginitis is based on an uncomplicated or complicated infection. Consider the following:

**Uncomplicated Infections**

**Option 1:** Fluconazole (oral) × 1 day

**Option 2:** Clotrimazole (intravaginal cream) × 3 to 7 days

**Option 3:** Miconazole (intravaginal cream) × 3 to 7 days

**Option 4:** Terazol (intravaginal cream) × 3 to 7 days

### Complicated Infections

**Option 1:** Fluconazole (oral) × total of 2 doses on day 1 and then on day 3

**Option 2:** Clotrimazole (intravaginal cream) × 7 to 14 days

### Follow-Up:

Patients with comorbid conditions (eg, poorly controlled diabetes, HIV) may require a follow-up if symptoms persist. Patients may require risk factor modification (eg, improve glycemic control) and cultures if not previously performed. It should be noted that *Candida species* other than *Candida albicans* are often resistant to azole-based antifungal agents.

### Pearls:

- Sexual partners of affected women do not have to be treated.

- Low-dose estrogen oral contraceptives do not appear to increase the risk of Candida vulvovaginitis.

- Caution is advised in using boric acid for recurrent Candida vulvovaginitis. Boric acid can lead to a fatal outcome if ingested. Since it can be toxic if absorbed systemically, the medication is encapsulated and given via suppository.

- **Foundational point**—*Candida glabrata* generally does not form hyphae or pseudohyphae, but rather buds on KOH prep.

- **On the CCS,** "Candida smear, vaginal secretions" and "wet mount, vaginal secretions" are both available in the practice CCS, but they are considered two distinct orders.

- **On the CCS,** you should be able to know when to use the "continuous" or "one time/bolus" mode of frequency when prescribing a medication.

# BREAST

## ▌ BREAST CANCER

Breast cancer is the second leading cause of cancer death in women in the United States. Most breast cancers arise from malignant proliferation of the epithelial cells lining the ducts or lobules of the breast. Breast cancer can be classified as invasive or noninvasive (in situ) which depends on whether the cancer cells have infiltrated surrounding tissue or are confined by their natural boundaries, respectively (see Table 9-1).

### Risk Factors:

Early menarche (<12 years old), late menopause (>55 years old), advancing age, nulliparity, late age of first term pregnancy (>30 years old), oral contraceptive (current or prior use), current use of hormone replacement therapy (estrogen + progestin), family history of breast cancer (first-degree relatives, and the risk is even higher with additional first-degrees affected or an earlier diagnosis of breast cancer in the first-degrees), breast-ovarian cancer syndrome defined by BRCA1 and BRCA2 genes, personal history of invasive breast cancer, personal history of noninvasive breast cancer (DCIS or LCIS), personal history of

| Table 9-1 • Histologic Types of Breast Cancer | | |
|---|---|---|
| Type | High Yield Features | Foundational Points |
| **Noninvasive Disease** | | |
| Ductal carcinoma in situ (DCIS) | • Confined to the mammary ducts.<br>• Divided into comedo and noncomedo subtypes.<br>• Prognosis is worse for comedo types.<br>• Considered a precursor to invasive ductal carcinoma.<br>• Fivefold risk for invasive breast cancer.<br>• Subsequent invasive breast cancer is usually in the ipsilateral breast.<br>• May be detected as an incidental finding. | • Histologically, comedo DCIS typically have central necrosis in the duct, which can calcify. |
| Lobular carcinoma in situ (LCIS) | • Considered a marker for increased risk of breast cancer rather than a direct precursor lesion.<br>• White women >black women<br>• Average age at diagnosis is in the mid 40s.<br>• The risk of subsequent invasive breast cancer is approximately 1% per year.<br>• Subsequent invasive breast cancer occurs in 25%-35% of women with LCIS.<br>• Subsequent invasive breast cancer can be ductal or lobular in origin.<br>• Subsequent invasive breast cancer can be ipsilateral or contralateral.<br>• May be detected as an incidental finding. | • LCIS usually presents in the terminal ducts or ductules (acini).<br>• Signet-ring cells that contain mucin are frequently present. |

**Table 9-1 • (Continued)**

| Type | High Yield Features | Foundational Points |
|---|---|---|
| **Invasive Disease** | | |
| Infiltrating ductal carcinoma | • Most common invasive lesion (70%-80%).<br>• Tumor is usually hard (scirrhous carcinoma).<br>• Tendency to metastasize via lymphatics. | • Histologically, tumor cells can be seen in nests or cords that infiltrate the stroma. |
| Infiltrating lobular carcinoma | • Second most common type of invasive breast cancer (5%-10%).<br>• Seen in older women.<br>• Tend to be bilateral.<br>• Tend to be multicentric.<br>• Metastasize to odd places (eg, ovary, uterus, meninges, GI tract). | • Associated with E-cadherin mutations.<br>• Signet-ring cells are common.<br>• Usually ER-positive. |
| Paget's disease of the breast | • Accounts for approximately 1%-3% of breast cancers.<br>• Associated with an underlying in situ lesion (usually DCIS) and/or invasive breast cancer (usually HER2-positive) 85%-88% of the time. | • Histologically, the presence of malignant intraepithelial adenocarcinoma cells (Paget cells) within the epidermis of the nipple. |
| Inflammatory breast cancer | • Accounts for <2% of invasive breast cancers.<br>• Aggressive cancer.<br>• High risk for metastases.<br>• Black women >white women<br>• Early age of diagnosis in women, but older age of diagnosis in men. | • Histologically, dermal lymphatic invasion by malignant cells. |

benign breast disease (ie, atypical hyperplasia or proliferative lesions with atypia), dense breast tissue compared to women of the same age category, tall women, obesity in postmenopausal women (BMI ≥30 kg/m²), alcohol (>2 drinks/dy), ionizing radiation to the chest (especially at a young age).

## Clinical Features:

Patients may be asymptomatic, especially in the early stages of breast carcinomas or in DCIS and LCIS. In advanced lesions, a breast mass may be apparent. The classic presentation may be described as a hard, irregular, fixed breast mass with skin tethering. **Metastatic lesions** may present with bone pain, coughing or shortness of breath (lung involvement), nausea and jaundice (liver involvement), headache and altered cognition (brain involvement), or lymphadenopathy. **Paget's disease of the breast**, which is the presence of malignant cells within the epidermis of the nipple that can spread to the areola, may present as a scaly, ulcerated, oozing, erythematous, raw lesion involving the nipple and areola. Bloody discharge may be present. Paget's disease is usually unilateral, but bilateral cases have been reported. **Inflammatory breast cancer (IBC)**, which is the presence of malignant cells within the dermal lymphatics, may present with the classic peau d'orange (see Figure 9-2 and Color Plate 10). IBC may also appear as an "inflamed breast" that has a pink-red or purplish hue discoloration of the skin, a warm breast, nipple crusting, and nipple retraction may be present. Since IBC is an aggressive cancer, there is usually lymph node involvement and metastases at the time of presentation.

## Next Step:

**Step 1)** Breast cancer screening recommendations with mammography vary from several different organizations. The overall consensus is that screening should definitely begin by 50 to 69 years of age. The controversy lies within routine screening at 40 to 49 years of age, ≥70 years of age, and the frequency of screening.

In this area of controversy, cancer screening should be individualized, with shared decision-making, and risk and benefits should be discussed. The efficacy of breast self-examination (BSE) is unproven, and the clinical breast examination (CSE) is not standardized. Patients with known genetic predisposition for BRCA1 or BRCA2 mutation should be referred to genetic counseling.

**Step 2)** The screening mammography provides two views of the breast, and if a suspicious lesion is seen, a diagnostic mammography that provides supplemental views may be able to characterize the lesion better. In addition, the ultrasound may be ordered to differentiate between a cyst and a solid mass. A malignant lesion on ultrasound will typically demonstrate irregular borders, solid mass, and internal echoes.

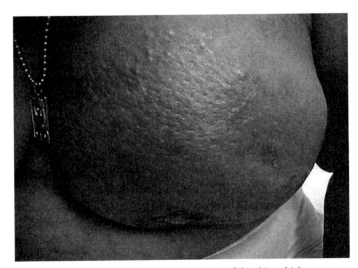

**FIGURE 9-2 • Peau d' orange.** Note the texture of the skin, which appears as an "orange peel." The skin is thickened with enlarged pores secondary to lymphedema. (Reproduced with permission from Usatine RP, Smith MA, Mayeaux EJ Jr, et al. *The Color Atlas of Family Medicine.* 2nd ed. New York: McGraw-Hill; 2013:553.)

**Step 3)** Tissue is the issue. There are many types of biopsy procedures (eg, FNA, core needle biopsy, stereotactic, MRI-guided, wire localization, excisional, incisional, skin punch biopsy), and the choice is dependent on the treating physician. However, it should be noted that additional biopsies are required for Paget's disease (biopsy of the nipple), inflammatory breast cancer (full thickness skin biopsy), and metastases (biopsy of a metastatic lesion). Once the tissue is obtained, the pathologist will look for histologic evidence of malignant disease and assay for estrogen (ER) and progesterone (PR) receptors and human epidermal growth factor 2 (HER2) receptor expression (see Table 9-1). Consider the following common biopsy procedures:

**Fine needle aspiration biopsy (FNA)**—FNA involves a syringe and a needle that essentially draws out the tissue specimen. Unfortunately, FNA cannot differentiate between in situ lesions and invasive cancer.

**Core needle biopsy (CNB)**—Core needle biopsy can be performed instead of the FNA, and the advantage of CNB is that it can differentiate between in situ and invasive cancer.

**Excisional biopsy**—Excisional biopsy can be performed as the initial procedure, but it can also be performed if the core needle biopsy is negative or nondiagnostic but the clinical suspicion is high.

**Step 4)** When 3 assessments (ie, clinical examination, radiographic evaluation, needle biopsy) are used to diagnosis breast cancer, it is referred to as the triple test, and when all three parameters are positive, it is said to be concordant. Patients should proceed to a staging workup to assess the extent of the disease. Typically, patients are staged preoperatively (clinical stage) and postoperatively (pathologic stage). Patients should initially have laboratory studies (eg, CBC, LFTs, alkaline phosphatase). There are no standardized imaging studies, but evaluation for bone, lungs, and liver may be pursued for patients suspected of metastases or locally advanced breast cancers (eg, PET scan, CT, CXR, liver ultrasound, bone scan).

**Step 5)** The treatment approach to patients with breast cancer vary. Consider the following:

### Lobular Carcinoma In Situ (LCIS)

**Step 1)** If LCIS is identified on core needle biopsy, the next best step is to perform an excisional biopsy to exclude an associated malignancy.

**Step 2)** Since LCIS is not viewed as a direct precursor to breast cancer, but rather as a marker of increased risk for invasive breast cancer, it is not necessary to perform a local excision with negative margins. Instead, treatment options include surveillance, chemoprevention with tamoxifen, or bilateral prophylactic mastectomy.

### Ductal Carcinoma In Situ (DCIS)

**Step 1)** Breast-conserving therapy (wide excision with negative margins + radiation). Axillary staging is generally not indicated in DCIS.

**Step 2)** ER-positive patients can be treated with tamoxifen for 5 years. ER-negative patients should have counseling on the use of tamoxifen since the benefits are unclear in this group of patients.

### Early Stage Breast Cancer

Patients in this category can have a tumor size that can potentially be >5 cm, but there is definitely no evidence of tumor extension to the chest wall or skin, fixed or matted nodes, or metastases.

**Step 1)** Preoperatively, in a clinically detected axillary node, an FNA or core biopsy should be taken from the node. If the node is positive, then an axillary node dissection is undertaken at the time of surgery. If the node is negative, then a sentinel lymph node dissection (ie, injecting a dye and radioactive tracer near the lesion, which will identify one or more sentinel lymph nodes) is undertaken at the time of surgery.

**Step 2)** Breast-conserving therapy (BCT) or mastectomy ± radiation. The following are absolute contraindications for BCT:

- Pregnancy
- Prior radiation to the affected breast
- Persistent positive margins
- Diffuse malignant microcalcifications on mammography
- Multicentric disease (ie, ≥2 tumors outside the breast quadrant from the primary tumor)

**Step 3)** Adjuvant systemic therapy may be given. Consider the following:

**Chemotherapy**—Considered in patients that are node-positive, tumor size >1 cm, node-negative of tumor size >0.5 cm plus hormone receptor–negative, node-negative of tumor size >0.5 cm plus HER2-positive, or node-negative of tumor size >0.5 cm plus triple-negative breast cancer (ie, ER/PR-negative and HER2-negative).

**Biologic therapy**—Patients should be given trastuzumab as an IV infusion for patients that are HER2-positive.

**Hormonal therapy**—ER/PR-positive breast cancers may be given tamoxifen for premenopausal women (preferred approach) or an aromatase inhibitor (eg, letrozole, anastrozole, exemestane) for postmenopausal women (ie, improves survival outcomes compared to tamoxifen).

### Locally Advanced Breast Cancer

Patients in this category can have a tumor size that can potentially be >5 cm, may or may not have tumor extending to the chest wall or skin, may or may not have fixed or matted nodes, and definitely no evidence of metastases.

**Step 1)** Neoadjuvant (preoperative) chemotherapy should be given to patients with locally advanced disease. Trastuzumab may be added to the chemotherapy in patients that are HER2-positive.

**Step 2)** Surgery with either a mastectomy or breast-conserving surgery (ie, lumpectomy), which depends on the treatment response from the neoadjuvant therapy and patient preference.

**Step 3)** Postoperative radiation therapy.

**Step 4)** Adjuvant systemic therapy may be given. Adjuvant (postoperative) chemotherapy is generally not given if neoadjuvant chemotherapy was administered. Biologic therapy (eg, trastuzumab) may be resumed postoperatively for 1 year in patients that are HER2-positive, and hormonal therapy may be given to patients that are hormone receptor–positive.

### Metastases

Treatment is not aimed at a curative attempt but rather to improve the quality of life since the median survival is approximately 2 years. Patients have been treated with chemotherapy, hormonal therapy, biologics, surgical intervention (eg, thoracentesis for a pleural effusion), and bisphosphonates (eg, zoledronic acid) for bony metastases.

### Paget Disease of the Breast

Treatment approach is similar to any other invasive breast cancer. Mastectomy has been the traditional standard treatment, but breast-conserving therapy (ie, removal of the lesion plus nipple areolar complex + radiation) is gaining wider acceptance. Patients with an underlying DCIS do not have to undergo axillary node investigation, but patients with an underlying invasive cancer that is node-negative should undergo a sentinel lymph node biopsy, while those with a node-positive should undergo axillary node dissection.

### Inflammatory Breast Cancer

**Step 1)** Neoadjuvant chemotherapy and add trastuzumab to the chemotherapy if HER2-positive.

**Step 3)** Mastectomy (ie, usually modified radical mastectomy that includes axillary dissection since sentinel node biopsy is contraindicated in this breast cancer).

**Step 4)** Postoperative radiation therapy.

**Step 5)** Adjuvant biologic therapy (eg, trastuzumab) may be resumed postoperatively for 1 year in patients that are HER2-positive, and adjuvant hormonal therapy may be given to patients that are hormone receptor–positive.

### Follow-Up:

The cornerstone of surveillance includes the clinical examination and mammography. Asymptomatic cancer survivors do not require an aggressive surveillance that includes laboratory testing (eg, CBC, tumor markers) and radiographic imaging (eg, CXR, ultrasound, PET scans, CT). The 5-year survival rates for early stage breast cancer (stage I-IIB) range from 70% to 95%, local advanced breast cancer (stage IIIA-IIIB) range from 48% to 52%, and metastases (stage IV) is 18%. The 5-year survival for Paget's disease of the breast range from 20% to 60% with an associated palpable mass and 75% to 100% without a palpable mass. The 5-year survival rate for inflammatory breast cancer ranges from 30% to 55%, which is noticeably worse compared to noninflammatory advanced breast cancer.

### Pearls:

- Common sites for breast cancer metastases involve the bone, liver, and lungs. Less than 5% of cases will have CNS involvement as the first site of metastases.

- Premenopausal woman with a BMI $\geq 30$ kg/m$^2$ have a lower risk of breast cancer.

- MRI is not routinely used as a screening modality for breast cancer. The indications for breast MRI are still evolving; however, it is being used as an adjunct to mammography in patients that are at high risk for breast cancer (eg, BRCA mutation). Because of the high cost, MRI is typically used in select cases (eg, patient with axillary adenopathy with an occult tumor).

- The goal of neoadjuvant therapy is to improve surgical outcomes.

- Breast irradiation is contraindicated in pregnancy.

- Patients that generally have an unfavorable prognosis include black women >white women, young or old age at diagnosis, HER2 overexpression in the untreated, nodal involvement, or metastases.

- In the first 5 years following initial diagnosis of breast cancer, it appears that ER-negative cancers have a higher rate of recurrence compared to ER-positive cancers.

- There is a higher risk of recurrence in patients who receive only breast-conserving surgery (eg, lumpectomy) without radiation compared to breast-conserving therapy (BCT).

- The breast-cancer survival rate is nearly equivalent in patients receiving breast-conserving therapy (ie, lumpectomy + radiation) or total mastectomy.

- Simple mastectomy involves removal of the entire breast without removal of the axillary contents or pectoral muscles.

- Modified radical mastectomy involves removal of the breast, underlying fascia of the pectoralis major muscle, and axillary contents, but sparing the pectoralis major muscle.

- Radical mastectomy involves removal of the breast, pectoralis major and minor muscles, and axillary contents.

- Tamoxifen is a selective estrogen receptor modulator (SERM) that is an estrogen receptor antagonist on tumor cells in the breast. However, it may act as an estrogen agonist on the uterus.

- Tamoxifen is approved for breast cancer treatment and breast cancer prevention in premenopausal and postmenopausal women at high risk.

- Tamoxifen can reduce the risk of developing hormone receptor–positive breast cancer in both premenopausal and postmenopausal women, but does not affect improved survival rates.

- Tamoxifen is associated with an increased risk of endometrial cancer, thromboembolic events, hot flashes, vaginal discharge, cataracts, sexual dysfunction, and liver dysfunction, but a protective effect on bone mineral density (BMD) in postmenopausal women.

- Tamoxifen is contraindicated in patients on warfarin therapy and in patients with DCIS or high risk for breast cancer who have a history of thromboembolism. Tamoxifen should also be avoided in pregnancy (category D).

- Raloxifene is a SERM that is an estrogen receptor antagonist on the breast and uterus, but has estrogenic effects on the bone ($\uparrow$ bone density) and lipids ($\downarrow$ LDL).

- Raloxifene is approved for postmenopausal osteoporosis and breast cancer prevention in postmenopausal women at high risk for invasive breast cancer.

- Raloxifene can reduce the risk of developing hormone receptor–positive breast cancer, but does not affect improved survival rates.

- Raloxifene is associated with hot flashes and thromboembolic events, but no increased risk in endometrial cancer.

- Raloxifene is contraindicated in patients with a history of thromboembolic disorders.

- Aromatase inhibitors (eg, letrozole, anastrozole, exemestane) lead to a reduction in circulating estrogen by inhibiting the peripheral conversion of androgens to estrogens.

- Aromatase inhibitors are approved for breast cancer treatment but not for breast cancer prevention.

- Aromatase inhibitors demonstrate improved outcomes in hormone receptor–positive postmenopausal women compared to tamoxifen.

- Aromatase inhibitors are associated with an increased risk of fractures, decrease bone mineral density (osteoporosis), hypercholesterolemia, hot flashes, and cardiac events (eg, MI, angina).

- Aromatase inhibitors are associated with a lower risk of endometrial cancer and venous thrombosis compared to tamoxifen.

- Aromatase inhibitors are contraindicated in pregnancy (category X).

- Trastuzumab is a monoclonal antibody that binds to extracellular HER2 protein, which then mediates antibody-dependent cellular cytotoxicity in cells that overexpress HER2.

- Trastuzumab is approved for breast cancer treatment in patients that are HER2-positive.

- Adding trastuzumab to adjuvant chemotherapy has been shown to have a survival benefit in HER2-positive patients.

- Trastuzumab is associated with cardiomyopathy (ie, CHF and decreased left ventricular ejection fraction [LVEF]).

- There are no contraindications to use trastuzumab.

- Common chemotherapy agents used in breast cancer include doxorubicin, cyclophosphamide, and paclitaxel.

- Ovarian function cessation is an alternative to tamoxifen therapy in women who defer the risks associated with tamoxifen. Ovarian cessation can be accomplished by ovarian ablation (eg, oophorectomy or pelvic radiation) or ovarian suppression via GnRH agonists (eg, goserelin) with the end goal of reducing estrogen levels. When considering childbearing, ovarian suppression would be the better choice for women who want to continue to have children, while ovarian ablation would be acceptable for women who have completed childbearing.

- **On the CCS,** remember to order an oncology consult if you're going to use chemotherapy. You are managing the patient through the eyes of a primary care physician.

- **On the CCS,** upon establishing a diagnosis of breast cancer, remember to "advise patient, cancer diagnosis."

# ENDOCRINE DISORDERS

## ENDOMETRIOSIS

Endometriosis is characterized by the presence of endometrial glands and stroma at extrauterine sites. The ectopic implants can occur at almost any place within the body. The ovaries are the most common site, but other locations include the anterior and posterior cul-de-sac, posterior broad ligaments, uterosacral ligaments, uterus, fallopian tubes, sigmoid colon, appendix, round ligaments, vagina, cervix, cecum, abdominal scars, kidney, ureter, and bladder. The etiology is unclear.

Risk Factors:

**Increased risk**—Early menarche, nulliparity, late menopause, prolonged menses, short menstrual cycles, family history (first-degree relatives)

**Decreased risk**—Late menarche, increased parity

Clinical Features:

Approximately one-third of patients will be asymptomatic. Symptomatic patients may present with a pattern recognition of secondary dysmenorrhea, deep dyspareunia, subfertility, heavy or irregular bleeding, chronic fatigue, or back pain. Keep in mind that the cyclic pain that the patient feels is correlated with menses. Since endometriosis can affect almost any organ, clinical manifestations can vary such as the gastrointestinal tract (eg, dyschezia, hematochezia, diarrhea, constipation, abdominal pain, bloating) or the urinary tract (eg, dysuria, hematuria, urinary frequency). On examination, possible findings include tender nodules along the uterosacral ligament or posterior cul-de-sac. Thickening of the uterosacral ligaments. The uterus may be painful upon movement, and it may be fixed in the retroverted position. The ovaries may be enlarged, tender, and fixed. Prior surgical scars may be tender at the time of menstruation.

Next Step:

**Step 1)** A presumptive clinical diagnosis of endometriosis can be initially managed with empiric medical therapy. It should be noted that the primary modality for diagnosing endometriosis is by direct visualization of the implants via laparoscopy. However, since the procedure is invasive, it is often limited in the initial management. Asymptomatic patients can be managed expectantly. NSAIDs and/or oral estrogen-progestin contraceptives can be attempted for mild pelvic pain for 3 to 6 months.

**Step 2)** Patients that continue to have pain despite NSAIDs or OCPs can be managed with other hormonal therapies. Consider the following:

**GnRH agonists**—Leuprolide can be given as an IM injection once a month or every 3 months (ie, higher dosage) for a 6-month course of treatment. Retreatment can be extended to another 6-month course of treatment if add-back therapy with estrogen-progestin is given. Alternatives to leuprolide include nafarelin, which is administered intranasally, or goserelin, which is administered SubQ every 28 days for a maximum treatment duration of 6 months.

**Progestins**—Progestins induce decidualization and atrophy of the endometrial tissue. Medroxyprogesterone can be given as an IM injection every 3 months for up to 12 months, or norethindrone acetate can be administered orally for 6 to 9 months.

**Steroid analogue**—Danazol has antigonadotropic activity. It suppresses FSH and LH, which causes atrophy of the endometrial tissue. It is administered orally and can be given for up to 9 months. Since there are adverse side effects (eg, acne, oily skin, hirsutism, weight gain, hot flashes, depression, emotional lability, breast atrophy), it has fallen out of favor as a first-line agent.

**Step 3)** Patients that are refractory to medical management are candidates for a diagnostic laparoscopy and therapeutic treatment. Upon laparoscopy, the diagnosis can be confirmed by visualizing the implants and obtaining a biopsy. The classic lesions are described as a "powder-burn" or "gunshot" lesions. However, the lesions can vary in their color from blue-black, red, white, brown, yellow, clear, or pink. Surgery can be divided into conservative (eg, lysis of adhesions, implant resection) or definitive (eg, TAH-BSO). Definitive surgical therapy would be ideal in patients that have completed their childbearing and who continue to have unbearable symptoms despite other forms of treatment.

### Follow-Up:

Endometriosis is typically a chronic and progressive disease that can cause significant morbidity. Patients may require ongoing follow-ups since the duration of medical therapy is restricted (eg, GnRH agonists, progestins, danazol) except for oral contraceptives. In addition, patients that elect to do conservative surgery may have recurrence of their endometriosis, and postoperative adhesion formation can occur.

### Pearls:

- Most patients with endometriosis have elevated CA-125 levels.
- The degree of visible endometriosis is not correlated with the severity of symptoms.
- Patients with endometriosis are not completely infertile. Problems with fertility may be attributable to pelvic adhesions, distorted anatomy, or endometriomas. Management of subfertility involves a multi-interventional approach (eg, clomiphene, in vitro fertilization, intrauterine insemination, expectant management, surgery).
- Medical treatment of minimal to mild endometriosis does not lead to a higher rate of pregnancy compared to expectant management.

- Symptoms of endometriosis often improve during pregnancy and menopause. However, symptoms can recur after menopause, but most are related to postmenopausal hormone replacement therapy.
- *Endometriomas* refers to ovarian endometriosis that becomes cystic. The cysts contain a brown thick fluid, sometimes referred to as a "chocolate cyst." Patients can be asymptomatic, or the cysts can be painful with the potential to rupture.
- Imaging studies are not very helpful in the primary diagnosis of endometriosis. Ultrasound may be helpful in detecting an endometrioma. CT scans and MRI are not routinely performed because of nonspecific findings on CT and the questionable cost-effectiveness of an MRI.
- **Foundational point**—On histology, the two major findings are the presence of endometrial glands and endometrial stroma. Sometimes, hemosiderin-laden macrophages may be present.
- **On the CCS**, if you decide to treat with oral contraceptives for endometriosis, an acceptable option is with the "OCP, low estrogen/low progestin" in the continuous mode of frequency.

## ▌POLYCYSTIC OVARIAN SYNDROME

Polycystic ovarian syndrome (PCOS) is characterized by a complex, diverse group of disorders of uncertain etiology. The principal features include hyperandrogenism, menstrual dysfunction, ovarian abnormalities, and metabolic abnormalities.

### Risk Factors:

Family history (first-degree relatives), diabetes mellitus type 1 and type 2, insulin resistance, antiepileptics (eg, valproic acid).

### Clinical Features:

Patients with PCOS can present with a variety of clinical manifestations. Consider the following:

**Hyperandrogenism**—Patients can develop hirsutism (excessive hair) along the upper lip, chin, periareolar, or linea alba. Excessive androgen can also result in male pattern baldness (ie, androgenetic alopecia), acne, voice deepening, clitoromegaly, or increased muscle mass.

**Menstrual dysfunction**—Patients can develop secondary amenorrhea, oligomenorrhea, anovulation, or ovulation-related infertility. Menstrual irregularities frequently present at the time of menarche (ie, teenage years).

**Ovarian abnormalities**—Polycystic ovaries with multiple peripheral follicles may be seen in patients with PCOS, but not all patients.

**Metabolic abnormalities**—Patients may develop type 2 diabetes, hyperinsulinemia, insulin resistance, acanthosis nigricans (possible sign of insulin resistance), dyslipidemia, metabolic syndrome, or obesity (approximately 50% of patients with PCOS are obese).

**Sleep apnea**—Sleep apnea is a common finding in PCOS. Patients should be asked about excessive daytime somnolence.

## Next Step:

**Step 1)** The Rotterdam criteria can be used to make the diagnosis of PCOS. It requires 2 out of 3 of the following:

- Oligo-ovulation and/or anovulation
- Clinical and/or biochemical signs of hyperandrogenism
- Polycystic ovaries (by transvaginal ultrasound)

**Step 2)** Disorders that mimic PCOS should be excluded; this principal is based on the NIH criteria. Consider the following adjunctive testing to rule out other conditions:

**TSH**—Rule out thyroid disorders

**β-hCG**—Rule out pregnancy in a female with amenorrhea or oligomenorrhea

**Serum prolactin level**—Rule out hyperprolactinemia as a cause of menstrual irregularities

**Serum IGF-1**—Rule out acromegaly as cause of menstrual irregularities or hirsutism

**24-hour urine cortisol level + low-dose dexamethasone suppression test**—Rule out Cushing's syndrome

**Total and free testosterone level**—Elevated levels indicate androgen excess

**Serum DHEA-S level**—Elevated levels suggests an adrenal androgen-secreting tumor

**Serum 17-hydroxyprogesterone level**—Elevated levels suggest nonclassic (late-onset) congenital adrenal hyperplasia secondary to 21-hydroxylase deficiency, which typically presents with hirsutism, acne, and menstrual irregularities.

**ACTH (cosyntropin) stimulation test**—Elevated 17-hyroxyprogesterone confirms the diagnosis of nonclassic congenital adrenal hyperplasia.

**Step 3)** Once the other disorders are excluded, the next best step is to assess the patient's risk for diabetes and dyslipidemia.

**Fasting lipid profile**—Patients typically demonstrate a high LDL, low HDL, and high triglycerides.

**Two-hour OGTT**—A 75-gram oral glucose tolerance test should be performed. A fasting glucose or hemoglobin A1C are acceptable alternatives.

**Step 4)** Treatment of PCOS depends on the specific clinical problem that the patient presents. Consider the following:

### Hyperandrogenism

**Step 1)** Estrogen-progestin contraceptives are considered first-line agents for patients that do not want to become pregnant. The estrogen component can increase sex-hormone binding globulin (SHBG) levels, which can ultimately decrease free testosterone levels.

**Step 2)** Patients that do not respond to OCPs in 6 months may add an antiandrogen to the regimen such as spironolactone or finasteride.

### Menstrual Dysfunction

Patients with anovulation, oligomenorrhea, or amenorrhea are at risk of endometrial cancer because of chronic unopposed estrogen. Endometrial protection should include progestin to prevent endometrial hyperplasia. Consider the following options:

**Option 1:** Estrogen-progestin contraceptives can provide endometrial protection, contraception, and reduce symptoms of hyperandrogenism.

**Option 2:** Progestin-only (eg, medroxyprogesterone acetate) can be given to patients that have a contraindication to estrogen-progestin contraceptives. It may be given intermittently as an oral administration for 7 to 10 days every 1 to 2 months. However, it will not provide contraception in this format of administration. Neither will it provide relief of hyperandrogenism since it lacks the estrogen component, but it will provide endometrial protection.

### Anovulatory Infertility

**Step 1)** Weight loss.

**Step 2)** If no response, clomiphene citrate.

**Step 3)** If no response, consider exogenous gonadotropins, laparoscopic ovarian surgery, or metformin in patients with coexisting glucose intolerance.

### Obesity

Diet, exercise, and weight loss.

### Type 2 Diabetes Mellitus

Management is similar to patients without PCOS.

### Dyslipidemia

Management is similar to patients without PCOS (see Table 3-3).

## Follow-Up:

PCOS is a complex disorder that usually requires ongoing follow-ups for complications and sequelae associated with the condition. Patients that were initially negative for impaired glucose tolerance or type 2 diabetes should be periodically reassessed. Unfortunately, there is no consensus on monitoring endometrial hyperplasia, but physicians should be cognizant of any abnormal uterine bleeding. Finally, physicians should also be aware of any eating disorders, depression, or anxiety, which patients with PCOS are prone to experience.

## Pearls:

- Patients with PCOS have low levels of sex hormone binding globulin (SHBG) secondary from hyperandrogenism and hyperinsulinemia.
- Patients with PCOS are at risk of developing gestational diabetes during pregnancy.
- OCPs can decrease luteinizing hormone (LH) secretion resulting in a decrease in ovarian androgen secretion.

- Patients with PCOS typically have elevated LH levels and an FSH that may be normal or low, which can lead to an elevated LH:FSH ratio greater than 3:1. It is unnecessary to order an LH nor an LH:FSH ratio in the diagnostic evaluation of PCOS.
- Normal LH levels do not exclude the diagnosis of PCOS.
- **Foundational point**—Elevated levels of LH can induce secretion of androstenedione from ovarian theca cells. Androstenedione is a precursor to testosterone. Once it is converted to testosterone, the testosterone can be converted to the more potent androgen dihydrotestosterone (DHT) by the enzyme 5α-reductase.
- **Foundational point**—Finasteride is a 5α-reductase inhibitor.
- **Foundational point**—On cut section of a polycystic ovary, the ovary is usually enlarged, there is a dense stroma, and follicular cysts are arranged along the periphery of the ovary.
- **Connecting point** (pg. 68)—Know the other causes of hyperprolactinemia.
- **Connecting point** (pg. 66)—Know the management of acromegaly.
- **Connecting point** (pg. 76)—Know the workup for Cushing's syndrome.
- **Connecting point** (pg. 79)—Know how to make the diagnosis of diabetes mellitus.
- **Connecting point** (pg. 23, 24)—Know how to manage a patient with hyperlipidemia and know the components of the metabolic syndrome.
- **On the CCS**, this type of case would be a complicated case, but remember that a thorough and comprehensive approach does not necessarily reduce your score unless you order something that poses a risk to your patient. Keep in mind that there are multiple correct algorithms to achieving a good score, but you want to try to manage your patients by ordering relevant items based on the history, physical exam, patient updates, or updated lab or imaging findings.

# Hematology

## KEYWORDS REVIEW

**Acanthocytes**—Also referred to as spur cells, which are spiculated red cells with irregular projections of varying sizes distributed throughout the cell and seen in liver disease and abetalipoproteinemia.

**Anisocytosis**—Variation in the size of red blood cells as seen on peripheral blood smear.

**Aplastic anemia**—Aplastic anemia can be characterized as bone marrow failure resulting in pancytopenia and bone marrow hypocellularity.

**Basophilic stippling**—Blue granules seen in the RBC representing ribosomal precipitates that occur in lead poisoning, thalassemias, and alcohol abuse.

**Bite cells**—The appearance of a "bite" on the RBC due to the removal of Heinz bodies by spleen phagocytes.

**Echinocytes**—Also referred to as burr cells, spiculated red cells with more uniform, evenly spaced projections compared to acanthocytes, seen in liver disease and end-stage renal disease.

**Heinz bodies**—Denatured hemoglobin found in RBCs, commonly seen in patients with G6PD deficiency following oxidative stress.

**Hemosiderin**—The intracellular storage of iron as opposed to circulating in the blood.

**Howell-Jolly bodies**—Cytoplasmic inclusions within RBCs representing nuclear remnants that are normally removed by the spleen. Howell-Jolly bodies are often found after a splenectomy or splenic dysfunction.

**Hypochromic**—Pertaining to low hemoglobin content in the RBCs.

MCHC—Mean corpuscular hemoglobin concentration reflects the hemoglobin concentration per given volume of RBCs. A low MCHC will usually have cells that are *hypochromic*, normal MCHC levels will have cells as *normochromic*, and elevated MCHC levels will have cells as *hyperchromic*.

Poikilocytosis—Variation in red blood cell shapes such as a spur cell, target cell, sickle cell, or schistocyte.

Rouleaux—RBCs "stacking" on top of each other as seen in the peripheral blood smear of multiple myeloma patients.

RPI—Reticulocyte production index is a doubly corrected reticulocyte count, which corrects for the anemia and reticulocyte maturation time. An RPI value close to 1.0 is considered normal.

Schistocyte—Fragmented helmet-shaped RBCs seen in microangiopathic hemolytic anemia, artificial heart valves, and malignant hypertension.

Sideroblastic anemia—Production of ringed sideroblasts (ie, a ring of iron deposits along the nucleus of an erythroblast as seen with Prussian blue stain) from the bone marrow which can be due to acquired or congenital causes.

Smudge cells—When fragile lymphocytes are smeared on a glass slide, the cells appear "smudged," which is characteristic of chronic lymphoid leukemia (CLL).

Spherocyte—RBCs that are sphere-shaped without central pallor, commonly seen in hereditary spherocytosis or autoimmune hemolytic anemia.

Target cell—RBCs with a central hyperchromic density with a halo of pallor that appears as a "bull's-eye," commonly seen in thalassemia, iron deficiency, liver disease, post splenectomy, and hemoglobinopathies (eg, Hb D).

Tear-shaped RBC—Also referred to as a dacrocyte, can be seen in myelofibrosis, myelodysplastic syndromes, severe iron deficiency, thalassemias, and hemolytic anemias.

# ANEMIA

## OVERVIEW OF ANEMIA

Anemia is an important indicator of disease. There are a variety of underlying causes and several ways to classify anemia. It may be helpful to broadly divide anemia into problems of production or problems of destruction and accelerated blood loss (hemorrhage). See Figure 10-1.

## IRON-DEFICIENCY ANEMIA

A finding of iron-deficiency anemia can be due to an **increase in iron loss** (eg, blood loss from menses, GI tract, or blood donation), **decrease in iron intake** (eg, inadequate diet, malabsorption, iron sequestration such as pulmonary hemosiderosis), or an **increase in demand for iron** (eg, pregnancy, infancy, adolescence).

Clinical Features:

Patients with iron-deficiency anemia may present with the anemia itself such as fatigue, pallor, reduced exercise tolerance, or poor feeding (infants). Commonly associated signs and symptoms of iron-deficiency anemia include:

**Neurologic**—Behavioral and neurodevelopmental disturbances seen in the young.
**Mouth**—Fissures at the corner of the mouth (cheilosis or angular stomatitis).
**Tongue**—Glossitis will present as a smooth tongue.
**Nails**—Koilonychia will present as spooning of the fingernails.

**Pica**—Patients may have an unusual appetite for certain substances such as ice (pagophagia), dirt (geophagia), hair (trichophagia), or starch (amylophagia).

Next Step:

**Step 1)** Diagnosis of iron-deficiency anemia is primarily a laboratory diagnosis. Order a **CBC**, which will also include the MCV, MCHC, and RDW, but not the reticulocyte count. In addition, order an **iron panel**, which will include serum iron, total iron binding capacity (ie, transferrin), and ferritin levels (see Table 10-1).

**Step 2)** Management of iron-deficiency anemia is to identify and treat the underlying cause of the iron-deficiency anemia. First-line treatment for iron-deficiency anemia is with **oral iron therapy** (eg, ferrous sulfate). With the appropriate dosage, the reticulocyte count should increase within 4 to 7 days after starting therapy, and the hemoglobin level should increase 1 g/dL every 2 to 3 weeks while on iron therapy. Intravenous iron therapy should be limited to patients with intolerance to oral iron, refractory to oral iron, dialysis patients, and patients with inflammatory bowel disease. In the pediatric population, if the anemia is not severe (ie, Hb <7) and a presumptive diagnosis of iron-deficiency anemia is made along with laboratory studies indicating a microcytic anemia, a therapeutic trial of iron therapy can be started.

Follow-Up:

It can take up to 2 to 4 months for iron stores to return back to baseline while on oral iron therapy. Deciding to continue for another 3 to 6 months of iron therapy should be individualized with each patient. Children on a therapeutic trial of iron should be seen in 4 weeks. If the microcytic anemia fails to respond to iron therapy, further workup is warranted (eg, stool hemoccult, reticulocyte count, peripheral blood smear, vitamin $B_{12}$ levels, folate levels, Hb electrophoresis).

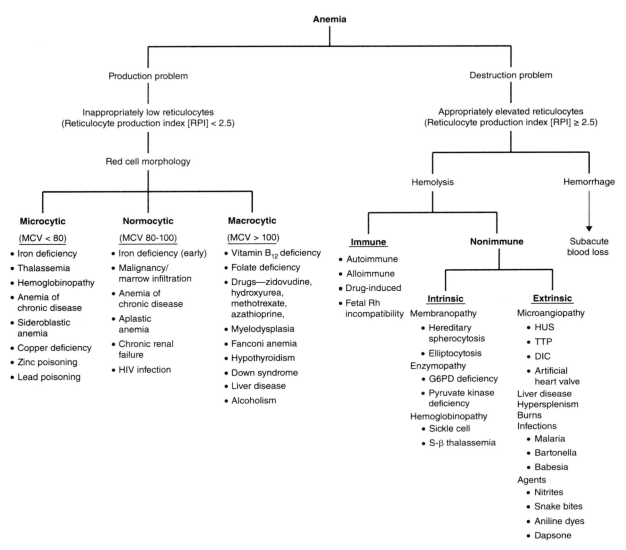

**FIGURE 10-1 • Overview of anemia.**

Pearls:

- Iron absorption occurs at the level of the duodenum and proximal jejunum.
- Iron absorption is reduced in the presence of tannates (eg, tea), phytates (eg, bran, cereal, oats, rye fiber), phosphates, and medications (eg, proton pump inhibitors, antacids, histamine H2 blockers).
- Iron absorption is enhanced in the presence of ascorbic acid, meat, fish, and poultry.

- Serum ferritin is the most useful indicator of iron-deficiency anemia because it has a very high sensitivity and specificity. However, interpretation should be adjusted accordingly in the setting of infectious or inflammatory conditions because ferritin is an acute-phase reactant. In some cases, a C-reactive protein (CRP) is added to the order to validate the results of the ferritin levels.
- Plummer-Vinson syndrome, also referred to as Paterson-Kelly syndrome, can be characterized by **iron-deficiency anemia**, and **esophageal webs** causing **dysphagia**.

| Table 10-1 • Laboratory Differentiation from Iron-deficiency Anemia | | | | |
|---|---|---|---|---|
| Parameter | Iron-deficiency Anemia | Anemia of Chronic Disease | Sideroblastic Anemia | Thalassemia |
| Serum Iron | ↓ | ↓ | Normal to high | Normal to high |
| Serum Ferritin | ↓ | Normal to high | Normal to high | Normal to high |
| TIBC (Transferrin) | ↑ | Normal to low | Normal | Normal |
| % Transferrin Saturation | ↓ | Normal to low | Normal to high | Normal to high |

- Transferrin is a protein that binds to iron and circulates in the plasma. The TIBC is a laboratory test that indirectly measures the transferrin.

- Serum transferrin receptor (sTfR) is a protein released into circulation, with elevated levels are seen in iron-deficient states.

- Protoporphyrin is involved in the intermediate steps to heme synthesis. Elevated levels of protoporphyrin are seen in iron deficiency and lead poisoning.

- Red cell volume distribution width (RDW) is a measure of the variation in RBC size (anisocytosis). An elevated RDW is commonly seen in deficiencies in iron, vitamin $B_{12}$, and folate.

- The Mentzer index (ie, MCV/RBC count) is sometimes used to differentiate between iron-deficiency anemia and thalassemia. A Mentzer index >13 suggests iron-deficiency anemia, while a value <13 suggests a thalassemia.

- Iron-deficiency anemia during pregnancy is mainly due to plasma volume expansion relative to hemoglobin mass. Although most prenatal vitamins contain iron, sometimes iron is given in the second or third trimester to augment maternal hemoglobin.

- **Connecting point** (pg. 186)—Part of the presumptive diagnosis in children with iron-deficiency anemia is to determine if the child (<1 years old) is consuming whole cow's milk because it can cause intestinal bleeding and it is low in iron content.

- **On the CCS**, if you want the iron panel, you have to order it separately such as "Iron, serum with/TIBC" and "Ferritin, serum." The practice CCS software does not recognize "iron panel" in the order menu.

- **On the CCS**, the practice CCS software will recognize an order for "reticulocyte count" but does not recognize "reticulocyte production index (RPI)."

- **On the CCS**, the "CBC with differential" will provide you results of the CBC, WBC differential, and peripheral blood smear.

- **On the CCS**, consider a stool hemoccult in an adult since the premise of iron deficiency in an adult is a GI bleed until proven otherwise.

- **On the CCS**, any child who presents with iron deficiency should have a blood lead level to screen for lead toxicity if it was not already completed by routine screening.

- **On the CCS**, remember to "advise patient, side effects of medication" since oral iron can cause nausea, vomiting, GI upset, constipation, and diarrhea.

# HEMOGLOBINOPATHIES

## ▌ ALPHA THALASSEMIA

Alpha ($\alpha$) thalassemia is due to a deletion or mutation in one or more of the four alpha globin genes (ie, aa/aa). This results in an underproduction of alpha globin chains, but a relative excess of gamma ($\gamma$)-globin chains in the fetus and newborn and beta ($\beta$)-globin chains in children and adults.

### Clinical and Hematologic Features:

The signs, symptoms, and test results will differ, depending on how many alpha alleles are affected:

**1 alpha defect** (−a/aa)—Also referred to as a silent carrier, alpha thalassemia minima, or alpha thalassemia-2 trait. These patients will be asymptomatic and hematologically are normal. Hemoglobin electrophoresis will be normal (ie, normal levels of HbA, HbA2, HbF).

**2 alpha defects** (cis deletion aa/−−, or trans deletion a−/a−)—Also referred to as alpha thalassemia minor or alpha thalassemia-1 trait. Asians will commonly carry the cis deletion, while people of African origin will carry the trans deletion. Most patients will have **mild anemia** with the blood smear demonstrating **microcytosis**, **hypochromia**, and **target cells**. Hemoglobin electrophoresis will be normal.

**3 alpha defects** (a−/−−)—Also referred to as hemoglobin H (HbH) disease, which is composed of 4 beta chains forming an unstable tetramer. In the later stages of erythropoiesis, HbH will precipitate and form inclusion bodies within the red blood cells, which will result in moderate to severe **chronic hemolytic anemia**. Other findings may include **variable bony changes**, **splenomegaly**, and **neonatal jaundice**. Hemoglobin electrophoresis will typically demonstrate a higher percentage of Hb Barts ($\gamma_4$) at birth, but a higher percentage of HbH ($\beta_4$) in older children and adults.

**4 alpha defects** (−−/−−)—Also referred to as alpha thalassemia major or hydrops fetalis with Hb Barts. At this point, there are no alpha chains. Instead, there is an excess of gamma ($\gamma$) globin chains forming tetramers or Hb Barts ($\gamma_4$) that will have such a high oxygen affinity that it shifts the oxygen dissociation curve to the left. As a result, almost no oxygen is delivered to the fetus, which causes asphyxia, massive total body edema (hydrops fetalis), high-output congestive heart failure, and **death in utero** or shortly after birth. Hemoglobin electrophoresis will show the presence of Hb Barts ($\gamma_4$), HbH ($\beta_4$), Hb Portland ($Z_2\gamma_2$) and the complete absence of HbA, HbA2, and HbF.

### Next Step:

**Step 1)** Diagnosis of alpha thalassemia is usually one of exclusion. However, begin with laboratory testing such as a CBC and ferritin levels (see Table 10-1). Alpha thalassemia is commonly mistaken for iron-deficiency anemia, and it is important to differentiate the two conditions because supplemental iron therapy can cause iron overload resulting in secondary hemochromatosis in patients with alpha thalassemia. Other diagnostic testing includes a peripheral blood smear and staining with a supravital dye such as brilliant cresyl blue to detect inclusion bodies as seen in HbH disease.

**Step 2)** Hemoglobin electrophoresis may be helpful when alpha thalassemia is still suspected.

**Step 3)** There is no specific therapy for silent carriers or alpha thalassemia minor. Alpha thalassemia major is incompatible with extrauterine life. Similar to G6PD deficiency, HbH disease may have exacerbations of hemolytic anemia when exposed to oxidant stress such as infection or drugs (eg, sulfa). During these periods, transfusions may be required along with iron chelation (eg, deferoxamine). In time, patients with HbH disease may require a splenectomy if transfusion requirements are increased or if there is excessive anemia.

**Step 4)** Genetics counseling should be offered.

### Follow-Up:

Patients undergoing chronic transfusion therapy should have close follow-up to ensure that the patient is not iron overloaded.

### Pearls:

- **Foundational point**—Hemoglobin F (ie, $\alpha_2\gamma_2$) is the predominant hemoglobin during fetal development and decreases significantly after 6 months of life. It is only 1% to 2% of the hemoglobin in adults.

- **Foundational point**—Hemoglobin A (ie, $\alpha_2\beta_2$) is the predominant form of hemoglobin in adults and children >6 months of life.

- **Foundational point**—Hemoglobin A2 (ie, $\alpha_2\delta_2$) is composed of two alpha chains and two delta chains. It is a minor component of hemoglobin and is <3% of the total hemoglobin found in adults.

- **Foundational point**—Fetal hemoglobin has a higher affinity for oxygen and will therefore shift the oxygen-hemoglobin dissociation curve to the left.

- **Connecting point** (pg. 176)—Fetal hydrops can also be seen in rhesus incompatibility.

- **Connecting point** (see next section)—HbH disease can resemble beta thalassemia intermedia.

- **On the CCS,** when you order "hemoglobin electrophoresis" in the practice CCS, you will get results of the HbA, HbA2, HbS, and HbF.

## ▌BETA THALASSEMIA

Beta (β) thalassemia is due to a mutation or rarely a deletion of one or both of the two beta globin genes (ie, β/β). This results in an underproduction of beta globin chains, but a relative excess of unstable alpha globin chains. The severity of the anemia depends on whether there is complete absence of beta globin chains ($\beta^\circ$) or decreased production of beta globin chains ($\beta^+$), as well as the gene dosage (ie, homozygous or heterozygous).

Beta thalassemia is commonly found in those of Mediterranean, African, and Asian descent.

### Clinical and Hematological Features:

The signs, symptoms, and test results will differ depending on the quantity and severity of affected beta globin alleles.

**Beta thalassemia minor**—Also referred to as β-thalassemia trait. These patients have one normal beta globin allele and one defective beta globin allele (eg, $\beta/\beta^\circ$ or $\beta/\beta^+$). The majority of these heterozygotes will be **asymptomatic**. Hematologically, they will have a normal RDW, and the peripheral blood smear may demonstrate microcytosis, hypochromia, target cells, tear-shaped RBC, or basophilic stippling. Hemoglobin electrophoresis will classically reveal a predominant HbA, elevated HbA2, and occasional elevations of HbF.

**Beta thalassemia intermedia**—Beta thalassemia intermedia refers to a group of patients with a clinical severity that falls between beta thalassemia minor and beta thalassemia major. The genotype in this category is very heterogeneous because patients in this group can have mild forms of homozygosity (eg, $\beta^+/\beta^+$) to severe forms of heterozygosity (eg, $\beta/\beta^\circ$ or $\beta/\beta^+$). Patients may not have any symptoms until after the first year of life, when they may have moderate anemia with occasional blood transfusions (not necessarily regular blood transfusions). Some of the clinical features include skeletal changes, hepatosplenomegaly, leg ulcers, thrombosis, gallstones, osteoporosis, or pulmonary hypertension.

**Beta thalassemia major**—Also referred to as Cooley's anemia, this is the most severe form of beta thalassemia. At this point, there are no beta globin chains produced (ie, $\beta^\circ/\beta^\circ$) or very small amounts produced (ie, $\beta^+/\beta^+$). In addition, there is an excess of insoluble aggregates of alpha globin chains that precipitate within the cell (Heinz bodies) that ultimately lead to increased hemolysis and ineffective erythropoiesis. Symptoms do not appear in the first 6 month of life because of the presence of HbF. After 6 months, HbA would normally take over, but because there are no beta globin chains patients begin to experience **pallor**, **irritability**, **jaundice**, **abdominal swelling** due to **hepatosplenomegaly**, and **growth retardation**. Soon thereafter, ineffective erythropoiesis causes bone marrow expansion to occur which results in **"chipmunk facies," frontal bossing, prominent malar eminences**, and **"hair-on-end"** or **"crew haircut"** appearance on skull x-ray. Bone changes also occur on long bones, pelvis, and vertebrae. Ineffective erythropoiesis can also result in **extramedullary hematopoiesis** with a mass that can potentially cause a spinal cord compression. After the age of 10, patients will have complications related to chronic iron overload. Common manifestations include **diabetes, heart failure, bronzing of the skin, hypothyroidism**, and **hypogonadism** (ie, delayed onset of primary and secondary sexual development). Patients who have not been transfused regularly will typically die before the third decade of life, and most deaths are due to cardiac-related complications. Hematologically, the peripheral blood smear will be similar to beta thalassemia minor with the addition of increased nucleated RBCs and the presence of inclusion bodies (Heinz bodies), which can be appreciated at this stage with a supravital dye. Patients may have findings of hemolysis, which include ↑ LDH, ↑ indirect bilirubin, and ↓ haptoglobin. Hemoglobin electrophoresis will reveal absent to severely reduced HbA, variable levels of HbA2, and elevated levels of HbF.

### Next Step:

**Step 1)** Diagnosis of beta thalassemia minor may not always be apparent on routine CBC and can commonly be mistaken for iron-deficiency anemia. It should be noted that the MCV of beta thalassemia minor ranges from 55 to 75 fL, with a hematocrit almost always >30%. However, in iron deficiency an MCV is rarely <80 fL until the hematocrit is <30%. Obtaining iron studies (see Table 10-1) is helpful in differentiating between the two conditions and to avoid unnecessarily administrating iron supplements to patients with beta thalassemia. Diagnosis of beta thalassemia intermedia is often made clinically. Patients in this category should be able to maintain a hemoglobin ≥6 to 7 g/dL at the time of diagnosis and do not require regular blood transfusions. The diagnosis of beta thalassemia major is often made earlier because the signs and symptoms are presented earlier. Laboratory studies showing signs of hemolysis, abnormalities on the peripheral blood smear, and staining of inclusion bodies will begin to make the diagnosis of beta thalassemia major apparent.

**Step 2)** Hemoglobin electrophoresis is used to confirm the diagnosis of beta thalassemia. Bone marrow examination is usually not needed to make the diagnosis, but examination will reveal marked erythroid hyperplasia.

**Step 3)** Treatment of beta thalassemia is as follows:

### Beta Thalassemia Major

- **Blood transfusions** are given on a regular basis. Before the first transfusion, hepatitis B vaccination is given and red blood cell antigen typing is carried out.
- **Iron chelation therapy** (eg, deferoxamine) along with careful administration of vitamin C (improves iron chelation) is inevitable in this group of patients.
- **Hematopoietic cell transplantation** (HCT) should be considered in a select group of patients for the possibility of a cure.
- **Splenectomy** is usually required if the transfusion requirements increase >50% or there is growth retardation or symptomatic splenomegaly.

- **Vaccinations** with pneumococcal and Haemophilus vaccines should be given before a splenectomy is anticipated.
- **Prophylactic antibiotics** with penicillin are given to splenectomized patients.
- **Folic acid** supplementation.

### Beta Thalassemia Intermedia

- **Blood transfusions** may be occasionally given when patients become symptomatic (ie, usually Hb <7 g/dL) at such times as an aplastic crisis from parvovirus B19 infections. Eventually, the majority of patients will need chronic blood transfusions by their third or fourth decade of life, which would then classify them as beta thalassemia major.
- **Iron chelation therapy** may be needed when serum ferritin levels exceed 300 µg/L or there is evidence of iron deposition into organs from imaging.
- Splenectomy, vaccinations, prophylactic antibiotics, and folic acid may be needed for the same reasons as beta thalassemia major.

### Beta Thalassemia Minor

- There is no specific therapy for beta thalassemia minor.

**Step 4)** Genetic counseling should be offered since beta thalassemia is inherited in an autosomal recessive manner.

### Follow-Up:

Patients affected with beta thalassemia major need close monitoring that includes assessment of growth and development, ophthalmologic and audiologic exams, cardiac, thyroid, pituitary, and gallbladder evaluations, bone densitometry to assess for osteoporosis, and serum evaluations of ferritin, LFTs, and assessment of glucose intolerance.

### Pearls:

- Iron overload can still occur in patients with beta thalassemia intermedia even without blood transfusions because of increased intestinal absorption of iron secondary to ineffective erythropoiesis.
- **On the CCS**, in nonacute cases, you will be required to advance the time and schedule appointments for the patient; therefore, be sure to have enough practice with the CCS software to be able to advance the time, and yet be aware of the "Simulated time" and "Real time."

# BLEEDING DISORDERS

## ▌HEMOPHILIA

Hemophilia A (factor VIII deficiency) and hemophilia B (factor IX deficiency) are X-linked recessive disorders that occur almost exclusively in males since they have only one X chromosome.

### Clinical Features:

Patients will usually have a family history of hemophilia. Another indicator is excessive bleeding at the time of a circumcision. Hemophilia A and hemophilia B (ie, Christmas disease) are clinically indistinguishable other than therapy. Although bleeding can occur anywhere, common sites for bleeding are into the joints, muscle, and GI tract. However, consider the overall picture of the signs and symptoms, which include from a relative head to toe fashion:

**Neurologic**—Headache, vomiting, lethargy, stiff neck, intracranial hemorrhage (neonates).

**Head and Neck**—Epistaxis, oral bleeding from dental procedures, hemoptysis.

**GI**—Hematemesis, melena, abdominal pain.

**Genitourinary**—Hematuria, circumcision bleeding.

**Joints**—Hemarthrosis.

**Muscle**—Hematoma formation can occur in any of the muscles, with the iliopsoas as the most concerning because of the potential for large volume of blood loss and compression of the femoral nerve.

**Bone**—Pseudotumors may form in bones as a result of unresolved hematomas.

**Dermatologic**—Excessive bruising.

### Next Step:

**Step 1**) Diagnosis of hemophilia can be made by the clinical evaluation and laboratory testing. Expected lab findings include a **normal platelet count**, a **normal PT** (ie, extrinsic cascade), and **elevated activated partial thromboplastin time** (ie, intrinsic cascade). However, patients that have mild hemophilia (see below) may have normal aPTTs.

**Step 2**) A **mixing study** will help determine if the elevated aPTT is due to a clotting factor deficiency or an inhibitor of a factor (ie, IgG antibody). When the patient's blood is mixed with normal blood and the PTT does not correct, then it is most likely an inhibitor and a workup with an inhibitor assay such as the Bethesda assay should be pursued. When the patient's blood is mixed with normal blood and the PTT does correct, then it is most likely a clotting factor deficiency and a workup with factor VIII and IX assays should be pursued. For both hemophilia A and B, the severity of the hemophilia is based on the assay in which severe hemophilia is considered when there is <1% normal factor, moderate hemophilia is 1% to 5% normal factor, and mild hemophilia is >5% normal factor.

**Step 3**) Treatment for hemophilia A or B is with recombinant factor VIII or recombinant factor IX, respectively. Treatment for patients that have inhibitors is more difficult to manage. Since inhibitors are less commonly seen in hemophilia B compared to hemophilia A, further discussion will be based on hemophilia A. Patients that have low-titer inhibitors (ie, low responders) respond well to high doses of factor VIII. Patients that have high-titer inhibitors (ie, high responders) or demonstrate an anamnestic response can be treated with activated prothrombin complex concentrates (aPCC) or with a by passing agent such as activated Factor VII (FVIIa).

**Step 4**) Genetic counseling should be offered to families with a newborn who has hemophilia, especially if there was no family history.

### Disposition:

Admit patients from the ED if the patient is bleeding from the head and neck area or retroperitoneum (eg, iliopsoas bleeds).

### Pearls:

- Hemophilia A affects 1 in 5000 males, which is more common than hemophilia B affecting 1 in 25,000 to 35,000 males.
- Cryoprecipitate (ie, factor VIII, factor XIII, vWF, fibrinogen) is no longer used to treat hemophilia A because of concerns of blood-borne infections such as HIV and hepatitis C.
- Plasma-derived products emerged to reduce the risk of viral transmission, but viruses such as hepatitis A and parvovirus still pose a threat.
- Recombinant products are well-refined products that further reduce the risk of blood-borne infections, but their cost remains fairly high.
- aPCC have been associated with thrombosis, myocardial infarction, and DIC.
- Patients with mild hemophilia A can be treated with desmopressin (DDAVP) because it transiently increases the levels of factor VIII and vWF factor.
- Antifibrinolytics such as ε-aminocaproic acid and tranexamic acid are used to treat oral mucosal hemorrhage. These agents should be avoided in the presence of hematuria because they can cause obstructive uropathy.
- Avoid NSAIDs and aspirin for pain control; instead use acetaminophen.
- Patients should be treated with factor replacement therapy if they are going to have a central line or any other invasive procedure.
- Female carriers can have variable levels of factor VIII or IX and experience mild bleeding. Female carriers will transmit the disease to half of their sons, and half of their daughters will be carriers.
- **Connecting point** (pg. 163)—X-linked recessive disorders will show no male-to-male transmission.
- **CJ:** A patient is being treated with factor replacement therapy at therapeutic doses for a GI bleed, but the therapy does not seem to help. What do you think is wrong? **Answer:** Patients that fail to respond to factor replacement therapy most likely have an inhibitor problem rather than a factor deficiency.
- **On the CCS**, the practice CCS does not recognize "mixing study."
- **On the CCS**, both "plasma factor VIII" and "plasma factor IX" levels are available in the practice CCS.
- **On the CCS**, ordering "factor VIII, therapy" in the practice CCS will automatically be converted to "antihemophilic factor, therapy."
- **On the CCS**, if you want to order factor IX therapy, it will be viewed as "factor IX complex" in the practice CCS.

## VON WILLEBRAND DISEASE

Von Willebrand disease (vWD) is the most common inherited bleeding disorder. Von Willebrand factor (vWF) serves two important roles. First, in the event of vascular injury, vWF binds to the exposed subendothelium and subsequently binds to platelets through the Gp Ib-IX platelet receptor. Second, vWF binds and protects factor VIII from proteolysis within the plasma, thereby increasing the half-life of factor VIII. In essence, von Willebrand disease can affect both the **platelet function** and **coagulation pathway**. There are three inherited types and one acquired type of von Willebrand disease.

**Type 1**—An autosomal dominant disease that can be characterized as a partial quantitative vWF deficiency. Type 1 is the most common type.

**Type 2**—Mainly an autosomal dominant disease, but several subtypes can be autosomal recessive. There are 4 subtypes which include 2A, 2B, 2M, and 2N. Type 2 vWD can be characterized as a qualitative vWF deficiency.

**Type 3**—An autosomal recessive disease that can be characterized as complete vWF deficiency. Type 3 is a rare disease.

**Acquired vWD**—Occurs by several different mechanisms, but can be seen in patients with multiple myeloma, Waldenström's macroglobulinemia, polycythemia vera, MGUS, CML, CLL, SLE, valvular heart disease, and Wilms tumor. Acquired vWD is a rare disease.

### Clinical Features:

In most cases of vWD, symptoms are mild. A family history may be present, but not always (especially with acquired vWD). A medication history of taking aspirin or NSAIDs may precipitate a bleed that would normally not occur. A history of prolonged bleeding during specific events such as dental extractions, tonsillectomy, childbirth, or other medical procedures are clues that something is wrong. Common sites of bleeding include mucous membranes (eg, nosebleeds, gingival bleeds), uterus (eg, menorrhagia), and skin (eg, bruising). In types 2N and 3, factor VIII is appreciably low and will present similarly to hemophilia A, which includes joint bleeding, soft tissue bleeds, and hematuria. Although type 3 is fairly rare, it is a severe form and patients will present earlier in life such as at the time of a circumcision.

### Next Step:

**Step 1)** Diagnosis of vWD can be made by the clinical evaluation and laboratory testing. Initial lab testing should include a CBC, PT, and PTT. Expected findings include a **normal platelet count**, a **normal PT**, and **a normal to elevated PTT**. Certainly types 2N and 3 will have elevated PTT (ie, intrinsic cascade) because their factor VIII is significantly low.

**Step 2)** If the PTT is elevated or if all the initial lab tests are normal but there is suspicion for vWD, then order a screening test that includes a vWF antigen test, vWF activity test (ie, ristocetin cofactor test), and a factor VIII activity test (ie, FVIII coagulant assay). See Table 10-2 for expected results.

**Step 3)** If the vWD screening test demonstrates an abnormal result or if the lab tests are normal but there is still suspicion for vWD, then repeat the initial screening tests and refer to a specialist for further specialized vWD studies.

**Step 4)** Treatment of vWD is based on three approaches. First, promoting release of vWF into circulation from endothelial cells via desmopressin (DDAVP). Second, replacement of vWF with plasma-derived, viral-inactivated vWF concentrates. Third, controlling hemostasis with antifibrinolytics.

### Table 10-2 • Expected vWD Screening Results

| Type | vWF Antigen | Ristocetin Cofactor Activity | Factor VIII Activity |
|---|---|---|---|
| Type 1 | ↓ | ↓ | ↓ |
| Type 2A | ↓ | ↓ | ↓ |
| Type 2B | ↓ | ↓ | ↓ |
| Type 2M | ↓ | ↓ | ↓ |
| Type 2N | ↓ or normal | ↓ or normal | ↓ |
| Type 3 | ↓ or undetectable | ↓ or undetectable | ↓ |

### Desmopressin (DDAVP)

- DDAVP is a synthetic derivative of vasopressin.
- DDAVP is used in type 1 and in some patients with type 2.
- DDAVP can worsen thrombocytopenia seen in type 2B patients.
- DDAVP is not recommended in type 3 because it does not increase vWF levels.
- DDAVP can cause tachyphylaxis and water retention leading to hyponatremia.

### Plasma-Derived vWF Concentrates

- Humate-P and Alphanate are trade names that are FDA approved for treatment of vWD.
- Humate-P and Alphanate contain both factor VIII and vWF.
- Humate-P or Alphanate are used in patients who no longer respond to DDAVP, require long periods of DDAVP, type 3 patients, some type 2 patients, and those with significant bleeding or those having major surgery.
- Cryoprecipitate is no longer recommended because of concerns of viral transmission.

### Antifibrinolytics

- ε-aminocaproic acid or tranexamic acid are particularly useful in mucocutaneous bleeds.
- Antifibrinolytics can be used as monotherapy or adjunctive therapy to other medications.
- Both agents are contraindicated in patients with upper urinary bleeding because it can cause ureteral obstruction.

### Follow-Up:

Patients diagnosed with type 1 and most type 2s should be tested with DDAVP to assess their response with the medication.

### Pearls:

- Patients with blood type O have vWF levels that are 30% lower compared to the other blood types.
- Factor VIII and vWF are both acute phase reactants that can be elevated in times of stress, pregnancy, exercise, inflammation, and the use of estrogen or oral contraceptives.
- Patients with menorrhagia who do not want to become pregnant can use oral contraceptives for therapy, but those

who want to become pregnant are treated with DDAVP, antifibrinolytics, or vWF concentrates.

- Ristocetin is an antibiotic that is off the market because it causes thrombocytopenia, but now used in assays. In the presence of vWF factors, adding ristocetin will cause platelets to agglutinate.

- Bleeding time is not routinely performed because of the wide variation of the test, but for board purposes bleeding time can be normal to elevated in vWD.

- **Connecting point** (pg. 162)—Be familiar with the other autosomal dominant disorders.

- On the CCS, "von Willebrand factor antigen, plasma," "ristocetin cofactor," and "coagulation factor VIII, plasma" are available in the practice CCS.

- **On the CCS,** both "DDAVP" and "desmopressin" are available in the practice CCS.

- **On the CCS,** both trade names for "Humate-P" and "Alphanate" are available in the practice CCS.

- **On the CCS,** "aminocaproic acid" is available, but "tranexamic acid" is not available in the practice CCS.

# NEOPLASIA

## ▌MULTIPLE MYELOMA

Multiple myeloma is a malignant proliferation of plasma cells. The plasma cells can overproduce M proteins (ie, IgG, IgM, IgA, IgE, or IgD) depending on their heavy chain class and ultimately causing hyperviscosity. Myeloma cells can produce abnormal light chain proteins (ie, κ-kappa or λ-lambda) that can cause end-organ damage. Finally, myeloma cells can secrete cytokines that can stimulate osteoClast activity (ie, "bone-Crushing cells") while suppressing osteoblast activity (ie, "bone-forming cells"). The end result of osteoclast activity can be bone lesions, hypercalcemia, and osteoporosis. The etiology of multiple myeloma is still not fully understood.

### Clinical Features:

Multiple myeloma is a disease of older adults with the median age at diagnosis of 68 years. Men are more likely to have the disease compared to females, and blacks are twice as likely as whites to have multiple myeloma. Multiple myeloma can present in a variety of ways, and it can best be remembered by the mnemonic **"TIN-CRAB."**

**Thickened blood**—Hyperviscosity can cause headaches, blurry vision, retinopathy, fatigue, sensory loss, stroke, myocardial infarction, heart failure, or Raynaud phenomenon. One of the causes of hyperviscosity can be cryoglobulinemia, which is the presence of cryoglobulins (ie, immunoglobulins that can undergo reversible precipitation at low temperatures) in the serum.

**Infection**—Abnormal humoral immunity and leukopenia can cause recurrent infections. Common organisms include *Staphylococcus aureus*, *Streptococcus pneumoniae*, and *Klebsiella pneumoniae* in the lungs and *E coli* and other gram-negative bugs in the urinary tract.

**Neurologic—Spinal cord compression** can occur from a vertebral fracture or a plasmacytoma. As a result, patients can experience back pain, radiculopathy, or loss of bowel and bladder control. Patients with multiple myeloma can have **peripheral neuropathy** due to the infiltration of amyloid into peripheral nerves. Carpal tunnel syndrome is a common peripheral neuropathy seen in patients with multiple myeloma.

**Calcium**—Hypercalcemia can occur from the breakdown of bone. Patients can experience confusion, depression, polydipsia, nausea, or lethargy.

**Renal**—Renal failure is seen in almost 25% of patients with multiple myeloma, and at least 50% of patients with multiple myeloma have some type of renal pathology. The most common renal dysfunction is the "myeloma kidney," which is a light chain cast nephropathy seen in the tubules. Other pathologies are Fanconi's syndrome in the tubules, amyloidosis in the glomeruli, and interstitial nephritis in the interstitium.

**Anemia**—Approximately 80% of patients with multiple myeloma will have a normocytic, normochromic anemia. The anemia may be due to tumor cell replacement in the bone marrow and inhibition of hematopoiesis by factors released by the tumor cell. Patients will usually experience weakness, pallor, and malaise.

**Bone**—Bone pain is a common presenting symptom. The pain is usually in the back, chest, or ribs and less frequently in the arms and legs. The pain of multiple myeloma is precipitated by movement. The pain is usually not worse at night, compared to metastatic carcinoma where it is worse at night. The bone lesions are **lytic lesions**, and persistent localized pain usually signifies a pathologic fracture. Patients can actually lose height if there is a vertebral collapse from the fracture.

### Next Step:

**Step 1)** Routine laboratory testing in patients who initially present with multiple myeloma may show the following:

> **CBC with peripheral smear**—Anemia, Rouleaux formation
>
> **CMP**—↑ BUN, ↑ Cr, ↑ calcium, normal alkaline phosphatase (ie, no osteoblastic activity)
>
> **ESR**—Elevated
>
> **Uric acid**—Elevated
>
> **Urinalysis**—± protein (ie, UA will pick up albumin in urine, not Bence Jones protein).

**Step 2)** Further diagnostic testing should be conducted in patients with initial lab findings and overall clinical picture of multiple myeloma.

> **SPEP (Serum protein electrophoresis) with immunofixation**—SPEP screens for the presence of monoclonal (M) proteins (also referred to as paraprotein). Immunofixation

confirms the presence of M proteins and identifies the subtype of protein.

**UPEP (urine protein electrophoresis) with immunofixation**—UPEP can detect M protein, but it can also identify elevated light chains (κ or λ), which is also referred to as Bence Jones protein.

**Bone marrow aspiration and biopsy**—Smears will appear with a preponderance of plasma cells with an eccentric nucleus.

**Skeletal survey**—Plain radiograph is the modality of choice, and lytic lesions will appear as "punched-out" lesions. MRI is the preferred technique in patients with spinal cord compression or soft tissue plasmacytomas. Nuclear bone scans are *not* recommended because there is no osteoblastic activity.

**Step 3)** Diagnosis can now be made if all three of the following criteria are met:

1) Presence of serum or urinary M protein.
2) Presence of bone marrow plasma cells or plasmacytoma.
3) Presence of end-organ damage (**C**–↑ calcium, **R**–renal failure, **A**–anemia, **B**–bone lesions).

**Step 4)** Once the diagnosis is made, the patient is staged. The International Staging System (ISS) is a common staging system that incorporates serum albumin and serum $\beta_2$-microglobulin. Lower albumin levels and higher $\beta_2$-microglobulin are indicators of a poor prognosis. But know that the **$\beta_2$-microglobulin** is the single most useful and important predictor of survival.

**Step 5)** Patients that are asymptomatic may not require any treatment. However, once the patient becomes symptomatic and the disease becomes more progressive, therapeutic intervention is usually required. Treatment and management of multiple myeloma is as follows:

**Multiple myeloma**—Patients are evaluated on whether or not they are stem cell transplant candidates. Patients that are not candidates tend to have comorbidities such as NYHA III or IV, or are older and inactive and probably would not be able to withstand treatment. Patients that are not transplant candidates usually undergo a treatment of melphalan, prednisone, and thalidomide (MPT). Patients that are candidates for transplant can undergo vincristine, doxorubicin (Adriamycin), or dexamethasone (VAD), or they can undergo thalidomide plus dexamethasone. Patients that are candidates for transplant should not be treated with melphalan because it can cause stem cell damage and collection for stem cells will be diminished.

**Thickened blood**—Patients that are symptomatic from the hyperviscosity should be treated with plasmapheresis regardless of the viscosity level.

**Infections**—The use of prophylactic antibiotics is controversial, but initiate empiric antibiotics if an infection is suspected. Pneumococcal, Haemophilus, and influenza vaccines should be given despite a suboptimal response. Patients with serious recurrent infections may need IVIG.

**Neurologic**—Spinal cord compression is a medical emergency, and any patient suspected of having a spinal cord compression should have an emergency MRI. Initial treatment may include dexamethasone, while definitive therapy may include surgery or radiation therapy.

**Calcium**—Hypercalcemia can initially be treated with normal saline and steroids (eg, dexamethasone). Also add intravenous bisphosphonates (eg, zoledronic acid, pamidronate) because it can inhibit osteoclast activity and provide secondary prevention in bony complications.

**Renal**—Treat the underlying cause of the renal pathology. In general, patients should be well hydrated to excrete light chains and calcium. Avoid nephrotoxic agents such as NSAIDs and radiocontrast dye.

**Anemia**—Patients with significant symptoms should be treated with irradiated, leukoreduced blood transfusions. Erythropoietin therapy is also given to patients with hemoglobin ≤10 g/dL.

**Bone**—Bone pain can be controlled with opiates, and bone disease can be managed with radiation therapy, surgical procedures (eg, vertebroplasty, kyphoplasty), and intravenous bisphosphonates (eg, zoledronic acid, pamidronate).

**Follow-Up:**

One of the ways to determine the response of chemotherapy is to assess the M protein levels via SPEP or UPEP.

**Pearls:**

- The approximate survival rate in patients with multiple myeloma is 3 years.
- Smoldering multiple myeloma is also referred to as asymptomatic multiple myeloma and can be diagnosed if serum M protein is ≥3 g/dL and/or bone marrow plasma cells ≥10%, and there is no end organ damage.
- Monoclonal gammopathy of undetermined significance (MGUS) can be diagnosed if serum M protein is <3 g/dL, bone marrow plasma cells <10%, and there is no end organ damage.
- Although multiple myeloma arises de novo, it appears that MGUS can progress to multiple myeloma with a risk of progression of approximately 1% per year.
- Patients with smoldering multiple myeloma or MGUS usually require no therapy.
- **Connecting point** (pg. 73)—Review the clinical features section on hypercalcemia.
- **On the CCS**, the practice CCS recognizes "SPEP," "UPEP," and "bone marrow biopsy" in the order menu.
- **On the CCS**, immunofixation will be recognized as either "serum immunoelectrophoresis" or "urine immunoelectrophoresis" in the practice CCS.
- **On the CCS**, the practice CCS does not recognize "beta 2 microglobulin."
- **On the CCS**, remember to "bridge" your therapy by addressing any acute issues (eg, spinal cord compression) and addressing the long-term care (eg, chemotherapy).

# CCS: G6PD DEFICIENCY CASE INTRODUCTION

Day 1 @ 11:00
Office

A 20-year-old Greek man comes to the office because of weakness, back pain, dark urine, and jaundice.

## Initial Vital Signs:
Temperature: 37.0°C (98.6°F)
Pulse: 92 beats/min, regular rhythm
Respiratory: 17/min
Blood pressure: 116/75 mm Hg
Height: 182.9 cm (72.0 inches)
Weight: 77 kg (170 lb)
BMI: 23.1 kg/m$^2$

## Initial History:
Reason (s) for visit: Weakness, back pain, dark urine, jaundice

## HPI:
A 20-year-old college student presents to the office with weakness, back pain, dark urine, and "yellowing of the skin." He denies any sick contacts, travel, or trauma. He cannot recall any precipitating events, other than 4 days ago when he opened up a sealed container that contained strong vapors of mothballs. After removing his coat jacket from the sealed container and wearing the jacket, he noticed that he started to feel weak and had back pain several hours later. Approximately 2 days later, he noticed brownish-red urine and yellowing of his skin. The only other time that he had similar symptoms was when he consumed fava beans 15 years ago, but no further workup was done because of insurance reasons.

| | |
|---|---|
| **Past Medical History:** | Neonatal hyperbilirubinemia treated with phototherapy. |
| **Past Surgical History:** | None |
| **Medications:** | None |
| **Allergies:** | None |
| **Vaccinations:** | Up to date |
| **Family History:** | Father, age 48, and mother, age 45, are both healthy. One older brother is healthy and one younger sister is healthy. An uncle (mother's side) has a blood disorder. |
| **Social History:** | Does not smoke, drink, or do drugs. Single, no children. Full-time college student. Plays collegiate golf. |

## Review of Systems:
| | |
|---|---|
| General: | See HPI |
| Skin: | See HPI |
| HEENT: | See HPI |
| Musculoskeletal: | See HPI |
| Cardiorespiratory: | Negative |
| Gastrointestinal: | Negative |
| Genitourinary: | See HPI |
| Neuropsychiatric: | Negative |

Day 1 @ 11:10

## Physical Examination:
| | |
|---|---|
| **General appearance:** | Appears uncomfortable. |
| **Skin:** | Jaundice. Pallor. |
| **Lymph nodes:** | No lymphadenopathy. |
| **HEENT/Neck:** | Normocephalic. Scleral icterus; Pale conjunctivae. EOMI, PERRLA. Hearing normal. Ears, nose, mouth normal. Pharynx normal. Neck supple; trachea midline; no masses or bruits; thyroid normal. |
| **Chest/Lungs:** | Chest wall normal. Diaphragm moving equally and symmetrically with respiration. Auscultation and percussion normal. |
| **Heart/Cardiovascular:** | S1, S2 normal. No murmurs, rubs, gallops, or extra sounds. No JVD. |
| **Abdomen:** | Normal bowel sounds; no bruits. No tenderness. No masses. No hernias. No hepatosplenomegaly. |
| **Extremities/Spine:** | No joint deformity or warmth. No cyanosis or clubbing. No edema. Peripheral pulses normal. Spine examination normal. No paraspinal tenderness. |
| **Neuro/Psych:** | Mental status normal. Cranial nerve and sensory examination normal. Motor strength 4/5 throughout. Cerebellar function normal. Deep tendon reflexes normal. Gait normal. |

## First Order Sheet:
1) CBC with differential, stat

**Result:** WBC-8000, H/H-7/35%, Plt-250,000, Differential-WNL MCV-85, MCHC-37% (nl: 31-36%), RDW-12% (nl: 11.5-13.6)

2) Peripheral smear, stat

**Results:** Presence of bite cells and spherocytes. Normochromic normocytic erythrocytes; leukocytes and platelets normal in number and morphology.

3) BMP, stat

**Result:** Glu-100, Urea-14, Na-140, K-4.9, Cl-102, $HCO_3$-25, Cr-1, Ca-9.5

4) Reticulocyte count, blood, stat

**Result:** 4% (nl: 0.5-1.5)

5) LDH, serum, stat

**Result:** 500 IU/L (nl: 45-90)

6) LFT, stat

**Result:** AST-50, ALT-20, Alb-5, Protein-7, AlkP-65, Total Bil-4.0 (nl: 0.1-1.0), Direct Bil-0.3 (nl: 0-0.3)

7) PT/INR, stat

**Result:** 9 seconds (nl: <12 seconds), INR-1.0

8) PTT, stat

**Result:** 25 seconds (nl: <28 seconds)

9) Urinalysis, stat

**Result:** Appearance-brownish-red, Bilirubin-positive

**Actions:**
1) Change location to inpatient unit

**Second Order Sheet:**
1) IV access

2) NS, 0.9% NaCl, IV, continuous

3) Vital signs, q8 hrs

4) Urine output, routine, q8 hrs

5) Type and crossmatch, blood, stat

**Result:** O+

6) Transfuse, packed RBC's, routine

**Follow-Up History:**
"Hey Doc, I'm starting to feel better."

**Third Order Sheet:**
1) Haptoglobin, serum, routine

**Result:** 20 mg/dL (nl: 30-175)

2) Coombs' test, direct, routine

**Result:** Negative

3) G6PD, blood, quantitative, routine

**Result:** 12.5 U/g Hb (nl: 10.0-14.2)

4) Heinz body stain, routine

**Result:** Inclusion bodies detected.

**Vital sign is now available**

**Result:** 37°C, HR-88, RR-16, BP-120/78

**Urine output is now available**

**Result:** Voiding adequate amounts.

**Fourth Order Sheet:**
1) H/H, routine

**Result:** Hemoglobin-13.5 g/dL, Hematocrit-41%

**This case will end in the next few minutes of "real time."**
You may **add** or **delete** orders at this time, then enter a diagnosis on the following screen.

**Fifth Order Sheet:**
1) G6PD, blood, quantitative, routine
   Future date: In 90 days

**Result:** 12.0 U/g Hb (nl: 10.0-14.2)

2) Hemosiderin stain, urine, routine
   Future date: In 7 days

**Result:** Positive

3) Counsel family/patient, routine

**Please enter your diagnosis:**

G6PD Deficiency

**DISCUSSION:**

G6PD deficiency is the most common enzymopathy. It is an X-linked recessive disorder commonly affecting persons of Mediterranean, Middle Eastern, African, and Asian descent. The importance of G6PD is that it ultimately defends against oxidant injury within the blood cell. G6PD catalyzes NADP to its reduced form of NADPH. NADPH is an important cofactor in maintaining elevated levels of the reducing agent, glutathione (GSH), and thereby protecting the cell from oxidant injury. In the event that GSH is absent or very low, such as in G6PD deficiency, oxidants can accumulate within the cell and denature hemoglobin and form precipitates of inclusion bodies (Heinz bodies). The precipitates can eventually damage the membranes and cause intravascular hemolysis. Extravascular hemolysis can also occur outside the vascular compartment, and destruction can occur in the spleen, liver, and bone marrow. As the inclusion-bearing red cell passes through the spleen, the macrophages remove the Heinz bodies, which gives the cell a "bite cell" appearance on peripheral smear.

**Clinical Features:**

The majority of patients with G6PD deficiency will remain asymptomatic throughout their life. The two main clinical presentations that can occur in G6PD deficiency are **acute hemolytic anemia** and **neonatal hyperbilirubinemia**. The four triggers that can cause an acute hemolytic anemia are (1) infections, (2) fava beans, (3) DKA, and (4) agents (see Table 10-3). Once exposed to the offending trigger, patients will start to

## Table 10-3 • Triggering Agents of Acute Hemolytic Anemia in Persons with G6PD Deficiency

| Agents | Purpose |
|---|---|
| Naphthalene | Used in mothballs |
| Henna | Used in body art and hair dyes |
| Primaquine | Antimalarial |
| Dapsone | Antibiotic used to treat leprosy |
| Nitrofurantoin | Antibiotic used to treat UTIs |
| Nalidixic acid | Antibiotic used to treat UTIs |
| Sulfamethoxazole | Antibiotic (part of the TMP-SMX) |
| Sulfacetamide | Antibiotic used to treat acne or conjunctivitis |
| Sulfanilamide | Antifungal used to treat vulvovaginitis from C albicans |
| Phenazopyridine | Urinary analgesic |
| Methylene blue | Antidote to treat cyanide poisoning and drug-induced methemoglobinemia |

feel weak and may have abdominal or back pain. After 2 to 4 days from exposure, they will develop a sudden onset of jaundice, pallor, and dark urine. The hemolytic episode is self-limited even in the presence of the offending trigger because it is thought that the older erythrocytes (ie, greatest enzyme deficiency) have been hemolyzed, but the younger erythrocytes and reticulocytes (ie, near-normal enzyme activity) can sustain oxidative damage. There are several different variants of G6PD deficiency, but the two most common types include:

**G6PD Mediterranean**—Commonly affects people from Greek, Italian, Arabic, and Jewish (Kurdish) descent. Classified as a class II variant and according to the World Health Organization is described as severe enzyme deficiency, but with intermittent hemolysis associated with infection, drugs, or chemicals. Favism is more likely to occur in this variant. Symptoms of favism typically begin within 24 hours of fava bean ingestion, and symptoms include fever, chills, headache, nausea, and back pain, which is then followed by jaundice and hemoglobinuria.

**G6PD A– variant**—Commonly affects people of African descent. Classified as a class III variant and according to the World Health Organization is described as moderate enzyme deficiency (10%-60% of normal), but with intermittent hemolysis usually associated with infection, drugs, or chemicals. Favism is not as common in this group.

### Next Step Summary:

**Step 1**) When an acute hemolytic anemia develops, no treatment is needed in most cases. However, in this case, the patient's overall clinical condition appeared severe enough to warrant a blood transfusion (ie, symptomatic, vitals starting to become unstable, Hb of 7).

**Step 2**) The presence of jaundice, dark urine, and symptoms of anemia should make you think about a hemolytic process. Several laboratory studies were ordered during the CCS to give you

a better assessment. The following list describes issues to think about during the case:

**Intravascular hemolysis**—RBCs will release LDH, AST, hemoglobin, and potassium into circulation. Free hemoglobin will be bound to haptoglobin, and any remaining free hemoglobin will be filtered through the kidneys and appear as dark urine caused by the hemoglobinuria. As the hemoglobin passes through the renal tubules, some of the hemoglobin is taken up by the renal tubular cells and then broken down, and the iron is then stored as hemosiderin in the renal tubular cells. Approximately, one week later, the renal tubular cells will slough off and the iron can be detected by a Prussian blue stain and test positive for hemosiderinuria.

**Extravascular hemolysis**—The presence of bite cells on peripheral smear is an indication of extravascular hemolysis. The loss of membrane from the bite cells can induce further damage resulting in spherocytes. The presence of spherocytes is also an indication of extravascular hemolysis.

**G6PD Deficiency assessment**—The G6PD blood quantity level is falsely negative in this case. It is the older erythrocytes that have been hemolyzed, and thereby does not truly reflect the steady state. The normal value in this case reflects the reticulocytes and young erythrocytes that have normal or near-normal enzyme activity.

**Rule out liver and biliary disease**—The LFTs show a normal ALT but a modest increase in AST, most likely from the red blood cells. An elevated total bilirubin but a normal direct bilirubin indicates a problem with excess unconjugated bilirubin (ie, indirect bilirubin) most likely from the hemolytic anemia and not from an intrinsic liver disease problem. The indirect bilirubin can also be calculated by Indirect = Total – Direct. An indirect value >1.2 mg/dL and a direct bilirubin value <20% of the total bilirubin should make you think about excess unconjugation.

**Rule out a coagulopathy**—Both PT and PTT are within normal range.

**Rule out autoimmune hemolytic anemia**—Direct Coomb's test was negative in this case.

**Step 3**) Prevent another episode by identifying and avoiding the triggering factor.

### Follow-Up:

Patients should have a repeat G6PD level 3 months from the hemolytic episode because at that time, the patient will be in a steady-state condition with a true reflection of the red blood cells at different ages.

### Pearls:

- Both G6PD Mediterranean and G6PD A– variant are at risk of developing neonatal hyperbilirubinemia.

- Neonatal hyperbilirubinemia will usually not present at birth, but rather in 2 to 3 days after birth.

- Neonatal hyperbilirubinemia may require phototherapy or exchange transfusion.

- Severe neonatal jaundice can result in kernicterus.

- Acute hemolytic anemia can also occur in a G6PD deficient baby who is ingesting oxidizing drugs from a woman who is breastfeeding (see Table 10-3).

- Splenomegaly may not always be present in G6PD deficient patients.

- In the presence of many spherocytes, the MCHC can be elevated.

- Reticulocytosis should be seen within 5 days after a hemolytic episode.

- The presence of Heinz bodies can be detected with a supravital dye, but will disappear within 4 days after the hemolytic episode.

- Fava beans are also referred to as broad beans, pigeon beans, haba beans, bell beans, fever beans, horse beans, silkworm beans, tick beans, field beans, or English dwarf beans.

- **Foundational point**—G6PD deficiency involves the pentose phosphate pathway (also referred to as the hexose monophosphate shunt. The pathway ultimately produces NADPH, which then can convert oxidized glutathione to reduced glutathione. The reduced glutathione can now protect the cell from oxidant injury (eg, $H_2O_2$).

- **Connecting point** (pg. 194)—Sulfacetamide may be used to prevent an infection in corneal abrasions.

- **Connecting point** (pg. 48)—Sulfacetamide is used to treat mild acne.

- **On the CCS**, in this case the mother is most likely an X-linked carrier of the disease and her brother (patient's uncle) probably has the disease.

- **On the CCS**, the complete metabolic panel (CMP) will give you the total bilirubin level, but not the direct bilirubin level. Therefore, order the LFT to give you both total and direct bilirubin levels to assess the indirect bilirubin.

- **On the CCS**, be sure that whenever you provide treatment for the patient, you follow up with the appropriate monitoring parameters (eg, vitals, blood work, imaging).

# 11

# Neurology

## KEYWORDS REVIEW

**Abulia**—Inability to make decisions or act.

**Agnosia**—Inability to recognize and interpret sensory impressions from the visual, auditory, olfactory, gustatory, or tactile senses.

**Agraphia**—Inability to write.

**Anisocoria**—Unequal size of the pupils (eg, uncal herniation with CN III compression), which usually indicates a lesion in the efferent fibers innervating the pupillary sphincter muscles.

**Anosognosia**—Unaware or denial that a neurological deficit is occurring.

**Apractagnosia**—Inability to use objects (eg, pencil to draw) or to perform motor activities (eg, assembling a model airplane).

**Apraxia**—Inability to carry out learned purposeful movements.

**Bradykinesia**—Slowness of muscular movements.

**Choreoathetosis**—A condition characterized by choreic (rapid, jerky) and athetoid (slow, writhing) movements.

**Color anomia**—Inability to identify the name of colors, but can distinguish between colors.

**Desiccation**—Drying out or dehydration.

**Dyspraxia**—Partial loss of the ability to perform coordinated movements.

**Dystonia**—Sustained, involuntary muscular contractions that cause uncontrollable repetitive movements or distorted postures.

**Homonymous hemianopsia**—A visual field deficit affecting the right or left half of the visual field of both eyes. For example, a patient with a left homonymous hemianopsia will not be able to see on the left visual field (ie, temporal side of the left eye and nasal side of the right eye).

**Hypesthesia**—Decreased sensitivity to stimuli, also known as hypoesthesia.

**Myoclonus**—A brief, shocklike, involuntary contraction of a muscle or group of muscles.

**Oscillopsia**—Oscillating vision or the sensation that objects are moving back and forth.

**Romberg's test**—Mainly a test of proprioception or the integrity of the dorsal columns. To maintain balance, you need two of the three parameters (ie, vision, vestibular function,

proprioception). A positive Romberg test occurs when patients sway after closing their eyes with their feet together.

**Paraparesis**—Partial paralysis of the lower extremity.

**Paraplegia**—Paralysis of the lower extremity and lower trunk.

**Prosopagnosia**—Inability to recognize familiar faces, even the patient's own face.

**Scanning speech**—A type of ataxic dysarthria in which words are broken into separate syllables (ie, noticeable pauses between syllables).

**Scotoma**—An area of depressed vision in the visual field, but surrounded with normal vision.

**Spondylolisthesis**—The anterior or posterior displacement of a vertebra with respect to an adjacent vertebra.

**Spondylolysis**—A defect or crack at the pars interarticularis that can sometimes lead to spondylolisthesis.

**Spondylosis**—Degenerative spinal changes.

**Tactile aphasia**—Inability to name objects by tactile sensation.

---

# DEGENERATIVE DISEASE

## MULTIPLE SCLEROSIS

Multiple sclerosis (MS) is a demyelinating disorder that results in variable neurologic dysfunction. Although the etiology of MS is unknown, the primary mechanism involves inflammation, demyelination, and axon degeneration.

**Clinical Features:**

Multiple sclerosis usually affects more women than men, and the mean age of onset is between 20 and 40 years of age. The neurologic manifestations of MS can vary, and there is no single clinical feature that is pathognomonic for MS. It may be helpful to consider the features of MS in a relative head to toe fashion:

**Psych**—Depression, euphoria, mood swings

**Brain**—Seizures, cognitive dysfunction (eg, dementia, ↓ concentration, ↓ memory), vertigo, tremors, gait imbalance (due to cerebellar or corticospinal tract lesions), cerebellar dysarthria (scanning speech)

**Face**—Facial weakness (ipsilateral taste sensation is preserved), facial myokymia (twitching), facial paresthesia, trigeminal neuralgia

**Ocular**—Nystagmus, diplopia, optic neuritis (eye pain followed by central scotoma), Marcus Gunn pupil, internuclear ophthalmoplegia (INO), ocular dysmetria

**Spine**—Lhermitte's sign (electric shock radiating down the spine and sometimes into the legs upon neck flexion), acute transverse myelitis

**Bowel**—Constipation, incontinence

**Bladder**—Urinary urgency, incontinence

**Sexual dysfunction**—Erectile dysfunction, ↓ vaginal lubrication, ↓ libido

**Motor symptoms**—Spasticity, hyperreflexia, paraparesis, paraplegia, Babinski sign (reflecting upper motor neuron lesion), ↑ deep tendon reflexes

**Sensory symptoms**—Pain at any location that can change with time, paresthesias, ↓ vibration and position sense (posterior column pathways), ↓ pain sensation and light touch (spinothalamic tract)

**Systemic**—Fatigue

In addition to the above clinical features, MS also displays three unique characteristics (heat sensitivity, paroxysmal symptoms, and disease patterns). The neurologic signs and symptoms can be worsened with increasing body temperature or **heat sensitivity** (Uhthoff sign). For example, after a hot shower a patient may have urinary urgency. Patients with MS can also have **paroxysmal symptoms** of motor and sensory dysfunction (eg, ataxia, paresthesia, flashing lights), but these attacks do not represent true exacerbations. The paroxysmal symptoms can last for a few seconds to several minutes and can occur multiple times a day lasting for several weeks to months. Paroxysmal symptoms may be precipitated by sensory stimuli, movement, or hyperventilation. Patients with MS can also have different **disease patterns,** which can sometimes confuse the clinical picture. Consider the following different types of disease patterns:

**Relapsing-remitting MS**—Accounts for about 85% of cases and is characterized by discrete relapses (attacks) followed by periods of remission with either full recovery or residual deficits. However, there is no functional decline between the attacks.

**Primary progressive MS**—Accounts for about 10% of cases and is characterized by a steady functional decline from the onset with occasional plateaus, but without acute attacks.

**Secondary progressive MS**—Initially starts as a relapsing-remitting pattern, but then changes to a steady functional decline with or without attacks or plateaus. Secondary progressive MS causes the most neurological disability, and patients with the relapsing-remitting MS are at risk of developing secondary progressive MS.

**Progressive-relapsing MS**—Accounts for about 5% of cases and is characterized by a steady functional decline from the onset with superimposed attacks upon the declining course.

Next Step:

**Step 1**) Multiple sclerosis is a **clinical diagnosis**. Patients should have ≥2 symptomatic episodes that suggest white matter pathology in ≥2 distinct locations in the CNS. The attacks (paroxysmal episodes excluded) should last for more than 24 hours, and the episodes should be separated by at least 1 month or more. No single test is diagnostic, but rather supportive. Consider the following ancillary tests:

**MRI**—MRI is the best initial test and the procedure of choice for supporting the diagnosis of MS.

**CSF analysis**—CSF analysis via lumbar puncture may reveal a normal CSF pressure, normal or slightly elevated CSF protein, clear CSF fluid, and cell pleocytosis (↑ normal cell count). Patients with MS may also have an increase in intrathecal production of **IgG**, which would demonstrate as an **oligoclonal banding (OCB)** on gel electrophoresis. However, these findings are not specific for MS since OCBs can be found in other chronic CNS infections.

**Evoked potentials**—Evoked potentials (EPs) are not specific for MS, but any delays in latencies are suggestive of demyelination. The three most common EPs are visual (VEP), somatosensory (SSEP), and brainstem auditory (BAEP). At this time, the American Academy of Neurology does not recommend BAEP for diagnostic purposes.

**Step 2**) Treatment for multiple sclerosis mainly involves pharmacologic therapy. Unfortunately, the treatments for primary or secondary progressive MS are less well established compared to the relapsing-remitting disease. Consider the following treatments for the following conditions:

**Acute attacks**—The preferred treatment is with IV methylprednisolone for 3 to 7 days ± oral prednisone taper. Plasmapheresis (plasma exchange) can be considered for the relapsing forms of MS if patients have a contraindication or are refractory to glucocorticoid treatment.

**Relapsing-remitting MS (RRMS)**—The disease modifying agents are used for the relapsing forms of MS. The following are FDA approved drugs for treatment of RRMS:

- **Interferon beta-1b**—First agent approved for use in MS. IFN beta-1b can induce flulike symptoms. Administer SubQ.

- **Interferon beta-1a**—Similar effect and side effect as IFN beta-1b. Administer SubQ or IM.

- **Glatiramer acetate**—Similar to interferon betas, glatiramer is also considered a first-line agent. Side effects include injection site inflammation, flulike syndrome, chest pain, and anxiety. Administer SubQ.

- **Natalizumab**—Typically reserved for patients with active RRMS that are refractory to interferon betas and glatiramer. Natalizumab can result in progressive multifocal leukoencephalopathy (PML) due to an opportunistic infection with the JC virus. Administer as IV infusion.

- **Mitoxantrone**—Approved to use in patients with relapsing-remitting and secondary progressive MS. Mitoxantrone should not be used as a first-line agent, but rather for those who have failed other therapies. Mitoxantrone is associated with cardiac toxicity, acute leukemia, amenorrhea, and is a pregnancy category D drug (ie, positive fetal risk). Administer as IV infusion.

- **Teriflunomide**—Approved for relapsing forms of MS. Associated with hepatotoxicity and is a pregnancy category X drug (ie, contraindicated in pregnancy). Administer orally.

- **Fingolimod**—Approved for relapsing forms of MS. Associated with VZV infections, macular edema, cardiac adverse effects, and pulmonary dysfunction. Fingolimod is contraindicated in patients with prolonged QT at baseline, sick sinus syndrome, 2° or 3° AV blocks, treatment with Ia or III antiarrhythmics, or recent (past 6 months) TIA, stroke, MI, unstable angina, or decompensated HF. Administer orally.

- **Specific symptoms in MS**—The following symptoms may be ameliorated by different therapies:

  - **Depression**—SSRIs (eg, sertraline) or second-line agents such as tricyclics (eg, amitriptyline).

  - **Cognitive dysfunction**—No proven pharmacologic therapy to be of benefit. Mainly supportive.

  - **Seizures**—Antiepileptic drugs.

  - **Gait imbalance**—Potassium channel blocker (eg, dalfampridine).

  - **Optic neuritis**—IV methylprednisolone is the preferred approach. Oral prednisone has a risk of recurrent optic neuritis.

  - **Constipation**—Increase fluid intake and consider stool softeners or laxatives.

  - **Urinary urgency**—Oxybutynin or tolterodine.

  - **Erectile dysfunction**—PDE-5 inhibitors (eg, sildenafil, tadalafil).

  - **Spasticity**—Baclofen, dantrolene, or tizanidine.

  - **Fatigue**—Amantadine, methylphenidate, or SSRIs.

  - **Heat sensitivity**—Air conditioning and heat avoidance.

  - **Paroxysmal symptoms**—Low-dose anticonvulsants (eg, carbamazepine, gabapentin).

**Follow-Up:**

Patients with MS should be seen once a year at a minimum and more frequently when treated with disease modifying drugs.

**Pearls:**

- Whites, especially from Northern Europe, are at higher risk of developing MS compared to Asians and Africans.
- Patients that develop the relapsing form of MS typically have a better prognosis compared to the progressive disease.
- Some studies have found that there are fewer attacks during pregnancy (especially the third trimester), but an increase in attacks in the first 3 months postpartum. However, it is agreed that pregnancy does not affect the disease course of MS, and at the same time, MS does not affect the course of pregnancy, with the exception of treating with certain disease modifying drugs that are known teratogens.
- MRI T1-weighted images can sometimes demonstrate hypo-intense lesions that can appear as "black holes" that represents axonal damage.
- Some patients with MS can have Charcot's triad, which consists of nystagmus, dysarthria (scanning speech), and intention tremor.
- **Internuclear ophthalmoplegia (INO)** is a conjugate lateral gaze disorder caused by a lesion in the medial longitudinal fasciculus (MLF) of the brainstem. Upon horizontal gaze, there is impaired adduction of the affected eye that is ipsilateral to the MLF lesion, and at the same time, there is nystagmus of the contralateral eye that is in abduction. The cumulative effect is horizontal diplopia while looking to one side. Convergence is preserved. When bilateral INO is present, it is suggestive of multiple sclerosis (not pathognomonic), and vertical nystagmus is usually seen upon upward gaze.
- **Marcus Gunn pupil** is a relative afferent pupillary defect that can be seen in patients with optic neuritis and other optic nerve disorders. When light is directed in the affected eye with the afferent pupillary defect, a mild constriction will occur in both pupils (direct and consensual reflex), hence a "relative defect." When light is directed in the unaffected eye, both pupils constrict normally. In either case during illumination, both pupil sizes are the same because of an intact efferent pathway (unlike anisocoria). During the swinging flashlight maneuver, a penlight is rapidly moved between the left and right pupil, and if an afferent pupillary defect is present, the pupils will constrict normally but will also appear to dilate (ie, consider a normal constriction relative to a soft constriction).

- Progressive multifocal leukoencephalopathy (PML) is a progressive demyelinating disease affecting the white matter at multiple locations. PML typically results from reactivation of the JC virus in immunosuppressed individuals. Symptoms include visual disturbances, hemiparesis, ataxia, limb clumsiness, altered mental status, and sometimes seizures. Patients taking natalizumab for MS should discontinue the medication.
- Acute transverse myelitis is characterized by an inflammatory process that results in spinal cord injury in 1 or 2 segments of the cord. In MS, there is partial rather than total cord involvement in the transverse plane. Patients will present with sudden onset of symptoms below the level of the lesion. Common findings include lower extremity weakness, sensory disturbances, and sphincter (rectal and bladder) dysfunction.
- Acute disseminated encephalomyelitis (ADEM) should be part of the differential diagnosis and is characterized by multifocal demyelinating lesions in the CNS that are frequently seen in the setting of postvaccination or a viral infection. ADEM takes on a self-limited and monophasic course.
- Clinically isolated syndrome (CIS) is characterized by a single attack that is congruent with MS. CIS can take a self-limited course or disseminate into the diagnosis of MS.
- Once you understand this topic, you will have a better and broader understanding of MS that will sharpen your overall clinical judgment.
- **On the CCS**, if you decide to order a lumbar puncture, you also need to order the specific components of the CSF analysis (eg, CSF protein, CSF cell count, or CSF immunoelectrophoresis, which has the IgG and oligoclonal banding).
- **On the CCS**, remember to "advise patient, side effects of medication" if you decide to treat an MS patient.
- **On the CCS**, remember to always "bridge" your therapy. MS is a good example because in some cases you have to treat specific symptoms while treating acute exacerbations and at the same time treating the chronic or remitting portion of the disease. Other good examples of "bridging your therapy" (ie, addressing the acute stage along with the chronic stage of the disease) is with rheumatoid arthritis, gout, multiple myeloma, PTSD, panic disorder, nephrolithiasis, Meniere's disease, anaphylaxis, hyperthyroidism, primary hyperparathyroidism, hypoparathyroidism, third degree AV block, WPW, and torsades de pointes.

# SPINAL DISEASE

## LUMBAR SPINAL STENOSIS

Lumbar spinal stenosis (LSS) refers to narrowing of the spinal canal that can lead to neural compression on a single intervertebral disk level or on multiple levels. The most common cause of LSS is due to degenerative changes in the lumbar region or spondylosis. Other causes of LSS are acquired factors (eg, trauma, neoplasms, spondylolisthesis) or congenital conditions (eg, achondroplasia, spina bifida).

**Clinical Features:**

Patients with degenerative arthritis LSS are typically older people (>50 years). The classic presentation is **bilateral neurogenic claudication** or pseudoclaudication. Patients may report pain in the buttock, lower back, or radiating leg pain (unilateral or bilateral), or they may complain of numbness, tingling, or weakness in the legs, and not uncommonly, they may complain of a combination of everything. Symptoms are usually exacerbated by standing, walking, walking downhill, or maintaining spinal extension (eg, riding a bike in the extended position). However, climbing stairs or walking uphill does not exacerbate neurogenic claudication. Symptoms are often relieved by sitting, lying supine, or maintaining a flexed position (eg, leaning on a shopping cart). If there are unilateral radicular symptoms (eg, focal sensory loss, pain, or weakness), then consider the possibility of stenosis at the neural foramen or lateral recess. However, since the degenerative-type LSS affects multiple levels, it is not uncommon to have polyradiculopathy. On neurologic examination, patients with LSS usually have a normal exam with normal peripheral pulses and skin exam (ie, no pallor). In a small subset of patients, patients may have a positive (abnormal) Romberg test, wide-based gait, or a positive straight leg raise test.

### Next Step:

**Step 1**) The diagnosis of LSS is based on a thorough **clinical assessment** and neuroimaging. The imaging of choice for LSS is an **MRI**.

**Step 2**) The initial management approach is with conservative treatment such as pharmacologic therapy (eg, NSAIDs, analgesics) and physical therapy.

**Step 3**) When patients continue to have disabling symptoms despite conservative therapy, then surgical intervention is considered. The surgical procedure is usually a decompressive laminectomy ± lumbar fusion.

### Follow-Up:

Patients that decide to undergo surgery should continue to follow up with their primary care physician since approximately 25% of patients may develop recurrent stenosis after 5 years of the initial surgery.

### Pearls:

- Spinal stenosis can also occur at the cervical and thoracic levels.
- There is no strong correlation between the severity of the stenosis and the severity of the symptoms.

- As we age, there is disc desiccation with loss of disc height, and it is thought that the stress placed on the surrounding structures leads to segmental instability and therefore a compensatory change (eg, facet joint hypertrophy, osteophyte formation) that results in narrowing of the spinal canal and neural foramina.

- Epidural steroid injections are used to treat patients with LSS, but because of the limited evidence-based information, epidural injections is not routinely recommended.

- **Vascular claudication** is a result of peripheral vascular disease and can be easily confused with neurogenic claudication since both disorders are typically seen in the elderly population.

- Vascular claudication is exacerbated by walking (either uphill, straight, or downhill), and biking (either in the flexed or extended position). Symptoms are relieved by standing, sitting, or lying supine. Spinal flexion does not alleviate the pain, and spinal extension does not exacerbate the pain. In other words, when the patient is in the quiet state or "just chillin," then symptoms are not exacerbated.

- The terminal portion of the spinal cord has a tapered conical shape structure, the conus medullaris, that usually sits between T12 and L2 vertebral levels.

- Infrequently, compression of the conus medullaris (conus medullaris syndrome) or lumbosacral nerve roots (cauda equina syndrome) can be a complication of LSS. Patients may complain of motor and sensory abnormalities in the lower extremities and bowel and bladder dysfunction. Patients that present with rapidly progressive symptoms may require an emergent MRI and urgent surgical consultation.

- **Connecting point** (pg. 299)—Know how to manage peripheral arterial disease (PAD).

- **On the CCS**, "physical therapy" is available in the practice CCS.

- **On the CCS**, if you feel that you've completely managed the patient and the case does not end, you can advance the simulated time by selecting the "Call/see me as needed" option. The patient will then be sent home and the case will advance to the next pending result, patient update, or to the end of the case.

# CEREBROVASCULAR DISEASES

## ▌ISCHEMIC STROKE

A stroke is characterized by a sudden neurologic deficit that results from inadequate blood flow (ischemic stroke) or from brain hemorrhage (intracerebral or subarachnoid). Ischemic strokes result from embolism, thrombosis in situ, or systemic hypoperfusion. Approximately 80% of strokes are ischemic and 20% are hemorrhagic.

### Risk Factors:

Hypertension, diabetes mellitus, smoking, hyperlipidemia, atrial fibrillation, endocarditis, valvular disease, carotid stenosis, TIAs, cardiac structural anomalies, oral contraceptives, illicit drugs.

### Clinical Features:

Symptoms of ischemic stroke can be abrupt and maximal at onset, which would suggest an embolic stroke. Neurologic symptoms that are progressive with a waxing and waning pattern may suggest thrombosis, hypoperfusion, or recurrent emboli.

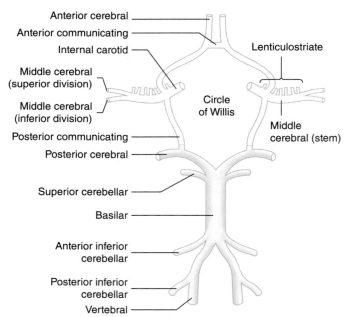

**FIGURE 11-1 • Cerebral vasculature.** Arteries of the anterior (white) and posterior (purple) cerebral circulation in relation to the circle of Willis. (Reproduced with permission from Aminoff MJ, et al. *Clinical Neurology.* 6th ed. New York: McGraw-Hill; 2005:288.)

There are various stroke syndromes that typically correlate with compromise to a specific arterial supply (see Figure 11-1). Consider the following, and keep in mind that not all patients will present the same:

**Anterior cerebral artery**—Contralateral hemiplegia and hemisensory loss (lower extremity > upper extremity and face); urinary incontinence; abulia; gait apraxia; dyspraxia of left limb; tactile aphasia in left limb; or grasp and sucking reflexes

**Anterior choroidal artery**—The anterior choroidal artery is a branch from the internal carotid artery. Features include contralateral hemiplegia, homonymous hemianopsia, and hemihypesthesia.

**Middle cerebral artery (MCA)**—Contralateral hemiplegia and hemisensory loss (upper extremity and face > lower extremity); homonymous hemianopsia; gaze preference toward the side of the lesion; dominant hemisphere (Broca's aphasia, Wernicke's aphasia); nondominant hemisphere (neglect, anosognosia, apractognosia); and proximal MCA give rise to penetrating vessels (lenticulostriate arteries) that can result in lacunar strokes (see below).

**Posterior cerebral artery (PCA)**—Homonymous hemianopsia; visual hallucinations; achromatopia (color blindness); color anomia; third nerve palsy; prosopagnosia; memory impairment; verbal dyslexia without agraphia (non-dominant hemisphere); choreoathetosis; sensory loss; contralateral hemiplegia (ie, cerebral peduncle affected)

**Basilar artery**—The **superior cerebellar artery (SCA)** is a branch of the basilar artery (see Figure 11-1) and occlusion of the SCA results in nausea, vomiting, ipsilateral cerebellar ataxia, dysarthria (slurred speech), or contralateral loss of pain and temperature. The **anterior inferior cerebellar artery (AICA)** is also a branch of the basilar artery and occlusion of the AICA can produce nausea, vomiting, ipsilateral cerebellar ataxia, facial weakness, vertigo, tinnitus, unilateral deafness, nystagmus, Horner's syndrome, conjugate lateral gaze paresis, or contralateral loss of pain and temperature. Basilar artery occlusion that results in bilateral ventral pontine damage can cause the "**locked-in syndrome**" that manifest as quadriplegia, spared consciousness, and preserved vertical eye movements and blinking. Occlusion of the rostral section of the basilar artery is typically due to an embolism and the syndrome is referred to as "**top-of-the-basilar syndrome.**" Manifestations include oculomotor and pupillary abnormalities, memory impairment, abulia, or hypersomnolence. Finally, occlusion of the lower basilar artery can be responsible for the medial medullary syndrome (see below).

**Vertebral artery**—Occlusion of the vertebral artery or lower basilar artery can result in the **medial medullary syndrome**, which consists of ipsilateral paralysis with atrophy of half the tongue, contralateral paralysis of arm and leg (sparing the face), and contralateral impairment of tactile and proprioceptive senses over half of the body. **Lateral medullary syndrome (Wallenberg syndrome)** can also occur, which is the result of an occlusion of the vertebral artery (majority of cases) or posterior inferior cerebellar artery (PICA), which is a branch of the vertebral artery (see Figure 11-1). Manifestations of the Wallenberg syndrome include vertigo, nausea, vomiting, nystagmus, diplopia, oscillopsia, Horner's syndrome, loss of taste, dysphagia, hoarseness, paralysis of vocal cord, ↓ gag reflex, hiccup, numbness of ipsilateral arm, trunk, or leg, ataxia of limbs, falling to side of lesion, ipsilateral pain, numbness, and impaired sensation over half the face, and contralateral impairment of pain and thermal senses over half the body (sometimes the face). The **posterior inferior cerebellar artery (PICA)** is also responsible for cerebellar infarctions. Common findings include occiput headaches, gait ataxia, vomiting, truncal dysfunction, hypotonia, or ipsilateral body tilt upon sitting or standing.

**Internal carotid artery (ICA)**—Not only does the ICA perfuse the brain, but also the optic nerve and retina through the ophthalmic artery, which is branch of the ICA. The central retinal artery is a branch of the ophthalmic artery that runs within the dural sheath of the optic nerve and emerges at the optic disc. For that discussion, patients with internal carotid disease (eg, carotid occlusion or small emboli to the central retinal artery) can present with transient monocular blindness (**amaurosis fugax**) prior to the onset of a stroke. Patients may complain of blurring, fogging, "graying," dimming, or a wedge of visual loss in one eye. At other times, patients may complain of a curtain or shade coming across the visual field in the affected eye. In most cases, symptoms are of short duration (a few minutes).

**Common carotid artery**—Atheromatous plaques can develop in the common carotids and result in occlusion of the vessel. Signs and symptoms of an occluded common carotid can be similar to signs and symptoms of an occluded ICA. Auscultation of the carotids may reveal a carotid bruit, which would suggest stenosis of the carotid artery.

**Lacunar strokes**—Lacunar strokes are small vessel strokes due to an occlusion of small penetrating vessels that arise from larger arteries at acute angles (eg, MCA, circle of Willis, basilar artery, vertebral arteries). Lacunar strokes are non-cortical infarcts that usually affect the basal ganglia, pons, and subcortical white matter (eg, internal capsule). Manifestations can include a pure motor hemiparesis (no sensory deficit), pure sensory stroke (no motor deficit), ataxic hemiparesis, sensorimotor stroke (both motor and sensory deficit present), or dysarthria–clumsy hand syndrome.

## Next Step:

**Step 1)** Patients suspected of having a stroke require an urgent evaluation because time is of the essence. The best first step is to assess **A**irway, **B**reathing, and **C**irculation.

**Step 2)** Place monitoring equipment on patient: pulse oximetry (check for hypoxia), continuous blood pressure cuff, continuous cardiac monitoring, and 12-lead EKG.

**Step 3)** Provide supplemental oxygen to maintain $O_2$ saturation >94% (do not give if nonhypoxic).

**Step 4)** Establish IV access with laboratory studies (eg, CBC, BMP, PT/INR, PTT, troponins, lipid profile) and in select patients order toxicology screen, blood alcohol level, HCG, or ABG (if hypoxia is suspected).

**Step 5)** Finger-stick glucose. Treat hypoglycemia (glucose <60 mg/dL) with slow IV push of 25 mL of 50% dextrose to reach normoglycemia. Oral glucose should be avoided because you want to keep the patient NPO. In addition, oral glucose takes longer to achieve normoglycemia compared to IV. Treating hypoglycemia is important right away because it is one of the exclusion criteria for IV fibrinolysis (see Table 11-1).

**Step 6)** Perform a focused history and physical. In addition, the NIH stroke scale can be performed at this time.

**Step 7)** Order an emergent noncontrast CT or MRI to exclude intracerebral hemorrhage and to determine hypodensity (on CT) or hyperintensity (on MRI). In most cases, a noncontrast CT is sufficient to make management decisions. Determining hypodensity is important on CT because it is part of the exclusion criteria for IV fibrinolysis (see Table 11-1). The goal of CT initiation is ≤25 minutes, and CT interpretation should be done in ≤45 minutes from the time of entering the ED.

**Step 8)** Determine if the patient is a candidate for fibrinolytic therapy since the goal of therapy (door-to-drug) should be ≤60 minutes. The inclusion and exclusion criteria to receive IV recombinant tissue plasminogen activator (rtPA) are based on the guidelines from the American Heart Association/American Stroke Association (see Table 11-1). Consider the following two scenarios:

### Table 11-1 • AHA/ASA Criteria for IV rtPA in Acute Ischemic Stroke within 4.5 Hours

**Indications (All Three Must Apply)**

1) Diagnosis of ischemic stroke causing measurable neurologic deficit.

2) Onset of symptoms within 3-4.5 hours; if the exact time is not known, then use the last time the patient was known to be normal.

3) Age ≥18 years.

**Major Contraindications (Any of the Following)**

**Vitals**
Elevated BP (systolic >185 or diastolic >110)

**History**
Hx of stroke or significant head trauma within the previous 3 months
Hx of arterial puncture at noncompressible site in previous 7 days
Hx of previous intracranial hemorrhage
Recent intracranial or intraspinal surgery
Intracranial neoplasm, AV malformation, or aneurysm

**Clinical picture**
Symptoms suggestive of subarachnoid hemorrhage
Active internal bleeding
Bleeding diathesis

**Labs**
Platelets <100,000/mm$^3$
Blood glucose <50 mg/dL
Anticoagulant use with INR >1.7 or PT >15 seconds
Heparin use within 48 hours resulting in ↑ PTT (greater than upper limit of normal)
Direct thrombin inhibitor use or direct factor Xa inhibitor use with ↑ lab tests (eg, PTT, INR, platelets)

**Imaging**
CT showing multilobar infarction (hypodensity > one-third cerebral hemisphere)

**Candidate for Fibrinolytic Therapy**

- Hold all anticoagulants and antiplatelets for 24 hours.
- Hypoglycemia should be treated (see step 5).
- Elevated BP (>185/110) should be treated with IV labetalol or IV nicardipine, and if unable to go below 185/110 mm Hg, then do *not* administer rtPA.
- If all criteria are met (see Table 11-1), administer **IV alteplase (rtPA)** followed by a transfer to a stroke unit or ICU.

**Noncandidate for Fibrinolytic Therapy**

- Administer aspirin followed by a transfer to a stroke unit or ICU.

**Step 9**) Continue with supportive care; further investigation may be considered to determine the cause of the stroke. Consider the following:

**Blood pressure**—Patients receiving IV fibrinolysis should have their BP checked every 15 minutes for the first 2 hours with a goal BP of <180/105. If elevated, IV labetalol or IV nicardipine can be given.

**Neuro checks**—Patients receiving IV fibrinolysis should have neuro assessments at least every 15 minutes during and after fibrinolytic therapy for at least the first 2 hours.

**Hyperglycemia**—Hyperglycemia is not uncommon in acute ischemic strokes and is associated with a worse outcome during the first 24 hours after a stroke compared to normoglycemic patients with a stroke. Treat hyperglycemia to a level within 140 to 180 mg/dL, and remember to monitor glucose levels with Accu-Cheks.

**Hyperthermia**—Temperatures >38°C should be investigated and treated with antipyretics.

**Fluid status**—Euvolemic patients can be given maintenance fluids, and hypovolemic patients should be given normal saline.

**Cardiac monitoring**—Monitor for at least 24 hours after a stroke to detect atrial fibrillation or other arrhythmias.

**Ancillary testing**—Other testing may be considered to search for the cause of the stroke such as carotid doppler ultrasound, TEE, TTE, CTA, MRA, or blood tests in younger patients without a clear underlying cause (eg, protein C, protein S, factor V Leiden, ANA, anti–double stranded DNA [anti-dsDNA] antibodies).

**Step 10**) Encourage secondary prevention, which may include any of the following:

**Lifestyle modification**—Smoking cessation, reduce heavy alcohol intake, and encourage physical activity (if able to perform).

**Hypertension**—Reduce blood pressure in patients who had an ischemic stroke or TIA and are beyond the first 24 hours.

**Hyperlipidemia**—Initiate a statin in patients who have evidence of atherosclerosis, LDL ≥100 mg/dL, and who are without known CHD.

**Diabetics**—Maintain glycemic control and keep BP <130/80.

**Noncardioembolic strokes**—Patients with noncardioembolic strokes should be given either aspirin alone, clopidogrel alone, or aspirin + dipyridamole. Do not give aspirin and clopidogrel together because it can increase the risk of hemorrhage. Ticlopidine is another antiplatelet agent that is used to prevent recurrence, but it is not a first-line agent and is generally reserved for patients who are intolerant of aspirin or clopidogrel. Also, remember not to give aspirin within 24 hours of IV rtPA therapy, but it should be given within 48 hours after a stroke (ie, it decreases mortality if given within 48 hours).

**Cardioembolic strokes**—Anticoagulation with warfarin should be given to patients with atrial fibrillation (paroxysmal or permanent), mechanical prosthetic heart valves, rheumatic valve disease, or in patients with an LV thrombus in the setting of an acute MI.

**Disposition:**

Patients generally have better outcomes in a stroke unit where there are systems of stroke protocols in place and where delivery of care is more efficient. Remember to obtain a CT or MRI at 24 hours after fibrinolytic therapy before starting antiplatelets or anticoagulants.

**Pearls:**

- Systemic hypoperfusion typically causes diffuse global cerebral deficits; common causes are cardiac arrest, PE, or acute MI.
- Thrombosis and embolism typically cause focal deficits.
- A rim of ischemic tissue that surrounds the core of infarcted tissue is referred to as the ischemic penumbra, which eventually can infarct if blood flow is not restored. Therefore, the goal is to "save the penumbra!"
- The medial and lateral medullary syndromes contain a number of signs and symptoms, and not all patients will present the same, but you should be able to "feel the pattern" of the manifestations (ie, pattern recognition becomes essential).
- The NIH stroke scale (NIHSS) is a validated scale that is composed of 11 items with a total score from 0 to 42 with a higher number indicating impairment.
- Patients that are within 3 hours of a stroke with a NIHSS score >22 generally have a poor prognosis.
- The **CHADS$_2$** score (**C**HF, **H**TN, **A**ge >75 years, **D**M, prior **S**troke or TIA) estimates the risk of a stroke in patients with nonvalvular atrial fibrillation and helps determine if antithrombotic therapy (ie, anticoagulant or antiplatelet therapy) is recommended. Each component is worth 1 point except for **S**, which is worth 2 points, for a total maximum score of 6 points. A score of 0 points indicates low risk and antithrombotic therapy is not necessary, but some physicians will give aspirin even though the benefit has not been proven in this category. A score of 1 point reflects intermediate risk, and either warfarin or aspirin can be given. A score ≥2 points reflects relatively higher risk, and oral anticoagulant therapy (eg, warfarin, dabigatran, Rivaroxaban) is generally recommended over antiplatelet therapy (eg, aspirin).
- Hypodensity seen on CT can potentially increase the risk of hemorrhage when fibrinolytic therapy is given.

- Obtain a lumbar puncture after a nondiagnostic CT (ie, negative finding for blood) for suspected subarachnoid hemorrhage.
- The use of emergent anticoagulation (eg, LMWH, UFH) is not recommended to prevent recurrent stroke.
- Anticoagulation is not recommended within 24 hours of IV rtPA therapy.
- An emergent carotid endarterectomy (CEA) in patients with acute ischemic stroke remains to be defined (ie, do not pick this on the test).
- Be aware that patients with hypertension or diabetes are predisposed to lacunar strokes because of small vessel disease.
- **Foundational point**—Lipohyalinosis can be seen in small vessel occlusion resulting in lacunar strokes. It is thought that lipohyalinosis is the result of hypertension.
- **Foundational point**—Broca's aphasia (nonfluent aphasia) is when speech is nonfluent, but comprehension for spoken language is intact (except for grammar). The impairment can be due to an occlusion (ie, embolism) of the superior division of the middle cerebral artery resulting in an infarction in the Broca's area (expressive language) of the dominant hemisphere located in the frontal lobe of the brain.
- **Foundational point**—Wernicke's aphasia (fluent aphasia) is when speech is fluent, but comprehension for spoken and written language is not intact. The spoken language is usually meaningless, contains neologisms, and may have a pattern of a "word salad." The impairment can be due to an occlusion (ie, embolism) of the inferior division of the middle cerebral artery resulting in an infarction in the Wernicke's area (receptive language) of the dominant hemisphere located in the temporal lobe of the brain.
- **Connecting point** (pg. 23)—Know the management of hyperlipidemia.
- **On the CCS**, "NIH stroke scale" is available in the practice CCS.
- **On the CCS**, "dextrose 50%" is available in the practice CCS.
- **On the CCS**, "alteplase" and "rtPA" are both available in the practice CCS, and if you order rtPA it will be converted to alteplase on the order sheet.
- **On the CCS**, if you decide to treat with rtPA, be sure to enter it in the continuous mode of frequency because the protocol recommends 10% of the rtPA should be given as a bolus over 1 minute and then infused over 60 minutes.
- **On the CCS**, "nicardipine" is not available in the practice CCS, but "labetalol" is available. If you need to treat the hypertension, order IV labetalol as a one time/bolus and check the blood pressure. The AHA/ASA recommends that you can repeat the bolus one more time if elevated BP persists.
- **On the CCS**, assume that consent is given to you for any procedure or treatment, and if not, you will be notified.
- **On the CCS**, you should able to order a noncontrast head CT within 25 minutes of the simulated time.
- **On the CCS**, suboptimal management would include ordering any test or procedure (eg, vascular imaging, TEE) that would delay treatment. Remember you want to give IV fibrinolysis within 60 minutes or less of the simulated time.

# TRANSIENT ISCHEMIC ATTACK

Transient ischemic attack (TIA) was originally defined as a transient neurologic deficit that resolved arbitrarily in <24 hours. However, the American Heart Association and American Stroke Association (AHA/ASA) has endorsed a new definition that a TIA is a transient episode of neurologic dysfunction caused by focal brain, spinal cord, or retinal ischemia, **without acute infarction**. The new tissue-based definition as opposed to the time-based definition reflects the fact that the end point is tissue injury rather than time since even a small amount of time (eg, <1 hour) of transient neurologic symptoms can result in infarction.

## Clinical Features:

TIAs can occur by the same mechanism (ie, embolism, thrombosis, hypoperfusion) and can affect the same vascular territories as ischemic stroke (see Clinical Features in Ischemic Stroke topic). TIAs can precede, accompany, or follow (rarely) a stroke or occur independently without leading to a stroke. **Large artery low flow TIAs** (ie, true TIAs) are brief (lasting just a few minutes to a few hours), stereotyped, and recurrent. **Embolic TIAs** are typically prolonged (lasting several hours) compared to true TIAs. **Lacunar TIAs** can precede lacunar strokes and can be characterized by their brief, repetitive motor or sensory deficits. On neurologic examination, patients can be completely normal between attacks. A classic ocular attack is **amaurosis fugax** (see ICA discussion under Clinical Features in the Ischemic Stroke topic).

## Next Step:

**Step 1)** Any patient suspected of having a stroke requires a prompt evaluation. Remember that embolic TIAs can have a prolong episode (hours) of focal neurologic symptoms, and if you're evaluating that patient during that time you cannot be 100% sure that it is an embolic TIA or an ischemic stroke. For that reason, initially treat TIAs with urgent care and consider your first step by accessing **A**irway, **B**reathing, and **C**irculation.

**Step 2)** Place monitoring equipment on patient: pulse oximetry (check for hypoxia), continuous blood pressure cuff, continuous cardiac monitoring, and 12-lead EKG.

**Step 3)** Provide supplemental oxygen if hypoxemic.

**Step 4)** Establish IV access with laboratory studies (eg, CBC, BMP, PT/INR, PTT, troponins, lipid profile) and in select patients order toxicology screen, blood alcohol level, HCG, or ABG (if hypoxia suspected).

**Step 5)** Finger-stick glucose; treat if indicated.

**Step 6)** Perform a targeted history and physical. In addition, the NIH stroke scale can be performed at this time.

**Step 7)** Order an emergent noncontrast CT or MRI. The AHA/ASA guidelines recommend that patients with TIAs should have neuroimaging within 24 hours of symptom onset and that MRI with diffusion-weighted imaging (DWI) is the preferred modality, but head CT is acceptable if MRI is not available.

**Step 8)** Further investigation of the underlying cause should be considered.

**Neurovascular assessment**—The AHA/ASA recommends that noninvasive imaging (eg, CTA, MRA, transcranial Doppler ultrasound) of the cervical vessels should be routinely performed. Noninvasive imaging can also be performed to assess the intracranial vasculature if knowledge of an intracranial stenosis or occlusion would alter management. To confirm an intracranial stenosis, a catheter angiography is the procedure of choice because it is more accurate than noninvasive imaging.

**Carotid ultrasound (CUS)**—A carotid ultrasound can be considered to assess the carotids especially if a carotid bruit was heard on physical exam.

**Echocardiography**—A transthoracic echocardiography (TTE) can be considered in patients without a clear underlying cause. A transesophageal echocardiography (TEE) provides superior visualization of the posterior cardiac structures compared to the TTE and can be considered in patients with valvular disease, PFOs, or aortic arch atherosclerosis.

**Blood Tests**—Younger patients without clear vascular risk factors may have further blood workup, which may include protein C, protein S, factor V Leiden, ANA, or anti–double stranded DNA.

**Step 9**) The goal in treating patients with TIAs is to ameliorate any existing deficit and to prevent future strokes. However, patients with rapidly improving symptoms should not be given IV fibrinolytic therapy. Since approximately 4% to 10% of patients will have a stroke within the first two days after a TIA, it is important to emphasize stroke prevention treatment. The following preventive measures are based on the AHA/ASA guidelines and are the same as for ischemic stroke:

**Modifiable risk factors**—Smoking cessation, reduce heavy alcohol intake, and encourage physical activity (if able to perform).

**Treatable risk factors**—Reduce blood pressure in patients who had an ischemic stroke or TIA and are beyond the first 24 hours; initiate a statin in patients who have evidence of atherosclerosis, LDL ≥100 mg/dL, and who are without known CHD; diabetics should maintain good glycemic control and keep BP <130/80.

**Noncardioembolic TIAs**—Patients with noncardioembolic TIAs should be given either aspirin alone, clopidogrel alone, or aspirin + dipyridamole. Do not give aspirin and clopidogrel together because it can increase the risk of hemorrhage. Ticlopidine is another antiplatelet agent that is used to prevent recurrence, but it is not a first-line agent and is generally reserved for patients who are intolerant of aspirin or clopidogrel.

**Cardioembolic TIAs**—Anticoagulation with warfarin should be given to patients with atrial fibrillation (paroxysmal or permanent), mechanical prosthetic heart valves, rheumatic valve disease, and in patients with an LV thrombus in the setting of an acute MI.

**Carotid endarterectomy (CEA)**—CEA is recommended in patients with a recent TIA or ischemic stroke (past 6 months) that have severe carotid stenosis that is >70%, and the estimated risk of perioperative morbidity and mortality is <6%. CEA is not indicated when carotid stenosis is <50%. Between 50% and 69% stenosis, the indication is not as clear because it depends on various factors (eg, comorbidities, age, sex, estimated risk). The timing of CEA is also less clear, but some authorities recommend waiting between 2 and 6 weeks. Remember that an urgent CEA is not well established and not a good choice to pick on the exam.

**Disposition:**

The **ABCD²** score (**A**ge, **B**lood pressure, **C**linical features, **D**uration of symptoms, and **D**iabetes) is a tool that can estimate the risk of an ischemic stroke in patients who present acutely after a TIA. The AHA/ASA guidelines state that it is reasonable to hospitalize patients with a TIA who present within 72 hours of the event and either have an ABCD² score ≥3, an ABCD² score 0 to 2 and uncertainty that diagnostic workup can be completed within 2 days as an outpatient, or an ABCD² score 0 to 2 and other evidence that the event was caused by focal ischemia. Once the patient is in the hospital, it is also reasonable to place the patient in a telemetry unit or on Holter monitoring if the underlying cause is still unknown.

**Pearls:**

- In light of the new definition of a TIA, TIA essentially does not result in acute infarction, but ischemic strokes do result in infarction of CNS tissue leaving persistent neurologic deficits.
- Diffusion-weighted MRI imaging (DWI) can detect early ischemia and has a high sensitivity and specificity for detecting early infarction.
- Carotid angioplasty and stenting (CAS) is an alternative to CEA, but CEA is still considered gold standard.
- **On the CCS**, patients that have a carotid artery stenosis >70% should have a "vascular surgery consult."
- **On the CCS**, most patients with TIAs that are seen in the ED or in the office should be hospitalized because of the opportunity to give IV fibrinolysis if a stroke does occur and to assess any other stroke risk factors.

# INTRACEREBRAL HEMORRHAGE

Intracerebral hemorrhage (ICH) is the second most common cause of stroke. **Hypertension** is the most common underlying cause of spontaneous ICH. Other causes of ICH include amyloid angiopathy, arteriovenous malformations, vasculitis, coagulopathies, CNS infections, trauma, tumors, and drugs (cocaine, amphetamines, anticoagulants, thrombolytics).

**Risk Factors:**

Hypertension, older age, alcohol abuse, illicit drugs (ie, sympathomimetics).

**Clinical Features:**

The neurologic symptoms are usually of a gradual onset (ie, minutes to hours), unlike a subarachnoid hemorrhage where symptoms are abrupt. Symptoms alone in ICH may be indistinguishable from ischemic stroke. In addition, neurologic deficits vary depending on the site of hemorrhage. Consider the following locations in a relative superior to inferior direction:

**Lobar hemorrhage**—Lobar hemorrhages have a higher association with seizures. Consider the following lobes: frontal lobe (frontal headaches, contralateral hemiparesis), temporal lobe (aphasia), parietal lobe (contralateral hemisensory loss), occipital lobe (homonymous hemianopsia)

**Putamenal hemorrhage**—The putamen is the most common location for hypertensive hemorrhage. Features include contralateral hemiparesis, contralateral sensory loss, homonymous hemianopsia, or gaze palsy. With larger hemorrhages, stupor and coma ensue.

**Thalamic hemorrhage**—Contralateral hemiparesis, contralateral sensory loss, transient homonymous hemianopsia, vertical gaze palsy, eyes that are down and in (ie, looking at nose), miotic pupils, eyes unreactive to light, aphasia (dominant hemisphere), or neglect (nondominant hemisphere).

**Pontine hemorrhage**—Deep coma with quadriplegia, decerebrate rigidity, pinpoint pupils reactive to light, absent horizontal eye movements, or ocular bobbing.

**Cerebellar hemorrhage**—Vomiting, occipital headaches, gait ataxia, vertigo, gaze palsy, or facial weakness. Stupor and coma ensue in the presence of brainstem compression.

**Next Step:**

**Step 1)** ICH is a medical emergency, and it is important to assess **A**irway, **B**reathing, and **C**irculation.

**Step 2)** Place monitoring equipment on patient: pulse oximetry, continuous blood pressure cuff, continuous cardiac monitoring, and 12-lead EKG.

**Step 3)** Provide supplemental oxygen if hypoxemic.

**Step 4)** Establish IV access with laboratory studies (eg, CBC, BMP, PT/INR, PTT, troponins, lipid profile) and in select patients order toxicology screen, blood alcohol level, HCG, or ABG (if hypoxia suspected).

**Step 5)** Finger-stick glucose; treat if indicated

**Step 6)** Perform a targeted history and physical. In addition, the NIH stroke scale can be performed at this time.

**Step 7)** Order an emergent noncontrast CT or MRI. Patients that have a cerebellar hemorrhage >3 cm in diameter who are deteriorating, or those who have a brainstem compression, and/or those who have a hydrocephalus from ventricular obstruction require an urgent surgical removal of the hemorrhage.

**Step 8)** Change location to ICU and manage acute ICH in a monitored setting.

**Step 9)** Treat the following components of acute ICH:

**Hyperglycemia**—Target glucose levels in patients with ICH is yet to be defined, but treatment with insulin to maintain normoglycemia is reasonable. Remember to monitor glucose levels with Accu-Cheks.

**Fever**—Look for the underlying cause (eg, abscess) and treat with antipyretics.

**Seizures**—Routine prophylactic antiepileptics are not recommended, but if a seizure does occur, treat with a benzodiazepine (eg, IV lorazepam) for rapid control followed by a loading dose of either IV fosphenytoin or phenytoin to prevent recurrence.

**Anticoagulant-associated ICH**—Stop all anticoagulants and antiplatelet therapy. Short-term reversal of **warfarin-associated ICH** can be accomplished by either FFP, prothrombin complex concentrates (PCC), or recombinant factor VIIa (rFVIIa). Long-term reversal of warfarin-associated ICH can be achieved with intravenous infusion of vitamin K. There is no standardized protocol to reverse anticoagulation, but a recommended approach is to administer vitamin K as a slow intravenous infusion in conjunction with FFP plus PCC. In this approach, you bridge the short-term reversal with the long-term reversal. **Heparin-associated ICH** can be reversed with an intravenous infusion of protamine sulfate.

**Elevated intracranial pressure (ICP)**—ICP can result in a midline shift with subsequent neurologic dysfunction. Simple measures to lower ICP may include elevating the head of the bed to 30 degrees and providing appropriate analgesia and sedation. More aggressive approaches include osmotic therapy (eg, mannitol, hypertonic saline), barbiturate anesthesia, neuromuscular blockade, or ventriculostomy. Glucocorticoids are not used to lower ICP in patients with ICH. Hyperventilation ($PaCO_2$ of 25-30 mm Hg) is not routinely performed because the effects are rapid and transient.

**Blood pressure control**—The management of blood pressure is still inconclusive, and the AHA/ASA guidelines acknowledge that the evidence for the efficacy of BP management in ICH is currently incomplete. However, the guidelines state that it is probably safe to acutely lower the systolic BP to 140 mm Hg when the presenting systolic BP is between 150 and 220 mm Hg. IV labetalol, nicardipine, or hydralazine are suggested agents for the boards.

**Step 10)** Encourage secondary prevention such as smoking cessation, reduce heavy alcohol intake, quit illicit drugs, low-fat diet, reduce sodium intake, regular exercise, and a goal blood pressure of <140/90 or <130/80 in patients with diabetes or chronic kidney disease.

**Disposition:**

All patients with ICH should be monitored and managed in the ICU.

**Pearls:**

- Anticoagulant-associated ICH and amyloid angiopathy are usually lobar hemorrhages.

- Hyperglycemia is a common finding in patients with acute strokes and is usually associated with poor outcomes.

- When there is a suspicion for structural lesions (eg, vascular malformations, tumors) based on radiologic or clinical findings, further evaluation can be made by contrast CT, contrast

MRI, magnetic resonance angiography (MRA), contrast CT angiography (CTA), CT venography, or magnetic resonance venography.

- Surgical hematoma evacuation for supratentorial ICH remains controversial.

- In general, a lumbar puncture is not recommended in patients with ICH because it may induce a cerebral herniation or aggravate a midline shift.

- Patients with acute ICH should have pneumatic compression stockings to prevent venous thromboembolism (VTE).

- It can take >6 hours to reverse anticoagulation with vitamin K.

- The AHA/ASA does not routinely recommend rFVIIa as the sole agent for treating anticoagulation reversal in patients

with ICH. In addition, rFVIIa has been associated with thromboembolic events.

- **On the CCS**, "FFP" and "PCC" are both available on the practice CCS, but not "rFVIIa."

- **On the CCS**, PCC is also known as factor IX complex and if you order "PCC" in the practice CCS, the order will be converted to "factor IX complex" on the order sheet.

- **On the CCS**, ICH is a neurologic emergency, and therefore, your timing and sequence of actions will play an important part of your evaluation.

- **On the CCS**, if there are any CCS cases in which you determine the patient may have an adverse or fatal outcome, remember to obtain an "advance directive," which is available in the practice CCS.

# MOVEMENT DISORDER

## HUNTINGTON'S DISEASE

Huntington's disease (HD) is an autosomal dominant inherited disorder that results in expansion of a CAG trinucleotide repeat in the huntingtin gene located on the short arm of chromosome 4. The major pathology in HD is atrophy of the caudate nucleus and putamen.

**Clinical Features:**

Huntington's disease is a chronic progressive disease that can start as early as 2 years old to 80 years old, but typically begins in the fourth or fifth decade. HD can be characterized by abnormal movements, psychiatric symptoms, and cognitive deterioration.

> **Movements**—In the early stages, patients may appear fidgety or restless. Eventually, choreiform movements (ie, rapid, involuntary, arrhythmic movements) are pronounced and involve most of the musculature. In advancing disease, the **chorea** is gradually replaced with spasticity, bradykinesia, myoclonus, dystonia (eg, abnormal postures), or a parkinsonian akinetic-rigid state. Other movement abnormalities that may be present in HD include oculomotor dysfunction, dysarthria, dysphagia, gait disturbances, or hyperreflexia.

> **Psychiatric**—Patients can have depression with suicide tendencies, delusions, hallucinations, irritability, or paranoia at any point during the disease.

> **Cognitive**—Patients can develop dementia, lack insight of their cognitive deficits, and may have difficulty with concentration.

**Next Step:**

**Step 1)** The diagnosis of HD is based on typical clinical features and a family history of genetically proven HD. In the absence of a family history of HD, patients can undergo genetic testing

to confirm or exclude the diagnosis of HD. Neuroimaging (eg, brain MRI) is no longer used to confirm the diagnosis of HD, but can still support the diagnosis by showing atrophy of the caudate nucleus.

**Step 2)** There is no cure for Huntington's disease, and treatment is focused on symptom control and supportive care, which requires a multidisciplinary approach. Dopamine-blocking agents (eg, tetrabenazine) may control the chorea, antipsychotics (eg, quetiapine) may help with the psychosis, antidepressants (eg, SSRIs) can assist with depression, but there is no effective therapy for dementia.

**Follow-Up:**

Genetic counseling is recommended for patients and their families.

**Pearls:**

- If HD presents before age 20, the patient is considered to have juvenile HD (Westphal variant), and clinical features can be characterized by parkinsonism (eg, rigidity), seizures, cerebellar ataxia, and little to no chorea.

- Some patients may be mistakenly diagnosed with a psychiatric illness when in fact they have HD.

- **Foundational point**—The CAG trinucleotide repeat encodes for polyglutamine tracts in the protein products (ie, longer polyglutamine tracts with more CAG repeats). CAG trinucleotide repeats can be seen in other disorders (eg, spinobulbar muscular atrophy) other than Huntington's disease.

- **Foundational point**—In Huntington's disease, the CAG trinucleotide repeat mutation gives rise to a mutant huntingtin protein (with polyglutamine expansion) that is toxic to the neurons, and aggregation of the mutant protein is the pathologic hallmark of the disease.

- **Foundational point**—Anticipation can be seen in Huntington's disease. Anticipation is a genetic terminology that explains that the genetic condition becomes more severe and appears earlier as the disease is passed down to following generations.

- **Foundational point**—Neurotransmitters, GABA and acetylcholine, are reduced in the basal ganglia in patients with Huntington's disease.

- **Connecting point** (pg. 162)—Be familiar with the other autosomal dominant disorders.

- **On the CCS**, "genetics counseling" is available in the practice CCS.

# NEOPLASM

## MENINGIOMA

Meningiomas are one of the most common primary brain tumors that are predominately benign and are typically attached to the dura (extradural is uncommon). Meningiomas can be seen in patients with **neurofibromatosis type 2 (NF2)**, and there is a clear association in patients exposed to **radiation** followed by a latency period before the development of the tumor.

### Clinical Features:

Meningiomas are typically slow-growing lesions that present in older adults and are more common in women compared to men. Patients with NF2 typically have multiple meningiomas, and they develop the tumors at an earlier age. Most individuals with meningiomas are asymptomatic, but depending on the size and location, symptoms may vary. Consider the following locations and possible effect:

**Cerebral convexities**—Seizures

**Subfrontal**—Mental status changes

**Intraventricular (eg, choroid plexus)**—Obstructive hydrocephalus

**Posterior cranial fossa**—Headaches, cranial nerve palsies, brain herniation

**Parasagittal frontoparietal**—Extremity weakness or numbness

**Parasellar**—Visual field defects, panhypopituitarism

**Occipital**—Hemianopsia

**Optic nerve sheath**—Unilateral visual loss

**Olfactory groove**—Anosmia

**Cerebellopontine angle**—Sensorineural hearing loss, vertigo

**Cavernous sinus**—Cranial nerve III, IV, $V_1$, $V_2$, and VI deficits

**Spine**—Brown-Séquard syndrome (ie, hemisection of the spinal cord) that presents with weakness, loss of vibration and proprioception ipsilateral to the lesion, but contralateral loss of pain and temperature.

### Next Step:

**Step 1)** The best initial approach in a patient suspected of having a meningioma is with imaging studies. The preferred modality is with a **contrast-enhanced (gadolinium) MRI**, although a contrast-enhanced CT is also acceptable. The most accurate test is with tissue biopsy, but in some cases obtaining tissue is not feasible because of the risk of further neurologic damage.

**Step 2)** Complete surgical resection is the preferred approach because it is curative. However, in cases when the tumor is not surgically resectable, radiation therapy is the treatment of choice.

### Follow-Up:

Patients who undergo treatment should have surveillance with an MRI in the postoperative period and then annually to detect any recurrence.

### Pearls:

- To date, there is no association between cell phone use and meningiomas.

- Malignant meningiomas can occur, but they are rare tumors.

- Patients with NF2 also commonly have vestibular schwannomas.

- Brown-Séquard syndrome can also be seen with spinal trauma, spinal cord tumors, disc herniation, infarctions, infections, or hematomas.

- Brown-Séquard syndrome involves one-half of the spinal cord and affects the dorsal column, corticospinal tract, and spinothalamic tract.

- Sometimes a meningioma will show a "tail" adjacent to the tumor mass (dural tail sign) on contrast-enhanced MRI that represents dural thickening (keep in mind that this is not pathognomonic).

- Older patients with comorbidities that are found to have an incidental finding of a small asymptomatic meningioma can be initially followed radiologically.

- Stereotactic radiotherapy uses precise and focused radiation delivered to a tumor with the goal of minimizing injury to adjacent structures.

- **Foundational point**—Psammomatous meningioma is one of many subtypes of meningioma. Histologically, it is characterized by numerous cellular whorls with psammoma bodies (laminated calcific concretions). Psammoma bodies can also be seen in other carcinomas (eg, papillary thyroid carcinoma, papillary renal cell carcinoma, papillary serous carcinoma of the ovary).

- **Connecting point** (pg. 162)—Be familiar with the other autosomal dominant disorders.

- **On the CCS**, "radiation therapy" and "stereotactic radiotherapy" are both available in the practice CCS, and if you order stereotactic radiotherapy, it will be converted to radiation therapy on the order sheet.

- **On the CCS,** if you decided to use radiation therapy on a patient, remember to order a "radiation therapy consult," but keep in mind that the practice CCS does not recognize "radiation oncologist" under the consults.

- **On the CCS,** as soon as you confirm the diagnosis of cancer, remember to "advise patient, cancer diagnosis," which is available in the practice CCS. Try not to advise the patient at the end of the CCS case because you are tested on the sequence of your actions.

# TRAUMA

## ▌EPIDURAL HEMATOMA

Epidural hematoma (EDH) is characterized by bleeding into the potential space between the skull and dura mater. The primary mechanism of EDH is trauma to the temporoparietal area with injury to the middle meningeal artery. In a small subset of patients, injury can occur in the posterior cranial fossa region resulting in EDH from disruption of the dural sinuses.

### Clinical Features:

After trauma to the head, the patient may go into a coma, or there may be a momentary loss of consciousness followed by recovery of consciousness or the "lucid interval." As the hematoma expands, the patient can deteriorate and may experience vomiting, drowsiness, confusion, headaches, seizures, aphasia, or hemiparesis. Without intervention, the hematoma will continue to expand resulting in elevated intracranial pressures (ie, Cushing's reflex—HTN, bradycardia, respiratory depression) with possible transtentorial or uncal herniation that can result in an oculomotor nerve palsy (ie, ipsilateral dilated pupil; paralysis of adduction, elevation, and depression; eye rests in a "down and out" position). Following a comatose period, death will ensue.

### Next Step:

**Step 1)** The best initial test is with an **unenhanced head CT scan.** The classic finding on CT scan is a lens-shaped (ie, biconvex or lenticular-shaped) mass ± midline shift (see Figure 11-2). On head CT scan, epidural hematomas do not cross suture lines because of the firm attachment of the dura to the sutures.

**Step 2)** Symptomatic patients require emergent surgical hematoma evacuation usually by burr hole evacuation (trephination) or open craniotomy. In addition, ligation of the bleeding vessel should be considered during the procedure. Only in select patients (ie, small EDH and asymptomatic) can surgical evacuation be deferred, but close monitoring should be emphasized with serial brain imaging.

### Disposition:

After initial management in the ED, patients should be transferred to the ICU or sent for surgical evacuation.

### Pearls:

- Epidural hematomas evolve more rapidly compared to subdural hematomas.

- The lucid interval seen in EDH can be of shorter duration (several hours) if the EDH is due to a pumping arterial bleed, but if the culprit is a venous bleed the lucid interval can be several days to weeks.

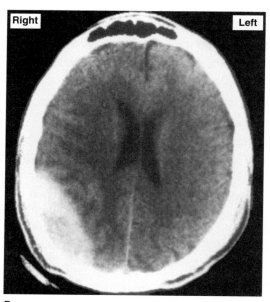

**FIGURE 11-2 • Subdural and epidural hematoma. A. Subdural hematoma.** Unenhanced CT scan demonstrating a large, hyperdense (white) crescent-shaped lesion that spans over most of the right cerebral hemisphere. Also note the shift of the lateral ventricles across the midline. **B. Epidural hematoma.** Unenhanced CT scan demonstrating a hyperdense (white) lenticular-shaped lesion over the right parieto-occipital region. Fracture of the occipital bone was seen on bone windows. (Reproduced with permission from Greenberg DA, Aminoff MJ, Simon RP. *Clinical Neurology.* 8th ed. New York: McGraw-Hill; 2012:54.)

- Elevated intracranial pressures (ICP) can also be seen with obstruction of the confluence of sinuses located in the posterior fossa.
- Not all patients will present with the classic lucid interval (ie, <20% of cases will demonstrate the lucid interval).
- Lumbar puncture is contraindicated in patients with suspected EDH since there is a risk of herniation.
- Spinal epidural hematomas may be related to trauma, coagulopathies, neoplasms, or vascular malformations. Patients may complain of pain, paresthesias, sensory loss, weakness, or bladder and bowel dysfunction. An MRI should be ordered in patients suspected of having a spinal epidural hematoma.
- **On the CCS**, ordering a complete physical exam would be considered suboptimal management since that would cost you extra time and delay treatment.
- **On the CCS**, "neuro checks" is available in the practice CCS, and it is an important monitoring parameter in patients with EDH since clinical deterioration can arise soon after the lucid (clear) period.

## ▌SUBDURAL HEMATOMA

Subdural hematoma (SDH) is characterized by bleeding into the space between the dura and the arachnoid membranes. The primary mechanism of SDH is a sudden acceleration or deceleration of the brain in relation to fixed dural structures resulting in tearing of the bridging veins. In a small subset of patients, arterial rupture (eg, small cortical arteries) can also result in SDH.

### Clinical Features:

Subdural hematomas can be classified as acute, subacute, or chronic. The time from onset is arbitrarily defined as acute (1-2 days after injury), subacute (3-14 days after injury), and chronic (>14 days after injury).

**Acute SDH**—Patients with significant cerebral atrophy (ie, elderly and alcoholic patients) are at high risk for acute SDH, especially if they have any coagulopathies. After trauma to the head, the patient may go into a coma, or there may be a brief "lucid interval" followed by progressive neurologic deterioration and eventually coma if there is no intervention. Subdural hematomas can also form in the posterior fossa causing elevated intracranial pressures (ICP) and resulting in vomiting, headaches, dysphagia, anisocoria, cranial nerve palsies, stiff neck, or ataxia.

**Chronic SDH**—Chronic SDH is commonly seen in older adults (especially if they are taking anticoagulants), but the traumatic etiology may not be as apparent. Patients may have insignificant head trauma that they may not remember. The clinical presentation is often insidious and may include headaches, apathy, drowsiness, lightheadedness, cognitive dysfunction, unsteady gait, or occasionally seizures.

### Next Step:

**Step 1**) The best initial test is with an **unenhanced head CT scan**. The SDH can be unilateral or bilateral and is commonly located over the frontotemporal region. Findings on CT scan will demonstrate a crescent-shaped lesion ± midline shift (see Figure 11-2), and unlike epidural hematomas, SDH can cross suture lines. The density of the lesion on CT scan can give us a relative time frame of the injury in that an acute SDH the lesion is hyperdense (white), subacute SDH the lesion is isodense (in relation to the brain), and chronic SDH appears as hypodense (dark).

**Step 2**) Patients with acute or chronic SDH who continue to have progressive neurologic deterioration and signs of increasing intracranial pressures (eg, Cushing's reflex, dilated pupil(s), decorticate or decerebrate posturing) should undergo urgent surgical hematoma evacuation either by burr hole or craniotomy. In addition, ligation of the bleeding vessel should be considered during the procedure. Only in select patients (ie, small SDH and asymptomatic) can surgical evacuation be deferred, but close monitoring should be emphasized with serial brain imaging.

### Disposition:

After initial management in the ED, patients should be transferred to the ICU or sent for surgical evacuation.

### Pearls:

- The evolution of a subdural hematoma develops more slowly compared to an epidural hematoma because of its venous origin.
- Venous bleeding is usually stopped by the rising intracranial pressures, which unlike arterial bleeds are steadily progressive.
- Lumbar puncture is contraindicated in patients with suspected SDH since there is a risk of herniation.
- A hygroma (fluidlike sac) can form from liquefaction of a chronic SDH or from separation of the dura from the arachnoid (eg, brain atrophy) resulting in an arachnoid tear allowing CSF to escape into the subdural space. Hygromas can be indistinguishable from chronic SDH on imaging studies. Hygromas that fail to resolve spontaneously and continue to expand require surgical evacuation.
- **CJ:** A 52-year-old alcoholic man complains of headaches in the emergency department. The patient vaguely states that he remembers hitting his head on the ground 9 days ago. The initial noncontrast head CT scan appears "normal" on preliminary results, but the index of suspicion for a subdural hematoma is high. What is your next best step? **Answer:** Patients with subacute SDH or chronic SDH will present with an isodense or hypodense lesion on noncontrast CT, respectively. These lesions can appear as normal findings on noncontrast CT, and therefore, the next best step is to consider an IV contrast CT or MRI. The contrast material will enhance the vascular capsule surrounding the hematoma.
- **On the CCS**, poor management would include failure to order any imaging study to identify the subdural hematoma.

# CCS: SUBARACHNOID HEMORRHAGE CASE INTRODUCTION

Day 1 @ 22:30
Emergency Room

A 55-year-old African American woman comes to the emergency department because of a headache.

**Initial Vital Signs:**
Temperature: 37.0°C (98.6°F)
Pulse: 80 beats/min
Respiratory: 16/min
Blood pressure: 147/92 mm Hg
Height: 172.7 cm (68.0 inches)
Weight: 54.5 kg (120 lb)
BMI: 18.2 kg/m$^2$

**Initial History:**
Reason(s) for visit: Headache

**HPI:**
A 55-year-old restaurant owner is brought into the emergency department by her husband because of a severe and sudden onset of a headache for the past 2 hours. She states that this is the "worst headache of my life" and rates her pain as 10/10 in severity. The pain is mainly over her right temporal area without radiation. She also has visual changes, photophobia, stiff neck, and nausea without vomiting. She denies any fevers, chills, recent trauma, or sick contacts. Over the past week, she has had two other episodes of sudden headaches without any relief from taking acetaminophen.

| | |
|---|---|
| **Past Medical History:** | Hypertension |
| **Past Surgical History:** | Cesarean deliveries at ages 22 and 24. |
| **Medications:** | HCTZ, amlodipine |
| **Allergies:** | None |
| **Vaccinations:** | Up to date |
| **Family History:** | Father died of lung cancer at age 70. Mother died of a subarachnoid hemorrhage at age 55. Older brother, age 57, has hyperlipidemia. |
| **Social History:** | Smokes one pack per day × 30 years; drinks two martinis every day and more on the weekends; Hx of cocaine abuse; married with two children; restaurant owner; enjoys cooking |

**Review of Systems:**

| | |
|---|---|
| General: | See HPI |
| Skin: | Negative |
| HEENT: | See HPI |
| Musculoskeletal: | See HPI |
| Cardiorespiratory: | Negative |
| Gastrointestinal: | See HPI |
| Genitourinary: | Negative |
| Neuropsychiatric: | See HPI |

Day 1 @ 22:38

**Physical Examination:**

| | |
|---|---|
| **General appearance:** | Well nourished, well developed; in pain and uncomfortable. |
| **HEENT/Neck:** | Normocephalic. Nontender to palpation over the right temporal area. EOMI, PERRLA. Subhyaloid retinal hemorrhages seen on funduscopic examination. Hearing normal. Ear, nose, and mouth normal. Pharynx normal. Neck supple; trachea midline; no masses or bruits; thyroid normal. |
| **Chest/Lungs:** | Chest wall normal. Diaphragm and chest moving equally and symmetrically with respiration. Auscultation and percussion normal. |
| **Heart/Cardiovascular:** | S1, S2 normal. No murmurs, rubs, gallops, or extra sounds. No JVD. |
| **Abdomen:** | Normal bowel sounds; no bruits. No tenderness. No masses. No hernias. No hepatosplenomegaly. |
| **Extremities/Spine:** | No joint deformity or warmth. No cyanosis or clubbing. No edema. Peripheral pulses normal. Spine exam normal. |
| **Neuro/Psych:** | GCS score of 13. Nuchal rigidity with positive Kernig's and Brudzinski's sign. Cranial nerve exam normal. Sensory exam normal. Pronator drift absent or other motor deficit absent. Cerebellar function normal. Deep tendon reflexes normal. |

**First Order Sheet:**
1) IV access
2) Ketorolac, IV, one time/ bolus

**Second Order Sheet:**
1) Head CT without contrast, stat

**Result:** No blood seen in the ventricles or inter-hemispheric fissures. No hydrocephalus. No mass effect. Normal findings.

**Third Order Sheet:**
1) Lumbar puncture, stat

**Result:** Opening pressure 210 mm $H_2O$ (nl: 70-180 mm $H_2O$); gross blood obtained.

2) CSF cell count, stat

**Result:** RBCs seen with a cell count of $7 \times 10^6/mm^3$

**Note:** Do not wait for the report time before transferring to the ICU.

**Actions:**
1) Change location to ICU

**Note:** Vitals are automatically ordered as q4 hrs in the practice CCS.

**Fourth Order Sheet:**
1) NPO
2) Urine output, routine, q8 hrs
3) Neuro checks, routine, q1 hr
4) Pneumatic compression stocking
5) Bedrest, complete
6) Omeprazole, oral, continuous
7) Docusate, oral, continuous
8) Pulse oximetry, stat — **Result:** 97%
9) Continuous cardiac monitor, stat — **Result:** Regular sinus
10) Continuous blood pressure cuff, stat — **Result:** 147/92 mm Hg
11) 12-Lead EKG, stat — **Result:** U waves present
12) Neurosurgery consult, stat — **Reason:** Suspected sub-arachnoid hemorrhage.
13) Nimodipine, oral, continuous
14) PT/INR, stat — **Result:** PT-10 seconds (nl: <12), INR-1.0 (nl: 1.0-1.3)
15) PTT, stat — **Result:** 26 seconds (nl: <28)
16) CBC with differential, stat — **Result:** WBC-9,000, H/H-14/38%, Plt-200,000, Differential- normal
17) BMP, stat — **Result:** Glu-90, Urea-12, Na-134, K-3.9, Cl-103, HCO3-26, Cr-1, Ca-9.3

**Fifth Order Sheet:**
1) NaCl tablets, oral, one time/bolus
2) Isotonic saline solution, IV, continuous
3) BMP, routine, q6 hrs

**BMP result is now available** — **Result:** Glu-90, Urea-12, Na-138, K-3.9, Cl-103, HCO3-26, Cr-1, Ca- 9.3

**Vitals are now available** — **Result:** Temp-37°C, HR-80, RR-16, BP-147/92

**Neuro signs available** — **Result:** Alert, PERRLA, moves all 4 extremities.

**Sixth Order Sheet:**
1) Check cardiac monitor — **Result:** Regular sinus
2) Pulse oximetry — **Result:** 97%

**Seventh Order Sheet:**
1) Cerebral angiography, stat — **Result:** Right middle cerebral artery (MCA) aneurysm detected.

**Neurosurgery consult recommendations:** Based on a favorable clinical grade along with a multidisciplinary decision, the recommendation is neurosurgical clipping. After discussion with the patient regarding alternative treatments, risks and benefits with surgery, the patient agrees with surgery. Thank you for the consult.

**This case will end in the next few minutes of "real time."**
You may **add** or **delete** orders at this time, then enter a diagnosis on the following screen.

**Eighth Order Sheet:**
1) Type and crossmatch, blood, stat
2) Chest x-ray, PA/lateral, stat
3) Counsel family/patient
4) Advise patient, no smoking
5) Advise patient, limit alcohol intake
6) Advise patient, no illegal drug use
7) Advise patient, advance directive

**Please enter your diagnosis:**
Subarachnoid Hemorrhage

**DISCUSSION:**
Subarachnoid hemorrhage (SAH) refers to bleeding into the subarachnoid space that is between the arachnoid membranes and pia mater. Most causes of SAH are due to a rupture of a saccular aneurysm. Other causes of SAH can be from nonaneurysmal mechanisms such as arteriovenous malformations or intracranial arterial dissection. Approximately 20% of strokes are hemorrhagic, with 10% accounting for SAH and 10% accounting for intracerebral hemorrhage. Unfortunately, about 10% of patients with SAH will die prior to reaching the hospital.

## Risk Factors:

Hypertension, smoking, heavy alcohol intake, sympathomimetic drugs (eg, cocaine), very low BMI, family history of aneurysmal SAH (especially first-degree relatives), autosomal dominant polycystic kidney disease, Ehlers-Danlos syndrome type IV, glucocorticoid-remediable aldosteronism (GRA)

## Clinical Features:

Aneurysmal SAH is more likely to be seen in patients between 40 and 60 years of age, with a higher incidence seen in women compared to men. All ethnic groups are at risk of SAH, but blacks have a higher risk compared to whites. The classic presentation is a sudden onset of severe headaches (ie, thunderclap headache) that patients often describe as the "worst headache of my life." Approximately 30% of these sudden headaches occur at night, and 30% of headaches will lateralize to the side of the aneurysm (eg, right-sided headaches with a right-sided MCA). A second presentation to be aware of in patients with SAH is prodromal signs and symptoms prior to the rupture of the aneurysm or the major SAH. Prodromal events can be due to sentinel leaks, emboli, or a mass effect. Sentinel leaks are "warning leaks" where patients lose a small amount of blood from the aneurysm resulting in sentinel headaches. Embolization from a thrombus within an aneurysm can result in TIAs. A mass effect from an expanding aneurysm can result in neurologic dysfunction that is based on the location of the aneurysm. For example, anterior communicating artery (hemiparesis, abulia), middle cerebral artery (face and upper extremity paresis, aphasia, retro-orbital pain), internal carotid artery or large aneurysms (cavernous sinus compression affecting CN III, IV, $V_1$, $V_2$, and VI), PICA or AICA (occipital pain), and at the junction of the posterior communicating artery and internal carotid artery (CN 3- oculomotor nerve palsy). Finally, the last presentation to be aware of in patients with SAH is immediate loss of consciousness (LOC) soon after the rupture. Keep in mind that other associated features of SAH that may or may not be present are nausea, vomiting, seizures, subhyaloid retinal hemorrhages, or meningismus (ie, signs and symptoms of meningeal irritation but without actual infection).

## Next Step Summary:

**Step 1)** SAH is a medical emergency, and as you approach this case you want to consider your differential diagnosis, which includes meningitis, ischemic stroke, intracerebral hemorrhage, TIA, encephalitis, migraine, and cluster headache.

**Step 2)** Perform a targeted physical exam.

**Step 3)** Address any pain issues, and in this case, the patient was complaining of a 10/10 pain.

**Step 4)** The best initial diagnostic test is with a **noncontrast head CT**. The sensitivity of the CT is highest if performed within 12 hours of symptom onset. The sensitivity of the CT remains fairly high in the first 3 days, and then progressively declines until after the fifth to seventh day the CT shows an increase in negative CT scans for SAH. By the 10th day, most of the blood in the subarachnoid is resorbed. If the head CT is normal (ie, no

blood on CT) then the next best step is to perform a **lumbar puncture (LP)**. The classic finding on LP for SAH is an elevated opening pressure and an elevated RBC count that can reach >1 million/mm³. The next question you have to consider is whether an elevated RBC count is due a traumatic LP or SAH. There are 3 ways you can differentiate between a traumatic LP and SAH. First, you can collect the CSF in 4 tubes, and if the RBC count is consistently elevated in all 4 tubes, it would suggest an SAH, but if the last tube has a lower RBC count, it would suggest a traumatic LP. However, counting RBCs in the tubes is not always reliable since there are cases where there is a lower RBC count in the later tubes of SAH. The second way of differentiating between a traumatic LP and SAH is to quickly take your CSF samples and spin them down (centrifugation) to look for xanthochromia. If the supernatant appears pink or yellow, xanthochromia is present because the color reflects the breakdown of RBCs. Keep in mind that if xanthochromia is present, it means that blood has been in the CSF for at least 2 hours. On the other side, if you don't have xanthochromia it would imply that there is no blood in the CSF or there was not enough time for RBCs to break down (which suggests a traumatic LP). Therefore, it is important to centrifuge your samples quickly. Finally, the last way of differentiating between a traumatic LP and SAH is to look at the opening pressure. A traumatic LP will generally have a normal opening pressure since the puncture was probably a local vessel, but bleeding into the CSF from a SAH would elevate the opening pressure.

**Step 5)** All antiplatelet and anticoagulant therapy should be discontinued in patients with SAH until definitive treatment of the aneurysm. Remember to look at the patients medication(s) to determine if you want to discontinue them in all of your CCS cases.

**Step 6)** Admit suspected patients with SAH to the ICU for continuous monitoring and basic ICU care (eg, GI prophylaxis, stool softeners, bedrest, I/Os, pneumatic compression stocking, neuro checks). At this point, you can order your basic labs and a baseline EKG, but you do not want to wait for the report time on the CCS before ordering the treatment. Also be aware that EKG abnormalities are common in SAH, which is thought to represent myocardial injury from autonomic stimulation or release of catecholamines. Possible EKG abnormalities include ST depressions, T wave inversions, prominent U waves, QT prolongation, tachycardia, or bradycardia.

**Step 7)** Consider the following treatment management of SAH:

**Blood pressure control**—Hypertension should be controlled from the time of SAH symptom onset until the time of aneurysm obliteration. It is thought that lowering the blood pressure will reduce the risk of rebleeding, but it can also lead to cerebral ischemia. The target blood pressure is yet to be defined, but the AHA/ASA guidelines recommend a decrease in systolic BP <160 mm Hg to be reasonable. For the boards, you can use IV labetalol but avoid nitroglycerin and nitroprusside because they can increase the intracranial pressure (ICP).

**Aneurysm Repair**—The goal of aneurysm repair is to prevent rerupture. Aneurysm obliteration can be accomplished by "clipping" the aneurysm (via neurosurgeon) or "coiling" embolization of the aneurysm (via endovascular specialist).

The choice of procedure depends on the location of the aneurysm, the grade of the patient, and availability of the resources to perform the procedure.

**Vasospasms**—Vasospasms are a complication of SAH that can lead to cerebral ischemia and infarction. Vasospasms are the leading cause of mortality and morbidity after aneurysm rupture. Vasospasms typically peak 7 to 10 days after a rupture and spontaneously resolve after 21 days. Transcranial Doppler (TCD) can monitor for the development of a vasospasm. The calcium channel blocker nimodipine was initially used to prevent vasospasms, but there is no substantial evidence that the drug affects the incidence of the vasospasms. However, since nimodipine has been shown to improve the neurological outcomes, the use of the drug is still recommended and should be instituted within 96 hours (4 days) of the SAH.

**Hyponatremia**—Hyponatremia is fairly common following SAH. Hyponatremia is typically due to SIADH and less commonly from cerebral salt-wasting. Cerebral salt-wasting results in volume depletion that eventually leads to the release of ADH. Treatment of cerebral salt-wasting can be accomplished by infusing isotonic saline, which will restore the volume status to euvolemia, eventually inhibiting the release of ADH. Treatment of SIADH is usually with fluid restriction, but in patients with SAH, you do not want to restrict fluid because hypovolemia can result in cerebral ischemia. Salt tablets coupled with isotonic saline can initially be attempted, but eventually 3% hypertonic saline solution may be required if hyponatremia persists. Remember not to correct the sodium too quickly as it could result in central pontine myelinolysis.

**Hydrocephalus**—Acute symptomatic patients can be managed by either lumbar CSF drainage or with a ventriculostomy, which has an infectious risk but does have the benefit of direct measurement of the ICP.

**Seizures**—Management of seizures that are related to SAH is an area of controversy. Avoid prophylaxis or treatment of seizures on the boards.

**Step 8)** Once the patient is medically stabilized, then cerebral angiography (ie, digital subtraction angiography [DSA] with 3-dimensional rotational angiography) should be performed in patients with SAH to determine the location(s) of the aneurysm, assess the anatomy, and to help guide treatment (ie, coiling vs. clipping). The timing of the cerebral angiography will usually depend on the surgical considerations, but the timing of the surgery is still under debate. For board purposes, do not delay life-saving treatment for the sake of a cerebral angiography (eg, obtaining cerebral angiography before treating an acute hydrocephalus).

Disposition:

Patients should be managed in the ICU, and those who undergo clipping or coiling should have a follow-up vascular imaging.

Pearls:
- SAH is frequently misdiagnosed, and if it's in your differential diagnosis for headache, be sure to work it up because it is a medical emergency.

- Pregnancy does not appear to be a risk factor for the development of aneurysmal SAH.
- Screening patients for an intracranial aneurysm is not recommended for the general population. In addition, routinely screening individual family members of an affected person with an intracranial aneurysm is not well established, but may be considered on an individual basis.
- Subhyaloid retinal hemorrhages can be seen in approximately 20% of SAH cases.
- In the majority of cases, if xanthochromia is truly present in the CSF it will show by 12 hours after the SAH event.
- Xanthochromia can last in the CSF for >2 weeks.
- Xanthochromia can be detected either by the naked eye (common method) or by spectrophotometry (more sensitive).
- Spectrophotometry can detect breakdown products of blood with bilirubin as the end product of heme degradation. Bilirubin levels peak at 48 hours after an SAH event and can last for 4 weeks in the CSF.
- Digital subtraction angiography (DSA) is a fluoroscopy technique that involves taking images before and after contrast dye that results in subtracting bone and soft tissue from the images permitting clearer visualization of the blood vessels.
- Patients with SAH can have elevated troponin levels, especially if there are EKG abnormalities or LV dysfunction.
- Patients with SAH can also have elevated BNP levels, although the cause is still unclear.
- Perimesencephalic nonaneurysmal SAH is a type of nonaneurysmal SAH where blood is isolated to the cisterns that are anterior to the brainstem. In the majority of cases, the underlying cause is unknown, but the clinical course is milder, fewer complications, and overall better outcome compared to aneurysmal SAH. On imaging, CT may show blood in the interpeduncular cistern that is anterior to the midbrain, and patients will have a normal cerebral angiography. However, you should be aware that perimesencephalic aneurysmal SAH can also occur in a small subset of patients, and the aneurysm typically arises in the posterior circulation. Therefore, any patient with perimesencephalic SAH should undergo angiographic evaluation.
- Glucocorticoid therapy is not routinely used in SAH because there is little evidence that demonstrates a beneficial or adverse effect from therapy.
- Rebleeding is a complication of SAH, and the risk of rebleeding is greatest in the first 2 to 12 hours. Early rebleeding typically has a worse outcome compared to later rebleeding.
- In most cases, CSF taken from the LP should give you a normal WBC-to-RBC ratio of approximately 1:700 to 1000. But be aware that in some cases there may be a brisk CSF leukocytosis that occurs within 48 hours secondary to chemical meningitis which is caused by the breakdown products of subarachnoid blood, thereby altering the WBC-to-RBC ratio. There may also be lowered CSF glucose and slightly elevated CSF protein levels.
- Meningismus seen in SAH is typically caused by the breakdown products of blood with signs and symptoms appearing after several hours of the event.

- The mechanism of nimodipine's beneficial effect is still unknown.
- Treatment for symptomatic vasospasms (ie, not prevention) has been attempted with the triple-H therapy, which includes hypervolemia, induced hypertension, and hemodilution. Triple-H therapy is typically pursued after aneurysm obliteration to prevent the risk of rebleeding. However, triple-H therapy is not routinely recommended because there are no randomized clinical trials on this type of intervention.
- **On the CCS**, "CSF xanthochromia" is not available on the practice CCS.
- **On the CCS**, "spectrophotometry" is not available on the practice CCS.
- **On the CCS**, "transcranial Doppler" is not available on the practice CCS.
- **On the CCS**, "DSA, cerebral" is not available on the practice CCS, but "cerebral angiography" is available.
- **On the CCS**, "coiling" or "clipping" are not available on the practice CCS, but "aneurysm repair, intracranial" is available.
- **On the CCS**, "ventriculostomy" is not available on the practice CCS, but "ventriculocisternostomy" is available, which is the same thing (don't be thrown off, just piece the words together).
- **On the CCS**, do not assume that any orders will be written for you (eg, vitals) during the CCS cases.
- **On the CCS**, "nimodipine" is available in the practice CCS. The medication should be given orally or by NG tube. Do not give as IV since it has been associated with serious adverse events (eg, death, significant hypotension). Also, you want to order it as a continuous mode of frequency because it is given as q4 hrs for 21 days.
- **On the CCS**, suboptimal management would include delaying treatment (eg, waiting for the report time of labs before ordering a neurosurgery consult or nimodipine).
- **On the CCS**, poor management would include failure to order a noncontrast head CT or to follow that up with an LP if the CT was negative.

# 12

# Obstetrics

## KEYWORDS REVIEW

**Aneuploidy**—Abnormal number of chromosomes most commonly from an extra chromosome (eg, trisomy) or from a loss of chromosome (eg, monosomy).

**Argyll-Robertson pupil**—Pupil that does not constrict to light but can constrict to accommodation. This is pathognomonic for tertiary or late syphilis.

**Braxton-Hicks contractions**—Sporadic uterine contractions usually felt in the third trimester, most commonly described as nonrhythmic or irregular contractions.

**Chadwick's sign**—Bluish discoloration of the vulva, vagina, and cervix secondary from venous congestion that occurs between the 8th and 12th weeks of gestation.

**Colostrum**—The first milk produced after delivery, which is a yellowish milky substance that contains more proteins and minerals with less fat and carbohydrates compared to mature breast milk. It also contains IgA, which offers the newborn immune protection.

**Fetal hydrops**—Accumulation of fluid in fetal tissue.

**Goodell sign**—Softening of the cervix occurring in the 6th week of gestation.

**GP**$_{TPAL}$—Gravid, Para, Term, Preterm, Abortions, Living

**Gravid**—Total number of pregnancies.

**Gumma**—Central "gummy" necrotic lesion seen in tertiary or late syphilis.

159

Hegar sign—Softening of the uterus occurring in the sixth week of gestation.

Holoprosencephaly—Failure of the forebrain to develop into two hemispheres.

Latent syphilis—The stage of syphilis after untreated secondary syphilis. Latent syphilis is characterized by no clinical manifestations but positive serology for the infection. It is further divided into early latent (<1 year after secondary syphilis) or late latent (>1 year after secondary syphilis or time of infection is unknown).

Linea nigra—Hyperpigmented vertical line that runs from the pubis to the umbilicus.

Melasma—Also referred to as chloasma and known as the "mask of pregnancy" or hyperpigmentation of the face. The exact cause is still unknown.

Para—Number of pregnancies that led to viability.

Post-term—Delivery after 42 weeks, also referred to as post dates.

Preterm—Delivery of a baby of less than 37 weeks gestational age.

Tabes dorsalis—Degeneration of the posterior columns, characterized by weakness, shooting pains, ataxia, or impaired vibratory and position sense. This condition is seen in tertiary or late syphilis.

Term—Delivery from 37 to 42 weeks.

# ANTEPARTUM

## ANTEPARTUM MANAGEMENT

Antepartum is a period of many developmental and physiological changes in the mother and growing fetus (see Table 12-1). The health of the unborn child and pregnant woman is one of the greatest concerns and therefore, it is imperative to identify any problems through prenatal testing and fetal surveillance to achieve the best possible outcome (see Tables 12-1 and 12-2).

## CONGENITAL ABNORMALITIES

Congenital abnormalities are a common cause of neonatal morbidity and mortality and can occur in 2% to 4% of live births. Genetics, environment, and multifactorial factors contribute to birth defects.

**Genetic Disorders**

Common causes of genetic disorders can be broken down into **single gene disorders** (see Table 12-3) and **chromosomal abnormalities** (see Table 12-4). Genetic counseling is an integral

## Table 12-1 • Antepartum Logistics

**Maternal Physiologic Changes**

**Dental**—No increased incidence of dental caries. Occasionally, epulis gravidarum (ie, violaceous pedunculated lesions on gum line), which can bleed easily when brushing teeth.

**Cardiovascular**—↑ Cardiac output, ↑ stroke volume, ↑ heart rate, ↓ systemic vascular resistance

**Pulmonary**—↑ Tidal volume, ↑ minute ventilation, ↑ vital capacity, ↑ inspiratory capacity, ↓ expiratory reserve volume, ↓ residual volume, ↓ total lung capacity, respiratory rate is the same as prior to pregnancy

**Renal**—↑ Renin-angiotensin system, ↑ GFR, ↓ BUN, ↓ Cr, (Note: ↑ GFR reduces Na level, but it is then compensated by renin-angiotensin system.)

**GI**—Nausea, vomiting, gastric reflux, ↓ gastric motility, constipation, ↑ alkaline phosphatase, gallbladder dilates

**Hematology**—↑ Plasma volume resulting in dilutional anemia, ↑ RBC volume, ↑ ESR, ↓ hematocrit, ↓ serum iron

**Endocrine**—↑ HPL, ↑ progesterone, ↑ estradiol, ↑ cortisol, ↑ aldosterone, ↑ prolactin, ↑ ACTH, ↑ TBG, ↑ Total $T_3$ and $T_4$, no change in TSH

**Skin**—Linea nigra, palmar erythema, spider angiomata, melasma (chloasma)

| Important Timelines of Gestation | Standard Prenatal Vitamin Formulation |
|---|---|
| 30 days gestation—Fetus develops red blood cell antigens.<br>4th-5th week—Gestational sac can be detected by transvaginal ultrasound.<br>5th-6th week—Fetal cardiac activity begins and cardiac motion can be visualized by transvaginal ultrasound.<br>10th-12th week—Fetal heart tone can be heard by Doppler ultrasound.<br>17th-20th week—Fetal activity felt by mother or "quickening" at 20 weeks, and fundus is approximately at the umbilicus in a normal size woman.<br>24th-25th week—Surfactant production begins. | Iron<br>Zinc<br>Calcium<br>Vitamin B$_6$ (pyridoxine)<br>Vitamin C<br>Vitamin D<br>Folate—**Routine supplements contain 0.4mg/dy but should increase to 2-4mg/dy for patients with history of neural tube defects.** |

## Table 12-1 • (Continued)

### Routine Prenatal Testing and Procedures

| | Initial Visit and First Trimester | Second Trimester | Third Trimester |
|---|---|---|---|
| Blood related | CBC<br>Blood type<br>Rhesus type and antibody screen[c]<br>Serum free β-hCG (11-14 weeks)[a]<br>Serum PAPP-A (11-14 weeks)[a] | "Triple screen" (15-20 weeks)[a]<br>"Quad screen" (15-20 weeks)[a] | Glucose screen (24-28 weeks)[b]<br>RhoGAM (28-30 weeks)[c]<br>Repeat CBC (35-37 weeks) |
| Urine related | Urinalysis<br>Urine culture | | |
| ID related | Chlamydia/Gonorrhea cervical culture<br>Syphilis with RPR or VDRL<br>HIV screen with ELISA<br>Hepatitis B surface antigen<br>Rubella titer<br>Varicella titer | | GBS rectovaginal culture (35-37 weeks)<br>Repeat STD testing in high-risk groups<br>(28-36 weeks) |
| Procedures | Pap smear<br>US-Nuchal translucency (11-14 weeks)[a]<br>CVS (10-12 weeks)[a]<br>Hemoglobin electrophoresis[d] | US-Assess for fetal abnormalities (18-20 weeks)<br>Amniocentesis (15-20 weeks)[a] | |

BUN—blood urea nitrogen; Cr—creatinine; CVS—chorionic villus sampling; ESR—erythrocyte sedimentation rate; GBS—group B streptococcus; GFR—glomerular filtration rate; HPL—human placental lactogen; ID—infectious disease; US—ultrasound.

[a]Refer to "Congenital Abnormalities" section; [b]Refer to "Gestational Diabetes" section; [c]Refer to "Rhesus Incompatibility" section, [d]Indicated in patients with a history of thalassemias or hemoglobinopathies, generally cultures from Southeast Asia and Mediterranean regions

## Table 12-2 • Antepartum Surveillance

| Test | Why? | When? | How? | Comments |
|---|---|---|---|---|
| **Amniocentesis** | • Commonly used to karyotype fetal cells to determine chromosomal abnormalities. AFP and acetylcholinesterase obtained to detect neural tube defects. | For genetic analysis between the 15th-20th week of gestation. | Inserting a needle trans-abdominally through ultrasound guidance and aspirating amniotic fluid for analysis. | • Complications can occur such as fetal loss or clubbed foot in the new-born if the procedure is performed earlier such as the 11th-13th week. |
| **Chorionic villus sampling (CVS)** | • Genetic analysis.<br>• Advantage to CVS compared to amniocentesis is the ability to perform the procedure earlier in pregnancy permitting earlier decision-making regarding pregnancy termination or relieving parental anxiety when results are normal. | Between 10th-12th week of gestation. | Inserting a needle trans-abdominally or inserting a catheter transcervically under ultrasound guid-ance and aspirating pla-cental cells for analysis. | • Complications include fetal loss, limb defects, or oromandibular malfor-mations if the procedure is performed earlier than 10 weeks.<br>• CVS has a higher risk of fetal loss compared to a second trimester amniocentesis. |
| **Percutaneous umbilical blood sampling (PUBS), also known as cordocentesis** | Fetal blood can be used to assess fetal blood gases, karyotype, infections, meta-bolic evaluation, and can serve to diagnosis and treat fetal anemia with an intrauterine transfusion. | Typically ≥20 weeks gestation but depending on the clinical situation such as suspicion for fetal anemia or metabolic concerns. If karyotyping results are needed earlier, results can be available within 1-2 days. | Transabdominal needle aspiration of fetal vein under ultrasound guidance. | • Complications include, cord hematoma, fetoma-ternal hemorrhage, or fetal bradycardia second-ary to vasovagal response from puncturing the fetal artery instead of vein. |

(Continued)

## Table 12-2 • Antepartum Surveillance (Continued)

| Test | Why? | When? | How? | Comments |
|---|---|---|---|---|
| **Nonstress test (NST)** | To test for fetal well-being by assessing fetal heart rate (FHR) to fetal movement. | Typically after 32 weeks gestation. | Mother is in left decubitus position, with external fetal monitor on abdomen that records FHR. Mother reports fetal movement, which is noted on monitor strip and then correlated with FHR. | • A normal reactive test is ≥2 accelerations of FHR each lasting 15 beats above baseline for at least 15 seconds in a 20-minute period.<br>• A nonreactive test should be followed up with either a CST or BPP. |
| **Contraction stress test (CST)** | To test for uteroplacental function. | Typically in the second or third trimester when there is a nonreactive or nonreassuring NST. | Mother wears external monitor on abdomen and either spontaneous or induced contractions with oxyctocin are assessed along with the FHR. | • A negative test (normal) has no late decelerations on FHR.<br>• A positive test (abnormal) has late decelerations following ≥50% of contractions. |
| **Biophysical profile (BPP)** | To test for fetal well-being. The test can give us an indication of fetal acidemia in a noninvasive way based on five parameters, which are four ultrasound assessments and NST. | Can be used as early as 26-28 weeks gestation. | Two points per parameter for total of 10 points.<br>1) Fetal breathing<br>2) Fetal body movements<br>3) Fetal tone<br>4) Amniotic fluid index<br>5) NST | Point scale:<br>8-10 points—Reassuring<br>6 points—Concerning, needs further investigation.<br>0-4 points—Needs some intervention, most likely fetal acidemia. |

*AFP—Alpha-fetoprotein (Note: AFP is obtained from amniotic fluid in the amniocentesis.)*

part of prenatal care and should be offered to patients in the following cases:

- Pregnant woman ≥35 years old
- Consanguinity
- Family history of known or suspected hereditary diseases
- History of recurrent spontaneous abortions
- Previous child born with birth defects or growth abnormalities
- Abnormal screening results from first or second trimester
- Ethnicity: People of Mediterranean, Asian, and African descent have a risk for hemoglobinopathies. Eastern Europeans

(Ashkenazi Jews) have a risk for cystic fibrosis, Tay-Sachs, and Gaucher disease. Non-Jewish Caucasians with a family history of cystic fibrosis (CF) are at risk for CF.

### Single Gene Disorders

Single gene disorders are genetic conditions with a mutation or alteration in a specific gene that can be passed down into the next family generation. Modes of inheritance can be described as autosomal dominant, autosomal recessive, X-linked recessive, X-linked dominant, and mitochondrial, to name a few.

## Table 12-3 • Single Gene Disorders

| Autosomal Dominant | Autosomal Recessive | X-linked | Mitochondrial |
|---|---|---|---|
| Achondroplasia<br>ADPKD<br>Ehlers-Danlos syndrome<br>FAP<br>Huntington disease<br>HCM<br>Marfan syndrome<br>Neurofibromatosis type 1 and 2<br>von Willebrand disease | ARPKD<br>Cystic fibrosis<br>Cystinuria<br>Gaucher disease<br>Hemochromatosis<br>Phenylketonuria (PKU)<br>Sickle cell anemia<br>Tay-Sachs disease<br>Thalassemia syndromes<br>Wilson disease | **X-linked recessive**<br>• Androgen insensitivity syndrome<br>• Duchene muscular dystrophy<br>• G6PD<br>• Hemophilia A and B<br>• XLA<br>**X-linked dominant**<br>• Fragile X syndrome (most common form of familial mental retardation) | Kearns-Sayre syndrome<br>Leber-optic atrophy |

*ADPKD—autosomal dominant polycystic kidney disease, ARPKD—autosomal recessive polycystic kidney disease, FAP—familial adenomatous polyposis, HCM—hypertrophic cardiomyopathy*

## Table 12-4 • Chromosomal Abnormalities

| Genetic Disease | Clinical Features | Chromosomal Abnormality |
|---|---|---|
| Trisomy 21 (Down syndrome) | Mental retardation, epicanthal folds, slanted palpebral fissures, flat nasal bridge, transverse palmar crease, speckled iris (Brushfield spots), ASD, VSD, PDA, tetralogy of Fallot, duodenal atresia, celiac disease, Hirschsprung's disease, TEF, leukemia, sleep apnea, asthma, thyroid disease, atlantoaxial instability with possibility of C1-C2 dislocation, females are fertile, males typically infertile, hearing loss, ↑ risk of Alzheimer's, life span is shorter than general population but can live up to 50 y, ↑ maternal age increases risk of meiotic nondisjunction. | Three copies of chromosome 21, Robertsonian translocation, or mosaicism |
| Trisomy 18 (Edwards syndrome) | Clenched fist with overlapping fingers, mental retardation, omphalocele, VSD, ASD, PDA, rocker bottom feet; 50% die within first week. | Three copies of chromosome 18 |
| Trisomy 13 (Patau syndrome) | Mental retardation, holoprosencephaly, deafness, cleft lip ± palate, extra fingers or toes, VSD, ASD, PDA, rocker bottom feet; 80% die within first month. | Three copies of chromosome 13 |
| 45,X0 (Turner's syndrome) | Webbed neck, broad chest with widely spaced nipples, short stature with squarelike appearance, horseshoe kidney, coarctation, bicuspid aortic valve, HTN, hypothyroidism, celiac disease, premature ovarian failure/"streaked gonads," most are infertile, scoliosis, sausagelike fingers and toes from lymphedema, absent Barr bodies, intelligence is typically normal, ↑ maternal age does not increase risk of Turner's syndrome. | Loss of one of the sex chromosomes |
| 47,XXY (Klinefelter's syndrome) | Tall, gynecomastia, ↑ risk of breast cancer and germ cell tumors, small testes, infertile, hypogonadism/↓ testosterone levels, ↑ FSH, ↑ LH, intelligence is typically normal and is not in the disability range but still may have academic difficulties from other causes such as poor attention, ↑ paternal age has been associated with increased risk of Klinefelter's syndrome. | Nondisjunction of the sex chromosome resulting in an extra X chromosome in each male cell |

*ASD—atrial septal defect; HTN—hypertension; PDA—patent ductus arteriosus; TEF—tracheoesophageal fistula; VSD—ventral septal defect*

### Autosomal Dominant

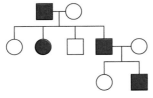

- 50% chance of obtaining the affected condition.
- Affected condition seen in every generation.
- Can affect men and women equally.

### Autosomal Recessive

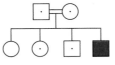

- 25% chance of obtaining the affected condition.
- 75% chance of being asymptomatic.
- Consanguinity commonly found.

### X-Linked Recessive

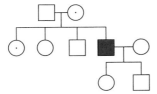

- 50% chance of each son being affected and 50% chance of each daughter being a carrier from the mother carrier.
- There is no male-to-male transmission

### Mitochondrial Inheritance

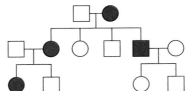

- Transmission is only through females.
- Children of affected males will be unaffected.
- Can affect both men and women.

 Female,  Affected female,  Carrier female,  Male,  Affected male,  Carrier male,  Consanguineous mating

## Table 12-5 • Prenatal Risk Assessment

| Abnormality | First Trimester | | | | Second Trimester | | | | | |
|---|---|---|---|---|---|---|---|---|---|---|
| | hCG | PAPP-A | US | CVS | hCG | MSAFP | uE3 | Inh A | US | Amniocentesis |
| Trisomy 21 (Down syndrome) | ↑ | ↓ | Look for an increase in nuchal translucency and absent nasal bone. | Women who undergo 1st trimester screen and test positive can have fetal karyotype determination by CVS (10-12 weeks gestation) for definitive diagnosis. | ↑ | ↓ | ↓ | ↑ | Look for an increase in nuchal fold. | Women who undergo 2nd trimester screen and test positive can have fetal karyotype determination by amniocentesis (15-20 weeks gestation) for definitive diagnosis. |
| Trisomy 18 (Edwards syndrome) | ↓ | ↓ | Structural anomalies can be detected in the 1st or 2nd trimester. | | ↓ | ↓ | ↓ | — | Structural anomalies can be detected in the 1st or 2nd trimester. | |
| Trisomy 13 (Patau syndrome) | ↓ | ↓ | | | — | — | — | — | | |
| Neural tube defects (NTD) | — | — | — | — | — | ↑ | — | — | US along with MSAFP are good 2nd trimester screens. | Can be performed if ultrasound is equivocal. Elevated amniotic AFP and AChE indicates an open NTD. |

AChE—acetylcholinesterase; AFP—alpha fetoprotein; Inh A—inhibin A; MSAFP—maternal serum alpha fetoprotein; US—ultrasound

## Prenatal Risk Assessment

Prenatal risk assessment is performed during the first or second trimester to detect genetic or structural abnormalities of the fetus (see Table 12-5). Consider the following screening parameters:

**PAPP-A**—Pregnancy associated plasma protein A can be measured between the 11th and 14th weeks of gestation. Often this specific marker is combined with the hCG, ultrasound (US), and maternal age to give a specific risk and is referred to as the "combined test" for the first trimester.

**MSAFP**—Maternal serum alpha-fetoprotein is measured in the second trimester and is part of the triple and quad screening. A common cause of abnormal MSAFP readings is an incorrect gestational age. On the boards, the next best step is to order an ultrasound to verify gestational age. Open neural tube defects (ie, skin is not covering the defect), ventral wall defects (eg, omphaloceles, gastroschisis), multifetal gestations, and fetal death have been associated with elevated MSAFP levels. Gestational trophoblastic disease and chromosomal trisomies have been associated with lower levels of MSAFP. MSAFP is expressed in multiple of the median (MoM). Essentially the MoM normalizes the value allowing for differences in labs and the population. A value above 2.0 to 2.5 is considered elevated but is still within the upper limits of normal.

**uE3**—Unconjugated estriol is a marker for a viable fetus, functioning placenta, and mother well-being.

**Inhibin A**—Inhibin A is a protein produced by the placenta and corpus luteum that is a marker used in the "quad screen."

**Triple screen**—Triple screen consists of the hCG, MSAFP, and uE3, which is performed between 15 and 20 weeks gestation.

**Quad screen**—Adding inhibin A to the triple screen comprises the quad screen and can also be performed between 15 and 20 weeks gestation.

### Environmental Factors

Environmental factors such as drugs, physical agents, maternal medical conditions, and infections can potentially harm the developing fetus (see Table 12-6). The US Food and Drug Administration (FDA) has produced a drug safety pregnancy classification based on fetal risk from pharmaceuticals. The system was intended to help guide physicians with the appropriate use of medications during pregnancy (see Table 12-7).

### Perinatal Infections

#### Neonatal Gonococcal Conjunctivitis

**Transmission:**

The primary mode of transmission is during vaginal delivery from infected mothers, although in utero infection can occur after ruptured membranes.

**Clinical Features:**

Gonococcal conjunctivitis usually presents 3 days after birth and should be differentiated from chemical conjunctivitis (ie, secondary from silver nitrate solution), which presents on the first day of life and resolves by the second or third day of birth. Babies will usually have bilateral purulent conjunctival discharge with swelling of the eyelids. Further progression can lead to corneal edema and ulceration.

## Table 12-6 • Common Teratogens

| Drugs | Result |
| --- | --- |
| Alcohol | Fetal alcohol syndrome, growth restriction, microcephaly, congenital heart disease |
| ACE inhibitor | Fetal hypotension, renal and skull defects |
| Aminoglycosides | Hearing defects |
| Androgens | Virilization of females |
| Carbamazepine | Neural tube defects, intrauterine growth restriction (IUGR), facial dysmorphology |
| Cocaine | Cerebral infarctions, IUGR, risk for placental abruption |
| Diethylstilbestrol (DES) | Clear cell adenocarcinoma of the vagina or cervix in adolescence |
| Fluoroquinolones | Cartilage damage |
| Iodide | Goiter |
| Lithium | Ebstein anomaly |
| Methotrexate | Fetal death, CNS and cardiac defects |
| Penicillamine | Cutis laxa (ie, loose redundant skin that hangs in folds) |
| Phenobarbital | Vitamin K deficiency/bleeding diathesis |
| Phenytoin | IUGR, facial dysmorphology, mental retardation, ventral septal defect (VSD) |
| Propylthiouracil | Goiter, hypothyroidism |
| Streptomycin | Hearing defects |
| Sulfonamides | Kernicterus |
| Tetracycline | Teeth discoloration, enamel hypoplasia |
| Thalidomide | Phocomelia (limbs look like "flippers") |
| Valproic acid | Neural tube defects |
| Vitamin A and isotretinoin | Cleft lip/palate, CNS and cardiac defects, facial dysmorphology. (Note: Topical retinoids have no known risk, only systemic formulas. Also, high-dose vitamin A has been implicated in malformations.) |
| Warfarin | Nasal hypoplasia, stippled bone epiphyses, IUGR, mental retardation |
| **Physical Agents** | **Result** |
| Ionizing radiation | Microcephaly, growth retardation |
| Lead | Stillbirths in high exposures |
| Organic mercury | Microcephaly, mental retardation, seizures |
| Tobacco smoke | IUGR, stillbirth |
| Toluene | Mental retardation, facial dysmorphology |
| **Maternal Conditions** | **Result** |
| Diabetes—uncontrolled | Macrosomia, sacral anomalies, but most common are cardiac abnormalities |
| Drug addiction | IUGR, neonate withdrawal |
| Grave's disease | Transient thyrotoxicosis |
| Hypertension (HTN) | IUGR, fetal demise |
| Phenylketonuria (PKU) | Microcephaly, mental retardation, VSD |
| Lupus (SLE) | Congenital heart block, thrombocytopenia, neutropenia, anemia |

## Table 12-7 • Food and Drug Administration (FDA) Pregnancy Categories

| | |
| --- | --- |
| Category A | Adequate human studies show no risk to fetus in any of the trimesters. |
| Category B | Animal studies show no risk to fetus and there are no adequate human studies *or* animal studies have shown harm but adequate human studies have failed to show risk to fetus. Benefit may outweigh risk. |
| Category C | Animal studies show harm to fetus and there are no adequate human studies *or* no animal studies conducted and there are no adequate human studies. Benefit may outweigh risk, but risk cannot be ruled out. |
| Category D | Positive evidence of human risk to fetus but benefit may outweigh risk in life-threatening situations. |
| Category X | Contraindicated in pregnancy. |

## Next Step:

**Step 1)** Definitive diagnosis is by culturing the exudate on a Thayer-Martin medium, which will demonstrate a gram-negative diplococci.

**Step 2)** Treat with 1 dose of intravenous (IV) or intramuscular (IM) ceftriaxone. However, IV or IM cefotaxime × 1 dose should be administered instead of ceftriaxone in the presence of hyperbilirubinemia. Topical antibiotics can be used on the eyes immediately after birth as prophylaxis but not for treatment.

## Pearls:

- If the neonate develops gonococcal arthritis or sepsis → Treat with IV or IM ceftriaxone. IV or IM cefotaxime may be administered instead of ceftriaxone in the presence of hyperbilirubinemia. Duration of treatment with either antibiotic is for 7 days, but extend therapy to 10 to 14 days if the neonate develops gonococcal meningitis.
- Evaluate the neonate for coinfection with chlamydia.
- **Foundational point**—*Neisseria gonorrhoeae* comes in pairs (diplococci) that look like two kidney beans facing each other. These bacteria contain pili that adhere to the host cell. They can evade the immune system by altering the antigens in the pili (ie, antigenic variation). Antigenic variation can also occur on the surface proteins called Opa (protein II or opacity related proteins). Since they are gram-negative bacteria, the endotoxin is within the LPS (ie, lipid A).
- **Connecting point** (pg. 2)—Know the definition of endotoxin and exotoxin.

### Neonatal Chlamydial Conjunctivitis and Pneumonia

## Transmission:

The primary mode of transmission is during vaginal delivery from mothers with *Chlamydia trachomatis* infection.

## Clinical Features:

**Conjunctivitis**—Usually presents 5 to 14 days after birth. Babies may have watery eye discharge that can become purulent. Other symptoms include pseudomembrane formation, eyelid swelling, and red conjunctivae.

**Pneumonia**—Respiratory symptoms may not occur until after 2 to 3 weeks of birth. Babies will present with a staccato cough and may be in respiratory distress.

## Next Step:

**Step 1)** The gold standard for diagnosing neonatal *Chlamydia trachomatis* is by culturing the conjunctiva and nasopharyngeal secretions. Ancillary testing includes a chest x-ray, which will typically reveal hyperinflation of the lungs with bilateral interstitial infiltrates.

**Step 2)** Treatment is with oral **erythromycin** for 14 days for either conjunctivitis or pneumonia. Remember to initiate antibiotic treatment without delay for suspected pneumonia based on clinical evaluation and x-ray findings (ie, do not wait for the culture results to come back).

## Pearls:

- *Chlamydia trachomatis* is the most common sexually transmitted genital infection.
- Do not be confused with the other types of *Chlamydophila* (formerly *Chlamydia*) species (eg, *Chlamydophila pneumoniae* and *Chlamydophila psittaci*) that can cause pneumonia (ie, atypical pneumonia).
- Conjunctivitis developed via infectious or noninfectious means in newborns is also referred to as ophthalmia neonatorum (ie, neonatal conjunctivitis).
- There is a risk of pyloric stenosis with the use of oral erythromycin.
- Do not forget to treat both the mother and her partner if they have a chlamydia infection.
- **Foundational point**—*Chlamydia trachomatis* (serotypes A, B, and C) can cause trachoma. Trachoma is a contagious eye infection that is the leading cause of blindness worldwide by infectious means. A key finding in active trachoma is follicles in the tarsal conjunctiva. With recurrent conjunctival inflammation, patients can progress to cicatricial disease, which includes eyelid scarring, trichiasis (ingrown eyelashes), and blindness.
- **Foundational point**—*Chlamydia trachomatis* (serotypes D-K) primarily causes neonatal infections (eg, neonatal conjunctivitis, neonatal pneumonia) and genital disease in adults (eg, cervicitis, PID, urethritis).
- **Foundational point**—*Chlamydia trachomatis* (serotypes L1, L2, and L3) can cause lymphogranuloma venereum, which is a genital ulcer disease.
- **Foundational point**—Chlamydiae do not have a peptidoglycan layer and have no muramic acid. Muramic acid is a component in many bacterial cell walls.
- **Foundational point**—Chlamydiae are gram-negative, obligate intracellular bacteria that rely on the host ATP since they cannot make their own.
- **Foundational point**—The life cycle of chlamydiae exists in two forms. First, they infect cells (affinity for columnar epithelial cells) as **elementary bodies**. Once inside the cell, they transform into **reticulate bodies** (also called initial body). From there, some transform back into elementary bodies, and then they are released from the cell where they can infect more cells.
- **Connecting point** (pg. 255)—Know the features of *Chlamydophila pneumoniae* and *Chlamydophila psittaci*.

### ToRCH Infections Related to Pregnancy

The acronym ToRCH (Toxoplasmosis, others [varicella, parvovirus B19, syphilis], Rubella, Cytomegalovirus, Herpes simplex) represents a group of pathogens that are responsible, but not limited to, intrauterine and perinatal infections that can lead to significant neonatal morbidity and mortality.

**Toxoplasmosis**

Transmission:

A pregnant woman can contract toxoplasmosis by ingesting the protozoan cysts from undercooked meats, raw meats, or cured meats. The other way of contraction is by fecal-oral transmission of the cysts from infected cat feces by cat litter, water, or soil. Once the mother is infected, the parasites can travel hematogenously to the placenta transmitting the infection to the baby.

Clinical Features:

**Mother**—Most infected mothers will be asymptomatic. However, symptoms will usually present with a mononucleosis-like syndrome that include fatigue, cervical lymphadenopathy, sore throat, and will be heterophile antibody negative.

**Baby**—Infected neonates will usually be asymptomatic at birth; however, the classic triad includes **intracranial calcifications, chorioretinitis,** and **hydrocephalus**. Late sequelae may include hearing loss, mental retardation, and seizures.

Next Step:

**Step 1**) Diagnosis for maternal toxoplasmosis infection can be made with serology. Test the serum for *Toxoplasma*-specific IgG and IgM antibodies. An IgG positive, IgM positive result suggests that the mother has immunity and has been infected within the past year, respectively. In this case, the next best step is to test the serum for IgG avidity. A low IgG avidity suggests a recent infection. A prenatal diagnosis for fetal toxoplasmosis infection can be made by obtaining amniotic fluid (via amniocentesis) for *Toxoplasma* PCR. In addition, fetal ultrasound may be helpful for detecting fetal abnormalities (eg, intracranial calcifications, ventricular dilatations).

**Step 2**) Initiate **spiramycin** in a pregnant woman if an acute infection is suspected as this medication can reduce the maternal-fetal transmission, but not actually treat established fetal infection.

**Step 3**) Administer **pyrimethamine**, **sulfadiazine**, and **folinic acid** once fetal infection has been established.

Pearl:

- It is important during pregnancy to avoid eating uncooked meats, avoid feeding cats undercooked meats, wear gloves or delegate the duty to clean cat litter, wash fruits and vegetables, and to have good hand hygiene.

- **Foundational point**—*Toxoplasma gondii* is an obligate intracellular protozoan that can exist in three forms (ie, oocysts, bradyzoites, tachyzoites). Humans can be infected by ingesting the oocysts (shed only in cat feces) or by ingesting uncooked meats that contain the bradyzoites. Infection to the fetus occurs by a transformation into tachyzoites that can travel into the bloodstream and into the placenta.

**Rubella (German Measles)**

Transmission:

The virus is spread by airborne droplets that can then replicate in the lymph tissue and spread hematogenously to the placenta transmitting the infection to the baby. Adults are considered infectious 7 days before and 4 days after the appearance of the rash. Babies are considered contagious for several months to one year after delivery as they can shed the virus from the pharynx.

Clinical Features:

**Mother**—Infected mothers will have prodromal symptoms prior to the onset of the rash such as cough, coryza, conjunctivitis, low-grade fever, suboccipital and posterior auricular lymphadenopathy, or rose spots on the soft palate (Forchheimer spots). A maculopapular rash will then start on the face and spread toward the trunk and extremities.

**Baby**—Infected fetuses who acquire the infection during the first trimester are at risk of a spontaneous abortion or developing the congenital rubella syndrome. After 20 weeks gestation, congenital rubella syndrome is uncommon. Some of the features of congenital rubella syndrome include **"blueberry muffin" rash, cataracts, patent ductus arteriosus, pulmonary artery stenosis,** and **radiolucent bone lesions**. Late sequelae include hearing loss, mental retardation, encephalitis, diabetes, and thyroid disease.

Next Step:

**Step 1**) Diagnosis for maternal rubella infection can be made with a rubella culture or serology. A positive result for rubella-specific IgM or a significant rise in rubella-specific IgG between the acute and convalescent phase indicates an acute infection. Prenatal diagnosis for fetal rubella infection can be made by rubella PCR via CVS or amniocentesis.

**Step 2**) There is **no specific treatment** that targets the rubella virus, only supportive care.

**Step 3**) Remember that rubella serum evaluation is part of the prenatal care. If the patient is nonimmune, give her the MMR vaccination after delivery since it is a live attenuated virus. Contraception should be used for one month following postpartum immunization.

Pearls:

- Immune globulin does not prevent or mitigate the infection.

- The mother can still have subclinical rubella "reinfection" despite previous rubella immunization.

- **Foundational point**—Rubella virus comes from the family Togaviridae of the genus *Rubivirus* and contains a positive-sense, single-stranded RNA.

**Cytomegalovirus**

Transmission:

Cytomegalovirus (CMV) transmission can occur from infected saliva, nasopharyngeal secretions, cervical secretions, semen, blood, urine, or breast milk. The following are examples of transmission:

- Transplacentally during pregnancy

- Hand-to-hand contact (eg, day care centers)

- Vaginal delivery

- Sexual transmission
- Blood transfusions
- Organ transplantation
- Breastfeeding (Remember, it's *not* a contraindication if infected.)

## Clinical Features:

**Mother**—Most infected mothers will be asymptomatic. However, symptoms will usually present with a mononucleosis-like syndrome that includes fatigue, cervical lymphadenopathy, and sore throat and will be heterophile antibody negative.

**Baby**—Most infected neonates will also be asymptomatic. However, features to look for include **periventricular calcifications, chorioretinitis, microcephaly, "blueberry muffin rash," IUGR,** and **hepatosplenomegaly**. Late sequelae include sensorineural hearing loss, mental retardation, and seizures.

## Next Step:

**Step 1)** Diagnosis for maternal primary CMV infection can be made with serology. Seroconversion of CMV specific IgG in acute and convalescent sera is diagnostic for an acute infection. CMV specific IgM has a limited role in diagnosis since it may be present in recurrent infection, reactivation infection, and primary infection, may be positive for 1 year after infection, and is only found in 75% to 90% of women with acute infection. A prenatal diagnosis for fetal CMV infection can be made by obtaining amniotic fluid (via amniocentesis) for CMV PCR. In addition, fetal ultrasound may be helpful for detecting fetal anomalies.

**Step 2)** There is **no specific treatment** for the pregnant mother, only supportive. Ganciclovir has been used in neonates when there are signs of end organ damage.

## Pearls:

- CMV is the most common congenital infection.
- **Foundational point**—The cells that CMV infect become enlarged, hence "cyto-megaly." Within the cells, intranuclear inclusions surrounded by a clear halo can be stained and an appearance of an "owl's eye" can be seen on microscope.
- **Foundational point**—CMV belongs to the family of Herpesviridae. Other members in this family include EBV (infectious mononucleosis), HSV-1 ("cold sores"), HSV-2 (genital herpes), VZV (chickenpox, shingles), HHV-6 (roseola infantum/sixth disease), HHV-7 (role in human disease is unknown), and HHV-8 (Kaposi's sarcoma). The members of this family contain a double-stranded linear DNA and can form intranuclear inclusion bodies.

## Herpes Simplex Virus

### Transmission:

Herpes simplex virus (HSV) transmission can occur from an ascending infection from the genital tract, transplacental transmission, or by direct contact with the genital lesions during vaginal delivery.

## Clinical Features:

**Mother**—Infected mothers will present with the characteristic tender genital vesicles with ulceration. Mothers may also have fever, dysuria, and tender inguinal lymphadenopathy. Prodromal symptoms such as pain, pruritus, or tingling may occur before the onset of genital lesions in mothers with recurrent disease.

**Baby**—Infected neonates can have the lesions on the skin, eyes, and mouth. The infection can also affect the nervous system (eg, seizures) and multiple organs (ie, disseminated disease).

## Next Step:

**Step 1)** Diagnosis for maternal HSV infection can be made by HSV culture of the vesicular fluid or HSV PCR.

**Step 2)** Treatment for first-episode genital herpes is with **oral acyclovir** for 7 to 10 days. Recurrent HSV infection during the first 35 weeks is not typically treated since the infection is short lived. However, suppressive antiviral therapy may be offered to patients with a history of genital HSV infection at 36 weeks gestation through delivery to reduce the risk of recurrence at term.

**Step 3)** Perform a cesarean section in mothers with **active HSV lesions** or mothers with **prodromal symptoms** at the time of delivery. Do not perform a prophylactic cesarean section in a woman with a history of recurrent genital HSV infection and without active genital HSV lesions.

**Step 4)** After delivery, neonates suspected of HSV infection should be given intravenous acyclovir until the infection is confirmed. In addition to acyclovir, add trifluridine eye drops if the neonate develops HSV keratitis.

## Pearls:

- Avoid fetal scalp electrode (FSE) monitoring during labor in women who have active genital herpes or history of HSV infection.
- HSV-2 has been the main causative agent for genital herpes in the past, but now HSV-1, which is the common agent for oropharyngeal herpes, has now increased in frequency for genital herpes.
- Asymptomatic viral shedding can occur up to 12 months after acquiring HSV-2.
- **Foundational point**—The Tzanck smear involves removing the blister roof and scraping the base of the vesicle and spreading it onto a glass slide to look for multinucleate giant cells. The Tzanck smear aids in the diagnosis (ie, not a first-line test) of HSV-1, HSV-2, and VZV, which contain these cells.

## Other Infections in Pregnancy
### Varicella

### Transmission:

The primary mode of transmission is by direct contact with the vesicular lesion and by airborne droplets. The mother is considered contagious 1 to 2 days before the onset of the rash until the lesions crust over. It is thought that fetal infection is via transplacental transmission.

## Clinical Features:

**Mother**—Infected mothers will present with a flulike prodrome 1 to 4 days prior to the onset of a pruritic vesicular rash. The lesions can appear on the face, trunk, and extremities and will appear in groups or "crops." The lesions will then take on different stages of evolution and then crust over in 7 to 10 days.

**Varicella pneumonia** can occur and is considered an emergency because of the relatively high mortality rate (40%) in untreated women. Symptoms will usually occur within one week of the rash and include fever, dry cough, and tachypnea.

**Baby**—Infected fetuses that acquire the infection before 20 weeks gestation can develop the congenital varicella syndrome, which includes **chorioretinitis**, **microphthalmia**, **cortical atrophy**, **IUGR**, **cutaneous scarring**, or **limb hypoplasia**. Congenital varicella syndrome after 20 weeks is uncommon, but perinatal infection just before or during delivery can result in **neonatal varicella**, which poses a serious threat. Manifestations can range from vesicular eruptions to the development of CNS disease (eg, meningoencephalitis) and disseminated visceral involvement (eg, varicella pneumonia).

## Next Step:

**Step 1)** Diagnosis for maternal varicella infection is made clinically. Fetal varicella infection can be assessed by VZV PCR and fetal ultrasound to detect fetal anomalies.

**Step 2)** Consider the following management approach:

**Exposed to chickenpox**—Pregnant women exposed to chickenpox should have their varicella IgG titers taken. If they are IgG positive, they are immune. If they are IgG negative, they should receive passive immunization with the varicella-zoster immune globulin (Trade name VariZIG) within 96 hours (4 days) of exposure to attenuate the infection.

**Evidence of chickenpox**—Neonates should be given varicella-zoster immune globulin (Trade name VariZIG) with a mother that has clinical evidence of chickenpox 5 days before or 2 days after delivery because of concern for neonatal varicella. If neonatal varicella develops, then treat with IV acyclovir.

**Step 3)** Remember that varicella serum evaluation is part of the prenatal care. If the mother is nonimmune, give her the varicella vaccine (Trade name Varivax) after delivery since it is a live attenuated virus. The second vaccine dose should be given 4 to 8 weeks later. Contraception should be used for one month following each dose of the vaccine.

## Pearls:

- A nodular infiltrative pattern can be seen on chest x-ray in mothers with varicella pneumonia.
- A pregnant mother who develops varicella pneumonia should be hospitalized and treated with intravenous acyclovir.

- Varicella-zoster immune globulin (VariZIG) should be given to premature infants >28 weeks from mothers known to have no immunity to varicella and premature infants <28 weeks regardless of the mother's immune status.
- Herpes zoster does not cause congenital malformations.
- Herpes zoster is considered contagious when the blisters are broken. Treat pregnant women with acyclovir if there is eye involvement (herpes zoster ophthalmicus) or if there is severe dermatomal pain.
- **Foundational point**—The varicella-zoster virus can establish latency in the sensory ganglia, and upon reactivation, there is intense inflammation of the dorsal root ganglion that can be accompanied by hemorrhagic necrosis of the nerve cells.

## Parvovirus B19

### Transmission:

The primary mode of transmission is respiratory. Maternal viremia will result in fetal infection via transplacental transmission (vertical transmission). Infected blood products can also harbor parvovirus B19.

### Clinical Features:

**Mother**—Infected mothers will usually present with flulike symptoms prior to the onset of a red rash on the face giving a "slapped cheek" appearance (although not as common in adults compared to children). Subsequently, a symmetric rash will occur on the trunk or extremity with central clearing producing a "lacy-reticulated" rash. Adults will commonly present with symmetrical polyarthralgias that usually resolve within 2 weeks. Transient aplastic crisis can occur in adults with chronic anemia (eg, sickle cell, thalassemia).

**Baby**—Infection in fetuses can result in fetal loss or fetal anemia leading to nonimmune **hydrops fetalis** (ie, accumulation of fluid in fetal tissues).

### Next Step:

**Step 1)** Diagnosis for maternal B19 infection can be made by serology. An IgG positive result indicates a prior infection with immunity. An IgM positive result is consistent with a recent infection, but be aware that IgM can be positive for several months or longer. However, to aid in the diagnosis, obtaining maternal serum for B19 PCR may be useful. A prenatal diagnosis for fetal B19 infection can be made by obtaining amniotic fluid (via amniocentesis) for B19 PCR.

**Step 2)** There is no specific vaccine or antiviral therapy for parvovirus B19 infection. The concern with infection is parvovirus-associated anemia in the fetus. If severe anemia is present, there will usually be an elevated middle cerebral artery (MCA) peak systolic velocity on MCA Doppler, and signs of hydrops will usually be present on fetal ultrasound. In such cases, fetal blood sampling and possible intrauterine blood transfusion may be warranted via percutaneous umbilical cord sampling (PUBS).

## Pearls:

- Transient aplastic crisis will usually resolve on its own in pregnant women, but IVIG has been used for women that have chronic anemia with chronic parvovirus B19 infection.
- **Foundational point**—Parvovirus B19 belongs to the family of Parvoviridae and contains a linear single-stranded DNA. The virus is most contagious during the shedding phase, which usually occurs 5 to 10 days after exposure.

## Syphilis

### Transmission:

The major mode of syphilis infection is by sexual transmission (horizontal transmission). Direct contact with abraded skin gives a portal entry for the pathogen. Transplacental transmission is the most common route for fetal infection, but direct contact with the lesion during delivery can also occur (vertical transmission). Transplacental transmission can occur at any time during pregnancy, but untreated mothers that are in the primary, secondary, or early latent stages of syphilis have a higher rate of transmission because of a higher spirochete load to transmit compared to the late latent stage and tertiary (late) stages of syphilis.

### Clinical Features:

**Mother**—Untreated mothers can present in any of the four stages of syphilis:

**Primary**—Painless chancre, lymphadenopathy

**Secondary**—Maculopapular rash on palms and soles, condyloma lata, mucous patches

**Latent** (early)—Asymptomatic, but positive serology; (late)—asymptomatic, but positive serology.

**Tertiary** (late)—Neurosyphilis (eg, Argyll-Robertson pupils, tabes dorsalis), aortic aneurysm, aortic insufficiency, gumma formation

**Baby**—Untreated mothers can result in fetal loss, IUGR, preterm birth, or fetal infection. Infected infants can develop early or late congenital syphilis:

**Early (<2 years)**—Rhinitis or "snuffles" (contagious), maculopapular or vesicular rash (contagious), condyloma lata (contagious), hepatosplenomegaly, hydrops fetalis, pseudoparalysis (ie, no extremity movement because of bone pain), periostitis, jaundice.

**Late (>2 years)**—Hutchinson triad (1) Hutchinson teeth, which are small, notched, widely spaced teeth; (2) sensorineural hearing loss; (3) interstitial keratitis, frontal bossing, perforated hard palate, saddle nose, Saber shins (ie, anterior bowing of the tibia), Clutton joints (ie, symmetrical joint swelling, painless arthritis), Mulberry molars (ie, multiple cusps on the crown surface of the first molar giving it the appearance of a berry).

### Next Step:

**Step 1)** Syphilis screening is performed at the first prenatal care visit with a nontreponemal test such as **VDRL** or **RPR**. A reactive test is then confirmed with a specific treponemal test such as **FTA-ABS, MHA-TP,** or **TP-PA.**

**Step 2)** Treatment is based on the stage of infection of the pregnant mother:

- Primary, secondary, or early latent → Benzathine penicillin G intramuscularly (IM) × 1 dose.
- Late latent or tertiary (late) → Benzathine penicillin G intramuscularly (IM) × 1 dose per week for a total of 3 doses.
- Neurosyphilis → Aqueous crystalline penicillin G (IV) × 10 to 14 days or procaine penicillin G (IM) + probenecid (PO) × 10 to 14 days.

**Step 3)** VDRL or RPR titers are taken at 1, 3, 6, 12, and 24 months after therapy to see if there is an appropriate decline. A fourfold decline should be seen by the 6 month, and by 2 years the titers should be nonreactive. A fourfold rise or an inappropriate decline suggests treatment failure or reinfection, which may then warrant retreatment.

## Pearls:

- Treatment management for penicillin-allergic patients that are pregnant: skin testing → penicillin desensitization → penicillin treatment.
- Penicillin treatment is associated with the Jarisch-Herxheimer reaction, which may cause uterine contractions, preterm labor, or fetal heart rate decelerations.
- Diagnosis can also be made by **darkfield microscopy** showing the corkscrew motile spirochete or by **direct fluorescent antibody test** obtained from the lesion or exudate, but both require a fluorescent microscope.
- Specific treponemal tests (eg, FTA-ABS) do not reflect disease activity, and once they test positive, it remains positive for life, but it does not mean that the patient is immune.
- Women at high risk for syphilis should be retested with a nontreponemal test (eg, RPR) in the third trimester and at delivery.
- Women with syphilis should have HIV testing because of the high risk for coinfection.
- Pregnancy does not alter the course of syphilis.
- *Treponema pallidum* is not secreted in breast milk.
- Upon vaginal delivery, a large edematous placenta and umbilical cord will be a clue that the mother was infected with syphilis.
- **Foundational point**—Tabes dorsalis (also known as locomotor ataxia) affects the posterior columns and dorsal roots.
- **Foundational point**—Syphilis is caused by the spirochete *Treponema pallidum*. The spirochete has a corkscrew-shaped appearance that cannot be cultured by ordinary media and is too small to see with light microscope.

# PREGNANCY CONCERNS

### Spontaneous Abortion

Spontaneous abortion (ie, miscarriage), is the nonelective termination of a pregnancy before the fetus can reach viability, or in other words **<20 weeks gestation** or **<500 grams**.

First trimester abortions are commonly caused by chromosomal abnormalities. Second trimester abortions are often due to maternal conditions such as infections, systemic diseases (eg, lupus, diabetes), anatomic abnormalities (eg, bicornuate uterus), or environmental factors (eg, smoking, radiation).

Clinical Features:

There are different categories of abortion. See Table 12-8 for the classification.

Next Step:

**Step 1**) Evaluate a first trimester bleed with a **speculum examination**, with attention to the cervical os (see Table 12-8).

**Step 2**) An **ultrasound** should be performed to assess for products of conception and the presence of fetal cardiac activity, which should be visualized by the 6th week of gestation.

**Step 3**) If the uterus is empty on ultrasound, obtain a **quantitative β-HCG** to determine if the discriminatory level has been reached (refer to page 190, CCS—Ectopic Pregnancy).

**Step 4**) Refer to Table 12-8 for specific treatment management.

**Step 5**) Administer anti-D immune globulin (RhoGAM) in an unsensitized Rh(D)-negative woman after a D&C, D&E, or upon diagnosis if medical or expectant management is planned.

**Step 6**) Offer grief counseling.

### Table 12-8 • Classification of Spontaneous Abortion

| Categories | Definitions | Clinical Features | Next Step Treatment |
|---|---|---|---|
| **Threatened** | Think of this type as a "threat"; approximately 50% of these pregnancies will abort. | **Vaginal bleeding?** Yes, usually in the first half of pregnancy. **Abdominal/pelvic pain?** Mild cramping. **Cervical os?** Closed. **Passage of POC?** No, still retained. | There is no effective therapy. Bed rest is usually recommended, but it does not alter the course. |
| **Inevitable** | Think of this type as an abortion that is unavoidable. | **Vaginal bleeding?** Yes. **Abdominal/pelvic pain?** Yes, crampy pelvic pain and even uterine contractions may be present. **Cervical os?** Open. **Passage of POC?** No, still retained. | Evacuation with a D&C. Medical (ie, misoprostol) and expectant management are acceptable alternatives if the patient is stable, without infection, and there is no heavy bleeding. |
| **Incomplete** | Think of this type as the incomplete passage of POC. POC may be found at the level of the cervical canal. | **Vaginal bleeding?** Heavy. **Abdominal/pelvic pain?** Yes, usually intense crampy pain. **Cervical os?** Open. **Passage of POC?** Partial expulsion. | Evacuation with a D&C, especially in the presence of profuse bleeding. If there is fever, administer antibiotics before curettage. |
| **Complete** | Think of this type as the complete passage of POC. | **Vaginal bleeding?** Scant. **Abdominal/pelvic pain?** Mild to absent. **Cervical os?** Closed **Passage of POC?** Complete expulsion. | No specific treatment. |
| **Missed** | Fetal death <20 weeks gestation with retention of the fetal tissue for ≥4 weeks after fetal death. | **Symptoms?** After fetal death, women may or may not have any symptoms other than persistent amenorrhea. **Cervical os?** Closed. **Passage of POC?** No, still retained. **Ultrasound?** Gestational sac without fetal cardiac activity. | Treatment options include surgical (eg, D&C, D&E), medical (eg, misoprostol), or expectant management. |
| **Septic** | Evidence of infection | **Signs and symptoms?** Fever, chills, vaginal bleeding, foul discharge, leukocytosis, tachycardia, tachypnea, abdominal pain/tenderness, uterine tenderness, and malaise. | Step 1) Treat with broad-spectrum antibiotics to cover gram-positives, gram-negatives, and anaerobes. **Option 1:** IV ampicillin + IV gentamicin + IV clindamycin **Option 2:** IV ampicillin + IV gentamicin + IV metronidazole **Option 3:** IV levofloxacin + IV metronidazole Step 2) Uterine evacuation (eg, D&C) |

*D&C—dilatation and curettage; D&E—dilatation and evacuation; POC—products of conception*

**Follow-Up:**

Follow up in the office in 6 weeks, as menses should resume by this time. If no menses, obtain a serum β-HCG level and consider a new pregnancy, gestational trophoblastic disease, or intrauterine adhesions (ie, Asherman's syndrome).

**Pearls:**

- Differentials for first trimester bleeds include ectopic pregnancy, molar pregnancy, vaginal or cervical lacerations, polyps, infection, and postcoital bleed.

- When assessing for viability, a gestational sac should be visualized by approximately 5 to 6 weeks of gestation. If no sac is visualized within the uterus but the patient has appropriate hCG levels for viability, consider an ectopic pregnancy.

- Only the words *inevitable* and *incomplete* abortions have the prefix *in-*, which can help you remember that the cervical os is open only in these two conditions because "you can only go **in** if it is **open**" (see Table 12-8).

- A dilatation and evacuation (D&E) is a procedure that is generally performed in the second trimester since the fetus is larger. A curette is used to scrape the walls of the uterus and forceps are used to remove parts of the fetus.

- **On the CCS**, both "D and C" and "D and E" are available in the practice CCS.

- **On the CCS**, "HCG, beta" is available in the practice CCS, but you have to pick either "qualitative" or "quantitative." A qualitative will give you a negative or positive result, but a quantitative will give you a number to analyze.

## Cervical Incompetence

Cervical incompetence is a condition in which the cervix begins to dilate and efface (ie, thin out) during pregnancy before reaching term.

**Risk Factors:**

History of gynecologic procedures (eg, LEEP, conization, curettage), history of DES exposure, history of cervical lacerations during delivery, uterine anomalies

**Clinical Features:**

Most women with an incompetent cervix will present with **painless cervical dilatation** in the second trimester (15-28 weeks) with absent to mild contractions. Also, some women may experience cramping, lower abdominal pressure, and vaginal discharge. Without intervention, the cervical dilatation can lead to prolapse or bulging fetal membranes through the external cervical os with subsequent ruptured membranes and active uterine contractions leading to the expulsion of the fetus.

**Next Step:**

**Step 1)** Diagnosis is based on history (ie, recurrent second trimester losses, preterm birth), physical exam (ie, advanced cervical dilatation or effacement), and transvaginal ultrasound.

**Step 2)** One course of treatment is with a transvaginal cervical **cerclage**, which is a surgical procedure that involves suturing in and around the cervix to reinforce and strengthen a weaken cervix. There are three different scenarios to consider when a cerclage is placed:

**Elective cerclage**—Performed when there is a history of ≥3 unexplained second trimester losses or preterm births. Also, ultrasound evaluation should show a viable pregnancy without fetal anomalies. The procedure is performed between 13 and 16 weeks gestation.

**Emergent cerclage**—Emergent or rescue cerclage has been used in cases of advanced cervical dilatation or effacement with bulging membranes. The procedure has been performed up to 26 weeks gestation.

**Urgent cerclage**—Urgent or therapeutic cerclage has been used with caution in cases of ultrasound changes consistent with a shorten cervix or funneling (ie, membranes filling the internal os but with a closed external os giving the cervix an appearance of a funnel). However, it is not recommended to perform a cerclage in the mother who has no history of recurrent pregnancy losses or early preterm births. In these cases, transvaginal ultrasound surveillance would be the more judicious approach.

**Step 3)** Cerclage removal is typically at 36 to 37 weeks gestation, if there is suspicion for infection, or in the event of preterm labor.

**Follow-Up:**

After cerclage placement, patients are followed up with cervical exams and ultrasound evaluation as needed.

**Pearls:**

- Women diagnosed with cervical incompetence usually have a shorten cervix, but having a shorten cervix is not diagnostic of cervical incompetence.

- Transabdominal cerclage is a surgical procedure (via laparotomy) that involves placing a suture higher up at the cervicoisthmic junction (ie, at the level of the internal os). The procedure is usually reserved in cases when previous transvaginal cerclage has failed or when there are severe anatomical cervical defects.

- Transabdominal cerclage can be performed prior to pregnancy or at 11 to 14 weeks gestation.

- C-section is the mode of delivery after transabdominal cerclage placement.

- Contraindications to transabdominal or transvaginal cerclage include infections, bleeding, ruptured membranes, uterine contractions, or fetal anomalies.

## Dermatoses of Pregnancy

Pregnant women may undergo normal physiological skin changes (eg, melasma) and sometimes specific dermatoses of pregnancy (see Table 12-9). Dermatoses of pregnancy represents a heterogeneous group of skin diseases that is exclusively associated with pregnancy and/or postpartum.

## Table 12-9 • Dermatoses of Pregnancy

| Disorder | Clinical Features | Next Step Management |
|---|---|---|
| **Pruritus gravidarum (also known as intrahepatic cholestasis of pregnancy)** | There are **no primary** skin changes except for excoriations from scratching. Patients will have severe generalized pruritus, characteristically on the palms and soles of the feet. Symptoms are worse at night. Other possible features include: jaundice, steatorrhea, and signs of vitamin K deficiency. Symptoms and lab values normalize several days after delivery. Symptoms can recur in subsequent pregnancies.<br>**When?** Usually in the 2nd or 3rd trimester but sometimes 1st trimester.<br>**Labs?** ↑ serum bile acids, ↑ alkaline phosphatase, ↑ AST/ALT, ↑ to normal levels of GGT, ↑ total and direct bilirubin, ↑ cholic/chenodeoxycholic acid ratio. | 1) Diagnosis is based on exclusion of other diseases along with a history of pruritus and elevated lab values.<br>2) Treatment is with ursodeoxycholic acid (↑ bile flow), cholestyramine (↓ ileal absorption of bile salts), or hydroxyzine (antipruritic). |
| **Pruritic urticarial papules and plaques of pregnancy (PUPPP)** | Initially, erythematous papules and plaques start within the abdominal striae and then spread toward the extremities forming urticarial plaques while sparing the periumbilical area, face, soles, and palms. Small vesicles may be seen but not large bullae. The lesions are pruritic. Symptoms generally resolve spontaneously postpartum.<br>**When?** Usually in the 3rd trimester and sometimes postpartum.<br>**Labs?** No abnormalities. | 1) Diagnosis is made clinically.<br>2) Initial treatment is with topical steroids. For severe pruritus, oral steroids (eg, prednisone) may be needed. |
| **Herpes gestationis (also known as pemphigoid gestationis)** | Initially, erythematous urticarial plaques or papules begin on the trunk, usually **periumbilical**. The lesions progress to tense blisters and even bullae formation. The lesions can spread peripherally, affecting the palms and soles. Usually the face is spared, but mucosal lesions can be affected. The lesions are pruritic. Symptoms resolve within weeks to months after delivery. Symptoms can recur in subsequent pregnancies, after oral contraceptive use, or during menses.<br>**When?** Usually in the 2nd or 3rd trimester.<br>**Labs?** May see the presence of antithyroid antibodies.<br>**Direct immunofluorescence?** Should see the classic linear C3 band at the dermal-epidermal junction ± IgG.<br>**Pearl:** This is an autoimmune disorder with an HLA association and not related to the herpes viral infection. This disorder can also occur with trophoblastic diseases. | 1) Diagnosis is made clinically along with biopsy of the lesion for direct immunofluorescence. Direct immunofluorescence helps differentiate between PUPPP and herpes gestationis.<br>2) Initial treatment is with topical steroids. In most cases, it is not effective and oral steroids (eg, prednisone) are given. |
| **Impetigo herpetiformis (also known as pustular psoriasis of pregnancy)** | Sterile pustules **studded** on the margins of an erythematous patch that then coalesce forming lakes of pus. The lesions begin at the flexures and spread peripherally. Mucous membranes are usually involved. Constitutional symptoms usually occur such as nausea, vomiting, or fatigue. The lesions are typically nonpruritic. Symptoms resolve within weeks to months after delivery. Symptoms can recur in subsequent pregnancies, after oral contraceptive use, or with menses.<br>**When?** Usually in the 3rd trimester.<br>**Labs?** Hypocalcemia, hypoalbuminemia, leukocytosis.<br>**Pearl:** Not related to herpes infection, and patients do not have a history of psoriasis. | 1) Diagnosis is made clinically.<br>2) Treatment is with oral steroids and sometimes antibiotics for secondary infections from ruptured pustules. |

GGT—Gamma glutamyl transpeptidase

## Endocrine Disorder

### Gestational Diabetes

Diabetes diagnosed during pregnancy is referred to as gestational diabetes. Pregnancy can be characterized as a state of insulin resistance and hyperinsulinemia. Gestational diabetes occurs in a subset of pregnant women who cannot compensate for the insulin resistance, which is predominately caused by certain hormones such as human placental lactogen (HPL), growth hormone, progesterone, and corticotropin releasing hormone.

### Complications

**Mother**—Perineal injury from a macrosomic baby

**Baby**—Macrosomia and birth injury from the macrosomia (eg, brachial plexus injury)

**Antepartum Management:**

**Screening**

Oral glucose challenge test is performed between 24 and 28 weeks gestation.

Step 1) 50 gram oral glucose load given without regard to time of day or time of last meal.

Step 2) Plasma glucose level is measured in 1 hour.

Step 3) Plasma glucose level <130 mg/dL is normal and requires no further workup, but a glucose level ≥130 mg/dL is considered abnormal and is followed up by an oral glucose tolerance test (OGTT) for definitive diagnosis of gestational diabetes.

Oral glucose tolerance test (OGTT)

Step 1) Fasting plasma glucose level is measured.

Step 2) 100 gram oral glucose load given to a fasting pregnant woman.

Step 3) Plasma glucose level is measured at 1, 2, and 3 hours after ingestion.

Step 4) Two or more abnormal values indicate gestational diabetes: fasting glucose ≥95 mg/dL; 1 hour glucose ≥180 mg/dL; 2 hour glucose ≥155 mg/dL; 3 hour glucose ≥140 mg/dL.

**Treatment Management**

**Diet**—First-line therapy for gestational diabetes is dietary modification.

**Exercise**—Moderate exercise may improve tissue sensitivity to insulin.

**Glucose monitoring**—Home glucose monitoring should be checked at least 4 times a day. Glucose goals for women with gestational diabetes are:

Fasting glucose: ≤95 mg/dL

1 hour postprandial glucose: <130 to 140 mg/dL

2 hour postprandial glucose: ≤120 mg/dL

**Medications**—Pharmacotherapy is indicated when euglycemia cannot be achieved by nutritional therapy and exercise. First-line agents are the insulins. Oral hypoglycemic agents are not approved by the FDA for gestational diabetes, although there is increasing support for glyburide.

**Fetal Surveillance**—Women with gestational diabetes who are on insulin are managed similarly to women with pregestational diabetes. Fetal surveillance is not required in gestational diabetics who are well controlled on diet alone.

- Nonstress test (NST)—Twice weekly testing starting at 32 weeks gestation.
- Amniotic fluid index (AFI)—Twice weekly testing starting at 32 weeks gestation.
- Biophysical profile (BPP)—Can be used in place of NST or AFI since it includes both components.
- Obstetrical ultrasound—Assess fetal size, especially for the presence of macrosomia between 34 and 37 weeks gestation.

**Intrapartum Management:**

**Delivery Type and Timing**

**Induction of labor**—Performed in patients with well-controlled gestational diabetes between 39 and 40 weeks gestation. Poorly controlled gestational diabetes or other maternal-fetal indications are offered earlier delivery between 37 and 38 weeks gestation after confirmation of fetal lung maturity via amniocentesis. A lecithin-sphingomyelin (L/S) ratio ≥2.0 or the presence of phosphatidylglycerol indicates fetal lung maturity.

**C-section**—A scheduled cesarean section is offered to patients when the estimated fetal weight (EFW) is ≥4500 g (ie, macrosomia) to avoid risk of shoulder dystocia and related birth injuries.

**Glycemic Control**

**Glycemic goals**—Achieve glucose levels between 70 and 110 mg/dL.

**Glucose monitoring**—Finger sticks every 1 to 2 hours to allow for adjustments in infusion rates.

**Intravenous infusions**—Five percent dextrose and short-acting insulins are administered and adjusted to maintain glycemic goals during the intrapartum period.

**Postpartum Management:**

**Early postpartum**—Immediately after placenta delivery, the levels of HPL begin to diminish rapidly because of the short half-life, and the state of insulin resistance begins to decrease. As a result, the majority of patients with gestational diabetes do not require further insulin therapy. Routine finger-stick checks and insulin sliding scale are appropriate in this setting.

**Late postpartum**—An OGTT is performed between 6 and 12 weeks postpartum to detect any persistent diabetes in both diet-controlled and pharmacotherapy-controlled gestational diabetes.

Step 1) Fasting plasma glucose level is measured.

Step 2) 75 gram oral glucose load given to a fasting woman.

Step 3) Plasma glucose level is measured at 2 hours after ingestion.

Step 4) A fasting plasma glucose level ≥126 mg/dL or a 2-hour glucose level ≥200 mg/dL indicates **overt diabetes**. A fasting plasma glucose level between 100 and 125 mg/dL or a 2 hour glucose level between 140 and 199 mg/dL indicates glucose impairment or **prediabetes**.

**Pearls:**

- Patients with gestational diabetes are at risk for developing type 2 diabetes within 5 to 10 years.
- A patient with gestational diabetes is at risk for developing gestational diabetes again in subsequent pregnancies.
- **On the CCS**, you can type in "ogtt" in the order sheet to obtain the OGTT. Both the 1 hour and 3 hour OGTT are available in the practice CCS, but the results do not give you the normal reference values.

- **On the CCS,** if you need to refer to prior test results during the CCS, click on the "Review Chart" tab and then look for the "Lab Reports" or "Other Tests" tabs to find what you're looking for.

## Pregestational Diabetes

Diabetes diagnosed prior to pregnancy is referred to as pregestational diabetes (ie, overt, type 1, or type 2 diabetes).

## Complications

The incidence of complications is higher among patients with pregestational diabetes, especially those with poorly controlled diabetes, compared to gestational diabetes.

**Mother**—↑ risk of infections especially urinary tract infections (UTI), hypertension/preeclampsia, polyhydramnios, spontaneous abortion, preterm delivery, DKA, gastroparesis, worsening of diabetic retinopathy.

**Baby**—Congenital heart defects (eg, septal defects, tetrology of Fallot), neural tube defects, caudal regression syndrome/caudal agenesis (ie, abnormal development in the caudal region), respiratory distress syndrome (RDS), IUGR, renal agenesis, hypoglycemia, hypocalcemia, hyperbilirubinemia, polycythemia, stillbirth, macrosomia and related birth injuries.

## Antepartum Management:

**Maternal Care**—In addition to the routine prenatal testing, several additional tests and recommendations are advocated in pregestational diabetics. Consider the following tests in a relative head to toe fashion:

**Ophthalmology**—Refer to ophthalmologist for a dilated eye examination to evaluate for retinopathy.

**Cardiac**—Obtain an EKG at the first prenatal visit. Patients that are hypertensive should be off ACE inhibitors and ARBs because they are teratogenic. Consider methyldopa, amlodipine, or nifedipine to treat hypertension.

**Renal**—Obtain a baseline renal function and assess protein levels with a 24-hour urine collection or a spot urine protein-to-creatinine ratio (ie, more convenient for the patient).

**Endocrine**—Obtain a HbA1C at the first prenatal visit. A HbA1C ≥10% in the first trimester is associated with a higher risk of congenital malformations. Also, obtain a TSH with free T4 at the first prenatal visit.

## Treatment Management

**Diet**—Caloric requirements are based on the patient's body weight and activity level. Carbohydrate composition should be approximately 55%, protein 20%, and fat 25%.

**Exercise**—Patients that were able to exercise prior to pregnancy and are not deconditioned during pregnancy may continue to exercise.

**Glucose monitoring**—Home glucose monitoring should be done 5 to 7 times a day. HbA1C should be obtained at every trimester. Glucose goals for women with pregestational diabetes are:

HbA1C: ≤6%

Fasting glucose: ≤95 mg/dL

Preprandial glucose: ≤100 mg/dL

1 hour postprandial glucose: ≤140 mg/dL

2 hour postprandial glucose: ≤120 mg/dL

Bedtime: Keep glucose levels ≥60 mg/dL

**Medications**—Type 1 diabetics should continue with their insulin, although it should be noted that the insulin requirements will increase by the second half of pregnancy. Type 2 diabetics who are not glycemic controlled by diet alone or are on oral hypoglycemic agents should be treated with insulin during pregnancy.

**Fetal surveillance**—The goal of fetal surveillance is to assess for fetal well-being, fetal growth, and to detect congenital anomalies, which occur more commonly in pregestational diabetics.

- Nonstress test (NST) or biophysical profile (BPP)—Twice weekly testing starting at 32 weeks gestation or 26 weeks gestation if there are complications with the pregnancy (eg, preeclampsia).
- Ultrasound and fetal echocardiogram at 18 weeks gestation to assess for congenital anomalies, especially congenital heart defects.
- Ultrasound and maternal serum alpha-fetoprotein (MSAFP) in the second trimester to screen for neural tube defects (NTDs) since the prevalence is higher with pregestational diabetes. Levels of MSAFP in diabetics are naturally lower, and adjustments have to be made in order to interpret the results.
- Ultrasound exam at 32 weeks to assess for fetal growth and again at 38 weeks for an estimated fetal weight (EFW) to determine the type of delivery.

## Intrapartum Management:

Management is the same as gestational diabetes (see "Intrapartum Management").

## Postpartum Management:

**Type 1 diabetes**—Insulin is reduced to approximately one-third to one-half of the prepartum dose once the patient is able to eat.

**Type 2 diabetes**—Oral hypoglycemic agents can be resumed 1 to 2 days after delivery, but in the interim treat with insulin if the patient is eating.

## Pearls:

- Diabetes does not increase the risk for fetal chromosomal abnormalities (ie, aneuploidy).
- Diabetes does lower the levels of MSAFP, uE3, and inhibin A. Interpretation of the "triple" or "quad" screen should be adjusted accordingly.
- Postpartum depression is common among patients with pregestational and gestational diabetes.
- Offspring of women with pregestational diabetes are at risk for developing diabetes and obesity later in their lives.

## Hematologic Disorder

### Rhesus Incompatibility

There are many blood group systems, but the rhesus (Rh) system is the most frequently involved. Within the Rh system, there are several different types of antigens—in particular, the big D antigen on the red blood cells, which is also referred to as Rh(D) positive. Keep in mind there is no little d in the nomenclature.

### Clinical Progression:

When an Rh(D) negative woman is exposed to Rh(D) positive blood cells (eg, fetomaternal hemorrhage, blood transfusions, transplantation), the woman will develop antibodies to the D antigen (ie, isoimmunization). Anti-D IgG antibodies in the maternal circulation can then cross the placenta into the fetal circulation. Antibodies can then bind to the D antigens on the fetal erythrocyte cells of an Rh(D) positive fetus leading to cell destruction. If the mother is in her first pregnancy, the fetal effect is less severe such as **anemia** and **hyperbilirubinemia**. However, in subsequent pregnancies there is an anamnestic response of the immune system that can result in **erythroblastosis fetalis**. Clinical features of erythroblastosis fetalis may include anemia, jaundice, heart failure, enlarged spleen and liver, or **fetal hydrops**.

### Next Step:

**Step 1)** Rh(D) typing and antibody screen via **indirect Coombs test** is performed at the first prenatal visit. The indirect Coombs test is a very accurate way to determine antibody titer levels.

**Step 2)** There are two clinical scenarios to consider in the management of an Rh (D) negative mother. Determine whether she has developed antibodies (ie, sensitized) or no antibodies (ie, unsensitized). Consider the following:

**Unsensitized**—Determine if there are antibodies at the initial visit. If the there are no antibodies, the antibody screen is performed again at 28 weeks gestation and at delivery. If the mother is still unsensitized at 28 weeks gestation, **anti-D immune globulin** (RhoGAM) is given intramuscularly (IM). After delivery, fetal rhesus type is performed, and if the baby is Rh(D) negative, no further action is required. If the baby is Rh(D) positive, then anti-D immune globulin (RhoGAM) is provided again to the mother preferably within 72 hours of delivery. Keep in mind that anti-D immune globulin (RhoGAM) can be given up to 28 days after delivery.

**Sensitized**—If the mother develops antibodies from her first pregnancy, the next best step is to check her antibody titer level. If a critical titer level is reached, which is a value ≥1:16, then this indicates enough maternal antibodies to cause **severe fetal anemia**. Checking a titer level in later pregnancies from previously affected infants is not needed because fetal anemia will be certain and tracking the severity of anemia is not helpful. Keep in mind that providing anti-D immune globulin (RhoGAM) is not effective once the mother is sensitized. If a sensitized Rh (D) negative mother has reached her critical titer level, then the next best step is to determine the fetal rhesus type because if the fetus is Rh(D) negative, then there is no risk for fetal complications.

The least invasive way is by **paternal Rh type and zygosity**. If the father's Rh type is Rh(D) negative, then there is no further workup since the fetus will be Rh(D) negative. If the father is Rh(D) positive, then determine the zygosity (ie, homozygous or heterozygous). Consider the following:

**Homozygous**—If the father is homozygous, there is a 100% chance that the fetus will be Rh(D) positive, and therefore, there is no need to do fetal genotyping. At this point, you can manage the patient as a "sensitized pregnancy," and it is important to institute fetal surveillance to detect fetal anemia. Amniotic fluid bilirubin level assessment (via amniocentesis), fetal middle cerebral artery Doppler (MCA) assessment, and fetal blood sampling are techniques used to check for fetal anemia. If there is severe fetal anemia, an intrauterine blood transfusion via PUBS may be indicated.

**Heterozygous**—If the father is heterozygous, the father is unavailable, or the identity of the father is in question, then there is a chance that the fetus may be Rh(D) positive. Therefore, the next best step is to do fetal genotyping, which can be performed by either obtaining fetal blood, amniocytes (via amniocentesis), or cell-free fetal DNA from maternal blood.

### Follow-Up:

In a woman who is in her first pregnancy that is Rh(D) negative and sensitized, but does not reach the critical titer level, the next best step is to repeat titer levels every month until 24 weeks gestation and then every 2 weeks until delivery.

### Pearls:

- Remember that an Rh(D) positive woman does not require anti-D immune globulin at any time.

- Fetal middle cerebral artery (MCA) Doppler is a noninvasive way to detect fetal anemia. In an anemic fetus, blood will be shunted to the brain to maintain oxygenation and a **peaked systolic velocity** will be seen on Doppler because of an increased cardiac output and decreased blood viscosity.

- **Foundational point**—Rh(D) antigens are only present on red blood cells, and the D antigen is considered a potent alloantigen.

- **Connecting point** (pg. 3)—Know the principle actions of the other immunoglobulins.

- **CJ:** A 25-year-old $G_1P_0$ at 17 weeks gestation who is Rh(D) negative and unsensitized is in the ED because of a blunt trauma to the abdomen from an automobile accident. There is concern for fetomaternal hemorrhage. What is your next step? **Answer:** The best initial step to determine fetomaternal hemorrhage is to screen with the **Rosette test**. If the result is negative, you still give the standard dose of anti-D immune globulin. If the result is positive, you need to determine the amount of fetal red blood cells in maternal blood by the **Kleihauer-Betke test**. The Kleihauer-Betke test is valuable in determining if additional anti-D immune globulin is required from the standard dose. Other indications to give anti-D immune globulin (RhoGAM) in an Rh(D) negative woman who is **not** sensitized and has a fetus that is or possibly could be Rh(D) positive are:

- Procedures (eg, amniocentesis, chorionic villus sampling, fetal blood sampling)
- Trauma (eg, blunt trauma to the abdomen)
- First trimester spontaneous or elective abortion
- Second or third trimester bleeding (eg, abruption, previa)
- Third trimester rescreen at 28 weeks gestation
- Ectopic pregnancy
- Molar pregnancy (ie, hydatidiform mole)
- Fetal demise
- External cephalic version (ie, from breech to vertex presentation)

## Hypertensive Disorders

### Mild Preeclampsia

Preeclampsia is a condition in which **hypertension** and **proteinuria** arise after 20 weeks gestation in a previously normotensive woman. Preeclampsia can be further classified as mild or severe.

### Risk Factors for Preeclampsia:

Nulliparity, multiple gestation (eg, twins), age <20 or >40, previous history of preeclampsia, family history of preeclampsia, pregestational or gestational diabetes, antiphospholipid syndrome, chronic renal disease, chronic HTN, obesity.

### Clinical Features:

Most women with mild preeclampsia are asymptomatic. However, they can develop symptoms with progressive signs of end-organ damage (see Clinical Features under Severe Preeclampsia).

### Next Step:

**Step 1)** Diagnosis of mild preeclampsia is confirmed when both HTN and proteinuria are present:

> **HTN**—Systolic pressure ≥140 or diastolic pressure ≥90 after 20 weeks measured on two occasions at least 6 hours but not more than 7 days apart.
>
> **Proteinuria**—≥0.3 g (300 mg) in a 24-hour urine collection. A random urine dipstick of 1+ or 30 mg/dL is not diagnostic but only suggestive of mild preeclampsia.

**Step 2)** Once the diagnosis is made, obtain a set of laboratory tests that should include CBC, CMP, uric acid level, LDH, and a coagulation profile (PT, PTT, fibrinogen). Laboratory tests should be repeated weekly if there is no progression of preeclampsia but more frequently if there is suspicion for progression.

**Step 3)** Assess the fetus with an ultrasound, nonstress test, or biophysical profile on a weekly basis once the diagnosis of preeclampsia is made.

**Step 4)** Delivery is the definitive treatment for preeclampsia. However, there are many factors to consider prior to delivery. Consider three different scenarios in the management of a patient with mild preeclampsia that may include delivery, inpatient care, or outpatient care.

> **Indications for delivery**—The following is adapted from the Working Group Report on High Blood Pressure in Pregnancy:

- Gestational age ≥38 weeks
- Deteriorating hepatic or renal function
- Platelet <100,000/mm$^3$
- Persistent headaches, visual changes, epigastric pain, nausea, or vomiting
- Suspected placental abruption
- Severe IUGR
- Oligohydramnios
- Nonreassuring fetal surveillance

**Inpatient care**—Admit to the hospital in these cases:

- Noncompliant patient
- Poor access to receive medical care
- Signs of progression (eg, SBP >150, DBP >100, proteinuria >1 g/24 hours)
- Patient care may include:

> **Anticonvulsants**—Anticonvulsant therapy is controversial for mild preeclampsia.
>
> **Antihypertensives**—Do not treat unless BP ≥160/100 (see Severe Preeclampsia).
>
> **Fetal lung maturity**—Administer steroids (ie, betamethasone or dexamethasone) intramuscularly (IM) in women <34 weeks gestation.
>
> **Monitoring**—Close monitoring with NST/BPP, ultrasound/AFI, lab testing, BP monitor, cervical exams, and laboratory testing as indicated in the inpatient setting.

**Outpatient care**—Patients that are compliant, have good access to receive medical care, and show no signs of progression can be managed as an outpatient. Patients are recommended restricted physical activity.

### Follow-Up:

Patients managed as an outpatient should be evaluated for weekly blood pressure checks, physical exams, and NST/BPP. Ultrasound and AFI measurements are performed every 3 to 4 weeks.

### Pearls:

- Since women without preeclampsia naturally have edema during pregnancy, edema is no longer used as a criterion for the diagnosis of preeclampsia.
- Remember that indications for delivery do not mean immediate C-section. Often, an induction of labor will be attempted first.
- **On the CCS,** "NST" or "Nonstress test" is available in the practice CCS, and once the external monitor is attached, then type in "check fetal monitor" for future readings.

### Severe Preeclampsia

Severe preeclampsia can be differentiated from mild preeclampsia by signs of end-organ damage.

**Clinical Features:**

Women may experience multiple end-organ signs or symptoms. It may be helpful to think from a relative head to toe fashion:

**Neurologic**—Visual disturbances, persistent headaches, altered mental status

**Cardiovascular**—Hypertension (ie, BP ≥160/110)

**Respiratory**—Shortness of breath

**Renal**—Oliguria

**GI**—Epigastric pain, RUQ pain, nausea, vomiting

**Pelvis**—Signs of placental abruption (ie, vaginal bleeding, uterine pain), ↓ fetal movements

**Heme**—Bruising

**Next Step:**

**Step 1)** A woman with severe preeclampsia should be hospitalized to confirm the diagnosis, assess the severity of the disease, monitor the progression of the disease, and intervene if indicated.

**Step 2)** Diagnosis of severe preeclampsia is confirmed in the presence of mild preeclampsia **plus** any of the following:

**HTN**—Systolic pressure ≥160 or diastolic pressure ≥110 after 20 weeks measured on two occasions at least 6 hours but not more than 7 days apart.

**Proteinuria**—≥5 grams in a 24-hour urine collection. A random urine dipstick of 3+ is not diagnostic but only suggestive of severe preeclampsia.

**Neurologic**—Visual disturbances, persistent headaches, or altered mental status

**Respiratory**—Pulmonary edema or cyanosis

**Renal**—Oliguria (ie, <500 mL in 24 hours)

**GI**—Epigastric pain, RUQ pain, nausea, vomiting, or twice normal serum transaminases

**Heme**—Platelets <100,000/mm³

**Fetus**—IUGR

**Step 3)** Once the diagnosis is made, initial management should include:

**Anticonvulsants**—Intravenous magnesium sulfate to prevent a first seizure.

**Antihypertensives**—

Treat: When BP ≥160/100

Goal: SBP 140 to 150 and DBP 90 to 100

Acute therapy: Intravenous labetalol or hydralazine

Long-term therapy: Oral methyldopa, labetalol, or nifedipine

Contraindicated drugs: ACE inhibitors and ARBs

**Fetal lung maturity**—Administer steroids (IM) in women between 24 and 34 weeks gestation.

**Labs**—CBC, CMP, uric acid level, LDH, coagulation profile (PT, PTT, fibrinogen).

**Monitor**—Close monitoring with NST/BPP, ultrasound/AFI, BP monitoring every 1 to 2 hours, urine output, and physical exams.

**Step 4)** Delivery is the definitive treatment for preeclampsia. However, there are many factors to consider prior to delivery. Consider three different scenarios in the management of a patient with severe preeclampsia patient that may include delivery, expectant management, or termination:

**Indications for delivery**

- Gestational age ≥34 weeks
- Signs of end organ damage: Neurologic (headaches, visual disturbances, altered mental status), cardiovascular (uncontrolled BP), respiratory (pulmonary edema), renal (oliguria), GI (epigastric pain, RUQ pain), heme (severe thrombocytopenia).
- Eclampsia
- HELLP syndrome
- Fetal concerns: nonreassuring fetal surveillance, oligohydramnios.
- OB concerns: placental abruption, PPROM, preterm labor.

**Expectant management**—Can be considered between 24 and 34 weeks gestation in select cases. Both mother and fetus conditions should be reassuring.

**Termination**—Should be considered when <24 weeks gestation.

**Follow-Up:**

Hypertension should resolve within 12 weeks postpartum in a patient with preeclampsia. Evaluate any women who continue to have hypertension beyond this time period.

**Pearls:**

- There is a greater risk of recurrence of developing preeclampsia in future pregnancies in women with severe preeclampsia who delivered prior to 30 weeks compared to patients with mild preeclampsia who delivered near term.
- Intravenous nitroprusside is sometimes used as a last ditch effort to control refractory hypertension, but caution is advised because it can cause fetal cyanide poisoning.
- **CJ:** A women with severe preeclampsia is given intravenous magnesium sulfate. Over a period of time, the patient's respiration has decreased to 8 per minute, the patient is bradycardic and shows loss of deep tendon reflexes. In addition, the fetal heart monitor shows decrease in FHR and baseline variability. What is your next step? **Answer:** The patient is showing signs of magnesium toxicity. First, discontinue magnesium sulfate administration then provide supplemental oxygen, and start intravenous calcium gluconate.
- **On the CCS,** remember to transfer patients from the office setting to the inpatient setting to monitor the progression of severe preeclampsia.

**Eclampsia**

Eclampsia is characterized by new onset **tonic-clonic seizure** and/or **coma** in a patient with a history of preeclampsia and without any other attributable causes of the seizure. The etiology of eclamptic seizures is still unknown.

## Clinical Features:

Eclampsia can occur during the antepartum, intrapartum, or postpartum period. However, it typically occurs after 20 weeks gestation. Patients may have headaches, altered mental changes, visual disturbances, or epigastric pain prior to the onset of a seizure. In a small subset of patients, there is no associated hypertension or proteinuria. The seizure itself can occur more than once, with each seizure lasting between 60 and 75 seconds. After the tonic-clonic phase is the postictal phase, which can last for several minutes to hours. During the maternal seizure, the fetus will show signs of fetal bradycardia and then compensatory fetal tachycardia after resolution of the seizure.

## Next Step:

**Step 1) Protect the airway!** Roll the patient to the left decubitus position to prevent aspiration and improve uterine blood flow. Other steps to do in this life-threatening emergency include: insert a padded tongue depressor to prevent lacerations, elevate padded bedside rails, apply oxygen face mask, obtain pulse oximetry readings, initiate cardiac monitoring, secure IV line, and suction oral secretions.

**Step 2)** Prevent another seizure with intravenous magnesium sulfate. In most cases, the initial seizure will have passed before therapy can even be given. Therefore, treatment is directed at preventing another seizure rather than "correcting" the seizure.

**Step 3)** Control the hypertension, if present, with intravenous labetalol or hydralazine (see step 3 under Severe Preeclampsia).

**Step 4)** Delivery is the definitive treatment for eclampsia in a woman at any gestational age and once the patient has been stabilized. Vaginal delivery can be considered in a patient >32 weeks gestation with a favorable cervix and in the absence of other complications (eg, fetal malpresentation). A cesarean section can be considered in women <32 weeks gestation with an unfavorable cervix.

## Follow-Up:

Follow up any patient within 1 to 2 weeks after delivery to reassess for residual effects of the seizure and to reassess the blood pressure.

## Pearls:

- The recurrence risk of eclampsia in future pregnancies is only 2%.
- **On the CCS**, once the patient is stabilized, you can perform a targeted physical exam and obtain your labs (eg, CBC, CMP, PT/PTT).
- **On the CCS**, essential monitoring parameters include a **fetal monitor** for the fetus and **urine output** for the mother.
- **On the CCS**, treatment of severe hypertension should include a "one time/bolus" of either intravenous hydralazine or labetalol. After each bolus, be sure to reassess the blood pressure by ordering vital signs. If the blood pressure does not drop after the first attempt, you may need to give another bolus every 10 to 15 minutes until you to see a response.
- **On the CCS**, magnesium sulfate is given to prevent another convulsion. It is typically given as an intravenous continuous infusion, therefore, select "continuous" for the mode of frequency.

- **On the CCS**, once you suspect an eclamptic episode, be sure to order an "Ob/gyn consult" for immediate delivery. This is an appropriate case to order a consult. Remember that you're ordering a consult from the point of view of a primary care physician.
- **On the CCS**, as with any acute cases, your timing is essential in simulated time.

## HELLP Syndrome

HELLP syndrome can be characterized by **H**emolysis, **E**levated **L**iver enzymes, and **L**ow **P**latelets. Some experts believe that the HELLP syndrome is a variant of severe preeclampsia, while other experts believe that it is a separate entity since a subset of patients will not have hypertension or proteinuria.

## Clinical Features:

HELLP syndrome is commonly seen in the **third trimester**, although it can occasionally occur in the second trimester or postpartum. Women may experience multiple end-organ signs or symptoms, and it may be helpful to consider them in a relative head to toe fashion:

**Neurologic**—Visual disturbances, headaches

**Respiratory**—Shortness of breath

**Cardiovascular**—Hypertension

**Renal**—Proteinuria

**GI**—Epigastric pain, RUQ pain, nausea, vomiting, jaundice

**Heme**—Bleeding

**Systemic**—Malaise

## Next Step:

**Step 1)** Diagnosis is made on findings based on the name HELLP:

Hemolysis: ↑ LDH, ↓ haptoglobin, ↑ indirect bilirubin, presence of schistocytes/helmet cells

Elevated Liver enzymes: ↑ AST, ↑ ALT

Low Platelets: <100,000/mm$^3$

**Step 2)** A patient with HELLP syndrome should be hospitalized for further management, which should include:

**Anticonvulsants**—Intravenous magnesium sulfate to prevent seizures.

**Antihypertensives**—Do not treat unless BP ≥160/100 (see Severe Preeclampsia).

**Fetal lung maturity**—Administer steroids if <34 weeks gestation if maternal and fetal conditions are reassuring, but do not delay immediate delivery in cases of rapid deterioration.

**Platelet transfusions**—Transfuse platelets when <20,000/mm$^3$ or when platelets are <50,000/mm$^3$ if cesarean section is scheduled.

**Step 3) Prompt delivery** is the definitive treatment for HELLP syndrome.

## Follow-Up:

Follow up any abnormal lab values that persist. Typically, lab values should normalize by approximately the sixth day postpartum.

**Pearls:**

- Complications of the HELLP syndrome include DIC, placental abruption, hepatic hematoma with rupture, hepatic infarction, ascites, renal failure, and pulmonary edema.

- **On the CCS,** to cancel an order, click on the item that you want to cancel in the order sheet, and another screen will automatically appear to confirm your cancellation.

# INTRAPARTUM

## ▌ STAGES OF LABOR

### Stage 1: Cervical Dilatation

**Latent phase**—Cervical dilatation from **0 to 4 cm**. Nulliparous—≤20 hours, multiparous—≤14 hours.

**Active phase**—Cervical dilatation from **4 to 10 cm**. Nulliparous—cervix dilating at least 1.2 cm/hr. Multiparous—Cervix dilating at least 1.5 cm/hr.

**Pearls:**

- Consider the **triple P's** if there is an arrest in the active phase (ie, >2 hours).

    **P**ower—Uterine contraction problems

    **P**elvis—Size or shape of the pelvis

    **P**assenger—Size or presentation of the infant

- Greater than 200 Montevideo units within 10 minutes is considered adequate contractions.

### Stage 2: Delivery of the Baby

**Epidural—**

Nulliparous—3 hours. Multiparous—2 hours.

**No epidural—**

Nulliparous—2 hours. Multiparous—1 hour.

**Pearl:**

- During this stage, the baby is undergoing the cardinal movements: Engagement → descent → flexion → internal rotation → extension → external rotation → expulsion

### Stage 3: Delivery of the Placenta

This stage can take up to 30 minutes.

**Pearl:**

- Signs of placental separation include a gush of blood, uterus feels firm and globular, uterine fundal rebound, and umbilical cord lengthening.

### Stage 4: Maternal Physiologic Adjustments

- Immediately postpartum lasting up to 2 hours after delivery of the placenta.

**Pearl:**

- Risk of uterine atony during this stage (ie, excessive vaginal bleeding, enlarged **boggy** fundus) → First step in management is bimanual massage of the uterus ± IV oxytocin.

## ▌ INTRAPARTUM SURVEILLANCE

The principal goal of intrapartum surveillance is to assess the fetal well-being and to prevent an adverse fetal outcome. Intrapartum fetal surveillance (see Table 12-10) includes both electronic methods and nonelectronic methods (eg, fetal scalp blood sampling).

| Table 12-10 • Intrapartum Surveillance | |
| --- | --- |
| **Test** | **Comments** |
| **Fetal scalp blood pH** | • Fetal blood pH can help clarify fetal acid-base status.<br>• Interpretation: Normal value—pH ≥7.25<br>   • Preacidotic—pH 7.20-7.24<br>   • Fetal acidosis—pH ≤7.19 on two collections 5-10 minutes apart → Immediate delivery |
| **Fetal scalp stimulation** | • Fetal scalp stimulation should elicit an FHR acceleration of 15 bpm lasting for 15 seconds, which corresponds to a scalp pH of ≥7.20. |
| **Electronic monitoring** | **External monitoring:**<br><br>**Fetal heart rate**—An external transducer similar to an ultrasound, strapped onto the woman's abdomen.<br><br>**Uterine contractions**—An external transducer (tocodynamometer) is strapped onto the abdomen.<br><br>**Internal monitoring:**<br><br>**Fetal heart rate**—A fetal scalp electrode (FSE) is directly applied to the fetal scalp through the cervix once the membranes have ruptured. FSE is more invasive compared to the external monitor, but it is more accurate in determining the beat-to-beat variability.<br><br>**Uterine contraction**—An intrauterine pressure catheter (IUPC) is inserted into the chorioamniotic sac once the membranes have ruptured. Similar to FSE, IUPC is used when external monitoring provides poor tracings or artifact. IUPC can provide accurate readings of the strength, duration, and amplitude of the contractions. |

# FETAL HEART RATE AND ACTIVITY

The FHR pattern is an important index of cardiac activity that is regulated through an interplay of the sympathetic and parasympathetic nervous system.

### Fetal Heart Rate

**Normal:** 110 to 160 bpm.

**Tachycardia:** >160 bpm. Causes: Maternal infection, maternal thyrotoxicosis, fetal anemia, medications (eg, atropine).

**Bradycardia:** <110 bpm. Causes: fetal congenital heart block, fetal anoxia, medications (eg, β-blockers).

**Sinusoidal heart rate:** A smooth undulating sinusoidal pattern that has been associated with fetal anemia. It should be noted that the sinusoidal pattern is not part of the definition of FHR variability since it is described as having a regular fluctuation (see Figure 12-1).

### Baseline Variability

Baseline variability describes an irregular fluctuation along the baseline of two cycles per minute or greater. The baseline variability gives us insight to the fetal cardiovascular function. See Figure 12-1 for the different patterns of FHR variability.

**Absent**—Undetectable, a flat appearance (ominous sign)

**Minimal**—Amplitude ≤5 bpm

**Moderate (Normal)**—Amplitude 6 to 25 bpm

**Marked**—Amplitude >25 bpm

### Acceleration

An abrupt increase in FHR above baseline. Adequate accelerations occur if:

**<32 weeks**—Accelerations ≥10 bpm above baseline for ≥10 seconds

**≥32 weeks**—Accelerations ≥15 bpm above baseline for ≥15 seconds

### Deceleration

A deceleration is visualized as a dip or decrease in the FHR. Consider four types of decelerations (see Figure 12-2):

### Early Deceleration

**Pattern:** The decelerations onset, nadir, and termination are coincident with the onset, peak, and termination of the maternal uterine contraction. Also, the FHR has a gradual decrease with return to baseline.

**Cause:** Fetal head compression

### Late Deceleration

**Pattern:** The deceleration is delayed and occurs after the termination of a contraction. Also, the FHR has a gradual decrease with return to baseline.

**Cause:** Uteroplacental insufficiency (ominous sign).

### Variable Deceleration

**Pattern:** The deceleration may start before, during, or after a uterine contraction. Also, the FHR has an abrupt decrease with a rapid return.

**Cause:** Umbilical cord compression

### Prolonged Deceleration

**Pattern:** A deceleration below the baseline of ≥15 bpm and lasting for at least 2 minutes but <10 minutes from onset to return to baseline.

**Cause:** Uterine hyperactivity, maternal hypotension, cord entanglement

### Summary of Nonreassuring Fetal Heart Patterns

- Bradycardia
- Absent variability
- Sinusoidal pattern
- Recurrent late decelerations
- Recurrent variable decelerations

# INDICATIONS FOR CESAREAN SECTION

The optimal mode of delivery is based on many factors to ensure the best possible maternal-fetal outcome. The decision to undergo a cesarean delivery is based on concerns of the mother, fetus, or a combination of the two (see Table 12-11).

# PRETERM PREMATURE RUPTURE OF MEMBRANES

Premature rupture of membranes (PROM) refers to rupture of fetal membranes prior to the onset of labor. When fetal membranes rupture prior to term (<37 weeks), it is referred to as preterm premature rupture of membranes (PPROM).

**Risk Factors:**

Smoking, intrauterine infection, history of PPROM, antepartum bleeding.

**Clinical Features:**

Some patients will experience a sudden gush of vaginal fluid, while others may notice a gradual leak of fluid. The vaginal fluid can appear as a clear color to a meconium-stained appearance.

**Next Step:**

**Step 1)** Avoid a digital cervical examination unless delivery is imminent because it can increase the risk of infection and decrease the time from rupture to delivery (ie, latency period).

**Step 2)** A sterile speculum exam should reveal pooling of the vaginal vault.

**Step 3)** Confirm the diagnosis with the **Fern test**, which should reveal a "ferning" pattern under a microscope. Also, the **Nitrazine test** is used to assess the pH of the fluid, which should reveal an alkaline pH of 7.0 to 7.3, or visually the nitrazine paper will turn blue.

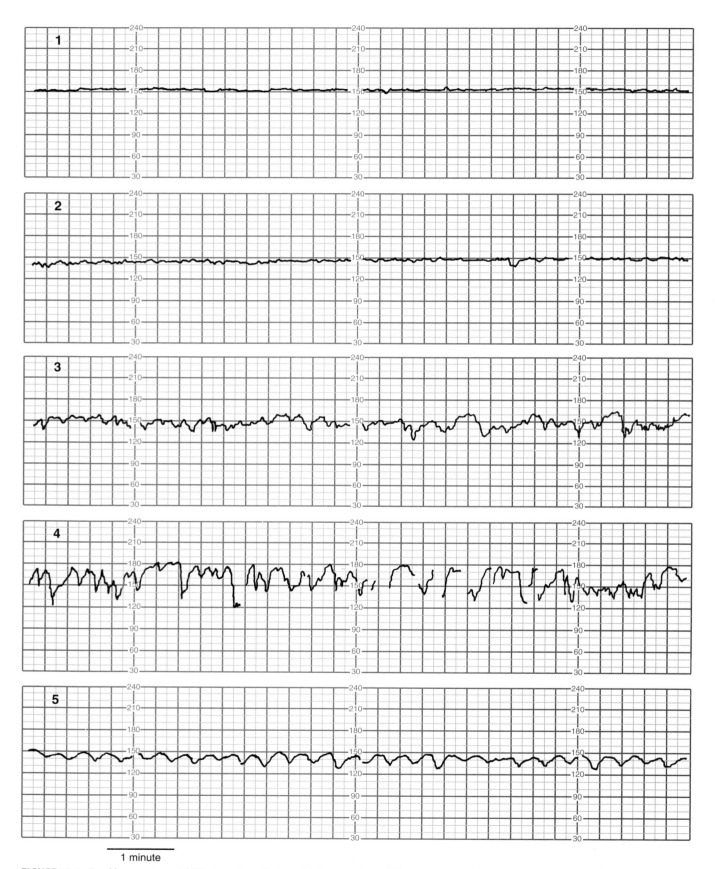

1 minute

**FIGURE 12-1 • Fetal heart rate variability (panels 1-4), sinusoidal pattern (panel 5).** 1. Absent variability. 2. Minimal variability, ≤5 bpm. 3. Moderate (normal) variability, 6-25 bpm. 4. Marked variability, >25 bpm. 5. Sinusoidal pattern is excluded from the definition of fetal heart rate variability. Note the smooth, sinelike pattern with regular fluctuation. (Reproduced with permission from Cunningham FG, et al. *Williams Obstetrics*. 23rd ed. New York: McGraw-Hill; 2010:418.)

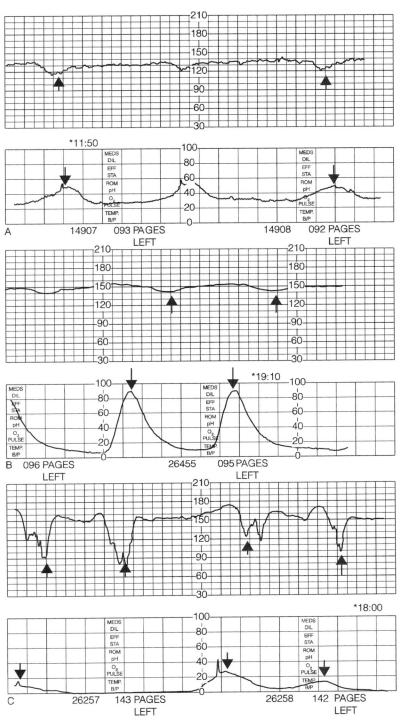

**FIGURE 12-2 • Decelerations. A. Early deceleration**—Note that the nadir of the FHR (top panel) and the peak of the uterine contractions (lower panel) occur at about the same time (see arrows). **B. Late deceleration**—Note that the nadir of the deceleration (top panel) occurs after the peak of the uterine contractions (lower panel). **C. Variable deceleration**—Note the abrupt decrease in FHR (top panel) compared to the gradual decrease in FHR in A and B. The onset, duration, and depth of the decelerations vary with successive uterine contractions, hence the term *variable*. (Reproduced with permission from Callahan TL, Caughey AB. *Blueprints Obstetrics and Gynecology*. 6th ed. Philadelphia, LWW; 2013:46.)

## Table 12-11 • Indications for Cesarean Section

| Maternal | Fetal | Maternal-Fetal |
|---|---|---|
| • Abdominal cerclage<br>• Active herpes simplex virus infection<br>• HIV infection<br>• Previous C-section<br>• Previous uterine surgery including myomectomy<br>• Cervical cancer<br>• Eclampsia with unfavorable cervix <32 weeks gestation<br>• Birth canal obstruction:<br>  • Condylomata<br>  • Ovarian tumors<br>  • Fibroids | • Fetal distress<br>  • Fetal acidemia<br>  • Bradycardia<br>  • Absent variability<br>• Fetal malpresentation<br>  • Breech<br>  • Transverse lie<br>• Fetal anomalies<br>  • Hydrocephalus<br>  • Macrosomia<br>  • Osteogenesis imperfecta<br>• Twins<br>  • Nonvertex first twin<br>  • Conjoined twins<br>• Cord prolapse | • Failed induction of labor<br>• Cephalopelvic disproportion<br>• Placenta abruption<br>• Placenta accreta<br>• Placenta previa<br>• Vasa previa |

**Step 4)** Obtain cultures for chlamydia, gonorrhea, and Group B streptococcus.

**Step 5)** Laboratory testing: CBC, urinalysis with urine culture.

**Step 6)** Obtain amniotic fluid from the vaginal vault to assess for fetal lung maturity.

**Step 7)** Ultrasound to assess for AFI, fetal presentation, gestational age, and potential cord prolapse.

**Step 8)** Consider three scenarios for the management of PPROM, and in all three cases, admit to the hospital.

### Immediate Delivery

- Infection
- Fetal distress
- Placental abruption
- Cord prolapse

### 24 to 33 Weeks Gestation

**Delivery**—Expectant management, but okay to deliver at 33 weeks if fetal lungs are mature.

**Fetal lungs**—Administer steroids.

**GBS ppx**—Yes, if GBS positive or status unknown.

**Prolong latency**—Yes, with antibiotics: IV ampicillin + IV erythromycin × 2 days, then PO amoxicillin + PO erythromycin × 5 days.

### ≥34 Weeks Gestation

**Delivery**—Proceed to deliver.

**Fetal lungs**—No steroids.

**GBS ppx**—Yes, if GBS positive or status unknown.

**Prolong latency**—No need.

### Follow-Up:

Close follow-up is warranted in patients being treated for infection (eg, chorioamnionitis) since intrauterine infections can be the source of a neonatal sepsis.

### Pearls:

- Approximately 90% of term patients and 50% of preterm patients who experience fetal membrane rupture will enter labor within 24 hours.

- A false positive result can occur with the nitrazine test if blood, semen, or alkaline soap is present in the vaginal fluid.

- Another test that can confirm ruptured membranes is a placental alpha microglobulin-1 protein assay (Market name: AmniSure). AmniSure is a rapid, noninvasive test that does not require a speculum exam, but does require inserting a sterile swab into the vagina to obtain a sample of the fluid. The results are not affected by the presence of blood, semen, or soap.

- An amniotic fluid index (AFI) <5 cm is considered oligohydramnios, which would be suggestive of fetal membrane rupture.

- The use of antibiotics can prolong the time from rupture to delivery and reduce the chance of infection.

- Tocolytics (eg, terbutaline) can be used for the first 48 hours when administering steroids if the patient is having a contraction. However, in the setting of chorioamnionitis, tocolysis should not be used.

- Complications of PPROM include infections, prematurity, cord prolapse, oligohydramnios, and pulmonary hypoplasia.

- **On the CCS**, both "Nitrazine test" and "Fern test" are available in the practice CCS.

- **On the CCS**, pay attention to the initial vital signs as fever and tachycardia will point you toward an infectious etiology and help you take the appropriate and timely actions of administering antibiotics.

# POSTPARTUM

## BREASTFEEDING CONCERNS

Breastfeeding problems is not uncommon in the postpartum period. It is important to recognize some of these problems to prevent early termination of breastfeeding and to maintain the associated health benefits for the infant (see Table 12-12).

## MENTAL HEALTH CONCERNS

See Table 12-13.

## POSTPARTUM FEVER

Postpartum febrile morbidity is defined as a temperature of 38.0°C (100.4°F) or higher, on at least two occasions of the first 10 days postpartum, **exclusive** of the first 24 hours (see Table 12-14).

| Table 12-12 • Breastfeeding Concerns | |
|---|---|
| **Concerns** | **Comments** |
| **Breast engorgement** | Bilateral breast engorgement can occur in a woman who does not breastfeed or those with ineffective breastfeeding techniques. Engorgement can be seen 3-5 days after delivery. Pain and "milk fever" are common. However, the fever usually resolves within 24 hours.<br>**Next step**—Frequent breastfeeding, cold ice packs, acetaminophen or ibuprofen for pain control (safe to use). Breast pumps can be used but should be avoided if possible since they are inefficient and can actually stimulate milk letdown. |
| **Cracked nipples** | Poor breastfeeding technique is a common cause for cracked nipples. In most cases, the infant is sucking only on the nipple and sucking harder to extract more milk.<br>**Next step**—Reevaluate latch-on technique, allow the baby to suck on both the nipple and areola thereby compressing the milk ducts and stimulating milk letdown. Allow the baby to nurse on the less sore breast first before transitioning to the breast with the cracked nipple as the baby will usually suck less vigorously on the second breast. A nipple shield may be used on the affected breast to protect the nipple as it heals. |
| **Plugged ducts** | Plugged ducts can cause milk stasis in the ducts, which would appear as a tender lump from the outside. If ducts do not become unplugged, a galactocele or retention cyst can form. From the outside, the galactocele may appear as a fluctuant mass mimicking an abscess. A cheesy substance can be extruded from the nipple. However, there are no fevers or systemic symptoms with either a plugged duct or galactocele.<br>**Next step**—Reevaluate latch-on, frequent feedings, and possibly needle aspiration if the galactocele does not resolve on its own. |
| **Mastitis** | Patients will experience a red, tender, hard breast with fever.<br>**Next step**—Antibiotics with dicloxacillin or cephalexin, acetaminophen or ibuprofen for pain control, and continue breastfeeding during medical therapy. |
| **Breast abscess** | Patients will experience a tender, fluctuant mass, with fever.<br>**Next step**—Drainage, antibiotics (dicloxacillin or cephalexin pending culture results), analgesics, continue breastfeeding during treatment. |
| **Candidal infections** | Infants with thrush may be an indication that the mother has a candidal infection on her nipples.<br>**Next step**—Apply topical nystatin on the affected breast, then wash off the medication prior to breastfeeding. Oral fluconazole may be given to the mother if the condition is persistent despite topical nystatin. |
| **Breastfeeding jaundice** | Jaundice that occurs from inadequate milk intake that may result in dehydration, hypovolemia, slower elimination of bilirubin, and ↑ enterohepatic circulation with elevated bilirubin levels. Symptoms occur within the first 2-3 days of life or at least by the first week of life. Remember that jaundice within the first 24 hours of life is always pathologic and other causes such as sepsis, hemolysis, or hemorrhage should be considered.<br>**Next step**—Reevaluate breastfeeding technique, increase breastfeeding frequency, or briefly provide formula supplementation. |
| **Breast milk jaundice** | Jaundice that occurs beyond the physiologic jaundice period. Physiologic jaundice is due to ↑ RBC cell mass, shortened RBC life span, ↓ bilirubin clearance, and ↑ enterohepatic circulation. In term infants, indirect bilirubin increases by the 3rd or 4th day of life to levels >5 mg/dL and then resolves within 1-2 weeks after birth. In contrast, preterm infants' bilirubin levels are greater and prolonged. Breast milk jaundice persists beyond the normal physiologic period in either term or preterm infants. However, it is still unknown what is in the breast milk that causes breast milk jaundice. A brief discontinuation of breastfeeding results in a decline in bilirubin levels.<br>**Next step**—Formula supplementation may be provided during the interim. Discontinuation of breastfeeding is not recommended unless bilirubin levels are >20 mg/dL, in which case phototherapy or possibly exchange transfusion may be indicated.<br>**Pearl:** An easy way to differentiate breastfeeding jaundice from breast milk jaundice is that breastfeeding jaundice has something to do with the breastfeeding (ie, not feeding enough) while breast milk jaundice has something to do with the breast milk (ie, an unknown inhibitor or substance). |

*(Continued)*

| Concerns | Comments |
|---|---|
| **Bloody nipple discharge** | A bloody nipple discharge can be seen a few days postpartum and it is related to the vascularization effects of the ducts. The condition should resolve within days, but if not, consider a cracked nipple with bleeding or an intra-ductal papilloma, in which case, send the milk for cytology. |
| **Lactational amenorrhea method** | Lactational amenorrhea method is a form of contraception that is highly effective if the mother is exclusively breastfeeding, amenorrheic, and less than 6 months postpartum. Mean time ovulation in breastfeeding mothers is 190 days, and 45 days for non-breastfeeding mothers. |
| **Overactive letdown** | Forceful milk ejection can occur from overactive letdown resulting in the infant gagging. In some cases, the infant will be very upset and go on a nursing strike.<br>**Next step**—Upon letdown, catch the milk on a piece of cloth, and then put the infant back onto the breast as the flow will lessen. The goal is to reduce or control the flow of milk. |
| **Green frothy stools** | Infants who produce green frothy stools can be seen with mothers who produce large amounts of milk and have a habit of switching from one breast to the other without full completion of one breast before moving on to the next. The residual milk or the milk that's left behind has a higher fat content that retards gut motility allowing for normal digestion at the small intestine level. Without the higher fat content, lactose will be digested at the level of the large bowel where green frothy stools are produced.<br>**Next step**—Full completion of one breast before moving on to the next breast. |
| **Contraindications to breastfeeding** | • Mother has alcohol or street drug abuse.<br>• Mother has HIV infection in the United States, although in developing countries the benefits may outweigh the risk.<br>• Mother has T-cell lymphotropic virus infection (HTLV-1 or 2).<br>• Mother has active and untreated tuberculosis.<br>• Mother has active herpes lesions on the breast.<br>• Mother is on antiretroviral medications.<br>• Mother is on chemotherapy or antimetabolite agents.<br>• Mother is undergoing radioactive therapy.<br>• Infant has galactosemia. |
| **Acceptable conditions to breastfeeding** | • Mother has silicone breast implants.<br>• Mother smokes cigarettes.<br>• Mother had postpartum varicella vaccination.<br>• Mother had postpartum MMR vaccination.<br>• Mother contracted toxoplasmosis during pregnancy.<br>• Mother contracted CMV infection during pregnancy.<br>• Mother contracted measles (rubeola) during pregnancy.<br>• Mother has hepatitis C infection.<br>• Mother has hepatitis B infection—Provide the passive immunization with the hepatitis B immune globulin (HBIG) and first dose of the active immunization with the hepatitis B vaccine to the newborn. The second and third doses of the vaccine should be given at the appropriate times, but there is no need to delay breastfeeding until the baby is fully immunized. |
| **Weaning** | Exclusive breastfeeding can occur until 6 months of age. After that time, breast milk won't meet the energy or nutritional demands of the growing infant. In addition, the baby's iron stores are good for 4-6 months after delivery. Iron-fortified supplementation and solids can be introduced at that time. Remember not to give whole cow's milk prior to 12 months of age, as it is low in iron content and can cause intestinal irritation leading to microscopic bleeding, which can lead to iron-deficiency anemia. |

Table 12-12 • Breastfeeding Concerns (Continued)

## PUBIC DIASTASIS

Pubic diastasis is the separation of the pubic bones. In nonpregnant women, the normal pubic symphysis gap is between 4 and 5 mm. During pregnancy, the connecting pelvic ligaments loosen and can cause the gap to increase up to 10 mm.

**Clinical Features:**

Symptoms of pubic diastasis may include any of the following:

• Suprapubic pain at rest or with palpation
• Waddling gait
• Swelling around the suprapubic area
• Pain exacerbated with weight-bearing
• Radiating pain into the legs or back
• Palpable displacement

**Next Step:**

**Step 1)** Pubic diastasis is a clinical diagnosis. Obtaining pelvic x-ray or other imaging is unnecessary. However, a pubic symphysis gap ≥10 mm seen on x-ray, confirms the diagnosis.

**Step 2)** Treatment is conservative and includes bed rest in the lateral decubitus position and pelvic support with an appropriately fitted pelvic binder.

## Table 12-13 • Mental Health Concerns

|  | Postpartum Depression | Postpartum Blues | Postpartum Psychosis |
|---|---|---|---|
| **Onset** | Within 3-6 months after delivery | Within 3-5 days after delivery | Within several days to weeks after delivery and almost always within 8 weeks |
| **Duration** | Months to years if untreated | Days to weeks, but usually within 2 weeks postpartum | Variable |
| **History of mood disorder** | Yes | No | Yes |
| **Clinical features** | • Indistinguishable from major depression.<br>• Anxiety, depressed mood, inadequacy, insomnia, anhedonia, appetite disturbance, suicidal thoughts, ambivalent feelings toward infant, decreased bonding with infant.<br>• High risk for future episodes. | • Less debilitating than postpartum depression.<br>• Mood swings, sadness, crying spells, anxiety, mild depressed mood, sometimes sleep disturbance, no suicidal thoughts. | • Mood swings, depressed mood, elated mood, delusions, hallucinations, suspiciousness, irrational statements, insomnia, suicidal thoughts, negative feelings toward infant.<br>• High rate of recurrence with subsequent pregnancies. |
| **Thoughts of harming infant?** | Yes | No | Yes |
| **Next step management** | • Psychosocial therapy in mild to moderate cases.<br>• Antidepressants + psychosocial therapy in moderate to severe cases.<br>• Consider electroconvulsive therapy (ECT) for rapid treatment when mother has active suicidal ideation. | Supportive care, the condition is self-limiting. | • This is considered a psychiatric emergency.<br>• Antidepressants, antipsychotics, mood stabilizers (eg, lithium).<br>• Discontinue breast-feeding.<br>• Possible psychiatric unit transfer.<br>• Consider ECT for rapid effective treatment. |

## Table 12-14 • Postpartum Fever

| Postpartum Day | 7 Ws | Comments |
|---|---|---|
| 0-1 | **W**ind—Atelectasis, pneumonia | Atelectasis and aspiration pneumonia are more common when general anesthesia is used. Encourage incentive spirometry and coughing. |
| 1-2 | **W**ater—UTI | Frequent bladder catheterizations secondary to epidural anesthesia or C-section deliveries can introduce bacteria into the lower urinary tract. |
| 2-3 | **W**omb—Endometritis | Endometritis is a common cause of postpartum fever secondary to prolonged labor, prolonged rupture of membranes, C-section, or manual placental removal. **Diagnosis** is mainly clinical and should be suspected when the mother has fever, foul lochia, uterine tenderness, and tachycardia. Endometrial cultures are not helpful. Leukocytosis may be seen but may be skewed by normal physiologic leukocytosis from pregnancy. **Treatment** is with IV clindamycin and gentamicin. If no response by 72 hours, add IV ampicillin and consider further workup with imaging (eg, pelvic ultrasound, CT abdomen, or chest x-ray). |
| 4-5 | **W**ound—Episiotomy infection, wound site infection | Consider in patients with a C-section. Look for signs of wound erythema or drainage. |
| 5-6 | **W**alk—DVT, PE, septic pelvic thrombophlebitis | Consider in patients with calf or thigh pain, dyspnea, cough, pleuritic pain, or pelvic tenderness. |
| 7-21 | **W**eaning—Breast engorgement, breast abscess, mastitis | Fever in breast engorgement is usually self-limiting, especially if the mother is breast-feeding. Breast abscess and mastitis may require antibiotics and drainage. |
| Anytime | **W**onder drugs—Drug fever | Common offending agents include aminoglycosides, anesthetics, anticholinergics, carbamazepine, cephalosporins, corticosteroids, heparin, macrolides, neuroleptics, penicillins, and vancomycin. |

**Step 3)** Surgery is sometimes performed with symphyseal separations ≥4 cm (ie, 40 mm).

**Follow-Up:**

Patients should been seen within 1 month postpartum as the pain typically subsides.

**Pearls:**

- It is thought that the hormones progesterone and relaxin loosen the pelvic ligaments during pregnancy along with the fetal head exerting pressure on the pelvic ligaments contribute to the separation of the pubic symphysis during vaginal delivery.

- Pubic diastasis can recur with subsequent pregnancies.

# CCS: ECTOPIC PREGNANCY CASE INTRODUCTION

Day 1 @ 10:00
Office

A 25-year-old African American woman presents to the office because of vaginal bleeding and abdominal pain. She also mentions that she missed her last two menstrual periods.

**Initial Vital Signs:**
Temperature: 37.0°C (98.6°F)
Pulse: 70 beats/min, regular rhythm
Respiratory: 15/min
Blood pressure: 120/70 mm Hg
Height: 160 cm (62.9 inches)
Weight: 59 kg (130 lb)
BMI: 23.0 kg/m$^2$

**Initial History:**
Reason(s) for visit: Vaginal bleeding, abdominal pain, missed periods.

**HPI:**
A 25-year-old $G_2P_{2002}$ sales associate has been having scant vaginal bleeding for the past 2 days. She describes the vaginal bleeding as a dark brownish-red color that occurs intermittently throughout the day. She also has lower abdominal pain for the past 4 weeks, which she describes as "on and off." The abdominal pain is described as a dull aching pain without radiation. When she experiences the pain she rates it 5/10 in severity with relief with acetaminophen. The patient states that her last menstrual period was 8 weeks ago with her previous menstrual cycles as "regular."

| | |
|---|---|
| **Past Medical History:** | History of PID |
| **Past Surgical History:** | Vaginal deliveries without complication at ages 21 and 24. |
| **Medications:** | None |
| **Allergies:** | None |

| | |
|---|---|
| **Vaccinations:** | Up to date |
| **Family History:** | Father, age 55, has hypertension. Mother, age 53, is healthy. No siblings. |
| **Social History:** | Smokes 1 ppd × 7 years; drinks 1 to 2 glasses of wine on the weekends; married; two children; sales associate; high school graduate; enjoys watching movies and reading. |

**Review of Systems:**

| | |
|---|---|
| General: | See HPI |
| HEENT: | Negative |
| Musculoskeletal: | Negative |
| Cardiorespiratory: | Negative |
| Gastrointestinal: | See HPI |
| Genitourinary: | See HPI |
| Neuropsychiatric: | Negative |

Day 1 @ 10:10

**Physical Examination:**

| | |
|---|---|
| **General appearance:** | Well nourished, well developed, appears to be in mild discomfort. |
| **HEENT/Neck:** | Normocephalic. EOMI, PERRLA. Hearing normal. Ears, nose, mouth normal. Pharynx normal. Neck supple; trachea midline; no masses or bruits; thyroid normal. |
| **Chest/Lungs:** | Chest wall normal. Diaphragm moving equally and symmetrically with respiration. Auscultation and percussion normal. |
| **Heart/Cardiovascular:** | S1, S2 normal. No murmurs, rubs, gallops, or extra sounds. No JVD. |

**Abdomen:** Normal bowel sounds; no bruit. Right lower quadrant tenderness. No masses. No hernias. No hepatosplenomegaly.

**Genitalia:** Labia normal. Scant dark brownish-red blood coming out from the cervical os. Cervix closed. Cervical motion tenderness. Mild uterine enlargement. No adnexal tenderness or mass appreciated.

**Rectal:** Sphincter tone normal. No mass or lesions. No occult blood.

**First Order Sheet:**
1) HCG, beta, urine, qualitative, stat — **Result:** Positive

**Second Order Sheet:**
1) Transvaginal pelvic ultrasound, stat — **Result:** Real time ultrasound shows no abnormal mass. Normal uterus, fallopian tubes, and ovaries.

**Third Order Sheet:**
1) HCG, beta, serum, quantitative, stat — **Result:** 1200 mIU/mL (nl: 0-3)
2) CBC with differential, stat — **Result:** WBC-8,000, H/H-12/40%, Plt-250,000, Differential-normal
3) Blood type and screen, stat — **Result:** Blood type O, Rh(D) negative, no antibodies detected
4) CMP, stat — **Result:** Ca-9.2, Glu-110, Urea-14, Cr-1, Prot-7, Alb-4, TBil-0.8, AlkP-60, AST-25, ALT-30, Na-140, K-4, Cl-102, HCO$_3$-25
5) Gonococcal culture, cervix, routine — **Result:** No *Neisseria gonorrhoeae* recovered
6) Chlamydia culture, cervix, routine — **Result:** No *Chlamydia trachomatis* isolated

**Actions:**
1) Change location to home
2) Schedule appointment: In 2 days

**Day 3**
The patient has arrived for the appointment.

**Recorded Vital Signs:**
Temperature: 37.0°C (98.6°F)
Pulse: 70 beats/min, regular rhythm
Respiratory: 15/min
Blood pressure: 120/70 mm Hg

**Physical Examination:**
**Chest/Lung:** Chest wall normal. Diaphragm moving equally and symmetrically with respiration. Auscultation and percussion normal.

**Heart/Cardiovascular:** S1, S2 normal. No murmurs, rubs, gallops, or extra sounds. No JVD.

**Abdominal:** Normal bowel sounds; no bruit. Right lower quadrant tenderness. No masses. No hernias. No hepatosplenomegaly.

**Genitalia:** Labia normal. Scant dark brownish-red blood coming from cervical os. Cervix closed. Cervical motion tenderness. Mild uterine enlargement. No adnexal tenderness or mass appreciated.

**Fourth Order Sheet:**
1) HCG, beta, serum, quantitative, stat — **Result:** 1800 mIU /mL (nl: 0-3)
2) Transvaginal pelvic trasound, stat — **Result:** Normal uterus and ovaries. Fallopian tube is normal on left. Right side demonstrates a tubal ring with a yolk sac but no cardiac activity. Tubal size is 2.0 cm on the right.

**Fifth Order Sheet:**
1) Methotrexate, IM, one time
2) RhoGAM, IM, one time

**Actions:**
1) Change location to home
2) Schedule appointment: In 4 days

**This case will end in the next few minutes of "real time."**
You may **add** or **delete** orders at this time, then enter a diagnosis on the following screen.

**Sixth Order Sheet:**
1) HCG, beta, serum, quantitative, routine
Future date: In 4 days — **Result:** 1440 mIU/mL (nl: 0-3)
**Note:** β-HCG level has decreased more than 15%

2) Advise patient, no smoking

3) Advise patient, no intercourse

4) Advise patient, no aspirin

5) Advise patient, side effects of medication

**Please enter your diagnosis:**

Ectopic pregnancy

## DISCUSSION:

Approximately 95% of ectopic pregnancies implant within the various parts of the fallopian tube. The remaining 5% can implant in the ovary, cervix, peritoneal cavity, and at cesarean scar locations.

### Risk Factors:

Previous ectopic pregnancy, tubal/pelvic surgery, IUD, PID, in utero DES exposure, infertility, multiple sex partners, and smoking. In this particular case, the patient had a history of PID and currently smokes.

### Clinical Features:

The classic presentation is abdominal pain, amenorrhea, and vaginal bleeding. Other features that may be present include cervical motion tenderness, adnexal tenderness, peritoneal signs, uterine enlargement, and early pregnancy symptoms (eg, breast fullness, nausea). Patients can also present with referred shoulder pain from diaphragmatic irritation secondary to blood leakage from a fallopian tube. Remember, a ruptured ectopic pregnancy will usually present with a clinically unstable person.

### Next Step Summary:

**Step 1)** Look at the vital signs because if the patient is hemodynamically unstable, you need start ordering IV access, continuous cardiac monitoring, continuous blood pressure cuff, pulse oximetry, type and crossmatch, CBC with differential, CMP, PTT, PT/INR, and an ob-gyn consult for presumed ruptured ectopic pregnancy. The ob-gyn will determine whether to do a laparotomy or a laparoscopic approach in addition to removing the entire fallopian tube (ie, salpingectomy) or creating a new opening (ie, salpingostomy).

**Step 2)** In this particular case, ectopic pregnancy may not be clearly apparent in the HPI. The best initial test is to rule out a pregnancy with a qualitative β-HCG. At this point, if you're still unsure of the diagnosis, keep the differentials broad: appendicitis, ovarian torsion, ovarian cyst, PID, UTI, fibroids, endometriosis, molar pregnancy, spontaneous abortion, and kidney stones.

**Step 3)** A positive β-HCG test should prompt you to look for an intrauterine pregnancy with a transvaginal ultrasound.

**Step 4)** If an intrauterine pregnancy cannot be visualized with an ultrasound, as in this case, a quantitative β-HCG is ordered to see if it exceeds the discriminatory level. The discriminatory level is the β-HCG level, at which a gestational sac should be visualized by an ultrasound by approximately 5 weeks gestation. If you're using a transvaginal ultrasound, the discriminatory level is ≥1500 mIU/mL, but if you're using a transabdominal ultrasound, the discriminatory level is ≥6500 mIU/mL. In this particular case, the initial β-HCG level was 1200 mIU/mL using a transvaginal ultrasound, which is below the discriminatory level and may indicate an ectopic pregnancy or an early intrauterine pregnancy. If the β-HCG level is above the discriminatory level without a pregnancy seen on ultrasound, then you still consider an ectopic pregnancy or multifetal gestation.

**Step 5)** When the discriminatory level is below 1500 mIU/mL and no pregnancy is seen on ultrasound, then repeat both ultrasound and quantitative β-HCG in 48 hours (2 days). A viable intrauterine pregnancy should have a β-HCG level doubling every 2 days until 6 to 7 weeks gestation. In our case, the patient was sent home and came back in 2 days with a repeat β-HCG of 1800 mIU/mL. We would expect a β-HCG level of 2400 mIU/mL from the initial 1200 mIU/mL in a viable intrauterine pregnancy. Since our case shows a suboptimal rise or possibly an HCG plateau, an ectopic pregnancy is most likely. In addition, a repeat transvaginal ultrasound in this case showed a right-sided tubal pregnancy. Keep in mind that an ultrasound is operator dependent and you may not always pick up an abnormality on the first evaluation as in this case.

**Step 6)** In a hemodynamically stable patient, the patient can undergo medical, surgical, or expectant management.

**Medical**—The patient can be treated with methotrexate with the following indications:

- Ectopic size <3.5 cm
- No fetal cardiac activity
- β-HCG level <5000 mIU/mL
- Absence of blood, kidney, and liver dysfunction.
- Patient is not breastfeeding.

**Surgical**—Patients can also be treated surgically if they have contraindications to methotrexate, failed medical therapy, or had a previous ectopic in the same fallopian tube. Remember to order an ob-gyn consult on the CCS with a reason for the consultation in 10 words or less.

**Expectant**—In select cases, patients can be offered expectant management if they are asymptomatic, unruptured ectopic pregnancy, and a β-HCG level <200 mIU/mL that is declining.

### Follow-Up:

Patients being treated with methotrexate should have a decrease in their β-HCG level between days 4 and 7. If β-HCG levels fall more than 15%, no further treatment is required and the patient can be followed weekly until β-HCG levels are undetectable. If the β-HCG level does not fall more than 15%, the patient may require an additional dose of methotrexate.

**Pearls:**

- In this particular CCS case, if the repeat β-HCG is doubling, an intrauterine pregnancy is still possible. The patient should be followed up with a transvaginal ultrasound to locate the pregnancy.
- Unsensitized Rh(D) negative patients should receive Rho-GAM.
- Be able to understand the concept of **type and screen**. The typing refers to the recipient's ABO and Rh status while screening for antibodies in the recipient's plasma that may react to the donor's blood. If the screen is positive for antibodies then further investigation with an antibody panel of the recipient's plasma may be warranted or the blood bank may proceed to identify compatible blood units. If the screen is negative for antibodies in the recipient's plasma, then the ABO and Rh status of the donor's blood is determined.
- The standard technique in the antibody screen is with the indirect Coombs test.
- Be able to understand the concept of **type and crossmatch**. Once the ABO and Rh type is determined in the recipient and donor, then a crossmatch is performed to detect ABO incompatibility as well as other significant antibodies by incubating the recipient's plasma with the donor's RBCs. Essentially, the crossmatch ensures optimal safety compared to the screen.
- In the event of a surgical procedure that is unlikely to require blood → order a type and screen.
- In the event of a surgical procedure that is highly likely to require blood → order a type and crossmatch.
- In the event that the patient is exsanguinating and there is an urgent need to transfuse blood but the patients ABO and Rh status is unknown and there is no time to complete compatibility testing → administer type O, Rh-negative blood.

- Obtaining serum progesterone levels is considered ancillary testing. However, a serum progesterone level >25 ng/mL most likely excludes ectopic pregnancy but a value <5 ng/mL suggests an ectopic pregnancy.
- **On the CCS,** "Type and screen," "Type and crossmatch," and "Type and Rh factor" are available in the practice CCS.
- **On the CCS,** "advise patient, no smoking" since it is a risk factor for ectopic pregnancy.
- **On the CCS,** "advise patient, no intercourse" until after β-HCG levels are undetectable while on methotrexate therapy.
- **On the CCS,** "advise patient, no NSAIDs" while on methotrexate because it can potentially increase the serum concentrations of methotrexate.
- **On the CCS,** "advise patient, side effects of medication" since methotrexate can cause nausea, vomiting, stomatitis, and pharyngitis.
- **On the CCS,** remember when you relocate patients from office to home or office to ED, the patients should always be stable or stabilized, respectively.
- **On the CCS,** the quantitative β-HCG measurements was managed as an outpatient basis in this particular case because the patient appeared stable and was judged to have low risk for an ectopic rupture. If you feel the patient is clinically unstable such as hypotension, tachycardia, fever, or apparent tubal mass >3.5 cm then admit and manage the patient in the hospital.
- **On the CCS,** always be aware of the "Report Time" when you order labs. If a report time for a lab result is 6 hours, you do not want your patient to be in your office for that long. In emergent cases, you will generally want to order your labs stat, but in routine office-based cases it is acceptable to send your patients home and then have them come back for a scheduled appointment.

# 13

# Ophthalmology

## KEYWORDS REVIEW

**Blepharitis**—Inflammation of the eyelids.

**Bulbar conjunctiva**—Membrane lining the sclera of the eye.

**Direct ophthalmoscope**—Commonly used during a routine physical exam; provides an upright image.

**Drusen**—Extracellular material that develops beneath the retinal pigment epithelium and can appear as yellow deposits on ophthalmoscopy.

**Hyperopia**—Farsightedness.

**Indirect ophthalmoscope**—Provides a larger view of the fundus compared to direct ophthalmoscope. The components include a light attached to a headband plus a handheld lens to view the fundus. The image is inverted, but it allows for

good depth perception (stereopsis) since you are viewing the image with binocular vision.

**Keratitis**—Inflammation of the cornea.

**Metamorphopsia**—Visual distortion of shapes or images.

**Miosis**—Pupil contraction.

**Mydriasis**—Pupil dilatation.

**Myopia**—Nearsightedness

**Optotype**—Letters (Snellen) or figures (Allen) used in testing visual acuity.

**Palpebral or tarsal conjunctiva**—Membrane lining the inner eyelid.

**Photopsia**—Flashes or sparks seen due to retinal irritation.

# CORNEA

## ▌CORNEAL ABRASION

Corneal abrasions occur when the integrity of the corneal epithelium has been disrupted. Abrasions may result from trauma, foreign body, contact lens, or spontaneous defects.

### Clinical Features:

Corneal abrasions can cause eye pain, tearing, blurring vision, photophobia, or an inability to open the eye. The type of injury can help delineate the etiology. Consider the following:

**Trauma**—Patients may have an abrasion from a fingernail, animal paw, paper, leaves, makeup applicator, or hand tool.

**Foreign body**—A foreign body sensation may be felt when material such as glass, plastic, rust, or vegetable material is embedded in the cornea.

**Contact lens**—Patients may a history of using contact lens. On eye exam, patients may have corneal white spots that reflect an ulcer or infiltrates.

**Spontaneous defects**—Patients typically do not have an immediate disruption of the cornea, but rather a history of a corneal abrasion that healed (also known as recurrent corneal erosion syndrome). Eye pain is usually felt in the middle of the night or upon awakening in the morning when they try to open their eyes.

### Next Step:

**Step 1)** Perform an eye examination. Most patients with a corneal abrasion will have a reactive miosis of the affected eye. If a patient has severe eye pain, a topical anesthetic (eg, proparacaine) may be given to facilitate visual acuity testing and the rest of the eye exam. Relief of the eye pain from the anesthetic is indicative of a corneal abrasion.

**Step 2)** Instill a drop of fluorescein into the eye and then visualize the eye with a cobalt blue filter or Wood's lamp. Any corneal defects will appear yellow-green. If a slit lamp with a cobalt blue light is available, look for leaking of the aqueous humor (Seidel sign), which is indicative of a penetrating ocular trauma.

**Step 3)** The treatment of corneal abrasions is based on the type of injury. Consider the following:

**Trauma**—Topical antibiotics (eg, erythromycin ointment or drops of ofloxacin, ciprofloxacin, polymyxin/trimethoprim, or sulfacetamide) may be given. Pain relief with topical cycloplegics (eg, cyclopentolate or homatropine) can also be given. Cycloplegics work by relaxing the ciliary body (ie, inhibit pupil constriction to light).

**Foreign body**—An attempt should be made to remove the foreign body with irrigation. If the foreign body cannot be removed, the patient should have a referral to an ophthalmologist. In the meantime, patients may be given topical antibiotics and cycloplegics (same as trauma) until they see the ophthalmologist.

**Contact lens**—Patients who wear contact lens are susceptible to infectious keratitis. If corneal white spots are seen on examination, the patient should have an urgent referral to an ophthalmologist. If there are no corneal white spots, but there are corneal defects via fluorescein stain, the next best step is to give topical antibiotics that are effective against *Pseudomonas* (eg, tobramycin, ofloxacin, or ciprofloxacin).

**Spontaneous defects**—The goal of recurrent corneal erosion syndrome is to restore the corneal epithelium. Small erosions may spontaneously heal on their own. For persistent cases, the management may include lubricant therapy (given at night), antibiotics, and cycloplegics. Further management with an ophthalmologist may include debridement, wearing soft contact lenses that act as a "bandage," or anterior stromal micropuncture.

### Follow-Up:

Most corneal abrasions heal on their own. Minor abrasions usually heal within 48 hours and do not require a follow-up if asymptomatic. For patients with larger abrasions, contact lens abrasion, or persistent symptoms (eg, recurrent corneal erosion syndrome) may require a follow-up within 48 to 72 hours.

### Pearls:

- Avoid treating patients with a topical anesthetic since it can potentially delay corneal healing.

- Avoid treating patients with topical atropine or scopolamine (ie, cycloplegic effects) since these agents can last for weeks.

- Do not treat corneal abrasions with topical steroids.

- Patching was a major treatment modality in the past for corneal abrasions. Studies are now showing the lack of benefit from patching and possibly harm (eg, infectious keratitis secondary to a nice and warm environment under the patch).

- Definitely do not patch an eye in a patient who wears contact lenses or is at high risk of infection (eg, vegetable matter, fingernails) because of the risk of infectious keratitis.

- **Foundational point**—The cornea is a very sensitive tissue that is richly innervated by the sensory nerve fibers of the ophthalmic division of the trigeminal nerve (CN $V_1$), so you can imagine the pain the patient feels with injury to the cornea.

- **On the CCS,** "corneal foreign body removal" is available in the practice CCS.

- **On the CCS,** poor management would include the failure to prescribe the appropriate antibiotics in patients with corneal abrasions secondary to contact lenses since infectious pseudomonas keratitis can result in vision loss.

# LENS

## CATARACT

A cataract is an opacity of the lens of the eye that is a common cause of visual impairment in children and is a leading cause of blindness in the world. Children and adults have different conditions and risk factors in the development of a cataract.

**Children**—Turner syndrome, Down syndrome (trisomy 21), Patau syndrome (trisomy 13), Edwards syndrome (trisomy 18), Alport syndrome, neurofibromatosis type 2, TORCH infections, galactosemia, type 1 diabetes, glucocorticoid use, ionizing radiation, trauma

**Adults**—Age, smoking, alcohol use, diabetes mellitus, glucocorticoid use, UV light, trauma

### Clinical Features:

Cataracts can present as a painless, gradual loss of vision. Common complaints include an increased glare and near-sightedness ("myopic shift"). In a preverbal child, there may be delays in the developmental milestones. On direct ophthalmoscope, the red reflex is usually diminished in the dilated or undilated eye. Patients may also have problems with visual acuity in the affected eye, which can be assessed by optotype (Snellen) testing.

### Next Step:

**Step 1)** An ophthalmologic examination usually makes the diagnosis. Further testing with a slit lamp examination may be indicated to rule out other pathology. The slit lamp exam can assess other ocular structures in the anterior segment of the eye (eg, conjunctiva, iris, cornea, anterior chamber, lens).

**Step 2)** Treatment involves cataract extraction with surgery and replacement with an intraocular lens (IOL) in adults and older children. Aphakic contact lenses may be given to children <9 months of age.

### Follow-Up:

As a primary care physician, it is important to do a good eye exam (ie, find the red reflex) since a delay in the diagnosis of a cataract can lead to amblyopia in children and possibly irreversible vision loss.

### Pearls:

- Adults may continue their aspirin or warfarin if cataract extraction is planned.

- If a white pupillary reflex (leukocoria) is seen in a child, the next best step is to promptly refer to an ophthalmologist to exclude the diagnosis of a retinoblastoma.

- Retinoblastoma is the most common ocular malignancy that results from a mutation in the retinoblastoma (RB1) gene mapped to chromosome 13q14. Other clues to a retinoblastoma include a family history, strabismus, and ocular inflammation.

- Leukocoria can be seen in a whole host of other conditions such as retinal detachment, cataracts, ocular trauma, Coats disease, and endophthalmitis.

- Galactosemia may present with cataracts, jaundice, hepatomegaly, failure to thrive, lethargy, and bruising.

- **On the CCS,** "slit lamp examination" is available in the practice CCS.

# RETINA

## RETINAL DETACHMENT

Retinal detachment is the separation of the neurosensory retina from the underlying retinal pigment epithelium (RPE) and choroid. The most common type of retinal detachment is the rhegmatogenous type (*rhegma* means "break" in Greek). In the rhegmatogenous retinal detachment, a retinal tear gives a portal entry for vitreous fluid to enter and separate the retina from the RPE. Other mechanisms of detachment include exudative (serous) retinal detachment (accumulation of subretinal fluid causing detachment but without a retinal break) and tractional retinal detachment (pulling of the retina from the RPE without a retinal break).

### Clinical Features:

Patients will often complain of **floaters** that may be described as "cobwebs." The sudden onset of floaters suggests a posterior vitreous detachment (PVD) with a retinal tear. Patients will also frequently complain of **photopsia** that is usually of short duration. The photopsia is often due to the tugging of the vitreous onto the corresponding retina (mechanical stimulation) which results in depolarization of the retina. If the patient complains of seeing many **black dots**, it is indicative of a vitreous hemorrhage. If the retinal detachment involves the macula or fovea centralis, visual acuity will be affected.

### Next Step:

**Step 1)** Retinal detachment is considered an ophthalmologic emergency, and patients should be seen by an ophthalmologist as soon as possible (<24 hours). An ophthalmologist will usually perform a **dilated indirect ophthalmoscopic evaluation** to assess the fundus of the eye. The fundal exam will typically reveal tentlike elevations of the retina (see Figure 13-1 and Color Plate 11). An ophthalmologist will also perform a slit-lamp biomicroscopy to assess the anterior segment of the eye. If retinal pigment epithelial cells ("tobacco dust") are seen behind the lens, it suggests that these cells have broken from the RPE layer and are floating in the vitreous.

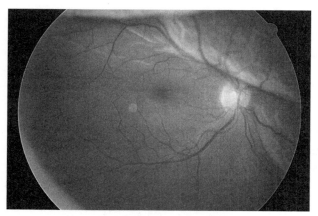

**FIGURE 13-1 • Retinal detachment.** Depicted is a superior retinal detachment with billowing or elevation of the retina with folds that can produce an inferior scotoma. Also, note that the fovea was spared, which led to normal visual acuity in this patient. (Reproduced with permission from Hauser SL, Josephson SA, et al. *Harrison's Neurology in Clinical Medicine.* 2nd ed. New York: McGraw-Hill; 2010:183.)

**Step 2)** Retinal detachments are treated by reattaching the retina through various techniques (eg, scleral buckling, pneumatic retinopexy, vitrectomy). In cases of a symptomatic retinal tear without a retinal detachment, most patients are treated with a barrier procedure such as laser photocoagulation or cryoretinopexy (ie, use of a cold probe to cause focal adhesion) to prevent a retinal detachment. In cases of only a posterior vitreous detachment (PVD) without a retinal tear, no specific therapy is indicated.

### Disposition:

An immediate ophthalmologic referral is warranted in patients suspected of having a retinal detachment.

### Pearls:

- Patients at risk of developing a retinal detachment include those with ocular trauma, myopia, or a history of cataract surgery.

- Common causes of tractional retinal detachment include proliferative diabetic retinopathy, sickle cell disease, penetrating trauma, and retinopathy of prematurity.

- Common causes of exudative retinal detachment include inflammatory conditions, neoplasms, and malignant hypertension.

- **On the CCS,** suboptimal management would include delaying the diagnosis of retinal detachment and getting the appropriate ophthalmology consult, stat.

- **On the CCS,** poor management would include the failure to order an eye exam and going straight to the ophthalmology consult.

## ■ MACULAR DEGENERATION

Age-related macular degeneration (ARMD) is a degenerative disease of the macula that results in central visual loss. Two

types of macular degeneration are wet (exudative) ARMD and dry (nonexudative) ARMD. The pathophysiology of dry ARMD is unknown, but it is associated with drusen formation underneath the retinal pigment epithelium (RPE). Wet ARMD is due to choroidal neovascularization that can result in leakage of fluid and blood into the subretinal space causing serous detachment of the fovea leading to vision loss.

### Risk Factors:

Smoking (major modifiable risk factor), increasing age, family history.

### Clinical Features:

Patients with ARMD will often complain of painless central visual impairment (central scotomas). Metamorphopsia may or may not be present in either type of ARMD. Dry ARMD usually has an insidious onset that can affect one or both eyes. Wet ARMD can have an insidious or acute onset that usually affects one eye, but both eyes can be affected. The cause for an acute onset in wet ARMD is usually the development of a subretinal hemorrhage.

### Next Step:

**Step 1)** An ophthalmologist will usually perform a dilated fundoscopic examination with slit lamp biomicroscopy that will reveal characteristic findings of ARMD (see Figure 13-2 and Color Plate 12). In addition, the following adjunctive tests may be performed to assess ARMD.

> **Amsler grid evaluation**—Amsler grid is a grid with horizontal and vertical lines with a dot in the middle. In normal vision, the lines will appear normal (straight) when focusing on the central dot. In ARMD, the lines will appear distorted (eg, wavy, bent) or absent when focusing on the central dot.

> **Retinal angiography**—Following a bolus of dye (fluorescein or indocyanine green) into a peripheral vein, an angiogram is taken of the eye. Consistent with wet ARMD is leakage of the dye (hyperfluorescence) secondary from the choroidal neovascular vessels.

> **Optical coherence tomography (OCT)**—OCT produces cross-sectional images of the retina that are useful in detecting subretinal fluid in wet ARMD.

**Step 2)** Smokers should be counseled to stop smoking.

**Step 3)** The clinical management depends on the type of ARMD. Consider the following:

> **Dry ARMD**—There is no effective therapy for dry ARMD. Oral supplements with vitamin C, vitamin E, beta-carotene, zinc, and copper are recommended in patients with moderate ARMD since it has been shown to lower the risk of progression to advanced ARMD. However, patients with mild ARMD do not seem to benefit from the supplements.

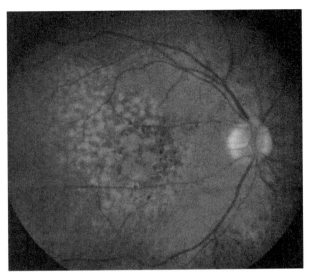
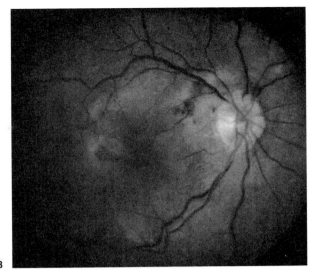

**FIGURE 13-2 • Macular degeneration. A. Dry ARMD**—Depicted are soft yellow drusen that are beginning to coalesce. **B. Wet ARMD**—A clearly evident subretinal hemorrhage over the macula may not always be present as in this case. However, further investigation with a fluorescein angiogram revealed leakage of fluorescein dye (hyperfluorescence) into the subretinal space of the macula in this patient. (Reproduced with permission from Gerstenblith AT, Rabinowitz MP, et al. *The Wills Eye Manual: Office and Emergency Room Diagnosis and Treatment of Eye Disease.* 6th ed. Philadelphia, LWW; 2012:323-324.)

**Wet ARMD**—Effective therapies for wet ARMD include VGEF inhibitors, photodynamic therapy, and thermal laser photocoagulation. Consider the following treatments:

**Vascular endothelial growth factor (VGEF) inhibitors:** VGEF plays an important role in ocular angiogenesis. Intravitreous injection of VGEF inhibitors (eg, ranibizumab, bevacizumab, pegaptanib, aflibercept) suppresses neovascularization.

**Photodynamic therapy:** Following an intravenous injection of verteporfin (photosensitive dye), a light of a certain wavelength is applied to the eye. The dye becomes activated by the light and induces occlusion via thrombosis of the abnormal vessels that usually retain most of the dye.

**Thermal laser photocoagulation:** Photocoagulation can destroy abnormal choroidal vessels, but it is not routinely used since it can cause a permanent blind spot in patients. It is generally reserved for patients who have abnormal vessels outside of the fovea.

**Supplements:** Similar to dry ARMD, patients are recommended vitamin C, vitamin E, beta-carotene, zinc, and copper to decrease the progression to advanced ARMD.

**Follow-Up:**

Patients are given an Amsler grid to take home to assess their vision on a regular basis. Patients should follow up with their ophthalmologist in the event of visual changes in daily activities or new changes with the Amsler grid.

**Pearls:**

- Dry (sometimes called atrophic) ARMD is more common than wet ARMD.
- Wet ARMD accounts for approximately 80% of legal blindness.
- Dry ARMD can sometimes progress to wet ARMD.
- Patients with a unilateral wet ARMD are at risk of developing neovascularization in the contralateral eye.
- Beta-carotene has been associated with an increased risk of lung cancer, therefore, advise patients who smoke to exclude beta-carotene from the recommended supplements.
- **Foundational point**—In wet ARMD, new vessels usually grow from the choroid through Bruch's membrane and into the subretinal or sub-RPE space.
- **On the CCS**, "advise patient, no smoking" if the patient smokes.

# GLAUCOMA

## ▌OPEN-ANGLE GLAUCOMA

Glaucoma is the second leading cause of blindness in the world following cataracts. Primary open-angle glaucoma (POAG) is a progressive optic neuropathy that may or may not be accompanied by an elevated intraocular pressure (IOP). Open-angle glaucoma results in optic nerve damage involving loss of retinal ganglion cells. The mechanism of optic nerve injury secondary to elevated IOP is unknown, nor do we know the cause of elevated IOP.

**Risk Factors:**

Increasing age (especially >40 years of age), blacks > whites, elevated IOP, family history.

## Clinical Features:

Open-angle glaucoma has an insidious onset, and patients may be asymptomatic until late in the disease when they will have visual complaints. Patients typically do not complain of any eye pain, unlike angle-closure glaucoma. The characteristic pattern of open-angle glaucoma involves peripheral visual loss followed by central field loss in which patients may have "tunnel vision." Once visual field loss occurs, it is irreversible. Open-angle glaucoma is usually bilateral, but frequently asymmetric. As the neural rim of the optic disc is destroyed, the cup within the optic disc becomes larger. This is referred to as "cupping," which appears as an excavation of the optic nerve. Over time, the cup-to-disc ratio may increase in glaucoma.

## Next Step:

**Step 1)** The diagnosis of open-angle glaucoma is based on the fundoscopic examination that demonstrates optic nerve damage (eg, cupping) and the presence of visual field defects. Consider the following adjunctive tests that are used to support the diagnosis.

**Automated perimetry**—This test evaluates the peripheral vision by having patients focus their eyes on a central point while light of varying intensities is displayed in their visual field.

**Tonometry**—Tonometry measures IOP. Normal IOPs are approximately 10 to 20 mm Hg.

**Pachymetry**—Pachymetry measures the corneal thickness. Patients with thin corneas are at risk in developing open-angle glaucoma.

**Gonioscopy**—Gonioscopy is performed to rule out angle-closure glaucoma.

**Slit-lamp exam**—Slit lamp may be used to examine the anterior segment (eg, cornea, iris, lens, anterior chamber) and posterior segment of the eye (eg, fundus, optic disc, vitreous).

**Step 2)** Treating patients with open-angle glaucoma is based on the clinical judgment of the ophthalmologist. There are no set criteria or IOPs that all ophthalmologist use to treat patients. For example, a patient with open-angle glaucoma with a normal IOP (also referred to as normal-tension or low-tension glaucoma) but with optic nerve changes (eg, thinning of the optic disc rim) and visual field defects are usually treated. On the flip side, patients with a onetime elevation in the IOP with a healthy optic nerve and normal visual field may not be treated unless the IOP is persistently elevated. If the decision is to treat, pharmacologic therapy with the goal of lowering the IOP is the initial choice before more invasive procedures are pursued. Consider the following therapies:

## Pharmacologic Therapy

**Beta-blockers**—Beta-blocker eye drops decrease aqueous humor production by the ciliary body. Agents that can be used include timolol, betaxolol, levobunolol, carteolol, or metipranolol. Beta-blocker drops should not be used in patients with heart blocks (unless they have a pacemaker), bronchospastic disease, bradycardia, or uncompensated heart failure.

**Alpha-2 adrenergic agonists**—Alpha agonist eye drops such as brimonidine can decrease aqueous humor production and increase uveoscleral outflow. Apraclonidine is another agent that can be used, but it functions to only decrease aqueous humor formation. Side effects include ocular pruritus, allergic conjunctivitis, contact dermatitis, and hyperemia.

**Prostaglandin analogs**—Prostaglandin eye drops increase uveoscleral outflow. Agents that can be used include latanoprost, travoprost, brimatoprost, or tafluprost. Side effects include discoloration of the iris, burning, stinging, blurring, and hyperemia.

**Cholinergic agonists**—Cholinergic eye drops increase aqueous outflow secondary to contraction of the ciliary muscle. Agents include pilocarpine or carbachol. Side effects include miosis, myopia, headaches, salivation, lacrimation, and hypertension.

**Carbonic anhydrase (CA) inhibitors**—CA inhibitors decrease aqueous humor production. This class of drug is considered second-line treatment. Topical agents that can be used include brinzolamide or dorzolamide. Oral (systemic) agents that can be used include acetazolamide or methazolamide. Topical side effects include bitter taste, burning, stinging, blurring, and superficial punctate keratitis. Oral side effects include myopia, taste alteration, decreased appetite, diarrhea, and agranulocytosis.

## Invasive Procedures

**Laser therapy**—A trabeculoplasty can be accomplished by laser therapy, which increase aqueous outflow.

**Surgery**—A trabeculectomy may be performed or placement of a shunt or "valve" may be attempted to release the aqueous fluid from the eye.

## Follow-Up:

The vast majority of patients will require long-term follow-up with their ophthalmologist because of the insidious and progressive nature of the disease. Most patients may also be noncompliant simply because they are asymptomatic or the side effects of the medications are troublesome.

## Pearls:

- Although not every patient with open-angle glaucoma will have an elevated IOP, those patients with an elevated IOP without characteristic findings of open-angle glaucoma (ie, cupping or visual field defects) should still be watched and evaluated carefully because they are still at risk in developing and progressing into open-angle glaucoma.

- Screening patients for open-angle glaucoma remains an area of controversy.

- Secondary glaucoma refers to glaucoma with an identifiable cause that can elevate the IOP resulting in optic nerve damage. Such causes include eye injury, inflammation (eg, uveitis), drug therapy (eg, glucocorticoid), tumors, advanced cataracts, or congenital conditions.

- **Foundational point**—Aqueous humor is produced by the ciliary process in the posterior chamber and passes through the pupil and into the anterior chamber. The fluid then passes through the trabecular meshwork (fenestrated structure) and then through the iridocorneal angle and into Schlemm's canal, where it drains into the episcleral vein.

- **On the CCS**, "tonometry" is available in the practice CCS and will give you the result with the normal values.
- **On the CCS**, remember to "advise patient, side effects of medication" if you prescribe any medications.

## ANGLE-CLOSURE GLAUCOMA

Angle-closure glaucoma is characterized by the narrowing of the anterior chamber angle. When there is greater contact between the lens and the iris, aqueous humor cannot flow through the pupil (pupillary block). Increasing IOPs will then close the anterior chamber angle and obstruct drainage of the aqueous fluid. Without treatment, elevated IOPs can damage the optic nerve and cause vision loss.

### Risk Factors:

Asians, Eskimos, females, increasing age (>40 years of age), family history, hyperopia, thick iris, dim lighting, medications (eg, anticholinergics, antidepressants, antipsychotics, anticonvulsants, sympathomimetics, decongestants, antihistamines, mydriatics).

### Clinical Features:

Angle-closure glaucoma has an abrupt onset, and patients typically complain of eye pain. Patients may see halos or blurry vision secondary to corneal edema. On examination, the cornea may be hazy or cloudy with a mid-dilated nonreactive pupil. The ocular globe may be hard. Conjunctival injection can also be present. Nonocular symptoms include headaches, nausea, and vomiting.

### Next Step:

**Step 1)** Angle-closure glaucoma is an ophthalmologic emergency. Provide analgesics for pain control and antiemetics (eg, ondansetron) for nausea and vomiting (ie, you do not want to have the patient to vomit on you while you're examining them). It should be noted that the pain and vomiting can potentially increase the already elevated IOP.

**Step 2)** The patient should be in the supine position because theoretically the lens will fall away from the iris and alleviate the pupillary block. Also, do not dim the lights or put a patch over the eye because mydriasis (pupillary dilatation) may exacerbate the condition. Perform an eye examination (eg, visual acuity, visual fields, ocular motility, fundus), but again, avoid dilating the eye for the fundus exam.

**Step 3)** Two important test to perform are **gonioscopy** (considered the gold standard) and **tonometry**. Gonioscopy will assess the angle of the anterior chamber while tonometry will typically reveal an IOP > 30 mm Hg in acute-angle glaucoma. Adjunctive testing with a slit lamp may also be useful in evaluating for corneal edema or abnormalities in the lens, iris, or pupil shape.

**Step 4)** Initiate treatment to lower the IOPs. Consider the following cocktail:

- IV or PO acetazolamide, stat, plus . . .
- Eye drop of timolol (if no contraindications exist), then
- Eye drop of apraclonidine (decreases aqueous production), then
- Eye drop of prednisolone (reduces ocular inflammation), then
- Reassess the IOP.

Now consider two scenarios. First, if the IOP is reduced then you can instill pilocarpine (pulls iris tissue away from the angle). However, instilling pilocarpine when the IOP is elevated is ineffective because the elevated pressures cause a pressure-induced ischemic paralysis of the iris. Second, if the IOP is persistently elevated despite the above cocktail, then the next best step is to consider an osmotic agent such as IV mannitol (reduces vitreous volume). Alternative osmotic agents include oral glycerol and isosorbide.

**Step 5)** Once the IOP is controlled, definitive treatment is with laser peripheral iridotomy. In this procedure, a tiny hole is made in the peripheral iris that allows the aqueous humor to flow through the hole, thereby creating a detour from the pupillary block. Prophylactic laser peripheral iridotomy may be offered to the patient in the other eye if a narrow angle is found on exam.

### Disposition/Follow-Up:

An ophthalmic consultation should be obtained as soon as possible in the ED since damage to the optic nerve is irreversible and can occur within hours. Ideally, systemic medications (eg, IV mannitol) should be given in conjunction with an ophthalmologist, but certainly an ED physician should initiate treatment without delay. Upon discharge, patients who received laser peripheral iridotomy may be seen in the office for reevaluation of the anterior chamber angle via gonioscopy.

### Pearls:

- Patients with angle-closure glaucoma can develop IOPs >60 mm Hg.
- Secondary angle closure refers to an underlying identifiable cause for narrowing of the anterior chamber angle (eg, tumor, trauma, surgery, displaced lens). If angle closure results in an elevated IOP that causes optic nerve damage, it is referred to as secondary angle-closure glaucoma.
- Patients with angle-closure glaucoma in one eye are at risk of developing an attack in the other eye. Therefore, it is important to exam both eyes and decide if the patient needs prophylactic laser peripheral iridotomy.
- **On the CCS**, this case is an emergency; move the simulated time judiciously.
- **On the CCS**, do not do a neurologic or GI workup in this type of case since that would delay treatment and would be considered suboptimal management.

# NEURO-OPHTHALMOLOGY

## AMBLYOPIA

Amblyopia ("dimness of vision" in Greek) is characterized by impaired visual acuity in the affected eye. It is thought that images are not properly projected onto the fovea and thereby fail to transmit information through the optic nerve and into the brain during a critical period of visual development. Therefore, the brain favors the visual input from the normal eye.

### Clinical Features:

Amblyopia is a common visual impairment in children. Consider the following causes and clinical findings of amblyopia.

**Strabismus**—Strabismus is ocular misalignment. The brain may favor visual input in one eye and suppress the other eye. One eye may move normally, while the other eye may point inward (esotropia), outward (exotropia), upward (hypertropia), or downward (hypotropia). Since patients are unable to use both eyes properly, depth perception (stereopsis) may be affected. It should be noted that strabismus does not always cause amblyopia, but it is a common cause.

**Anisometropia**—Anisometropia results in unequal refractive error between the eyes. The image that is clearer will usually become the dominant eye. Anisometropia can be a little tricky and easily missed because there are no obvious physical manifestations (ie, just by examining the eyes you cannot tell if there is a refractive error). However, an unequal red reflex (ie, one eye appears to be brighter than the other) may suggest unequal refraction.

**Visual deprivation**—The brain does not receive visual input from the affected eye. Common causes include cataracts, ptosis, or corneal opacities. Clinical exam may reveal a diminished red reflex or drooping of the eyelid.

### Next Step:

**Step 1)** Vision screening should be performed in children <5 years old beginning in the newborn period and at all well-child visits. Children ≥5 years old should also be periodically assessed at all health maintenance visits. Consider the following:

**Preverbal child**—Visual inspection of the ocular globe may reveal misalignment as seen in strabismus. The cover test can also evaluate for strabismus by having the child fixate on a distant object, then covering one of the eyes. If the uncovered eye is the strabismic eye, the eye will move and refixate on the object. However, if the uncovered eye is the normal straight eye, there will be no eye movement because the eye is already fixated on the object. Finally, another test can be performed to assess for amblyopia. Covering one of the eyes will cause a response. If the amblyopic eye is covered, the child may not be upset. However, covering the normal eye will cause the child to be agitated.

**Verbal child**—In older children, the diagnosis of amblyopia can be made when there is a ≥2 line difference in visual acuity between the eyes using a Snellen (letter) chart. However, the letters should be presented in rows (ie, crowding of letters will cause the amblyopic eye to do worse on visual acuity) because visual acuity is better when optotypes are presented in isolation (crowding phenomenon).

**Step 2)** Treatment of amblyopia begins with correcting any visual disturbances (eg, cataracts, ptosis) and refractive errors via glasses or contact lenses.

**Step 3)** The next step in management is to encourage the use of the amblyopic eye by occlusion therapy (ie, patching the good eye) or penalization therapy of the good eye. Penalization can be accomplished by spectacles or by cycloplegic eye drops (eg, atropine).

### Follow-Up:

The earlier amblyopia is detected during vision screening, the better the prognosis.

### Pearls:

- From the newborn period to 6 months of age, infants have the capacity to fix and follow an object. By 2 months of age and definitely by 6 months of age, infants should be able to shift their fixation across midline.

- **On the CCS,** long delays in the diagnosis of amblyopia would be considered suboptimal management because the patient is at risk of losing vision in the amblyopic eye. In general, with all your CCS cases, think about the consequence of delaying your diagnosis and not providing the appropriate treatment in a timely fashion. Remember, your goal is to use good sound judgment without delays.

# INFLAMMATORY CONDITIONS

## CHALAZION

Chalazion is a benign nodular lesion that develops from an obstruction of the meibomian gland or Zeis gland that are within the eyelid.

### Clinical Features:

Chalazia are usually rubbery, cystic, and **painless**. Patients may have a history of chalazia since they can recur.

### Next Step:

**Step 1)** A chalazion is a clinical diagnosis.

**Step 2)** Small chalazia often resolve on its own. For larger chalazia, warm compresses may be attempted. For persistent lesions (>4 weeks), a referral to an ophthalmologist may be indicated for an incision and curettage or glucocorticoid injection into the lesion.

### Follow-Up:

For persistent or recurring chalazia, a biopsy should be obtained for histologic evaluation since it may represent a carcinoma of the sebaceous cell, meibomian gland, or basal cell.

**Pearls:**

- Chalazia can be associated with rosacea and blepharitis.
- Both meibomian gland and Zeis gland are a type of sebaceous gland located within the palpebral conjunctiva, but the Zeis glands are near the margin of the eyelid since they keep the eyelashes clean.
- **Foundational point**—A chalazion is characterized by a chronic granulomatous inflammation. On histopathological examination, lipid-laden macrophages and lymphocytes can be observed.
- **On the CCS**, if you ever get "lost" during a CCS case, get yourself grounded again by quickly reviewing the case history and figure out what important steps to take in managing the patient. In this approach, you're hitting the "refresh" button in your mind.

# HORDEOLUM

Hordeolum is an acute focal infection (usually *Staphylococcus aureus*) that can affect the meibomian glands (internal hordeolum) or the Zeis glands (external hordeolum or stye).

### Clinical Features:

Patients with a hordeolum will generally have a swollen, **painful**, red eyelid. A stye will be near the lid-margin, but an internal hordeolum will be in the inner surface of the tarsal plate.

### Next Step:

**Step 1)** A hordeolum is a clinical diagnosis.

**Step 2)** Patients may benefit from warm compresses and erythromycin ophthalmic ointment. Systemic antibiotics are generally not indicated unless the hordeolum is associated with a preseptal cellulitis.

### Follow-Up:

If resolution does not occur within 2 weeks, the patient should be referred to an ophthalmologist.

### Pearls:

- A hordeolum can harden into a chalazion.
- **On the CCS**, "warm compresses" is available in the practice CCS.

# CONJUNCTIVITIS

Conjunctivitis is a common cause of "red eye" secondary to an inflammation of the conjunctiva from bacteria, virus, allergies, fungus, or irritants. When the cornea is also involved, it is referred to as keratoconjunctivitis.

### Clinical Features:

The clinical presentation of conjunctivitis can vary based on the etiology. Consider the following:

**Bacterial**—Bacterial conjunctivitis typically presents as a painless mucopurulent discharge that can be unilateral or bilateral. Often, the eyelids are stuck together upon awakening. Chemosis (conjunctiva edema) may be present. Common organisms in this category include *Staphylococcus aureus* (commonly seen in adults), *Streptococcus pneumoniae*, *Moraxella catarrhalis*, and *Haemophilus influenzae*. Patients are very contagious, and they can spread the infection from their secretions and from contaminated objects.

**Viral**—Viral conjunctivitis typically presents as a painless watery discharge. Often, one eye is infected and then the other eye becomes infected a couple of days later. Patients may report a gritty sensation in the eye. Patients will frequently have a prodrome (eg, upper respiratory infection, fever, pharyngitis, adenopathy) before viral conjunctivitis appears. On examination, there may be conjunctival injection, follicles ("bumps") on the tarsal conjunctiva, and a tender preauricular lymphadenopathy. Viral conjunctivitis is typically caused by adenovirus. Similar to bacterial conjunctivitis, adenovirus is very contagious. Adenovirus can also cause a unique condition called epidemic keratoconjunctivitis (EKC). As the name states, it occurs in epidemics. Patients with this condition will often have a foreign body sensation in the eye, photophobia, excessive tearing, and preauricular lymphadenopathy.

**Allergies**—Allergic conjunctivitis typically presents as painless watery discharge that is usually bilateral. The cardinal feature of allergic conjunctivitis is itchy eyes. Patients often have a history of atopy or allergies. On examination, the eyelids and conjunctivae may be edematous and erythematous. Similar to viral conjunctivitis, a bumpy appearance (cobblestone papillae) may be present on the tarsal conjunctiva.

### Next Step:

**Step 1)** Conjunctivitis is a clinical diagnosis. Cultures and sensitivities are generally not needed in bacterial conjunctivitis unless it is severe, recurrent, or resistant.

**Step 2)** Treatment is based on the type of conjunctivitis. Consider the following:

**Bacterial conjunctivitis**

**Option 1:** Erythromycin ophthalmic ointment × 5 to 7 days

**Option 2:** Polymyxin-trimethoprim eye drops × 5 to 7 days

**Option 3:** Patients who wear contact lenses and do not have corneal white spots can be treated with tobramycin, ofloxacin, or ciprofloxacin to cover Pseudomonas. In the presence of corneal white spots, an urgent referral to an ophthalmologist is warranted since an ocular perforation can occur.

**Viral conjunctivitis**—Viral conjunctivitis is a self-limited condition.

**Allergic conjunctivitis**—Allergic conjunctivitis is a self-limited condition. Avoid the allergen if possible. Patients may benefit from a topical antihistamine/vasoconstrictor (eg, naphazoline/pheniramine). The vasoconstrictor component alleviates chemosis (conjunctival edema).

Severe symptoms may require topical steroids, but administration should be under the guidance of an ophthalmologist since topical steroids can cause cataracts and glaucoma.

## Follow-Up:

Patients with bacterial conjunctivitis should respond to therapy within 5 days of administering antibiotics. Viral and allergic conjunctivitis may take 1 to 3 weeks. Patients should follow up with an ophthalmologist if symptoms persist beyond the expected time.

## Pearls:

- Emphasize hand washing to patients with bacterial and viral conjunctivitis since both conditions are very contagious. Treating physicians should also wash their hands since they are at risk of spreading the infection.

- Ideally, patients with bacterial or viral conjunctivitis should stay at home to prevent the spread of infection.

- **Foundational point**—Allergic conjunctivitis is a type I, IgE-mediated hypersensitivity.

- **Connecting point** (pgs. 164, 166)—Know how to manage neonatal gonococcal and chlamydial conjunctivitis.

- **On the CCS**, if you prescribe a medication for the patient to take home, remember to use the "continuous" mode of frequency because it takes into account the periodic administration. Keep in mind that there is no PRN.

# Orthopedics

## KEYWORDS REVIEW

Chondrolysis—Loss or lysis of articular cartilage.

Closed reduction—Manipulation of bone fragments without surgical exposure.

Comminution—Broken bone fragments.

Malunion—Union in a faulty position after a fracture.

Nonunion—An unhealed fracture.

Open reduction—Anatomic restoration of bone fragments with surgical exposure.

Paresthesia—An abnormal sensation such as tingling, prickling, or burning.

Shortening—Overriding of bone fragments.

# SPINE

## ▌ IDIOPATHIC SCOLIOSIS

Idiopathic scoliosis is the most common type of scoliosis, which is defined as an unknown cause for a lateral curvature of the spine usually with rotation. Idiopathic scoliosis can be further classified as infant (0-3 years), juvenile (4-9 years), and adolescent (≥10 years). Adolescent idiopathic scoliosis (AIS) is the most common of the three idiopathic types, and further discussion will be based on AIS.

### Clinical Features:

Idiopathic scoliosis is typically a painless disorder with a gradual curve progression. Patients usually do not complain of neurological symptoms such as bowel or bladder changes, numbness, or weakness. Patients may notice an unleveling of the shoulder or scapulae, forward rotation of a shoulder, or an asymmetric waistline. On exam, an **Adams forward bend test** is usually performed in which the patient bends forward allowing the arms to hang freely and the clinician observes from behind. The test assesses the rotational component of the scoliosis, and typically, a rib hump or lumbar prominence can be seen.

### Next Step:

**Step 1)** Diagnosis of AIS is made on clinical and radiographic evaluation. A scoliometer (inclinometer) is a screening device used in the office to assess trunk rotation. While the patient is in the Adams forward bending position, a scoliometer is placed on the back to measure the highest point of the curve providing measurements of the angle of rotation.

**Step 2)** Obtain a **PA and lateral x-ray** of the spine in the standing position if the angle of rotation from a scoliometer is ≥7° or obvious scoliosis noted on exam. Once the x-ray films are obtained, two pieces of information can be extracted, the degree of curvature, **Cobb's angle**, and the degree of skeletal maturity, the **Risser sign**. A Cobb's angle ≥10°, age ≥10, and exclusion of other causes for scoliosis confirms the diagnosis. The Risser sign has a grading system (0-5), with a grade 0 showing no ossification and grade 5 as skeletally matured.

**Step 3)** Refer to orthopedic surgeon with a Cobb's angle ≥20° or signs of progression of the Cobb's angle >5°. Treatment options for scoliosis can be broken down to the **triple O's**.

**Observe**—Skeletally immature patients (Risser 0-2) with a Cobb's angle <30° can be observed and followed up every 6 months for evaluation ± PA x-rays. There is no need to repeat lateral views if the initial films demonstrated normal configuration.

**Orthosis**—The basis of the bracing is to prevent curve progression and not necessarily correct the curvature. Therefore, bracing would not be appropriate for a skeletally matured patient (Risser 4-5). Skeletally immature patients (Risser 0-2) with a Cobb's angle between 30° and 40° or those with curve progression >5° at the 6-month visit from the observation phase can be braced.

**Operate**—A spinal fusion can be considered in skeletally immature patients with a Cobb's angle between 40° and 50°. Surgery should definitely be considered with a Cobb's angle ≥50° regardless of the skeletal maturity.

### Follow-Up:

Patients with scoliometer angle <7° can be followed up every 6 months without repeating x-rays.

### Pearls:

- Family history of scoliosis occurs frequently.
- Girls may be affected at a slightly higher rate than boys, but the risk of curvature progression is certainly higher in girls.
- Less common types of acquired or congenital scoliosis include **neuromuscular scoliosis**, which is associated with neurological conditions (eg, cerebral palsy, vertebral tumors), or **congenital scoliosis**, which can be due to vertebral malformations (eg, hemivertebrae). Unlike idiopathic scoliosis, findings of neurological symptoms, pain, or rapid progression can be seen with the less common types of scoliosis.
- **On the CCS**, an "X-ray, spine" is available in the practice CCS. However, you need to specify which part of the spine you want to evaluate (ie, cervical, thoracic, lumbosacral, or sacrum/coccyx).

# SHOULDER

## ▌ CLAVICLE FRACTURES

Most clavicle fractures occur from a direct blow to the shoulder such as a fall to the ground. Less common causes are indirect forces such as a fall onto an outstretched hand.

### Clinical Features:

There are three different types of clavicle fractures to consider:

**Proximal third**—Medial fractures are the least common types of clavicle fractures. However, it can be the most serious type of fracture because it is close to the sternum, which may result in intrathoracic injuries. Therefore, it is important to do a good neurovascular (eg, brachial plexus injury) and lung examination (eg, pneumothorax).

**Middle third**—Midshaft fractures are the most common types of clavicle fractures. Patients may have pain, tenderness, swelling, ecchymosis, or limited range of motion of the arm. Most often, patients will hear a "crack" at the time of injury.

**Distal third**—Distal third fractures have three subtypes, and they can sometimes be confused with acromioclavicular joint injuries. **Type I** are nondisplaced fractures with

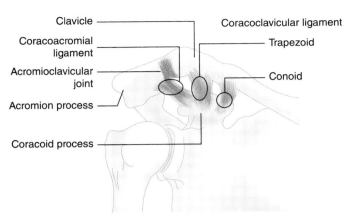

**FIGURE 14-1 · Anatomy of the shoulder.** The site for distal clavicle fractures. (Reproduced with permission from Tintinalli JE, Stapczynski JS, Ma OJ, et al. *Emergency Medicine: A Comprehensive Study Guide.* 7th ed. New York: McGraw-Hill; 2011:1832.)

intact ligaments holding the fragment in place. **Type II** are displaced fractures, which can occur by two mechanisms (Type IIA are displaced fractures with intact coracoclavicular ligaments and Type IIB are displaced fractures with a torn coracoclavicular ligament). It should be noted that the coracoclavicular ligament consists of two ligaments, the trapezoid and conoid. **Type III** involves articular surface injury at the acromioclavicular joint without displacement or ligament disruption (see Figure 14-1). In essence, type II fractures are displaced fractures and only type IIB fractures involve a torn ligament.

## Next Step:

**Step 1)** Along with your clinical assessment, an **AP x-ray** view of the clavicle will confirm the diagnosis. Sometimes when nothing is found on standard AP x-ray views, a 45° cephalic tilt view (ie, x-ray tube pointed at 45°) may provide a better assessment of the clavicle.

**Step 2)** The initial management steps is to provide pain relief (analgesics), ice, and upper extremity support. Consider the following management approach:

**Proximal third**—For nondisplaced medial fractures, patients can be managed with a sling to maintain immobi-

lization and healing usually occurs within 6 to 8 weeks. An urgent orthopedic referral should be obtained for neurovascular injuries, open fractures, or fracture displacement (for reduction).

**Middle third**—For nondisplaced midshaft fractures, patients can be managed with a sling or a figure of eight bandage until union occurs. An urgent orthopedic referral should be obtained for open fractures, displacement, or a "floating shoulder" (ie, glenoid neck fracture along with the clavicle).

**Distal third**—For types I and III, there is no displacement or minimal displacement. Therefore, patients can be managed with a sling for immobilization. An orthopedic referral should be obtained for type II fractures (displaced) since they may be prone to nonunion.

## Disposition:

Most nondisplaced or minimally displaced fractures will heal within 6 to 12 weeks with conservative management.

## Pearls:

- Open reduction internal fixation (ORIF) refers to open surgery and fixation with plates, screws, rods, or pins. ORIF may be required in displaced fractures with comminution that would not heal correctly with splinting alone.

- Patients with open fractures may require a tetanus shot and prophylactic antibiotics.

- When examining an x-ray of the clavicle, a general guideline for displacement is a clavicle that is displaced greater than one bone width from its original position.

- Complications of clavicle fractures include malunion, nonunion, arthritis (especially with proximal third fractures), and neurovascular injuries.

- Risk factors for malunion or nonunion include comminution, shortening, improper immobilization, and elderly patients.

- **On the CCS**, "sling, arm" is available in the practice CCS, but there is no "figure of eight bandage."

- **On the CCS**, an "X-ray, clavicle" is available in the practice CCS, but there is no option for a 45° cephalic tilt.

# ELBOW

## NURSEMAID'S ELBOW

Nursemaid's elbow (radial head subluxation) is a common elbow injury in children and typically occurs between the ages of 1 and 4 years old. The mechanism of injury is a sudden longitudinal traction on the arm with the forearm in pronation and the elbow in extension, which usually occurs while the child falls and is lifted up forcefully by the hand of another person.

During this event, a circular ligament (annular ligament) "slips" over the radial head.

### Clinical Features:

Children will usually be protective of the affected arm, holding the arm close to the body with a slightly flexed or extended elbow and the forearm in the pronated position. Patients will usually complain of pain with any attempt to supinate the forearm. Tenderness over the radial head (ie, elbow end) is typically present. Patients should be able to move their wrist or digits but reluctant to do so because of fear of reproducing the pain.

## Next Step:

**Step 1)** Nursemaid's elbow is a clinical diagnosis. X-ray is usually not required unless there is a suspicion for a fracture or failed attempts at reduction.

**Step 2)** Treatment is by reduction, which can be painful but does not require anesthesia. Two types of reduction procedures include:

**Supination-flexion technique**—Pressure is applied to the radial head with one finger with gentle traction of the forearm. The forearm is then supinated and the elbow is then fully flexed. A click is usually felt over the radial head during the reduction.

**Hyperpronation technique**—Pressure is applied to the radial head with one finger while holding the distal forearm and then subsequently hyperpronating the forearm. A click is usually felt over the radial head during the reduction.

## Disposition:

Patients will usually have immediate pain relief after a successful reduction and can go home and resume normal activity.

## Pearls:

- Nursemaid's elbow commonly affects more girls than boys.
- Nursemaid's elbow can recur but usually not after 4 years old because the radial head becomes more bulbous and the annular ligament becomes stronger.

# HAND

## ▌ SCAPHOID FRACTURES

Scaphoid fractures are common injuries involving the carpus and are typically due to a high-energy axial load on the wrist such as falling on an outstretched hand. Most scaphoid fractures go unnoticed, resulting in nonunion, delayed union, or avascular necrosis (AVN).

### Clinical Features:

Patients will often complain of pain and swelling along the radial side of the wrist. The scaphoid (navicular) bone is situated on the thumb side of the wrist and articulates with the radius. The scaphoid bone can be broken down to the distal third (ie, closest to the nail end), central third (ie, referred to as the waist), and proximal third (ie, closest to the radius). Palpating and eliciting point tenderness in the three different areas of the scaphoid bone can help determine the area of fracture. The scaphoid bone has a bony prominence (tubercle) at the distal end, and palpating in that specific area would indicate a distal fracture. Tenderness along the **anatomic snuffbox** would indicate a fracture at the waist of the scaphoid, while tenderness toward the radius would be a clue to a proximal fracture.

### Next Step:

**Step 1)** When a scaphoid fracture is suggested in the clinical assessment, obtain an **x-ray** in the PA, lateral, oblique, and scaphoid view (ie, wrist in ulnar deviation) of the wrist. Approximately 10% of initial x-rays will not detect a fracture, therefore if the initial x-ray films are negative, place the patient in a thumb spica splint and reimage in 7 to 10 days. For a rapid diagnosis and to avoid prolonged immobilization, a CT or MRI (MRI can also provide information on soft tissue injuries) are acceptable alternatives.

**Step 2)** Treatment for a **nondisplaced distal scaphoid fracture** is immobilization in a short-arm thumb spica cast for 4 to 6 weeks. Treatment for a **nondisplaced central or proximal scaphoid fracture** is immobilization in a long-arm thumb spica cast for 6 weeks then converted to a short-arm thumb spica cast for another 6 to 14 weeks. Referral to an orthopedic surgeon is indicated when there is an open fracture, associated neurovascular injuries, displacement more than 1 mm, AVN, nonunion, or carpal instability (eg, scapholunate dissociation).

### Disposition:

Patients seen in the ED with negative x-ray imaging for a scaphoid fracture should have close follow-up with their primary care physician to repeat the x-ray because delayed diagnosis and treatment results in an increased risk of nonunion.

### Pearls:

- Proximal scaphoid fractures have a greater risk of nonunion, delayed union, and avascularnecrosis (leading to degenerative joint disease) because the blood supply starts at the distal end of the scaphoid from the palmar carpal branch of the radial artery and finishes off at the proximal end of the scaphoid. A fracture can easily disrupt blood flow to the proximal segment.
- **On the CCS**, an "X-ray, wrist" will automatically give you radiographic readings of the AP, lateral, and oblique views, but not a scaphoid view in the practice CCS.
- **On the CCS**, both "splint extremity" and "cast extremity" are available in the practice CCS.

# HIP

## ▌HIP DISORDERS

See Table 14-1.

| Table 14-1 • Hip Disorders | Developmental Dysplasia of the Hip (DDH) | Transient Synovitis (TS) | Legg-Calvé-Perthes (LCP) Disease | Slipped Capital Femoral Epiphysis (SCFE) |
|---|---|---|---|---|
| **Age** | Infants | 3-8 years old | 3-12 years old | 8-15 years old |
| **Definition** | Acetabular dysplasia with hip joint instability. | Transient inflammation of the synovium of the hip. | Avascular necrosis of the proximal femoral head. | Epiphysis appears to "slip" posteriorly and inferiorly. |
| **Etiology** | Multifactorial | Unknown | Unknown | Unknown |
| **Clinical features** | • Asymmetric skinfolds of the upper thigh.<br>• Unequal leg length.<br>• Older children may have limping, toe-walking, or out-toeing. | • Appears nontoxic.<br>• Fever usually absent but can occur.<br>• URI usually present and precedes hip symptoms.<br>• Acute hip pain.<br>• May have referred knee or thigh pain. | • "Painless" limp.<br>• Decreased internal rotation and abduction of the hip.<br>• May have referred knee or thigh pain. | • Obese adolescents.<br>• Hip pain.<br>• Limp.<br>• Decreased internal rotation of hip, seen mainly in external rotation.<br>• May have referred knee or thigh pain. |
| **Next step** | **Step 1)** Perform the **Barlow** test, which attempts to dislocate the hip, and with the **Ortolani** test a "clunk" should be heard when you reduce the hip back.<br>**Step 2)** Ultrasound the hip for patients <6 months, or an AP and frog lateral x-rays for patients >6 months.<br>**Step 3)** Treat patients <6 months of age wth **Pavlik harness** (ie, puts patient in a flexed and abducted position). Treat patients 6-18 months with **closed reduction** under anesthesia and hip spica casting. Treat patients >18 months with **open reduction**. | **Step 1)** Obtain CBC, ESR, and CRP. If labs are normal, patient is afebrile, and nontoxic then patient can be followed clinically. If patient is febrile, ESR >20, ↑WBC, or ↑CRP → obtain hip ultrasound to look for joint effusion and consider arthrocentesis to rule out septic arthritis.<br>**Step 2)** Treatment of TS is conservative with limited activities and NSAIDs. Full recovery is expected in 1-4 weeks. | **Step 1)** Obtain AP and frog lateral x-rays of the pelvis, which will show fragmentation, flattening, and sclerosis of the proximal femur.<br>**Step 2)** Treatment involves minimal weight bearing and containing the femoral head within the acetabulum by bracing or surgery. | **Step 1)** Obtain AP and frog lateral x-rays of pelvis with early signs of SCFE showing widening of the physis.<br>**Step 2)** Refer to orthopedic surgeon for in situ fixation of the hip. |
| **Pearls** | • DDH can be bilateral in 20% of patients.<br>• Risk factors include breech position, female, family history, firstborn.<br>• DDH commonly occurs in healthy infants and is usually referred to as typical DDH.<br>• DDH can occur with underlying neuromuscular disorders that occur in utero and is referred to as teratologic DDH. | • TS can be bilateral in 5% of patients.<br>• Any hip pathology can cause referred pain to the thigh or knee.<br>• A small number of patients with TS can develop Legg-Calvé-Perthes disease. | • LCP can be bilateral in 10%-20% of patients.<br>• Older children >10 years who develop the disease are at risk of developing osteoarthritis of the hip as an adult. | • SCFE can be bilateral in 20%-40% of patients.<br>• Complications of SCFE are AVN and chondrolysis.<br>• SCFE is associated with panhypopituitarism, hypothyroidism, GH supplementation, and hypogonadism. |

*AP—Anteroposterior; AVN—Avascular necrosis; GH—Growth hormone; URI—Upper respiratory infection*

# KNEE

## ■ ANTERIOR CRUCIATE LIGAMENT INJURY

Anterior cruciate ligament (ACL) injuries can occur from contact injuries (eg, a blow to the lateral knee) or more commonly from noncontact mechanisms such as sudden deceleration, cutting, or pivoting of the lower extremity.

### Clinical Features:

Patients with noncontact injuries will often complain of a "pop" at the time of injury, followed by pain and swelling of the knee. Most patients with acute injuries will develop a knee effusion secondary to hemarthrosis. Patients usually do not return to play because of the instability or giving-way of the knee. Patients with contact injuries will typically have associated injuries or the "**unhappy triad**," which includes ACL, medial collateral ligament (MCL), and meniscus tears (lateral > medial).

### Next Step:

**Step 1)** Evaluate the patient soon after the injury. The evaluation should include inspection, palpation, range of motion, gait, strength, and neurovascular examination. There are three knee maneuvers to help with the assessment of ACL injuries:

**Anterior drawer test**—The knee is flexed at 90° with anterior pulling of the proximal tibia to check for anterior translation, which would indicate a positive test for an ACL tear.

**Lachman test**—The knee is flexed at 30° with anterior pulling of the proximal tibia and assessing for the quality of the endpoint of anterior translation. An intact ACL will have a distinct endpoint in contrast to a torn ACL, which will have a vague or soft endpoint.

**Pivot shift test**—The knee is in extension while internally rotating the tibia, followed by placing a valgus (abduction) force on the knee. While maintaining the forces described, the examiner flexes the knee which causes a reduction in the subluxed tibia. If a "clunk" is sensed by the examiner, it constitutes a positive test for an ACL-deficient knee.

**Step 2)** Most ACL injuries are a clinical diagnosis, but MRI is the primary modality to confirm a torn ACL.

**Step 3)** Acute management for patients without obvious deformities can be initially treated with **RICE** (Rest, Ice, Compression, Elevation) and NSAIDs.

**Step 4)** Treatment options include nonsurgical or surgical.

**Nonsurgical treatment**—Patients with low activity level, low demand on the knee, or small partial tears may be treated nonoperatively. Bracing is sometimes used to protect the knee from instability.

**Surgical treatment**—Patients that place high demand on the knee, young athletes, or patients with associated torn ligaments (eg, "unhappy triad") generally undergo arthroscopic repair.

**Step 5)** A rehabilitation program is part of the management, regardless of surgical or nonsurgical treatment.

### Disposition:

It may take 6 to 12 months to return to full activity following surgical repair with a rehabilitation program.

### Pearls:

- Patients with an ACL rupture are at risk of developing osteoarthritis in the future even after a successful surgery.

- Surgical intervention is usually delayed soon after an ACL injury to prevent scar tissue (arthrofibrosis) from developing.

- Placing a valgus stress at the lateral knee while holding the medial ankle will cause the lower leg to move out laterally, as if a "knocked knee." (A good way to remember this is to associate the letter *L* in *valgus* with the letter *L* in *laterally*.) Excessive medial laxity would suggest a medial collateral ligament (MCL) tear.

- Placing a varus stress at the medial knee while holding the lateral ankle will cause the lower leg to be adducted, as if a "bowlegged" person. Excessive lateral laxity would suggest a lateral collateral ligament (LCL) tear.

- **On the CCS,** an "arthroscopy" is available in the practice CCS, but you will be redirected to a "Prerequisite Order" screen to order a consult with "orthopedic surgery."

- **On the CCS,** you are evaluated in knowing when to order an appropriate consult. Do not assume that the CCS will always redirect you to the appropriate consultant when a procedure is ordered.

# NEOPLASM

## ■ OSTEOSARCOMA

Osteosarcoma (osteogenic sarcoma) is the most common pediatric bone tumor. Osteosarcoma is a primary malignant bone tumor that can be characterized by the production of osteoid (unmineralized bone) by the malignant cells. The etiology of osteosarcoma is unknown.

### Risk Factors:

Prior irradiation or chemotherapy, Paget's disease, hereditary retinoblastoma (RB1 gene mutation), Li-Fraumeni syndrome (p53 mutation), Rothmund-Thomson syndrome, bone dysplasias, bone infarcts.

## Clinical Features:

Osteosarcoma can occur in all age groups but usually has a bimodal age distribution with peaks in adolescence and in adults older than 65 years. In the pediatric population, osteosarcoma usually arises in a sporadic fashion and is considered a primary cancer. In adults, osteosarcoma is thought to arise as a secondary neoplasm (eg, Paget's disease, bone dysplasias). Osteosarcoma can affect any bone, but it has a predilection for the metaphysis of long bones and common sites include the distal femur, proximal tibia, and proximal humerus. Other possible sites include the pelvis, proximal femur, and jaw (seen in elderly patients). The most common symptom is localized pain that be present for months. In children, the pain may be dismissed as "growing pains." Signs and symptoms of fever, night sweats, weight loss, or regional lymphadenopathy is usually absent. On examination, a soft tender mass may be present. Distant metastases usually involve the lungs, and patients can develop respiratory symptoms.

## Next Step:

**Step 1)** The best initial test is to obtain a **plain x-ray** of the involved bone. The x-ray may reveal a lytic lesion (radiolucent) mixed with a sclerotic appearance (radiodense). However, there is no single feature that is diagnostic for osteosarcoma. Other ancillary testing may include a CBC, LDH, and CMP. Within the CMP, you want to look closely at the renal function, LFTs, electrolytes, and alkaline phosphatase. Be aware that the alkaline phosphatase and LDH are usually elevated in osteosarcoma. In addition, an elevated LDH usually indicates a poor outcome.

**Step 2)** Confirm the diagnosis with a biopsy (ie, "tissue is the issue").

**Step 3)** Once the diagnosis is confirmed, the patient should have a staging workup, which should include an MRI with gadolinium, CT chest to detect lung metastases, and a radionuclide bone scan with technetium to detect metastases to the bony skeleton.

**Step 4)** Treatment of osteosarcoma involves surgery and adjuvant chemotherapy. There is no standard chemotherapy regimen, but most include cisplatin and doxorubicin.

## Follow-Up:

Patients should have surveillance after initial treatment. Follow-ups usually include physical exams, blood work, and imaging. Survival has improved significantly to >70% (5-year survival rate) with the addition of adjuvant chemotherapy. Prognosis is lower (<50%) in patients with pulmonary metastases and an even poorer prognosis when metastases affect the bone.

## Pearls:

- Males are affected more than females.
- Osteosarcoma tends to metastasize to **bone** as well as **lung**.
- The most common site for disease relapse is the lung.
- Survival benefit appears to be similar when using neoadjuvant (preoperative) chemotherapy compared to adjuvant (postoperative) chemotherapy.
- Radiation therapy is not part of the routine management of osteosarcoma because they are radioresistant.
- Ewing sarcoma is radiosensitive, and radiation therapy is part of the management.
- Ewing sarcoma can produce the "Codman's triangle" on x-ray and multiple layers of the periosteal reaction can produce an "onion peel" appearance. Other descriptive terms used to describe Ewing sarcoma is a "moth-eaten" or "permeative" appearance that reflects the destructive nature of the lesion.
- Doxorubicin is cardiotoxic.
- Cisplatin is neurotoxic.
- Osteosarcoma has a predilection for areas with high activity for bone cell mitosis.
- **Foundational point**—The neoplastic bone appears to have a lacelike architecture on histology.
- **Foundational point**—There are different histologic types of osteosarcoma. The most common type is the conventional (intramedullary) osteosarcoma. Another type is the telangiectatic (vascular) osteosarcoma, which is mainly a lytic lesion without sclerosis and appears cystic (ie, sometimes confused with an aneurysmal bone cyst).
- **Foundational point**—The tumor in osteosarcoma can elevate the periosteum resulting in the "Codman's triangle" on x-ray. With further extension of the tumor through the periosteum, the mass may be ossified resulting in the "sunburst" appearance on x-ray.
- **On the CCS**, a "bone scan" is available in the practice CCS, but there is no option for "radionuclide bone scan."
- **On the CCS**, if you type in "biopsy" in the order sheet, the CCS practice software will provide you with a full list of body sites to take the biopsy.
- **On the CCS**, remember to "advise patient, cancer diagnosis" once the diagnosis is established.
- **On the CCS**, do not give chemotherapy by yourself. Remember you are the primary care physician. You need to have an oncology consult.
- **On the CCS**, remember you should be doing most of the workup before ordering an oncology consult.
- **On the CCS**, remember to "advise patient, side effects of medication" if it's decided to give chemotherapy to the patient.

# CCS: CARPAL TUNNEL SYNDROME CASE INTRODUCTION

Day 1 @ 14:00
Office

A 50-year-old white female comes to the office because of pain and tingling in her right hand.

**Initial Vital Signs:**
Temperature: 37.0°C (98.6°F)
Pulse: 75 beats/min, regular rhythm
Respiratory: 17/min
Blood pressure: 125/75 mm Hg
Height: 154.9 cm (61.0 inches)
Weight: 59 kg (130 lb)
BMI: 24.6 kg/m$^2$

**Initial History:**
Reason(s) for visit: Pain and tingling in her hand.

**HPI:**
A 50-year-old computer assistant comes to your office because of pain and tingling in her right hand. The patient states that her symptoms had been intermittent for the last 6 months but has become more persistent over the last 2 weeks. She has a dull aching pain over the ventral aspect of her right wrist with radiation into her forearm. Tingling is felt predominately over her right index finger, middle finger, ring finger, and thumb but sparing the thenar eminence. The patient states that her symptoms are exacerbated when she drives, types on the computer, and reads the newspaper. Her symptoms are worse at night and often wakes her up as she has to "flick" her wrist to alleviate her pain. She states that NSAIDs provides no relief. Over the last 2 weeks, she feels more "clumsy" since she has been dropping objects on the ground and has difficulty opening doors.

| | |
|---|---|
| **Past Medical History:** | None |
| **Past Surgical History:** | Cesarean deliveries at ages 27 and 30. |
| **Medications:** | None |
| **Allergies:** | None |
| **Vaccinations:** | Up to date |
| **Family History:** | Father died of a heart attack at age 67. Mother died of COPD complications at age 62. One sister, age 53, has diabetes. One brother, age 48, has hypertension. |
| **Social History:** | Does not smoke; drinks one glass of wine with dinner; married; two children; computer assistant for 25 years; high school graduate; enjoys reading and karaoke. |

**Review of Systems:**

| | |
|---|---|
| General: | See HPI |
| HEENT: | Negative |
| Musculoskeletal: | See HPI |
| Cardiorespiratory: | Negative |
| Gastrointestinal: | Negative |
| Genitourinary: | Negative |
| Neuropsychiatric: | See HPI |

Day 1 @ 14: 04

**Physical Examination:**

| | |
|---|---|
| **General appearance:** | Well nourished, well developed; in no apparent distress. |
| **Skin:** | Normal turgor. No lesions. Hair and nails normal. |
| **Extremities/Spine:** | Tenderness over the ventral aspect of the right wrist. No joint deformity or warmth. No cyanosis or clubbing. No edema. Peripheral pulses normal. Spine exam normal. |
| **Neuro/Psych:** | Mental status normal. Cranial nerve normal. Cerebellar function normal. Deep tendon reflexes normal. Sensory deficits noted over the palmar and dorsal aspects of the right thumb, index, middle, and ring finger. Normal sensation over the thenar eminence and hypothenar eminence. Motor exam demonstrates weakness in right thumb abduction and opposition. Moderate flattening over the right thenar eminence. Tinel sign-Positive, Phalen test-Positive, Carpal compression test-Positive, Hand elevation test-Positive. |

**First Order Sheet:**
1) Wrist splint, routine     **Result:** Patient fitted for wrist splint

**Actions:**
1) Reevaluate case: In 30 days

Day 31
The patient has arrived for the appointment.

**Recorded Vital Signs:**
Temperature: 37.0°C (98.6°F)
Pulse: 75 beats/min, regular rhythm
Respiratory: 17/min
Blood pressure: 125/75 mm Hg

**Follow-Up History:**
The patient's wrist feels "better" since the last visit.

**Physical Examination:**
Extremities/Spine: Decrease tenderness over the ventral aspect of the right wrist since the last visit. No joint deformity or warmth. No cyanosis or clubbing. No edema. Peripheral pulses normal. Spine exam normal.

Neuro/Psych: Mental status normal. Cranial nerve normal. Cerebellar function normal. Deep tendon reflexes normal. Sensory deficits noted over the palmar and dorsal aspects of the right thumb, index, middle, and ring finger. Normal sensation over the thenar eminence and hypothenar eminence. Motor exam demonstrates weakness in right thumb abduction and opposition. Moderate flattening over the right thenar eminence. Tinel sign-Positive, Phalen test-Positive, Carpal compression test-Positive, Hand elevation test-Positive.

**Actions:**
1) Reevaluate case: In 30 days

Day 55
**Patient's Condition**—The patient's condition is not improving, the pain and tingling is getting worse.

**Actions:**
1) Stop clock now.
2) Change location from home to office.

Day 55
The patient has arrived for the appointment.

**Recorded Vital Signs:**
Temperature: 37.0°C (98.6°F)
Pulse: 75 beats/min, regular rhythm
Respiratory: 17/min.
Blood pressure: 125/75 mm Hg

**Physical Examination:**
Extremities/Spine: Very tender over the ventral aspect of the right wrist. No joint deformity or warmth. No cyanosis or clubbing. No edema. Peripheral pulses normal. Spine exam normal.

Neuro/Psych: Mental status normal. Cranial nerve normal. Cerebellar function normal. Deep tendon reflexes normal. Sensory deficits noted over the palmar and dorsal aspects of the right thumb, index, middle, and ring finger. Normal sensation over the thenar eminence and hypothenar eminence. Motor exam demonstrates weakness in right thumb abduction and opposition. Moderate flattening over the right thenar eminence flattening is observed. Tinel sign-Positive, Phalen test-Positive, Carpal compression test-Positive, Hand elevation test-Positive.

**Second Order Sheet:**
1) Nerve conduction study, routine — **Result:** Delayed latencies and slowed conduction velocities across the carpal tunnel.
2) Electromyography, routine — **Result:** Mild to moderate denervation.

**Third Order Sheet:**
1) Methylprednisolone, one time — **Note:** Methylprednisolone injected into the carpal tunnel.

**This case will end in the next few minutes of "real time."**
You may **add** or **delete** orders at this time, then enter a diagnosis on the following screen.

**Fourth Order Sheet:**
1) Advise patient, no aspirin
2) Refer patient, occupational therapy

**Please enter your diagnosis:**

Carpal tunnel syndrome

**DISCUSSION:**
Carpal tunnel syndrome (CTS) is a very common entrapment neuropathy involving compression of the median nerve with an unknown etiology.

**Risk Factors:**

Hypothyroidism, rheumatoid arthritis, diabetes, amyloidosis, sarcoidosis, obesity, female, pregnancy, trauma, mass lesions.

## Clinical Features:

The classic presentation is pain and paresthesia along the median nerve distribution. The **sensory branch** of the median nerve innervates the palmar side of the thumb, index, middle, and half the ring finger, as well as the dorsal side of the index, middle, and half the ring finger. Even though the median nerve innervates selected areas, patients will complain of pain and paresthesia in all fingers (ie, including the pinky finger). However, patients should not complain of sensory changes in the thenar eminence because a sensory branch (ie, palmar cutaneous branch) of the median nerve branches off proximally and superficially to the flexor retinaculum, thereby passing over the carpal tunnel to directly innervate the thenar eminence. Nighttime symptoms that awaken patients are usually specific for CTS. Flexing or extending the wrist can elicit CTS symptoms such as driving a car, typing, or reading the newspaper. Patients flicking their wrist to alleviate their pain is referred to as the "flick sign." Patients may also have radiation of their sensory symptoms to the forearm and shoulder. In the later stages of CTS, patients may have weakness and clumsiness in their hands with atrophy seen in the thenar eminence. The **motor branch** of the median nerve supplies the thenar muscles, and therefore, patients will usually have weakness in thumb abduction and opposition. Several hand maneuvers have been described to help with the assessment, but fair short of their reliability. A positive **Tinel test** involves pain or paresthesia when the median nerve is percussed. A positive **Phalen test** involves pain or paresthesia when the dorsums of the hands are placed against each other causing hyperflexion. A positive **carpal compression test** involves reproducing the symptoms after firm pressure over the carpal tunnel. A positive **hand elevation test** involves reproducing the symptoms when the hands are raised over the head for at least 1 minute.

## Next Step Summary:

**Step 1)** CTS is a clinical diagnosis. **Nerve conduction studies** (NCS) and **electromyography** (EMG) are used to confirm the diagnosis. In this particular case, the patient was doing well with wrist splints, but then apparently started to have problems in her second month wearing the splints. If the diagnosis becomes unclear as in this case, testing with NCS and EMG would be the next best step. Suboptimal management would be to order an MRI, unless you suspect a mass lesion.

**Step 2)** First line treatment begins with **wrist splinting**, particularly at night. Patients should continue nocturnal splinting for at least 1 to 2 months. If patients continue to be symptomatic during that time, another modality of treatment should be added. In this particular case, methylprednisolone was injected into the carpal tunnel. An alternative to steroid injection is to administer oral steroids (eg, prednisone) for 10 to 14 days. Patients that continue to have sensory symptoms, motor dysfunction, and are refractory to conservative treatment should consider surgical carpal tunnel release as the next best step.

## Follow-Up:

Patients should be seen in 4 to 6 weeks after treatment to reassess the patient's condition as in this case.

## Pearls:

- Bilateral CTS is common.
- Differential diagnosis for CTS may include cervical radiculopathy, flexor carpi radialis tenosynovitis, Raynaud phenomenon, or median nerve compression at the elbow.
- CTS may not always present in the classic median nerve distribution.
- Anomalous innervations do exist within the hand.
- Patients experiencing sensory changes over the ring and pinky finger should think about ulnar nerve entrapments.
- Obtain a TSH, rheumatoid factor (RF), or HbA1C in patients who you suspect as having hypothyroidism, rheumatoid arthritis, or diabetes, respectively.
- Repetitive hand maneuvers, especially in the workplace environment have been implicated as a cause for CTS, but the evidence is still inconclusive.
- NSAIDs (including aspirin), diuretics, and vitamin B6 (pyridoxine) have shown to have no significant benefits when compared to placebo.
- **Foundational point**—The median nerve originates from roots C6 and C7 (lateral cord) plus roots C8 and T1 (medial cord).
- **On the CCS**, you cannot order "corticosteroid" but rather the generic or trade names.
- **On the CCS**, there is no option in the practice CCS to inject the steroid into the carpal tunnel or beneath the flexor retinaculum.
- **On the CCS**, in nonacute, routine office-based CCS cases, you are expected to advance the clock in weeks or months to change the patient's condition.
- **On the CCS**, the "Interval Hx" tab has an "Interval/follow up" option that is basically asking how the patient is doing.
- **On the CCS**, sometimes a "PATIENT UPDATE" may pop up on the screen as you advance the clock. You have to decide if these messages will affect your management plans. In this case, the patient was asked to come back to the office for a reevaluation before the appointment day. Remember, you cannot assess a patient at home; you have to relocate the patient back to a medical setting. If the patient is at home, the practice CCS software will not allow you to do a physical examination.

# 15

Otolaryngology—
Head and Neck

## KEYWORDS REVIEW

Chemosis—Swelling of the ocular (bulbar) conjunctiva.

Coryza—Acute rhinitis usually associated with a runny nose.

Endolymph—Fluid within the membranous labyrinth of the ear.

Hyposmia—Decreased sense of smell.

Odynophagia—Painful swallowing.

Otalgia—Ear pain.

Perilymph—Fluid that resides in the bony labyrinth. The bony labyrinth surrounds the membranous labyrinth and within the membranous labyrinth is the endolymph. The endolymph is completely separate from the perilymph.

Trismus—Inability to fully open the mouth (lockjaw).

# EAR DISORDERS

## ▌ACOUSTIC NEUROMA

Acoustic neuroma (vestibular schwannoma) is a slow-growing intracranial tumor that is derived from the Schwann cell sheath that invests the vestibulocochlear nerve (cranial nerve VIII). In the majority of cases, the tumor arises from the vestibular division (superior and inferior branches) and rarely from the cochlear division of CN VIII. The tumor resides within the internal auditory canal, and as it grows, it can extend into the posterior fossa to occupy the cerebellopontine angle (CPA).

### Clinical Features:

Acoustic neuromas typically present in patients that are in their fifth or sixth decade of life. Patients will present with a chronic **unilateral sensorineural hearing loss**, although sudden hearing loss can sometimes occur. Other findings include **tinnitus** and **equilibrium disturbances** that are not like true spinning vertigo. As the tumor progresses, other cranial nerves can be affected. Impingement of the trigeminal nerve (V) can lead to facial pain, numbness, hypesthesia, or a decrease in ipsilateral corneal reflex (afferent limb). Impingement of the facial nerve (VII) can result in taste disturbances, facial weakness, or a decrease in ipsilateral corneal reflex (efferent limb). Larger tumors can cause cerebellum or brainstem compression resulting in ataxia and secondary hydrocephalus, respectively. On exam, a unilateral sensorineural hearing loss will demonstrate sound lateralization to the good ear in the Weber test. In the Rinne test, a sensorineural hearing loss will demonstrate air conduction (AC) > bone conduction (BC) in both the good and bad ear.

### Next Step:

**Step 1)** The best initial test is with a hearing test or **audiometry**. The most common abnormality is an asymmetrical (left versus right) high-frequency sensorineural hearing loss. In addition, the audiogram will typically demonstrate poor speech discrimination scores that are out of proportion to the pure tone average.

**Step 2)** An **MRI with gadolinium** is the next best step in patients suspected of having an acoustic neuroma with an abnormal hearing test. An MRI can help establish a diagnosis by detecting tumors as small as 1 to 2 mm in diameter. A CT with contrast is an acceptable alternative in patients that have a contraindication to an MRI, but may not be reliable in detecting tumors that are <15 mm.

**Step 3)** Treatment approach includes surgical removal, stereotactic radiation therapy, or observation with serial imaging and audiometry.

### Follow-Up:

Since acoustic neuromas are slow-growing tumors, patients that elect interventional treatment or observation require regular follow-ups with MRI imaging and audiometry (ie, if hearing preservation is a concern).

### Pearls:

- Approximately 80% to 90% of tumors found within the CPA are acoustic neuromas.

- Other lesions that occupy the CPA include meningiomas and dermoid cysts.

- Although most acoustic neuromas are slow-growing tumors (1-2 mm/yr on imaging), a rapidly growing tumor (>2.5 mm/yr on imaging) is an indication for therapeutic intervention.

- Normal hearing threshold levels should be between 0 and 25 decibels (dB) on the audiogram. Threshold levels greater than 25 dB are considered abnormal.

- Symmetrical hearing impairment is an uncommon finding on the audiogram in patients with acoustic neuroma; however, it does not exclude the diagnosis (ie, infrequently, patients may present with a symmetrical sensorineural hearing loss).

- Bilateral acoustic neuromas can be seen in patients with neurofibromatosis type 2 (NF2). This can be easily remembered by "2 and 2" (ie, NF2 gives you 2 acoustic neuromas).

- Ancillary testing would include an auditory brainstem-evoked response (ABR/AER) that would demonstrate nerve conduction delays (ie, abnormal latencies) on the side of the tumor.

- A unilateral conductive hearing loss will demonstrate sound lateralization to the bad ear in the Weber test. In the Rinne test, a conductive hearing loss will demonstrate bone conduction > air conduction in the bad ear and air conduction > bone conduction in the good ear.

- Presbycusis (age-related hearing loss) is a progressive and symmetrical sensorineural hearing loss in elderly people that typically affects the high frequencies (eg, 4000-8000 Hertz), but with relative preservation of the speech discrimination scores.

- **Connecting point** (pg. 162)—Know that neurofibromatosis type 1 and type 2 are autosomal dominant disorders.

- **CJ:** A 77-year-old man with an acoustic neuroma is following up with annual MRIs for tumor surveillance. The last 2 years revealed a tumor growth rate of 1.9 mm/yr followed by 2.0 mm/yr. Last week his most recent MRI demonstrated a tumor growth rate of 2.8 mm/yr. The patient is concerned about the tumor progression and is worried about losing his hearing. He is willing to undergo surgery to preserve his hearing. He currently volunteers at the local library, drives his car, walks his dogs to the park, and has an active social life. What do you recommend? **Answer:** Age is not a contraindication to undergo surgery especially in this man with an active lifestyle. There is evidence of tumor progression, and the patient should undergo surgery with an attempt to preserve his hearing on the affected side.

- **On the CCS,** "audiometry" is available in the practice CCS.

- **On the CCS,** remember to counsel your patients once the diagnosis of cancer is made or "advise patient, cancer diagnosis," which is available in the practice CCS.

# MENIERE'S DISEASE

Meniere's disease is a disorder of the inner ear that is associated with an increase in endolymph resulting in distention of the endolymphatic system (endolymphatic hydrops). All patients with Meniere's disease will demonstrate endolymphatic hydrops on postmortem examination, but not all patients with endolymphatic hydrops will have signs or symptoms of Meniere's disease. The exact etiology of excessive endolymph in the endolymphatic system is still unknown.

## Clinical Features:

Meniere's disease can occur at any age but is frequently seen in the fifth decade of life. Patients will present with true spinning **vertigo** (rotational vertigo) that is episodic. The onset of vertigo is usually sudden, and it can last from several minutes to several hours and may vary in frequency (ie, sporadic or clusters). The vertiginous attacks can also vary in severity. In some cases, patients may experience a violent drop attack in which the patient falls, but does not lose consciousness. During acute attacks, a horizontal nystagmus with a rotary component can be observed. After the attack subsides, patients feel exhausted and may experience nausea and vomiting. A low-frequency fluctuating **sensorineural hearing loss** is typically seen early in the disease. With each successive vertiginous attack, there appears to be a progressive deterioration in hearing. Later in the course, all frequencies are usually affected and hearing loss is often permanent. A low-tone **tinnitus** that is described as a "roaring" or "blowing" sound and **aural fullness** may be continuous or intermittent during the course of the disease.

## Next Step:

**Step 1)** Meniere's disease is a clinical diagnosis, although further testing is often performed to rule out other conditions that may have symptoms that overlap with Meniere's disease. Consider the following ancillary testing:

**Labs**—BMP (assess electrolytes), TSH (rule out hyperthyroidism or hypothyroidism), hemoglobin A1C (rule out diabetes), RPR or VDRL (rule out neurosyphilis), or ANA (rule out autoimmune disease).

**Audiometry**—Hearing loss may be seen in the low frequencies (early in the disease) or with a mixed presentation (low and high frequencies). Later in the disease, the audiogram appears to flatten out affecting all frequencies.

**Electronystagmography (ENG)**—ENG, particularly the caloric testing (warm and cool water ear irrigation) may demonstrate a peripheral vestibular dysfunction (ie, thermally induced nystagmus is impaired on the affected side).

**MRI**—MRI can help rule out CNS abnormalities (eg, tumors, multiple sclerosis).

**Step 2)** Provide counseling and educate patients about the disease and treatment options.

**Step 3) Short-term management:** During an acute vertiginous attack, the patient should rest in bed since most patients will find a position that will minimize the vertigo. In the ED setting, you can provide the patient with an antihistamine (eg, IV/IM diphenhydramine) and an antiemetic (eg, IV/IM promethazine, prochlorperazine, ondansetron, or metoclopramide) for nausea and vomiting. At home, a patient can be given an anticholinergic agent such as a scopolamine transdermal patch that can be easily applied to the skin behind the ear. Treatment in the short-term management can be easily remembered by the **triple A's** (**A**ntihistamines, **A**ntiemetics, **A**nticholinergic).

**Step 4) Long-term management:** Long-term management is focused on controlling the vertigo since there is no effective therapy for the hearing loss, tinnitus, or aural fullness. Conservative therapy should be attempted first, and then patients can go onto more aggressive approaches for disabling and intractable vertigo. Consider the following approaches:

### Conservative Approaches

**Lifestyle modification**—Avoid possible triggers such as limiting high salt intake, caffeine, alcohol, nicotine, monosodium glutamate (MSG), or stress.

**Medical therapy**—When lifestyle changes are not effective, a diuretic (eg, HCTZ) along with prn (as-needed) vestibular suppressants (eg, meclizine, diphenhydramine, diazepam, clonazepam) and antiemetics (eg, ondansetron) can be used.

**Vestibular rehabilitation (VRT)**—VRT is an exercised-based program to promote central nervous system compensation for inner ear deficits.

### Invasive Approaches

- Intratympanic gentamicin
- Labyrinthectomy
- Vestibular nerve section
- Endolymphatic sac decompression
- Air pressure pulse generator

## Follow-Up:

Patients may need ongoing care since there is no cure for Meniere's disease and the disease pattern follows a period of remission that is speckled with periods of exacerbation.

## Pearls:

- Meniere's disease is usually unilateral, but it can be bilateral in approximately 15% to 20% of cases.

- Loop diuretics (eg, furosemide) should be avoided since it can be ototoxic to the ear.

- In a person with a normal vestibular system, an induced horizontal nystagmus can be obtained by caloric reflex testing. When cold water (or air) is irrigated into the ear, a fast-beating nystagmus should move away from the stimulated ear, while warm water (or air) will cause a fast-beating nystagmus to move toward the stimulated ear. The mnemonic **COWS** (**c**old-**o**pposite, **w**arm-**s**ame) is used to describe this effect, and another way to remember one of its effects is "cold-contralateral."

- Vertigo can be seen in other conditions such as benign paroxysmal positional vertigo (vertigo is provoked by head position and lasts <1 minute) and vestibular neuronitis (vertigo is spontaneous and lasts 24-48 hours).

- **On the CCS**, sometimes the diagnosis is clearly evident in the initial history. In other cases, the diagnosis may be ambiguous. In these types of situations, be sure to do appropriate physicals exams and order tests based on the initial history. Remember that an efficient approach will probably give you a higher score, but a thorough approach using your clinical judgment may not necessarily deduct from your score.
- **On the CCS**, remember to "bridge" your therapy by treating the acute issues (eg, vertiginous attack) along with the long-term care of the vertigo.

## ACUTE OTITIS MEDIA

Acute otitis media (AOM) is an acute bacterial infection of the middle ear. In the majority of cases, a viral upper respiratory tract infection is the triggering event that causes inflammation resulting in obstruction of the eustachian tube, thereby disrupting the aeration of the middle ear. Fluid accumulates in the middle ear and can become secondarily infected by bacteria. The most common bacteria in descending order are *Streptococcus pneumoniae* > nontypeable *Haemophilus influenzae* > *Moraxella catarrhalis*.

### Risk Factors:

Young age (strong risk factor), family history, pacifier use, absence of breastfeeding, altered immunity, day care, crowded conditions, tobacco smoke exposure, craniofacial abnormalities, fall or winter seasons, and race (Native Americans, Eskimos, Australian aborigine).

### Clinical Features:

AOM can occur at any age, but the peak incidence is between 6 and 18 months of age with a slightly higher incidence in boys than girls. Clinical manifestations may include fever, otalgia, otorrhea, rubbing of the ear, diminished hearing, or coexistent upper respiratory tract infection. In the young infant, feeding difficulties or irritability may be the presenting feature. Otoscopic examination may reveal several key elements. Consider the following:

**Color**—Marked redness of the tympanic membrane (TM) can be seen in AOM, which suggests acute inflammation.

**Translucency**—The tympanic membrane should normally be translucent, but if it appears opaque, it indicates fluid in the middle ear. In addition, an air-fluid level may be appreciated on exam. Consider AOM or otitis media with effusion (OME) (ie, **noninfected**) in patients with an opaque TM.

**Position**—A bulging tympanic membrane is a key finding in AOM and represents an important marker for acute inflammation.

**Mobility**—Pneumatic insufflation will demonstrate poor tympanic mobility with a fluid-filled middle ear.

### Next Step:

**Step 1)** AOM is a clinical diagnosis that is based on **signs and symptoms of middle ear inflammation** (eg, bulging TM, red TM not due to crying, otalgia, or fever) plus evidence of **middle ear effusion (MME)**. MME can be observed on otoscopic exam (eg, air-fluid level, bubbles, or opaque TM), pneumatic otoscopy (↓ TM mobility), or tympanometry (no peak or poor compliance at all frequencies).

**Step 2)** Treat the patient's pain with analgesics (eg, acetaminophen, ibuprofen).

**Step 3)** The initial management in AOM is to immediately treat with antibiotics or to observe for a period of 48 to 72 hours followed by antibiotics if there is no clinical improvement during that time. Based on the American Academy of Pediatrics (AAP)/American Academy of Family Physicians (AAFP) guidelines, the observation strategy can be offered to children 6 to 23 months of age with nonsevere unilateral AOM (ie, temperature <39°C [102.2°F] and mild ear pain for <48 hours) or in children ≥24 months of age with nonsevere unilateral or bilateral AOM. If the decision is to pursue antibiotics, there are several choices to consider. The typical duration of antibiotics can vary from 7 to 10 days.

> **Option 1:** Oral amoxicillin is a first-line agent that is recommended for most patients.
>
> **Option 2:** Amoxicillin-clavulanate for patients with a recent history of amoxicillin use (<30 days), unresponsive to amoxicillin in a patient with recurrent AOM, or patients with coexisting purulent conjunctivitis.
>
> **Option 3:** Cefuroxime, ceftriaxone, cefdinir, or cefpodoxime in patients with a penicillin allergy but without a type 1 hypersensitivity (ie, anaphylaxis, angioedema, bronchospasm, or urticaria).
>
> **Option 4:** Azithromycin, erythromycin, clarithromycin, or clindamycin with a type 1 hypersensitivity to a beta-lactam antibiotic.

**Step 4)** Administer a pneumococcal conjugate vaccine (PCV13) according to the recommended schedule of 2, 4, 6, and 12-15 months of age. Also, provide an inactivated influenza vaccine for children 6 to 23 months of age or either inactivated or live attenuated influenza vaccine for children ≥24 months of age. However, do not give a live attenuated influenza vaccine in patients who have asthma, are immunosuppressed, are in close contact with a severely immunocompromised patient, are in concomitant use with aspirin therapy, or have an anaphylactic reaction to chicken, egg, gelatin, gentamicin, or arginine.

### Follow-Up:

There are three important elements in the follow-up care. First, patients that are being observed and that fail to improve or worsen within 48 to 72 hours should begin antibiotics. Second, patients that were given antibiotics from the beginning but fail to improve after 48 to 72 hours should be reevaluated and possibly consider changing antibiotics to provide broader coverage (eg, amoxicillin-clavulanate or ceftriaxone). If ceftriaxone is given, it is given as IM or IV and up to 3 doses. If the patient responds to the first dose, then the second and third dose is not necessary. Finally, the AAP/AAFP guidelines recommend that patients may be offered tympanostomy tubes for recurrent

AOM, which is defined as ≥3 episodes within 6 months or ≥4 episodes within 12 months.

## Pearls:

- It is important to differentiate between AOM and OME (sometimes referred to as serous otitis media), since you do not want to unnecessarily give antibiotics to OME.

- OME and AOM may be part of a disease continuum in which OME precedes and predispose to AOM, or OME may be the result of AOM.

- Although both OME and AOM may demonstrate decreased tympanic mobility on pneumatic otoscopy, the tympanic membrane is usually retracted in OME but is bulging in AOM.

- Do not prescribe prophylactic antibiotics to reduce the frequency of AOM.

- Tympanocentesis (aspiration of the middle ear fluid) for culture is not routinely performed since treatment is with empiric antibiotics. Tympanocentesis may be considered in patients that have failed previous antibiotics.

- Otalgia in a nonverbal child may present as rubbing, tugging, or holding the ear.

- MME can last from several days up to several weeks, despite appropriate antibiotics for a resolved AOM (ie, sterilized effusion). The presence of an effusion does not indicate treatment failure.

- MME can cause hearing loss, but should resolve as the fluid is resorbed. If hearing loss is persistent, consider further evaluation with hearing and language testing.

- Tympanic membrane perforation (secondary to an increase in middle ear pressure) with associated otorrhea can be a complication of AOM. The preferred treatment in a patient with an acute perforation and AOM is with oral amoxicillin (rather than quinolone otic drops) since it covers the most likely pathogen in AOM (S pneumoniae), but it also has coverage against group A streptococci (GAS), which have been associated with a higher rate of TM perforation in AOM. Ironically, the perforation actually helps to alleviate the middle ear pressure by draining the fluid. The TM perforation will often heal on its own, but if it doesn't, it may lead to chronic otitis media (COM), which is defined as TM perforation in the setting of recurrent ear infections. COM with otorrhea through the perforation is referred to as chronic suppurative otitis media (CSOM) and it is treated with ciprofloxacin or ofloxacin otic drops.

- **On the CCS**, along with your clinical exams, remember to use the "Interval/Follow up" to see how the patient is doing in the follow-up visits.

- **On the CCS**, if the mother is the caretaker for a young infant with AOM, it is important to "counsel family/patient" which is in the practice CCS. This option will essentially educate the mother to care for her child since the child may not be able to understand any type of counseling.

## TYMPANIC MEMBRANE PERFORATION

Tympanic membrane (TM) perforation can be the result of middle ear infections (eg, otitis media), blunt trauma (eg, blow to the ear), penetrating trauma (eg, Q-tips), barotrauma (eg, scuba diving), slag burns (eg, welding), or lightening.

### Clinical Features:

Clinical manifestations typically include an acute onset of ear pain and a conductive hearing loss. In serious cases that include disruption of the inner ear, patients can experience vertigo, nystagmus, tinnitus, and a sensorineural hearing loss.

### Next Step:

**Step 1)** Tympanic membrane perforation is a clinical diagnosis. On otoscopic examination, a tympanic membrane perforation will be apparent with or without bloody otorrhea (see Figure 15-1 and Color Plate 13).

**Step 2)** An audiometry should be performed within 24 hours since a conductive hearing loss ≥35 dB may be associated with ossicular injury. Prompt otolaryngology consultation should be considered in patients with a hearing loss ≥35 dB, facial nerve paresis/paralysis, significant bleeding, or signs and symptoms of inner ear injury (ie, vertigo, nausea, vomiting, nystagmus, tinnitus, clear otorrhea).

**Step 3)** Most TM perforations will spontaneously heal. Larger perforations that do not heal completely may be repaired by an otolaryngologist. Otologic care includes educating the patient to avoid water entering the ears and forceful blowing of the nose, analgesics for pain, and antibiotic ear drops (eg, ciprofloxacin otic drops) for patients with contaminated injuries (eg, foreign material in the ear).

### Follow-Up:

Patients should have a follow-up audiometry in 4 weeks along with an evaluation of the tympanic membrane. Patients that

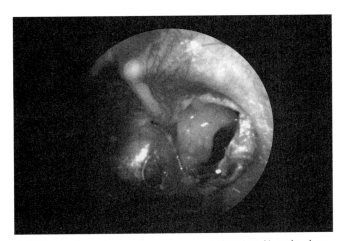

**FIGURE 15-1 • Acute tympanic membrane perforation.** Note the clean-cut margins of the perforation, which is commonly seen in traumatic cases. Also examine the hyperemic tympanic membrane, which suggests an acute process. (Photo Contributor: Richard A. Chole, MD, PhD. Reproduced with permission from Knoop KJ, et al. *The Atlas of Emergency Medicine*. 3rd ed. McGraw-Hill, www.accessmedicine.com.)

have persistent hearing loss or an unhealed tympanic membrane should be referred to an otolaryngologist.

Pearls:

- Patients that have a history of vertigo, nystagmus, tinnitus, and a sensorineural hearing loss are suggestive of an injury to the stapes footplate (footplate subluxation), which represents an otologic emergency.
- Do not perform ear irrigation in patients with a TM perforation since you may force more debris into the middle ear.

- Injury to the facial nerve will typically present with facial weakness and may include injury to the chorda tympani, a branch of the facial nerve that runs through the middle ear and is responsible for carrying sensory afferent fibers that provide taste sensation from the ipsilateral anterior two-thirds of the tongue.
- **On the CCS**, if a consult is needed, remember you are asking a consult from the point of view of a primary care physician.

# NOSE AND PARANASAL SINUSES

## ACUTE SINUSITIS

Acute sinusitis (or rhinosinusitis) is characterized by inflammation of the mucosal lining of the paranasal sinuses and nasal cavity. **Noninfectious causes** (eg, allergic rhinitis, polyp obstruction, Wegener's granulomatosis, cystic fibrosis) can result in impaired mucus clearance and obstruction of the sinus ostia. **Infectious causes** (eg, viruses, bacteria, fungi) can also result in acute sinusitis with viruses as the most common etiology. Bacterial sinusitis can be the result of a secondary infection following a viral infection. Most acute cases of fungal sinusitis occur in immunocompromised patients, patients with poorly controlled diabetes, transplant recipients, and patients receiving chronic steroids.

### Clinical Features:

Differentiating between viral and bacterial sinusitis is difficult based on clinical assessment. Viral sinusitis may present in close proximity to the time of a viral upper respiratory tract infection and usually symptoms of the sinusitis resolves within 7 to 10 days. Common clinical manifestations of sinusitis include nasal congestion, facial pain or pressure (worse when bending forward), fever, maxillary tooth pain, hyposmia, headache, halitosis, or ear pressure. On examination, there may be tenderness over the sinuses. Nasal speculum may demonstrate mucosal edema, discolored rhinorrhea, purulent discharge, or polyps. Symptom duration can be classified as acute (<4 weeks), subacute (4 to 12 weeks), or chronic (>12 weeks).

### Next Step:

**Step 1)** The diagnosis of uncomplicated acute sinusitis is made on clinical assessment. Imaging and cultures are not routinely performed in the initial evaluation of an uncomplicated case of acute sinusitis unless there is a reason to believe that there are complications (ie, orbital or intracranial extension of the infection).

**Step 2)** The best initial treatment approach in patients with mild symptoms is to recommend supportive care such as analgesics,

nasal saline (sterile) irrigation, proper fluid intake, and intranasal glucocorticoids (eg, mometasone) for patients with a history of allergic rhinitis. As mentioned before, uncomplicated viral sinusitis will resolve within 7 to 10 days and does not require antibiotics. Empiric antibiotics are indicated in patients with bacterial sinusitis. The key features to consider for a bacterial etiology include severe symptoms (eg, fever >39°C or >102.2°F, purulent discharge), persistent symptoms ≥10 days, or the patient was clinically improving following a viral upper respiratory tract infection and then turns the corner into an apparent worsening. Consider the following antibiotics for bacterial sinusitis:

> **Option 1:** Oral amoxicillin for 10 to 14 days is recommended as the initial therapy for most patients.
>
> **Option 2:** Doxycycline or a fluoroquinolone (levofloxacin or moxifloxacin) can be given to penicillin allergic patients.
>
> **Option 3:** High-dose amoxicillin-clavulanate or a fluoroquinolone (levofloxacin or moxifloxacin) can be given to patients with a recent history of antibiotic therapy within the past 4 weeks.

### Follow-Up:

Patients receiving antibiotic therapy for a bacterial sinusitis should respond to treatment after 3 to 5 days of initiating therapy. If there is no response to the initial treatment, consider changing to a different class of empiric antibiotics that will provide broader coverage (eg, amoxicillin-clavulanate, levofloxacin, or moxifloxacin). If patients respond from the change in antibiotics, then complete a 7- to 10-day course. If there is no improvement, consider obtaining cultures to redirect antibiotic therapy or order a CT scan.

### Pearls:

- The most common causes of community-acquired bacterial sinusitis are *Streptococcus pneumoniae*, nontypable *Haemophilus influenzae*, and *Moraxella catarrhalis*.
- The most common causes of viral sinusitis are rhinovirus, influenza virus, and parainfluenza virus.
- Mucormycosis (zygomycosis) is a fungal infection in the order of Mucorales that can infect the rhino-orbital-cerebral areas leading to a life-threatening condition.

- Thick purulent nasal discharge is suggestive of a bacterial infection, but it is not completely specific to a bacterial infection since it can sometimes occur in early viral infections.

- Cultures can be obtained by endoscopy-guided middle meatal cultures or by direct antral puncture (sinus aspirate culture).

- Obtaining cultures of purulent nasal secretions or nasal swabs of the nasal cavity is of limited value because of contamination by the normal bacterial flora.

- Although endoscopy-directed cultures can be contaminated by nasal flora, it is more commonly performed than direct sinus puncture because of the pain and discomfort associated with the sinus tap.

- Obtaining cultures is the most accurate test to determine the underlying bacterial pathogen, which can help guide antimicrobial therapy.

- Obtaining viral cultures is unnecessary.

- Transillumination of the sinuses is of limited value.

- A sinus CT scan or plain sinus x-ray is not routinely recommended in the initial evaluation of an uncomplicated case of acute sinusitis.

- A noncontrast sinus CT scan is the preferred imaging modality over plain sinus radiographs in cases of treatment failure.

- Typical findings seen in acute sinusitis are air-fluid levels and mucosal edema on sinus CT scan.

- A contrast head CT scan is indicated when complications are suspected such as cavernous sinus thrombosis, orbital cellulitis, osteomyelitis of the frontal bone (Pott puffy tumor), or brain abscess.

- Use sterile water for nasal irrigation since there have been reports of an amoeba infection from using tap water resulting in amebic encephalitis.

- Mucolytics (eg, guaifenesin) and antihistamines are not routinely recommended for acute sinusitis.

- Topical decongestants can be used for nasal congestion, but should not be used for more than 3 days since they can cause rebound congestion.

- **CJ:** A 35-year-old man with a history of sinusitis presents to the office with nasal congestion, runny nose, and a headache for the past 6 days. You recommend supportive therapy and ask that he come back in 1 week for a reassessment. The patient comes back in 4 days and complains of worsening headache, fever, diplopia, and right-sided eye swelling that was not there 4 days ago. On exam, the patient appears more distracted from the last visit. You note chemosis, ptosis, and lateral gaze palsy (ie, CN VI dysfunction). You suspect cavernous sinus thrombosis, so you decide to order an urgent head CT with contrast. The CT findings demonstrate a filling defect in the cavernous sinus with thickening of the vessel wall. What is your next best initial step? **Answer:** Prompt administration of broad-spectrum antibiotics should be given to patients with cavernous sinus thrombosis. Ideally, cultures should be obtained prior to antibiotics, but treatment should not be delayed. Empiric antibiotics should

include coverage against gram-positives with IV nafcillin (or IV oxacillin). If patients fail to respond to penicillin or MRSA is suspected, replace with IV vancomycin. Empiric antibiotics should also include broad gram-negative coverage with IV ceftriaxone (or IV cefepime). IV metronidazole should also be added to cover anaerobes if a sinus or dental infection is suspected. IV antibiotics are recommended for a minimum of 3 weeks.

- **Connecting point** (pg. 156)—An expanding intracranial aneurysm can result in compression of the cavernous sinus resulting in prodromal signs and symptoms prior to a subarachnoid hemorrhage.

- **On the CCS,** "Nasal C&S" is available in the practice CCS.

- **On the CCS,** remember to order "Advise patient, no smoking" if the patient smokes.

- **On the CCS,** if you're treating bacterial sinusitis with antibiotics, remember to set the antibiotic therapy in the continuous mode of frequency rather than a one-time/bolus. The "continuous" option takes into account periodic administration (eg, q6 hours).

# CHRONIC SINUSITIS

Chronic sinusitis (or rhinosinusitis) is an inflammatory condition of the paranasal sinuses and nasal cavity resulting in symptoms lasting >12 weeks. Most patients have undergone multiple treatments and unfortunately have suffered significant morbidity.

### Clinical Features:

The clinical manifestations of chronic sinusitis can vary. However, fever is usually absent in most patients. The following features are suggestive of chronic sinusitis:

1) Mucopurulent drainage
2) Nasal obstruction/congestion
3) Facial pain/fullness
4) Hyposmia

### Next Step:

**Step 1)** The diagnosis of chronic sinusitis is based on **TWO of the FOUR** suggestive features in the preceding list plus objective evidence of mucosal inflammation, which can be obtained by nasal endoscopy or CT imaging.

> **Nasal endoscopy**—Findings may reveal mucosal edema, purulent discharge, or polyps.

> **Noncontrast sinus CT**—Findings may reveal sinus opacification or mucoperiosteal thickening. Air-fluid levels are an uncommon finding in chronic sinusitis. Anatomic detail may also reveal sinus ostial obstruction, which may help guide future sinus surgery, if warranted.

**Step 2)** The goal of therapy is to control the inflammation, facilitate sinus drainage, and appropriately treat infections that may be present. In essence, this requires a multi-interventional approach that may require:

- Nasal saline (sterile) irrigation
- Intranasal glucocorticoids (eg, fluticasone, triamcinolone)
- Oral glucocorticoids (eg, prednisone)
- Oral antibiotics of 2 to 4 weeks duration (preferably culture-directed)

**Step 3)** When symptoms continue to persist despite maximal medical therapy, the patient should be referred to an otolaryngologist for functional endoscopic sinus surgery (FESS). FESS attempts to restore sinus health by improving drainage and facilitating normal mucociliary flow. FESS does not control the underlying inflammation; therefore, medical management needs to be maintained following surgery.

**Step 4)** Counsel patients with chronic sinusitis since their quality of life can be reduced if the condition is left untreated. Also, advise patients not to smoke since it can increase their risk of sinusitis.

### Follow-Up:

Patients often require regular follow-ups to reassess the patient's condition with the goal of improving quality of life since most cases of chronic sinusitis cannot be cured.

### Pearls:

- Allergic fungal rhinosinusitis can cause chronic fungal sinusitis, which is typically seen in immunocompetent patients that have an IgE-mediated allergy to a fungus. Patients can have nasal polyps, and they tend to have a very thick inspissated mucus (allergic mucin), which is usually identified at the time of surgery. Diagnosis is made by culturing the allergic mucin, which demonstrates fungal hyphae. Treatment involves surgical removal of the impacted mucus followed by oral and topical glucocorticoids.

- A 10- to 14-day course of antibiotics is typically given to patients with chronic sinusitis if a bacterial infection is suspected of causing an acute exacerbation.

- Patients are considered to have recurrent acute rhinosinusitis when there are ≥4 episodes per year of acute bacterial sinusitis without clinical manifestations of rhinosinusitis between the episodes.

- Allergy skin testing can be considered in patients with chronic sinusitis or recurrent acute rhinosinusitis.

- Nasal polyps can recur after surgical removal.

- Oral glucocorticoids can not only reduce inflammation, but also reduce the size of nasal polyps.

- Patients that have a combination of asthma, chronic rhinosinusitis with nasal polyposis, and sensitivity to aspirin or other COX-1 inhibiting NSAID (eg, ibuprofen, naproxen) have a condition referred to as aspirin exacerbated respiratory disease (AERD) or Samter's triad. Following ingestion of aspirin or COX-1 inhibiting NSAID, patients can develop ocular symptoms (eg, watery eyes), nasal symptoms (eg, nasal congestion), flushing, chest tightness, wheezing, cough, or headaches. Patients should avoid COX-1 inhibiting NSAIDS or undergo aspirin desensitization followed by aspirin therapy. Once desensitized, patients can ingest other COX-1 inhibiting NSAIDS, but patients must continue to take a daily aspirin or NSAID to maintain desensitization.

- **On the CCS**, if you decide to consult an otorhinolaryngologist, remember to implement a course of action before the consultant is able to see your patient.

# MOUTH AND THROAT DISORDERS

## ▌CROUP

Croup, also referred to as laryngotracheitis or laryngotracheobronchitis (ie, if the illness extends to the bronchi) is a respiratory illness that is typically caused by viruses. The most common type of virus is the **parainfluenza virus type 1**, which is responsible for most of the fall and winter epidemics. Other viruses that can cause croup include parainfluenza type 2 and type 3, RSV, influenza, rhinovirus, adenovirus, human bocavirus, and measles. Once the virus infects the nasal or pharyngeal mucosa, the infection progresses to the larynx and trachea. Inflammation can cause subglottic narrowing of the airway producing the classic "steeple sign" on x-ray.

### Clinical Features:

Croup is typically seen in children that are between 6 months and 3 years old. The clinical onset of croup is usually gradual. Patients may initially present with a prodrome of a low-grade fever, cough, sore throat, nasal congestion, or rhinorrhea. Within 1 to 2 days, patients will typically progress to the classic manifestations of croup, which include a "**barking (brassy) cough,**" **hoarseness**, and **inspiratory stridor**. On exam, two important features to be concerned about are **chest wall retractions** and **stridor at rest**, which indicates significant upper airway obstruction. Keep in mind that children have smaller airways compared to adults, and therefore children can rapidly deteriorate from an airway obstruction.

### Next Step:

**Step 1)** The best initial step is to approach the patient carefully since any anxiety can worsen the airway obstruction. Keep the child calm and comfortable by having him or her sit on the caretaker's lap.

**Step 2)** The diagnosis of croup is made on clinical assessment. Laboratory tests and imaging is usually unnecessary in the initial evaluation.

**Step 3)** Treatment of croup depends on the severity of the condition and the clinical setting (ie, ED, home, office). Consider the following management approach:

**Mild Disease**

- Patients with mild disease may have a brassy cough and hoarseness, but **without stridor at rest**.
- Patients managed at home may only require supportive care such as humidified air (mist therapy), antipyretics, and proper fluid intake.
- Patients seen in the ED or office may recommend supportive care as well as providing a single dose of oral dexamethasone.

**Moderate—Severe Disease**

- Patients with moderate to severe disease may appear more anxious, exhibit **stridor at rest**, or have chest wall retractions.
- Monitor patients with a pulse oximetry, and if hypoxemic ($O_2$ saturation <92% on room air), then provide humidified oxygen. If nonhypoxemic, then provided humidified air.
- Provide nebulized epinephrine to improve airway edema.
- Provide glucocorticoids in oral, intravenous, or intramuscular routes of administration.
- Dexamethasone is commonly used for croup and is available in the PO, IV, and IM forms. Inhaled steroids given as nebulized budesonide can be used as an alternative in patients who are vomiting.

**Disposition/Follow-Up:**

Patients should be observed in the ED for at least 3 hours after the last nebulized epinephrine since the effects of the epinephrine last less than 2 hours and patients can experience a "rebound phenomenon" where the patient appears to be worsening. Patients that fail to improve despite medical therapy (eg, more than 2 treatments of epinephrine) should be admitted to the hospital. Soon after discharge from the hospital, all patients should be seen by their primary care physician for a follow-up visit.

**Pearls:**

- Croup is usually a self-limited condition that resolves within 3 to 7 days.
- A biphasic inspiratory and expiratory stridor can be heard if there is a critically fixed airway obstruction.
- Leukocytosis can sometimes be seen in patients with croup. On the differentials, a lymphocytosis is suggestive of a viral cause, while elevated band neutrophils may indicate a bacterial etiology for the croup.
- All routes of administration (ie, PO, IV, IM) of dexamethasone to treat croup are equally effective. Inhaled budesonide has also been shown to be as effective as oral or parenteral dexamethasone.

- Patients with mild, moderate, or severe symptoms of croup all benefit from the use of steroids.
- The clinical efficacy of mist therapy (humidified air) is still unproven; however, the humidified air may provide a sense of comfort and may prevent the airway secretions from drying out.
- Mist tents (croup tents) should be avoided since they can increase the anxiety of the child.
- Nebulized epinephrine can be given as either racemic epinephrine (which has both D- and L-isomers) or as L-epinephrine. Either type is acceptable since there is no significant difference in the response to treatment between the two formulas.
- Decongestants and antitussives are not recommended because of their unproven benefit in the management of croup.
- Patients in the hospital that require ongoing epinephrine treatments should have cardiac monitoring.
- Spasmodic croup (recurrent croup) is characterized by croup-like symptoms but without fever, occurs at night, has an abrupt onset, abrupt cessation, short duration, and recurrent episodes, and patients usually feel okay between the attacks. The etiology is still unclear, but it is thought that a virus may still trigger the event or there may be an allergic mechanism in patients with atopic diseases. Treatment is usually focused on comforting the child with humidified air. Nebulized epinephrine and corticosteroids are generally not indicated.
- Impending respiratory failure can be a complication of croup. The child may appear cyanotic, with decreased consciousness, decreased chest wall retractions, and stridor at rest. Patients should be prepared for an emergent intubation.
- Patients with croup may demonstrate a distended hypopharynx during inspiration on a lateral neck x-ray. On posterior-anterior chest x-ray, the subglottic narrowing (steeple sign) may not always be seen and is not pathognomonic for croup since it can also be seen in bacterial tracheitis.
- **CJ:** A 3-year-old boy presents to the ED with stridor, fever, brassy cough, and hoarseness. On exam, the patient appears toxic, with no drooling, and the patient prefers to lie flat during the evaluation. You decide to administer nebulized epinephrine and a single dose of dexamethasone. The patient does not respond to the second treatment of nebulized epinephrine. You decide to order a lateral neck and AP x-ray that demonstrates subglottic narrowing and irregular tracheal margins. Your working diagnosis has changed to bacterial tracheitis, and you decide to consult an otolaryngologist. An otolaryngologist sees your patient and decides to go to the operating room with the patient for sedation, intubation, and bronchoscopy. Endoscopy reveals purulent secretions. Specimens for Gram's stain and cultures (aerobic and anaerobic) are obtained from suctioning of the tracheal membranes. Your next step is to treat with antibiotics, and the patient does not have any known drug allergies. What is the initial choice of antibiotics pending the results of the cultures? **Answer:** Bacterial tracheitis (bacterial croup) can be a primary or secondary infection (usually after a viral infection).

The most common cause of bacterial tracheitis is from *Staphylococcus aureus*. Clindamycin plus a third-generation cephalosporin (eg, ceftriaxone, cefotaxime) or clindamycin plus ampicillin-sulbactam are acceptable choices. In areas of increasing MRSA, vancomycin can be substituted for clindamycin.

- **Foundational point**—Epinephrine works by causing vasoconstriction of the precapillary arterioles, which leads to a decrease in capillary hydrostatic pressure causing fluid resorption with improvement of the mucosal edema.
- **On the CCS**, be cognizant about transferring the patient to the appropriate setting (ie, if the patient becomes intubated, be sure to transfer to the ICU for continued monitoring).
- **On the CCS**, "comfort patient" is available in the practice CCS.
- **On the CCS**, suboptimal management include delaying treatment in patients with croup that are in respiratory distress since neither laboratory tests nor imaging are necessary to make the diagnosis.
- **On the CCS**, keep in mind that if the patient has poor oral intake, consider other routes of administration of a medication other than the oral form.

# PERITONSILLAR ABSCESS

Peritonsillar abscess (PTA), also referred to as quinsy, is a polymicrobial accumulation of pus in the peritonsillar space. It is thought that the development of a PTA begins with an infection (ie, tonsillitis or pharyngitis) that progresses into a peritonsillar cellulitis and then into an abscess. In the absence of a preceding infection, obstruction of the Weber glands (ie, salivary glands that clear the tonsillar area of debris) resulting in a local cellulitis have been implicated in the formation of a PTA.

## Clinical Features:

Peritonsillar abscess commonly occurs in older children and adolescent, although it can occur at any age. Patients may present with a fever, unilateral sore throat for several days, trismus, muffled voice ("hot potato"), odynophagia, drooling (ie, difficulty swallowing their saliva), or ipsilateral referred otalgia (ie, secondary from neck swelling). On exam, findings may reveal a medial and inferior displacement of the tonsil, deviated uvula away from the involved side, and an edematous soft palate.

## Next Step:

**Step 1)** The diagnosis of peritonsillar abscess is usually made on clinical assessment. Laboratory tests and imaging are usually unnecessary in patients that have displacement of the tonsil with a deviated uvula.

**Step 2)** Treatment of a PTA involves supportive care (eg, antipyretics, analgesics, adequate hydration), antibiotics, and drainage of the abscess via needle aspiration, incision and drainage, or tonsillectomy. Cultures and gram staining of the abscess fluid should be obtained at the time of drainage followed by empiric antibiotics that can be altered pending the

results of the cultures and sensitivities. Acceptable choices of empiric antibiotics include either IV clindamycin or IV ampicillin-sulbactam. If the patient is able to tolerate oral intake, either oral clindamycin or oral amoxicillin-clavulanate can be given for a 14-day course.

## Disposition:

If the patient is discharged from the ED, arrange follow-up care within 24 hours of an aspiration to reassess any reaccumulation of pus and to assess the patient's well-being since further testing (ie, CT with contrast) or drainage procedures might be necessary.

## Pearls:

- Bilateral peritonsillar abscess is uncommon.
- Drooling or pooling of saliva is also seen in epiglottitis.
- CT with IV contrast will reveal a hypodense fluid collection with ring enhancement in patients with a PTA. CT may also reveal spread of infection into other deep neck spaces.
- A CT with IV contrast is a reasonable option in children that lack cooperation or who present with trismus that prevents an adequate intraoral examination.
- When comparing needle aspiration to I&D, there is no difference in outcome.
- Tonsillectomy is typically performed in patients with recurrent infections (eg, tonsillitis, pharyngitis, PTA) or upper airway obstructions (eg, sleep apnea).
- Although most PTAs are polymicrobial, the most common bacteria isolated is Group A Streptococcus (GAS). Other bacteria that are present include anaerobes, *Staphylococcus aureus*, and *Haemophilus* species.
- **CJ:** A 10-year-old boy presents to the ED with fever, right-sided sore throat for 7 days, drooling, and right-sided ear pain. On intraoral exam, there is marked erythema of the soft palate, but without uvula deviation or displacement of the tonsils. What is your next step? **Answer:** It is often difficult to differentiate a peritonsillar cellulitis from a peritonsillar abscess. A peritonsillar cellulitis will not form a discrete collection of pus, and you won't be able to palpate a fluctuant mass. The patient can be admitted to the hospital for a 24-hour treatment of IV antibiotics. Patients with a peritonsillar cellulitis will usually respond to antibiotics, but antibiotics alone are generally not sufficient to treat a true abscess.
- **On the CCS**, "ampicillin-sulbactam," "amoxicillin-clavulanate," and "clindamycin" are available in the practice CCS.
- **On the CCS**, the initial vital signs in every CCS case will give you a clue whether a case might be acute or non-life threatening.

# STREPTOCOCCAL PHARYNGITIS

*Streptococcus pyogenes* (Group A β-hemolytic Streptococcus, GAS) is the most common cause of bacterial pharyngitis, however, viruses are still the more common cause of acute pharyngitis.

## Clinical Features:

GAS is primarily seen in the age group of 5 to 15 years old and uncommonly seen in children <3 years old. The peak incidence of GAS typically occurs during the winter and early spring seasons. It should be noted that there is no single sign or symptom that can reliably predict the etiologic agent (ie, virus vs bacteria). However, the following features of GAS may include an abrupt clinical onset, fever, sore throat, lack of cough, nausea, vomiting, abdominal pain, or headache. On exam, there may be tonsillar exudates, tender anterior cervical lymphadenopathy, or palatal petechiae (petechiae can also be seen in viral infections).

## Next Step:

**Step 1)** The diagnostic approach for GAS pharyngitis is not definitively established. However, the diagnostic tests used to identify GAS are a rapid antigen detection test (RADT) or a throat culture. Both tests require specimens by swabbing the back of the throat. The throat culture is considered the gold standard, but results can take 24 to 48 hours, which would be more problematic for a culture follow-up in the ED setting. RADT can provide results in a shorter time and permit earlier administration of antibiotics if warranted. If the RADT result is positive for GAS, then proceed with antibiotic therapy. If the RADT result is negative for GAS, then proceed with a throat culture for children and adolescents (adults do not need a follow-up culture given the lower prevalence of GAS in this age bracket).

**Step 2)** Treatment of GAS pharyngitis is with antibiotics. Antibiotics can reduce the symptom duration, transmission, and complications (ie, acute rheumatic fever). Consider the following antibiotics:

> **Option 1:** Oral penicillin V × 10 days
>
> **Option 2:** Oral amoxicillin × 10 days
>
> **Option 3:** Single IM dose of penicillin G benzathine for potentially noncompliant patients.
>
> **Option 4:** Macrolides can be given to patients with allergies to beta-lactam antibiotics (ie, penicillin, cephalosporins). Consider oral erythromycin or clarithromycin for 10 days or azithromycin for 5 days.

## Follow-Up:

Clinical improvement should be seen within 3 days after initiating antibiotics. Patients that fail to respond to antibiotics should have a follow-up visit for further investigation.

## Pearls:

- Suppurative complications of GAS pharyngitis include mastoiditis, peritonsillar abscess, sinusitis, and otitis media.
- Nonsuppurative complications of GAS pharyngitis include post streptococcal glomerulonephritis and acute rheumatic fever.
- GAS pharyngitis is a self-limiting condition even without the use of antibiotic therapy. Symptoms typically resolve within 5 days, but antibiotics will hasten the recovery.

- Initiating antibiotic therapy for GAS pharyngitis can prevent acute rheumatic fever, but there is lack of evidence that it can prevent poststreptococcal glomerulonephritis.
- Group C and group G streptococci can also cause pharyngitis, but it does not cause acute rheumatic fever.
- Do not initiate empiric antibiotics prior to collecting your specimens since giving antibiotics before your collection may give you a false negative result.
- Clinical features that may indicate a viral pharyngitis include coryzal symptoms (rhinovirus, coronavirus), conjunctivitis (adenovirus), splenomegaly (EBV), ulcerations and vesiculations (HSV, Coxsackie A virus which can cause herpangina), stomatitis (HSV), or cough and myalgias (influenza).
- Continuous antimicrobial prophylaxis (penicillin V, penicillin G benzathine, or sulfadiazine) should be given to patients with a history of rheumatic fever or evidence of rheumatic heart disease (eg, rheumatic mitral stenosis) to prevent recurrent rheumatic fever (ie, secondary prevention).
- RADT has a high specificity (>95%) but variable sensitivities (70%-90%).
- Antistreptolysin O (ASO) streptococcal antibodies typically peak between the fourth and fifth weeks following a streptococcal pharyngitis. The ASO titers then begin to decline over the next several months.
- Serologic testing with the ASO titers may be useful when considering streptococcal sequelae (ie, rheumatic fever) but not in the evaluation of acute pharyngitis.
- **Foundational point**—*Streptococcus pyogenes* is a group A, beta-hemolytic, catalase-negative, bacitracin sensitive, facultative, gram-positive coccus that grows in chains. This organism is involved in skin infections (eg, necrotizing fasciitis, cellulitis, erysipelas, impetigo), streptococcal pharyngitis, scarlet fever, streptococcal toxic shock syndrome, rheumatic fever (type II hypersensitivity), and poststreptococcal glomerulonephritis (type III hypersensitivity).
- **Foundational point**—Microbiologic features of *Streptococcus pyogenes* include streptokinase (converts plasminogen to plasmin, which then degrades fibrin into fragments), hyaluronidase (hydrolyzes hyaluronic acid), DNAase (hydrolyzes DNA), NADase (hydrolyzes NAD), streptolysin S (lyses RBCs, nonantigenic, $O_2$ stable), streptolysin O (lyses RBCs, antigenic, $O_2$ labile), M-protein (helps evade phagocytosis, but antibodies can bind to M-protein and aid in opsonization), lipoteichoic acid (component of cell wall), protein F (adherence factor), and pyrogenic exotoxins (also called erythrogenic toxins).
- **Foundational point**—Similar to staphylococcal toxins (ie, TSST-1), pyrogenic exotoxins can act as superantigens by binding to both T cell receptors and MHC class II molecules on the antigen presenting cell and causing T cell proliferation and secretion of cytokines (IL-1, IL-6, IFN-gamma, TNF-alpha, and TNF-beta).
- **Foundational point**—*Streptococcus pyogenes* (pus-producing) and group C and G streptococci can produce streptolysin O, which is a membrane-damaging extracellular toxin.

The O stands for oxygen-labile, which is inactivated by oxygen but reactivated by thiol compounds. Streptolysin O can destroy red blood cells, hence β-hemolytic. On blood agar, a clear zone can be seen when *Streptococcus pyogenes* is cultured on the plate. Since streptolysin O is antigenic, antibodies will develop, hence, ASO antibodies.

- **Connecting point** (pg. 258)—Know the other types of streptococci.

- **Connecting point** (pgs. 8, 9)—Know the other types of hypersensitivity reactions.

- **Connecting point** (pg. 12)—Remember that if a test has a high specificity, it is most likely going to test negative for a disease with fewer false positive results. Therefore, if a test with high specificity comes back positive for a condition, it helps to establish a diagnosis. However, a negative test result does not rule out the condition.

- **Connecting point** (pg. 30)—Patients that have rheumatic mitral stenosis should receive prophylactic antibiotics to prevent rheumatic fever.

- **CJ:** An 18-year-old male comes to your office, and you strongly suspect streptococcal pharyngitis. You decide to do a throat culture and initiate empiric amoxicillin while the results of the culture are pending. After 2 days of antibiotic treatment, the patient notices a maculopapular rash over the trunk of his body. What does your clinical suspicion tell you? **Answer:** Patients with infectious mononucleosis can develop a rash following administration of amoxicillin or ampicillin. Obtaining a "Monospot" test would show reactive heterophile antibodies, which would be consistent with an EBV infection.

- **On the CCS**, keep a targeted physical exam in this type of case. An example in this case would be to do general appearance, lymph nodes, HEENT, chest, heart, and abdomen.

- **On the CCS**, "rapid strep screen" and "throat culture, Streptococcus" are both available in the practice CCS.

# 16

# Psychiatry

## KEYWORDS REVIEW

**Circumstantial speech**—A roundabout discussion, but eventually gets back to the original point.

**Coprolalia**—Obscene words.

**Copropraxia**—Obscene gestures.

**Countertransference**—A clinician's counter emotional reaction (usually unaware) to a patient's response when the

patient unconsciously transfers his or her feelings onto the clinician, usually based on unresolved childhood conflicts (eg, resentment toward parents).

**Echolalia**—Repeating a word or phrase just spoken by another person.

**Echopraxia**—Mimicking movements of another person.

Fugue—In Latin, it refers to "flight." As seen in dissociative fugue, a person takes flight to another location (similar to a "fugitive").

Global Assessment of Functioning (GAF)—GAF is part of the Axis V in the evaluation of patients and is given a score from 1 to 100. For a general guideline, a score of 1 represents danger to themselves or others, a score of 50 represents severe impairment in functioning, and a score of 100 represents superior functioning. (**DSM-5 Alert:** The multiaxial system is removed from the DSM-5 and has transitioned into a nonaxial documentation of diagnosis [formerly Axes I, II, and III] with separate notations for psychological and contextual factors [formerly Axis IV] and disability [formerly Axis V]. The GAF is removed from DSM-5 and is replaced with WHODAS for disability assessment. For board purposes, GAF is retained in this section because the transition to the DSM-5 might not have been implemented on the large pool of exam questions).

Hyperlexia—The precocious ability to read well without prior training. As seen in autism, individuals may read well, but with little comprehension.

Ideas of reference—The perception that the world is "referencing" the patient through special messages. *Delusions of reference* are similar in content, but the false beliefs are held with greater conviction.

Neologisms—Creating new words.

Palilalia—Repeating their own word or phrase.

Peregrinate—Travel

Stereotypy—Repetition of a meaningless act.

Tangential speech—The discussion is off-course and never gets back to the original point.

Trichotillomania—A compulsive urge to pull out one's own hair.

Word salad—Words thrown together that make no sense.

---

# ANXIETY DISORDERS

Anxiety disorders are serious mental illnesses that can be characterized by emotions of fear and anxiety.

**DSM-5 Alert:** Obsessive-compulsive disorder (OCD), posttraumatic stress disorder (PTSD), and acute stress disorder are no longer part of anxiety disorders.

## ❚ PANIC DISORDER

Panic disorder is an anxiety disorder than can be characterized by recurrent, spontaneous panic attacks.

**DSM-5 Alert:** Agoraphobia is now a separate codable diagnosis (ie, agoraphobia has diagnostic criteria and can occur irrespective of panic disorder). According to the DSM-5 criteria, diagnosis of agoraphobia can be made if (**1**) there is marked fear or anxiety about ≥2 of the 5 situations (public transportation, open spaces [eg, farmers' market], closed spaces [eg, theater], being in a crowd, being outside of the home alone), (**2**) fears or avoids situations because of thoughts that escape would be difficult or help would not be available in the event of developing symptoms, (**3**) fear or anxiety is always provoked from agoraphobic situations, (**4**) agoraphobic situations are avoided, tolerated with intense fear or anxiety, or require a companion, (**5**) fear or anxiety is out of proportion to the actual danger, (**6**) emotions (eg, fear, anxiety) or behavior (eg, avoidance) is ≥6 months, (**7**) the disturbance impairs functioning in important areas (eg, work, school, relationships), (**8**) emotions (eg, fear, anxiety) or behavior (eg, avoidance) is clearly excessive even in the presence of co-morbid conditions, and (**9**) the disturbance cannot be explained by another mental disorder.

Clinical Features:

Panic disorder can occur at any age but typically peaks in late adolescence or later in the third to fifth decade of life. The first panic attack is usually unexpected, with anticipatory anxiety for the following attacks. The panic attacks typically last 20 to 30 minutes, but rarely more than 1 hour. Panic disorder can be accompanied by agoraphobia, but they would be considered two separate diagnoses according to the DSM-5. A **panic attack** is characterized as having an intense fear for a discrete period of time with ≥4 of the following symptoms that develop abruptly and peak within minutes. It may be helpful to remember these symptoms in a head to toe fashion:

**Neuro**—Dizziness, trembling, paresthesias, chills or heat sensations, light-headedness

**Psych**—Fear of dying, fear of going crazy, sense of choking, sense of shortness of breath, derealization, depersonalization

**Cardiac**—Palpitations, chest pain, sweating, ↑ HR

**GI**—Nausea, GI upset

Next Step:

**Step 1)** A thorough history and physical is important to rule out any organic causes. Limited diagnostic testing may be appropriate and may include a TSH, CBC, BMP, EKG, CXR, urine toxicology screen, and pulse oximetry.

**Step 2)** The diagnosis of panic disorder is established when all of the following occur:

- Patient has recurrent, unexpected panic attacks
- Following the attacks, ≥1 month of having a maladaptive change in behavior, worried about the consequences, or persistent fear of having more attacks.

**Step 3)** Provide reassurance and educate patients that they are not "going to go crazy."

**Step 4) Short-term management:** Patients that are having a panic attack can be given benzodiazepines (eg, alprazolam, clonazepam). Benzodiazepines can be given for a short period of time and may serve as a bridge before a clinical response to SSRIs (can take 4-8 weeks). Caution is advised for patients who are elderly, are substance abusers, or have respiratory disorders.

**Step 5) Long-term management:** Cognitive behavioral therapy (CBT) **and/or** SSRIs. Alternatives to SSRIs include TCAs (eg, clomipramine, imipramine) and MAO inhibitors (eg, phenelzine). Patients that respond to pharmacotherapy should continue for at least 1 year after the symptoms are controlled.

### Follow-Up:

Panic disorder is a chronic illness with a variable course. Ongoing support and care is important as well as awareness of other comorbid conditions.

### Pearls:

- Panic disorder is associated with major depressive disorder, social phobia, specific phobia, generalized anxiety disorder, PTSD, OCD, substance abuse, personality disorders, and hypochondriasis.
- **On the CCS,** remember to "bridge" your therapy by addressing any acute issues along with the long-term care of the patient.
- **Clinical snapshot:** A 52-year-old woman develops recurrent chest pain, palpitations, tingling sensations in her fingers, and feeling extremely warm within several minutes every time she sits in her comfortable reclining chair. For the past 2 months, she now worries about having a heart attack if she sits in the reclining chair.

## ▌GENERAL ANXIETY DISORDER

General anxiety disorder (GAD) is characterized by excessive worrying about many things without a focus on specific items, which causes significant distress and impairment in important areas of functioning.

### Clinical Features:

The anxiety and worry that patients have with GAD are associated with symptoms that can be easily remembered into motor or cognitive domains. Consider the following symptoms:

**Motor**—Muscular tension, restlessness, fatigability

**Cognitive**—Poor concentration, irritability, sleep disturbances

### Next Step:

**Step 1)** A thorough history and physical are important with emphasis on ruling out caffeine intoxication, stimulant abuse, alcohol, and anxiolytic withdrawal. Limited diagnostic testing may be appropriate and may include a TSH, CBC, BMP, EKG, and urine toxicology screen.

**Step 2)** The diagnosis of GAD is established when all of the following occur:

- **Excessive anxiety and worry** about a number of events or activities for **at least 6 months**
- Difficulty controlling the worry
- **≥3 symptoms** (see Clinical Features)

**Step 3)** Management of GAD may include behavioral therapy **and/or** medications.

**CBT**—Components of CBT for GAD may include relaxation techniques, biofeedback, and education.

**SSRIs**—Onset of action is within 1 week, but a full response may not be evident for up to 4 to 8 weeks.

**Buspirone**—Buspirone can take up to 2 to 4 weeks for a clinical response.

**Benzodiazepines**—Benzodiazepines can be used as a short-term therapy and concomitantly with either SSRIs or buspirone to serve as bridge until the other meds take effect. Caution is advised for patients that are elderly, are substance abusers, or have respiratory disorders.

### Follow-Up:

GAD is a chronic illness that may be lifelong. Be aware that patients may seek many specialists for their complaints.

### Pearls:

- **GAD = Excessive worry + ≥3 symptoms + 6 months**
- Generalized anxiety disorder is associated with major depressive disorder, dysthymic disorder, social phobia, specific phobia, panic disorder, and substance abuse.
- **Clinical snapshot:** A 24-year-old premedical student has had difficulty concentrating in his premedical classes for the past year because he is worried about his academic performance. He is constantly tapping his legs on the ground during lectures, and he has difficulty falling asleep at night. He does not have any other medical condition and does not use caffeine or substances to keep him up. He lives 1 hour away from his family and is constantly worried about their well-being. He is also worried about his own health because of the demands of getting into medical school. He has tried exercising as an outlet to control his symptoms and to improve his health, but without success. He has seen his primary care physician and a neurologist for his sleep disturbances.

# TRAUMA- AND STRESSOR-RELATED DISORDERS

**DSM-5 Alert:** Trauma- and stressor-related disorders is a new category of mental disorders that include PTSD, acute stress disorder, reactive attachment disorder, disinhibited social engagement disorder, and adjustment disorders.

## ▌POSTTRAUMATIC STRESS DISORDER

PTSD is a mental disorder that develops from a traumatic stressor that results in psychological trauma.

**DSM-5 Alert:** The diagnostic criteria have changed significantly from the DSM-IV. Please refer to Step 1 to compare these changes. The following changes include (1) the diagnostic criteria can now be applied to children older than 6 years old with a different diagnostic criteria for children ≤6 years old, (2) the traumatic event is now explicit if the patient experienced directly, witnessed, or experienced indirectly (eg, learning of an event that occurred to somebody close to him or her), (3) the traumatic event no longer involves a response of intense fear, helplessness, or horror, (4) the traumatic event can now specifically include sexual violence, (5) the traumatic event can now include a recurring exposure that can be applied to first responders or police officers, (6) the numbing of general responsiveness is removed, (7) a new cluster is added that retains most of the numbing symptoms and is referred to as negative alterations in cognitions and mood (eg, feeling detached, loss of interest, inability to remember important information regarding the event, persistent negative emotions, persistent and exaggerated negative beliefs, inability to experience positive emotions, distorted cognitions about the cause), and (8) reckless or self-destructive behavior is added to heightened arousal. For board purposes, the DSM-IV criteria are retained in this section because the changes might not have been implemented on any given test.

### Clinical Features:

The onset of PTSD can occur shortly after the traumatic event or can be delayed as long as 30 years. Traumatic events may include war, physical abuse, sexual abuse, terrorist events, natural disasters, car accidents, plane crashes, severe physical injury, or medical complications.

### Next Step:

**Step 1)** The diagnosis of PTSD is established when all of the following occur:

- Experiencing a **traumatic event** that causes intense fear, helplessness, or horror. In addition, the individual experiences or witnesses an event that involves actual or threatened death or serious injury.
- Constantly **reexperiencing** the event (eg, images, dissociative flashbacks, symbolic cues, dreams).
- **Avoiding** anything associated with the event and **numbing of general responsiveness** (eg, feeling detached, loss of interest, restricted range of affect, inability to remember important information regarding the event, avoiding feelings, thoughts, or places related to the event).
- **Hyperarousal** (eg, startled, irritability, angry outbursts, hypervigilance, sleep disturbances, poor concentration).
- Duration of symptoms **>1 month**.
- **Impaired functioning** in important areas (eg, work, school, relationships).

**Step 2)** Following the traumatic event, support and education are important especially to destigmatize the idea that PTSD is an unworthy condition.

**Step 3) Short-term management:** Patients that have acute, severe symptoms of hyperarousal or anxiety immediately following the traumatic event can be temporarily treated with benzodiazepines (eg, lorazepam). Benzodiazepines should not be continued once the acute episode has resolved.

**Step 4) Long-term management:** Patients may require both pharmacologic therapy and psychotherapy when either modality is ineffective as a monotherapy. First-line pharmacologic therapies are the SSRIs (eg, sertraline, paroxetine). Remember that the clinical response to SSRIs can take up to 4 to 8 weeks. If medication is effective, the medication can be continued for at least 6 months to a year to prevent relapse. Psychotherapies may include CBT, psychodynamic psychotherapy, or eye movement desensitization and reprocessing (EMDR). In addition to the individual psychotherapies, family therapy and group therapy may be beneficial.

### Follow-Up:

PTSD is usually a chronic condition requiring ongoing support. Approximately one-third of patients with PTSD will never fully recover.

### Pearls:

- A good prognosis usually occurs in the setting of a good social support system, rapid engagement of treatment, short onset and duration of symptoms, good premorbid functioning, and absence of substance abuse and other psychiatric conditions.
- **Foundational point**—Benzodiazepines facilitate the inhibitory actions of GABA, which triggers the opening of chloride channels leading to an increase in chloride conductance.
- **On the CCS**, remember to "bridge" your therapy by treating the acute stages of PTSD with the long-term care of PTSD.
- **Clinical snapshot:** A 32-year-old Chicago firefighter sustained second and third degree burns over 80% of his body. He has been recovering over the past 3 months at a burn medical center. As he looks out his hospital room window, he sees hospital employees lighting up a cigarette with smoke over their heads. The patient becomes startled and quickly looks away. The patient knows exactly what time of day to avoid looking outside. He's had these symptoms for more than one month.

## ▌ ACUTE STRESS DISORDER

Acute stress disorder (ASD) is an anxiety disorder that develops within the initial month of a traumatic stressor and can potentially progress to PTSD after one month.

**DSM-5 Alert:** The diagnostic criteria have been updated. Please refer to Step 1 to compare these changes. The following changes include **(1)** the traumatic event is now explicit if the patient experienced directly, witnessed, or experienced indirectly (eg, learning of an event that occurred to somebody close to him or her), **(2)** the traumatic event no longer involves a response of intense fear, helplessness, or horror, **(3)** the traumatic event can now specifically include sexual violence, **(4)** the traumatic event can now include a recurring exposure that can be applied to first responders or police officers, **(5)** ≥9 symptoms from any of the five categories that include intrusion symptoms (eg, intrusive distressing memories, recurrent distressing dreams, flashbacks, reactions to internal or external cues), negative mood (eg, inability to experience positive emotions), dissociative symptoms (eg, dazed, inability to recall information from the event, having a different perspective from the environment or oneself), avoidance symptoms (eg, avoiding feelings, thoughts, or places related to the event), and arousal symptoms (eg, startled, irritability, angry outbursts, hypervigilance, sleep disturbances, poor concentration), and **(6)** duration of symptoms is 3 days to 1 month after the event. Keep in mind that acute stress disorder cannot be diagnosed until 3 days after the stressor. For board purposes, the DSM-IV criterias are left in place because the transition to the DSM-5 criteria might not have been implemented on the large pool of exam questions.

### Clinical Features:

The onset of ASD symptoms typically occurs within the first few days or weeks after the traumatic event. Similar to PTSD, the traumatic event can be a horrible experience for the patient. The two main differences between PTSD and ASD are the duration of symptoms (see step 1) and the presence of at least three dissociative symptoms.

### Next Step:

**Step 1)** The diagnosis of ASD is established when all of the following occur:

- Experiencing a **traumatic event** that causes intense fear, helplessness, or horror
- **Reexperiencing** the event

- **Avoidance** of stimuli
- **Hyperarousal**
- Onset of symptoms must occur **within 4 weeks** of the traumatic stressor, and the duration of symptoms occurs for **at least 2 days**, but **no longer than 4 weeks**.
- **Impaired functioning** in important areas (eg, work, school, relationships).
- Experience at least **3 dissociative symptoms** from the following "**5 D's**":
  1) **Detached** (ie, feeling numb)
  2) **Dazed** (ie, feeling "out of it,")
  3) **Derealization** (ie, feeling separated from the external environment)
  4) **Depersonalization** (ie, feeling separated from one's body)
  5) **Dissociative amnesia** (ie, inability to recall information)

**Step 2)** Following the traumatic event, provide support and education.

**Step 3)** First-line treatment is early intervention with trauma-focused CBT to reduce the likelihood of developing PTSD. Benzodiazepines can be given following the traumatic event to help with anxiety or sleep disturbances.

### Follow-Up:

Patients experiencing ASD should be seen closely for the first month to ensure that they are provided with therapeutic treatment.

### Pearls:

- It is not clear why some patients with ASD develop PTSD and others do not.
- **Connecting point** (pg. 231)—Know the different dissociative disorders and symptoms.
- **Clinical snapshot:** A 27-year-old woman was carjacked one week ago. Over the past week, she has had difficulty with reading newspapers, avoids driving, dreams of the event in her sleep, cannot recall the sequence of events while awake, feeling dazed, has flashbacks, easily startled, and avoids talking to friends or family about the event. She states to her therapist, "I feel a sense of cloudiness every day where I'm on top of the clouds."

# OBSESSIVE-COMPULSIVE AND RELATED DISORDERS

**DSM-5 Alert:** Obsessive-compulsive and related disorders is a new category of mental disorders that include OCD, body dysmorphic disorder, hoarding disorder, trichotillomania (hair-pulling disorder), excoriation (skin-picking) disorder, substance/medication-induced obsessive-compulsive and related disorder, and obsessive-compulsive and related disorder due to another medical condition.

## ▌ OBSESSIVE-COMPULSIVE DISORDER

It may be helpful to think of OCD as a "mental-behavior" disorder. The mental component is intrusive thoughts, and the behavior component is compulsive acts or repetitive behaviors to alleviate the distress associated with the thoughts.

**DSM-5 Alert:** OCD is no longer part of anxiety disorders. Changes to the OCD criteria include (1) the presence of obsessions, compulsions, or both to make the diagnosis of OCD, (2) the removal of "obsessions are not simply excessive worries about real-life problems" and the "individual recognizes that the obsession are a product of his or her mind" (see step 1), (3) different degrees on the spectrum of insight with specifiers described as poor insight (retained from DSM-IV), good or fair insight, or absent insight/delusional beliefs, and (4) addition of a tic-related specifier for OCD since patients may have a comorbid tic disorder.

Clinical Features:

The onset of obsessions or compulsions can occur together or separately. If the compulsions occur with the obsessions, the compulsion may not always alleviate the distress associated with obsession. Examples of concurrent obsessions-compulsions include fear of contamination—constantly washing, doubts—constantly checking, need for symmetry—constantly arranging, and unwanted sexual or aggressive thoughts—always praying.

Next Step:

**Step 1**) The diagnosis of OCD is established when all of the following occur:

- Presence of **obsessions *or* compulsions**.
- The obsessions are recurrent, the individual tries to suppress the obsessions, the obsessions are not simply excessive worries about real-life problems, and the individual recognizes that the obsessions are a product of his or her mind.
- The compulsions are acts of repetitive behaviors and the acts are aimed at reducing the distress.
- Patients recognize that the obsessions or compulsions are irrational.
- Impairment in normal life functioning (eg, work, school, relationships), the disturbance is time-consuming (>1 hour a day), and the disturbance causes marked distress to the individual.

**Step 2**) Management of OCD may include behavioral therapy **and/or** medications.

　　**CBT**—Components of CBT for OCD include exposure and prevention, cognitive therapy, and education.

　　**SSRIs**—SSRIs (eg, fluoxetine, fluvoxamine) are typically better tolerated than clomipramine.

　　**TCA**—Clomipramine can cause dry mouth, sedation, constipation, and orthostatic hypotension.

Follow-Up:

OCD is a chronic illness that requires ongoing care. Although symptoms may improve with treatment, patients may experience a waxing and waning of their symptoms during their lifetime.

Pearls:

- Side effects of SSRIs include sexual dysfunction, weight gain, agitation, insomnia, orthostatic hypotension, nausea, GI discomfort, and QTc prolongation.

- **Clinical snapshot:** A 32-year-old man is always late to work because he takes at least 2 hours to shave his face because he strives for extreme precision. He is preoccupied about the symmetry of how he shaves one side of his face compared to the other side.

# BODY DYSMORPHIC DISORDER

Body dysmorphic disorder can be characterized as having a preoccupation with a nonexistent bodily defect. However, if there is actually a slight defect, the concerns are overly excessive.

**DSM-5 Alert:** Body dysmorphic disorder is no longer categorized as a somatoform disorder. Changes to body dysmorphic disorder include (1) additional criterion that describes repetitive behaviors (eg, mirror checking, skin picking) and mental acts (eg, comparing appearance with others), (2) addition of degrees of insight specifiers (poor, good or fair, or absent insight/delusional beliefs), and (3) addition of a muscle dysmorphia specifier (preoccupied that his or her body build is too small or insufficiently muscular).

Clinical Features:

Patients with body dysmorphic disorder will feel some type of "ugliness" with some body part, even though they look completely normal. They may feel that other people are noticing their assumed flaw. The preoccupation usually involves the face (eg, ears, nose, chin, hair) or sexual parts (eg, breast, genitals). The body part may change during the course of the disorder. The preoccupations can be time consuming and can lead to social and occupational impairments.

Next Step Treatment:

**Step 1**) Physicians should know that reassurance or compliments will not alleviate the patients' concerns. Even dermatologic or plastic surgical procedures will typically be unsuccessful.

**Step 2**) Primary treatment usually consists of SSRIs (eg, fluoxetine) and CBT.

Follow-Up:

Patients on SSRIs should have monitoring of any side effects such as sexual dysfunction, sleep disturbances, nausea, diarrhea, agitation, or weight gain.

Pearls:

- Common age of onset is between 15 and 30 years old.
- Women are typically more affected than men.
- Patients are unlikely to get married.
- Body dysmorphic disorder is a chronic disease that typically waxes and wanes over time.
- **Clinical snapshot:** A 28-year-old woman who recently underwent a rhinoplasty still feels that there is a defect with her nose. She is homebound most of the time because she is worried about being ridiculed about her nose.

# DISSOCIATIVE DISORDERS

Dissociative disorders are a group of mental disorders that affect the patients' consciousness, memory, identity, or awareness of their environment (see Table 16-1). An easy way to remember dissociative disorders is that patients are dissociated from a sense of self or environment.

**DSM-5 Alert:** Changes to dissociative disorders include (1) dissociative fugue is no longer a separate diagnosis but rather a specifier to the diagnosis of dissociative amnesia, (2) derealization (feeling detached from the environment) is added to depersonalization disorder and the condition is now named depersonalization/derealization disorder, and (3) dissociative identity disorder may be reported or observed, gaps in the recall of events may occur for everyday events (not just traumatic events), and the disruption of identity may include descriptions in some cultures as an experience of possession. For board purposes, dissociative fugue is retained in Table 16-1 in the event that the exam continues to reflect DSM-IV.

## Table 16-1 • Dissociative Disorders

|  | Dissociative Amnesia | Dissociative Fugue | Dissociative Identity Disorder | Depersonalization Disorder |
|---|---|---|---|---|
| **Clinical features** | The inability to recall important personal information that is usually of a stressful or traumatic nature. Patients are usually aware that they have lost their memories. The memory loss can be short term (hours to days) or a lifetime experience. | **Sudden**, unexpected travel from home or one's workplace. When they arrive at the new location, patients assume a new identity or are confused about their personal identity. They forget everything in the past and are usually unaware of their forgetfulness. When they return to their former selves, they don't remember the fugue, but they can remember the time of onset of the fugue. | The presence of two or more identities within one person. There can be five to ten personalities, but at least two are taking control of the behaviors. Personalities can be of different ages, races, or sexes. Personalities can be aware of each other, and sometimes they can be friends or adversaries. Patients are unable to recall personal information. | **Recurrent** feelings of detachment from one's body or thought process, even in the presence of intact reality testing. Patients frequently encounter detachment from the external environment (derealization) such as normal-appearing objects that are changing shape. |
| **Next step treatment** | Treatment of choice is with psychotherapy augmented with either hypnosis or drug-assisted interviews (eg, thiopental). | Similar to dissociative amnesia, psychotherapy with hypnosis or drug-facilitated interviews. | Treatment involves insight-oriented psychotherapy. Antidepressants and antianxiety meds may serve as an adjunct to psychotherapy. Antipsychotics are rarely indicated. | There is no effective treatment. Antianxiety agents are sometimes used in these patients since anxiety usually accompanies this condition. |
| **Pearls** | • Occurs more often in women than in men.<br>• More common in young adults than older adults.<br>• Confabulation is an adaptive strategy to cover up their memory loss. | • Patients that have mood disorders, histrionic personalities, borderline personalities, and schizoid personalities are predisposed to the development of dissociative fugue.<br>• Travel is usually purposeful.<br>• Patients usually live quiet, modest lives.<br>• Patients often have experienced a traumatic event in their lives. | • This disorder is also known as multiple personality disorder.<br>• Women are affected more than men, but in children, boys are more likely to be affected than girls.<br>• Patients often have experienced a previous traumatic event, especially physical or sexual abuse. | • Usually occurs between the ages of 15 and 30 years.<br>• Comorbid conditions include anxiety disorders, OCD, depression, avoidant personality and borderline personality. |
| **Clinical snapshots** | A 22-year-old teacher was found on a park bench. She could not remember her home address. As a young girl, she would run to the park whenever there was domestic violence at home. | A 45-year-old video store clerk from Chicago suddenly left, leaving behind his wife and children. After several months, an anonymous tip found him in L.A. working in a bookstore. | During therapy, the therapist engages all seven personalities in a 37-year-old woman who was sexually abused by her uncle. The therapist can now reintegrate the different personalities to control her behaviors. | The patient replies to the therapist, "I feel like I'm in a dream. I'm here, but I'm really not here. My right hand feels ten times bigger than my left hand." |

# SOMATIC SYMPTOM AND RELATED DISORDERS

**DSM-5 Alert:** Somatic symptom and related disorders is a new category that includes factitious disorder, somatic symptom disorder, illness anxiety disorder, conversion disorder (functional neurological symptom disorder), and psychological factors affecting other medical conditions. The diagnosis of somatization disorder, hypochondriasis, and pain disorder have been removed in DSM-5, but for board purposes these topics will remain in this section in the event that the exam continues to reflect DSM-IV.

## ▌ FACTITIOUS DISORDER IMPOSED ON SELF

Factitious disorder imposed on self can be characterized by the perpetrator's deliberate act of causing deception by creating or exaggerating an illness.

**DSM-5 Alert:** Factious disorder imposed on self is a new term but it is still coded and diagnosed as a factitious disorder. In addition, the motivation for the behavior to assume the sick role that was seen in DSM-IV is now removed from DSM-5. For board purposes, the new terms seen in DSM-5 will be applied to this chapter to reflect the transition to include both DSM-IV and DSM-5 terminology on the exam.

**Clinical Features:**

The deceptive behavior is usually apparent even when the external rewards are not clearly evident (eg, money, shelter, avoiding legal responsibility). One of the motivations for the deceptive behavior is to assume the sick role. Perpetrators will **intentionally produce** medical or mental disorders, or they will **pretend** to have the disorders. The signs and symptoms of the intended disorder can be predominantly psychological or physical. If both types are present but neither predominates, then it is considered a mixed presentation. Examples of physical signs may include hematoma, hypoglycemia, hemoptysis, hematuria, rigid abdomen, intentional dehiscence, seizures, or self-trauma. Examples of psychological symptoms may include depression, conversion symptoms, suicide, homicide, or hallucinations. It should be noted that drug-seeking behavior may be part of the profile such as seeking psychoactive drugs or analgesics.

**Next Step:**

**Step 1)** Know that with every negative test that is returned to you, the patient may become more hostile.

**Step 2)** Request to interview the patient's reliable sources such as family or friends to uncover the nature of the patient's condition. If consent is not given, this may be a clue to the diagnosis.

**Step 3)** There is no specific therapy for factitious disorder. However, you should treat the self-induced injury and protect patients from self-harm or harm to others if they presented with suicidal or homicidal tendency.

**Follow-Up:**

Perpetrators will usually have familiarity with the medical jargon and will present the problem cleverly. However, an astute physician may have a sense that the patient is not truthful based on a careful history and prior diagnostic results (ie, clinical judgment).

**Pearls:**

- Munchausen syndrome is a chronic and dramatic variant of factitious disorder with predominantly physical signs and symptoms. These patients are characterized by having dangerous manipulations of the body (eg, surgery, excessive warfarin), move from place to place (peregrinate), and make false claims about their accomplishments or relationships with famous people (pseudologia fantastica).

- **Clinical snapshot:** A 25-year-old woman has punched herself in the face causing a black eye. She was seen in the emergency department and stated that a friend accidentally hit her with her elbow.

## ▌ FACTITIOUS DISORDER IMPOSED ON ANOTHER

Factitious disorder imposed on another can be characterized by the perpetrator's deliberate act of causing deception by creating or exaggerating an illness onto another person.

**DSM-5 Alert:** Factious disorder imposed on another replaced the previous term, factitious disorder by proxy. Factitious disorder by proxy was coded and diagnosed as factitious disorder not otherwise specified in DSM-IV, but it is now coded and diagnosed as a factious disorder in DSM-5.

**Clinical Features:**

The deceptive behavior is usually apparent even when the external rewards are not clearly evident. The victim is under the care of the perpetrator and is usually a child but may be an adult. The perpetrator will **intentionally produce** medical or mental disorders or will **pretend or fabricate** a disorder through the victim. The perpetrator usually appears concerned about the victim in the hospital, is well liked by the medical staff, and has familiarity with the medical terminology. Examples of induced conditions include bleeding, vomiting, diarrhea, seizures, apnea, fever, or rashes.

**Next Step:**

**Step 1)** Know that it can be difficult to prove that the perpetrator is causing the condition.

**Step 2)** Suspicion should arise when there is a discrepancy between the history and physical exam, the patient is not responding to treatment as expected, or additional problems occur after the perpetrator is told that the victim is improving.

**Step 3)** When factitious disorder imposed on another is suspected, the goal is to ensure the safety of the victim. Children may be admitted to the hospital to ensure their safety and to be treated for their induced condition. In addition, child protective services, social services, or law enforcement may be required to facilitate the safety of the victim.

**Follow-Up:**

Measures must be in place to prevent the perpetrator from fleeing with the victim once it has been revealed that factitious disorder imposed on another is present.

**Pearls:**

- When the perpetrator is separated from the victim, the problem usually resolves.
- The perpetrator is usually more concerned about his or her own welfare than about the actual victim.
- **Clinical snapshot:** A 37-year-old nurse who has diabetes has been crushing her metformin tablets into the food of her 10-year-old son. Her son has been having diarrhea, nausea, vomiting, and gas. After a negative medical workup, the primary care physician is still perplexed.

## CONVERSION DISORDER

Conversion disorder can be characterized as "converting" into a condition that is not "real" and causes considerable dysfunction in the patient.

**DSM-5 Alert:** Conversion disorder can now synonymously be called functional neurological symptom disorder. Modification to the conversion disorder criteria include **(1)** the incompatibility between the symptom and recognized neurological or medical conditions based on clinical findings, **(2)** the diagnosis can be specified with or without a psychological stressor, which demonstrates the importance that psychological factors may or may not be present at the time of diagnosis, **(3)** the diagnosis can be specified by the duration of symptoms (ie, <6 months is considered an acute episode and ≥6 months is considered persistent), and **(4)** the DSM-5 no longer requires that the symptom is not intentionally produced or feigned.

**Clinical Features:**

The symptoms or deficits typically affect voluntary **motor** or **sensory function**, which suggests a neurological component, but cannot be explained by a known neurological or medical disorder. A psychological component is usually associated with the symptoms or deficits. Common examples of conversion disorder include mutism, paralysis, blindness, pseudoseizures, anesthesia, paresthesia, deafness, tunnel vision, gait disturbances, tics, and tremors. The DSM-IV required that symptom is not intentionally produced or feigned.

**Next Step Treatment:**

**Step 1)** Know that the symptoms of conversion disorder usually resolve spontaneously.

**Step 2)** Maintain a therapeutic alliance with the patient and acknowledge the reality of the symptoms. Telling patients that their symptoms are imaginary often worsens their condition.

**Step 3)** Psychotherapy may be helpful.

**Follow-Up:**

In the majority of cases, the symptoms will resolve within a few days or in less than a month. However, the longer the symptoms persist, the worse the prognosis.

**Pearls:**

- The lack of concern about the impairment (la belle indifférence) has been associated with conversion disorder, but it is an inaccurate way to determine if the patient has conversion disorder because it is nonspecific for the condition.
- Approximately 25% of patients will have another episode in a setting of another stressor.
- Conversion disorder can sometimes be confused with somatization disorder because conversion conditions can be seen in somatization disorder.
- **Clinical snapshot:** A 17-year-old girl who was recently dumped by her boyfriend states that she feels a lump in her throat. After a negative examination, the physician acknowledges her symptoms and asks her to come back in a week for a follow-up visit.

## SOMATIZATION DISORDER

Somatization disorder is characterized by many somatic symptoms that are not medically explainable.

**DSM-5 Alert:** Somatization disorder is removed from DSM-5. A new disorder in DSM-5 is called somatic symptom disorder. Patients previously diagnosed with somatization disorder may meet the diagnosis for somatic symptom disorder if they also have maladaptive thoughts, feelings, and behaviors. The diagnostic criteria for somatic symptom disorder include **(1)** ≥1 somatic symptom causes significant disruption in his or her daily life, **(2)** the excessive thoughts, feelings, and behaviors of the somatic symptom cause a persistent high level of anxiety, take excessive time and energy devoted to the symptoms, or include persistent thoughts of the symptoms, and **(3)** persistent symptoms (ie, not all symptoms may be necessarily continuous) that usually last >6 months. In addition, the diagnosis can be specified with pain (previously pain disorder). For board purposes, somatization disorder is retained in this chapter because the changes might not have been implemented on any given test.

**Clinical Features:**

The onset of the physical complaints is **before the age of 30**. The following conditions can occur at any time and must meet the **"4-2-1-1"** (easily remembered by pager number 4-2-1-1):

**4 pain symptoms**—Examples include pain related to the head, chest, abdomen, back, joints, extremities, dysmenorrhea, dyspareunia, dysuria, dyschezia.

**2 gastrointestinal symptoms**—Examples include nausea, vomiting, diarrhea, gas, bloating (note that there is no pain-related symptom).

**1 sexual symptom**—Examples include erectile or ejaculatory dysfunction, irregular menses, excessive menstrual bleeding (note that there is no pain-related symptom).

**1 pseudoneurological symptom**—Conversion type conditions such as blindness, deafness, double vision, aphonia, hoarseness, seizures, amnesia, hallucinations, imbalance, paralysis, muscle weakness, fainting, lump in the throat.

**Next Step Treatment:**

**Step 1**) Establish a single physician as the primary caretaker.

**Step 2**) Acknowledge any new complaint and reassure that the most serious disease is ruled out.

**Step 3**) Limit diagnostic or therapeutic interventions unless they are clinically warranted.

**Step 4**) Educate patients on how to cope with their physical symptoms.

**Step 5**) Consider psychotherapy, especially CBT.

**Step 6**) Schedule relatively brief monthly visits.

**Follow-Up:**

Follow up with other physicians since most patients will go "doctor shopping" and unnecessary, costly tests will be ordered.

**Pearls:**

- There is **no pretending or intention** in somatization disorder.
- **Clinical snapshot:** A 20-year-old woman who has a history of back pain, menometrorrhagia, constipation, diarrhea, left leg pain, and pain during sexual intercourse is in your office following a negative workup for her chest pain. She was speaking to your office staff prior to going into the examination room. As you ask her questions, she is now completely mute.

# HYPOCHONDRIASIS

Hypochondriasis can be characterized as having a preoccupation with having a serious medical illness despite appropriate medical reassurance.

**DSM-5 Alert:** Hypochondriasis is removed from DSM-5. Patients previously diagnosed with hypochondriasis who have high anxiety about their health, but without moderate to severe somatic symptoms can now be diagnosed with illness anxiety disorder, which is a new DSM-5 disorder. For board purposes, hypochondriasis is retained in this chapter because changes might not have been implemented on the large pool of exam questions.

**Clinical Features:**

The fear of having a serious medical condition usually arises from a misinterpretation of bodily symptoms or functions. For example, normal abdominal pressure may be perceived as abdominal pain. Despite a negative medical workup, patients believe that they have a particular disease that will continue to persist. Over time, the belief may actually be transferred to another disease. The belief must last at least **6 months** for a diagnosis.

**Next Step Treatment:**

**Step 1**) Know that most patients may be resistant to psychiatric treatment.

**Step 2**) Establish a single physician as the primary caretaker.

**Step 3**) Acknowledge the patient's symptoms, provide consistent reassurance, and have a nonjudgmental stance.

**Step 4**) Psychotherapy is considered first-line treatment.

**Step 5**) Schedule regular visits to reassure patients that they are not being abandoned.

**Follow-Up:**

Follow up with other physicians since most patients will go "doctor shopping" and unnecessary, costly tests will be ordered.

**Pearls:**

- Patients will be convinced that they have a specific disorder, but their beliefs are not so rigidly fixed as to be a delusional disorder.
- **Clinical snapshot:** After a negative workup for colon cancer, a 55-year-old man is still convinced that he has colon cancer after 8 months. He states that he has "thin caliber stools" and he read somewhere on the Internet that people with colon cancer can have these kinds of stools.

# PAIN DISORDER

Pain disorder is characterized by having pain as the primary complaint in one or more body part that cannot be fully attributed to a known medical disorder. The pain is sufficient to cause social and occupational impairments.

**DSM-5 Alert:** Pain disorder is removed as a separate diagnosis and now used as a specifier for the diagnosis of somatic symptom disorder in DSM-5. For board purposes, pain disorder is retained in this chapter because the changes might not have been implemented on any given test.

**Clinical Features:**

Pain disorder can be divided into two main subtypes:

1) **Pain disorder with a psychological component**—The psychological component plays a major role in the onset, severity, exacerbation, or maintenance of the pain. The duration can be acute (<6 months) or chronic (>6 months).

2) **Pain disorder with a psychological component + general medical condition**—Both the psychological component and the general medical condition play important roles in the onset, severity, exacerbation, or maintenance of the pain. The duration can be acute (<6 months) or chronic (>6 months).

**Next Step Treatment:**

**Step 1**) Know that the patients' experience of their pain is real.

**Step 2**) Empathize with the patients' suffering, and do not confront them (ie, do not say, "Your pain is not real").

**Step 3)** Educate patients that there is a link between psychological factors causing psychogenic pain.

**Step 4)** Psychotherapy may be helpful.

**Step 5)** Treat comorbid conditions (eg, SSRIs for depression).

**Follow-Up:**

Maintain regular follow-ups since the pain disorder can be chronic and disabling. Ensure that patients have the coping skills to deal with their symptoms since the overall goal is bring them back to a functioning level by reducing their social and occupational impairments.

**Pearls:**

- There is **no pretending or intention** in pain disorder.
- Judicious use of analgesics should be maintained because long-term analgesic treatment can lead to substance abuse.
- Be vigilant in patients that might have a substance abuse problem since patients will use alcohol and other substances to reduce their pain.
- Associated conditions include anxiety disorders and depressive disorders (eg, major depression, dysthymia).

- Pain disorder can sometimes be confused with somatization disorder since pain is part of the "4-2-1-1." However, in pain disorder, the psychological component must be significantly involved in the pain symptoms.
- Pain disorder without a psychological component, but with an associated general medical condition is not considered a mental disorder.
- Examples of a psychological component may include trauma, abuse, stressors in the family, finance, occupation, or academics.
- **Clinical snapshot:** A 52-year-old restaurant manager has been seen in the office for low back pain for the past 10 months. He is becoming socially withdrawn and starting to skip work. He has a negative medical workup for any serious medical condition, and he has tried physical therapy, heating pads, massage therapy, and ibuprofen with minimal success. Upon questioning his family history, he reveals that his brother to whom he had been very close died 1 year ago. With every family gathering since his brother's passing, his back pain seems to worsen the following day.

# PERSONALITY DISORDERS

Personality disorders are grouped into three clusters, and these mental disorders reflect a deeply ingrained way of thinking and behaving that is very different from the patient's culture's expectations and that can lead to impaired functioning in work, school, or relationships (see Table 16-2).

## Table 16-2 • Personality Disorders

| Type | Clinical Features | Next Step Behavioral Approach | Clinical Snapshots |
|---|---|---|---|
| **Cluster A—"Eerie"** | | | |
| **Paranoid—"Distrust"** | • Suspicious<br>• Reluctant to confide in others<br>• Misinterprets benign remarks<br>• Bears grudges | Clinical interaction should be honest, straightforward, and apologetic if appropriate. | A 70-year-old woman is constantly accusing her husband of infidelity with another woman. |
| **Schizoid—"Detached"** | • No interest in relationships<br>• Appears cold and aloof<br>• Lacks friends and sex | The clinician should have a calm and reassuring stance. | A 32-year-old man lives in a rural area and has no friends in his town. |
| **Schizotypal—"Odd"** | • Magical thinking<br>• Eccentric behavior<br>• Odd speech<br>• Ideas of reference, but the false beliefs are not firmly fixed<br>• Paranoid ideation | Maintain a nonjudgmental stance. | A 45-year-old man wears a hat and sunglasses while watching TV because he believes that the messages are directed at him. |
| **Cluster B—"Emotional"** | | | |
| **Antisocial—"Trouble"** | • Disregard for others<br>• Deceitful<br>• Irresponsible, impulsive<br>• Conduct disorder before age 15<br>• Must be at least age 18 | Set firm behavioral limits. | A 22-year-old man who has been in and out of jail states that he has no remorse for stealing a woman's purse. |

*(Continued)*

## Table 16-2 • Personality Disorders (Continued)

| Type | Clinical Features | Next Step Behavioral Approach | Clinical Snapshots |
|---|---|---|---|
| **Borderline—"Splitting"** | • Splits (ie, sees people as all good or all bad)<br>• Intense and unstable relationships<br>• Inappropriate anger<br>• Impulsive (eg, sex, drugs, spending)<br>• Suicidal and self-mutilating behavior<br>• Feeling empty all the time | 1) Politely confront the patient that no one is all good or all bad.<br>2) Have good communication with all the medical staff.<br>3) Be aware of countertransference, which can impair clinical judgment.<br>4) Be able to establish clear boundaries with respect to treatment and behavior toward others. | A 35-year-old woman treats the nursing staff with disrespect but acknowledges the treating physician as a "superb doctor." |
| **Histrionic—"Dramatic"** | • Seductive<br>• Attention-seeking<br>• Speech lacks detail<br>• Emotionally labile | Be professional and avoid any close relationships. | A 25-year-old woman wearing a provocative dress is seen by a young male ED resident for knee pain. She is quick to draw up her dress to show her knee and begins to flirt with him. |
| **Narcissistic—"Entitlement"** | • Grandiosity<br>• Fantasies of success or ideal love<br>• Exploitative<br>• Envious<br>• Excessive admiration<br>• Empathy is lacking | Be professional, avoid being defensive, and be able to tolerate the patient's character. | A 59-year-old judge is requesting to be transferred to another inpatient room. He states that because he is a judge and has a "special" role in society, he demands a cleaner and better room. |
| Cluster C—"Edgy and Embarrassed" | | | |
| **Obsessive-compulsive personality disorder (OCPD)—"Perfectionist"** | • Preoccupied with orders and rules<br>• Organized<br>• Overconscientious<br>• Stingy and stubborn<br>• Devoted to work<br>• Reluctant to delegate tasks<br>• Unlike other personality disorders, OCPD patients are aware of their suffering.<br>• Unlike OCD, there are no obsessive thoughts or compulsive behaviors in patients with OCPD. | 1) Allow patients to be actively involved and take ownership of their healthcare.<br>2) Avoid being authoritative.<br>3) Be aware of countertransference. | A 45-year-old man is unable to discard his old socks that he has had for 3 years even though there is no sentimental value. |
| **Avoidant—"Shy"** | • Fear of disapproval or rejection<br>• Feeling inadequate<br>• Unlike schizoid, patients desire relationships but fear criticism. | Maintain a trusting doctor-patient relationship. Be accepting of the patient's fears of criticism. | A 38-year-old unmarried woman says she begins to tense up while interviewing for a job. She is afraid of being ridiculed for saying something wrong. |
| **Dependent—"Clingy"** | • Difficulty making decisions<br>• Difficulty expressing disagreement<br>• Fear of being alone<br>• Nonproactive because of low self-confidence<br>• Needs support from others<br>• Seeks new relationships when one ends<br>• Submissive | Be alert that patients may withhold information. | A 25-year-old woman is in an abusive relationship with her husband. The husband is the sole provider of the family and makes all the decisions in the household. The patient becomes tense when the clinician discusses her husband. |

# NEURODEVELOPMENTAL DISORDERS

**DSM-5 Alert:** Neurodevelopmental disorders is a new category of mental disorders that include intellectual disabilities, communication disorders, autism spectrum disorder, ADHD, specific learning disorder, and motor disorders (eg, Tourette's disorder, persistent motor or vocal tic disorder, provisional tic disorder). In addition, the term mental retardation used in DSM-IV is now replaced with intellectual disability (intellectual development disorder).

## ▌AUTISM

Autism is characterized by impairments of three major developmental domains: **communication**, **behavior**, and **socialization**. Autism is categorized as a pervasive developmental disorder, a classification that also includes Rett's disorder, childhood disintegrative disorder, and Asperger's disorder (see Table 16-3). The etiology of autism is still unknown.

### Table 16-3 • Pervasive Developmental Disorders (DSM-IV Terminology)

| | Rett's Disorder | Childhood Disintegrative Disorder (CDD) | Asperger's Disorder |
|---|---|---|---|
| **Clinical features** | • Occurs exclusively in **females**.<br>• Initially develops normally, then deteriorates.<br>• Head circumference is normal at birth, then over time there is **deceleration of head growth** that can then result in microcephaly.<br>• Height and weight eventually decline.<br>• **Loss of purposeful hand movements**, replaced by stereotypic hand movements.<br>• **Loss of acquired speech**.<br>• Deterioration in milestones.<br>• Psychomotor retardation.<br>• Poor coordination and gait abnormalities.<br>• Associated conditions include respiratory irregularities, seizures, dementia, scoliosis, cardiac abnormalities, sleep disturbances, and fractures. | • Initially **develops normally for at least the first 2 years** of life, then "disintegrates."<br>• Boys > girls.<br>• Minimum age of onset is 2 years old, with the vast majority occurring between 3 and 4 years old.<br>• Before the age of 10, there is loss of previously acquired skills in any of the following:<br><br>  • Bowel or bladder control<br>  • Language<br>  • Social skills<br>  • Motor skills<br>  • Play<br><br>• Similar to autism, CDD can affect **C**ommunication, **B**ehavior, and **S**ocialization ("**CBS**").<br>• Unlike autism, patients previously acquired normal development in CDD.<br>• Unlike Rett's, there are no hand stereotypies, and onset is usually a little later in CDD.<br>• The main associated condition is seizure disorder. | • Boys > girls.<br>• Asperger's is similar to autism, but the main distinction is the **lack of language delay**. In addition, there is no delay in cognitive development, adaptive behavior, or age-appropriate learning skills.<br>• Individuals can use single words by age 2 and communicative phrases by age 3. However, they have difficulty with a give-and-take conversation (ie, usually one-sided conversation).<br>• Functional use of language may be odd such as using sarcasm inappropriately.<br>• The tone and rhythm of language may be odd such as speaking in a theatrical manner.<br>• Individuals with a normal IQ and high-level social skills are likely to have the best prognosis.<br>• Associated conditions include ADHD, depression, mood disorders, tic disorders, anxiety, and oppositional defiant disorder. |
| **Next step treatment** | No specific therapy for Rett's disorder, but the goal is symptomatic intervention. Antiepileptics for seizures, physiotherapy for muscular dysfunction, medication and behavior therapy for behavioral problems. | Treatment of CDD is similar to autism. There is no known medication that specifically addresses CDD. A multidisciplinary approach is optimal. | Similar to autism, a multidisciplinary approach is required. Patients do better in a structured and organized environment. Initially address depression by nonpharmacologic methods (eg, counseling), if unsuccessful, consider medication. Consider risperidone for disruptive behavior when nonpharmacologic methods are unsuccessful. |
| **Clinical snapshots** | After the first 6 months of apparently normal development, an 18-month-old toddler can no longer say "mama." Her head growth has declined, and she now has frequent hand-wringing. | A 5-year-old boy who previously spoke in sentences can now only speak in fragments. He can no longer draw stick figures, is no longer toilet trained, and no longer accepts hugs from his parents. | A 9-year-old boy with a history of ADHD has repetitive hand flapping and has difficulty with normal reciprocal social interactions. There are no issues with language, but he sometimes speaks to his teachers in a professorlike tone. |

**DSM-5 Alert:** Autistic disorder, Asperger's disorder, Rett's disorder, childhood disintegrative disorder, and pervasive developmental disorder not otherwise specified are no longer separate disorders, but rather compose a new DSM-5 disorder called autism spectrum disorder. Patients previously diagnosed with autistic disorder, Asperger's disorder, or pervasive developmental disorder not otherwise specified can be given the diagnosis of autism spectrum disorder, but those disorders that do not meet the criteria for autism spectrum disorder (eg, Rett's disorder, childhood disintegrative disorder) may need to be evaluated for social (pragmatic) communication disorder, which is a new DSM-5 disorder. Diagnostic criteria for autism spectrum disorder include (1) deficits in social communication and social interactions, (2) restricted repetitive behaviors, interests, and activities, (3) symptoms are present in early development, (4) significant functional impairment (eg, social, work, school), and (5) the disturbance is not better explained by intellectual disability or global developmental delay. In addition, autism spectrum disorder can specified with or without an accompanying intellectual impairment or language impairment. For board purposes, autistic disorder, Rett's disorder, childhood disintegrative disorder, and Asperger's disorder are retained in this chapter because changes might not have been implemented on the large pool of exam questions.

## Clinical Features:

The onset of symptoms of autism occurs by the **age of 3**. Boys are 4 times more affected than girls. In the majority of cases, autistic individuals will have mental retardation with an IQ ≤70. However, in a subset of individuals, they can be "high functioning" with an IQ >70. Regardless of the level of intelligence, some individuals have very special skills (ie, "savant skills") such as an extraordinary ability in mathematics, calendar calculation, puzzles, hyperlexia, singing, playing music, or memorizing and reciting. The three major impairments in autism are **c**ommunication, **b**ehavior, and **s**ocialization, which can be best remembered by the mnemonic "**CBS.**" CBS is a major television network, which is a form of communication. In autism, communication is impaired, behavior is broadcasted in a stereotype pattern, and patients live in a socially isolated system.

### Communication

- Inability to use **language** to communicate
- Both expressive and receptive language are usually affected
- Inability to have a conversation
- Inability to make a sentence even if they have an expansive vocabulary
- Repetitive use of language such as echolalia
- Inability to engage in spontaneous imaginative play

### Behavior

- Preoccupation with a stereotype behavior
- Preoccupation with parts of an object
- Adherence to routines or rituals and resistant to changes or transition

- Stereotyped motor mannerisms such as rocking, hand flapping, or head banging

### Socialization

- Failure to develop peer relationships
- Failure to have normal reciprocal social interactions
- Failure to seek shared enjoyment or achievements with others
- Failure to show social relatedness with nonverbal behaviors such as normal eye-to-eye gaze, facial expressions, or body gestures

### Next Step:

**Step 1)** The diagnosis of autism is a clinical diagnosis that is based on impairments in three key areas: communication, behavior, and socialization, with the onset prior to age 3 years.

**Step 2)** In addition to a comprehensive evaluation, additional assessments may be indicated to identify comorbid conditions. The following conditions are associated with autism:

- Seizures
- Macrocephaly
- Phenylketonuria (PKU)
- Tuberous sclerosis complex (hypopigmented macules)
- Fragile X syndrome (large ears, long face, large testes)
- Angelman syndrome (happy appearance, ataxic gait, language delay)

**Step 3)** There is **no cure for autism**. Family education and counseling is essential since families are often distraught. Management of autistic individuals is with behavioral and educational interventions with the goal of improving overall function. Pharmacologic agents are only used if behavioral and educational interventions are ineffective, and the agents are used to target a specific type of condition (eg, irritability, aggression, self-injury). Only aripiprazole and risperidone are FDA approved for use in children with autistic disorders.

### Follow-Up:

Autistic individuals need ongoing care and require the same routine preventive and screening healthcare as other people.

### Pearls:

- Individuals with a higher IQ and those who can use language by 5 to 7 years of age are likely to have the best prognosis.
- High-functioning individuals can find employment and live independently, while low-functioning individuals usually require dependence and home or residential care.
- To date, there is no evidence to support the association between autism and vaccines, especially the measles, mumps, and rubella (MMR) vaccine.
- To date, there is no evidence to support the association between autism and the mercury-based preservative, thimerosal, which is found in some vaccines.
- **Connecting point** (pg. 162)—Autism can be associated with fragile X syndrome.

- **Clinical snapshot:** A 6-year-old boy with autistic disorder frequently looks from the corner of his eyes. He does not make eye-to-eye contact with anybody. He is preoccupied with shiny surfaces and the edges of a ruler. His parents were concerned about his language development when he was 18 months old because he could only say "mama." At home, he would repeat words that he heard during the school day. He also has a tendency to pinch himself and twist his torso and is resistant to being touched. Now, his parents have to lock the bathroom door because he would flush the toilet all day. At school, he played by himself in the corner of the room. He played with the same toy day after day, and if another child picked up the toy, he would have a tantrum. His parents are receiving family counseling, mostly because they don't feel the same reciprocal family love from him.

## ▌ TOURETTE'S DISORDER

Tourette's disorder is characterized by both involuntary **motor** and **vocal tics** with the onset usually in childhood.

**DSM-5 Alert:** The DSM-5 criteria no longer require a tic-free period of more than 3 consecutive months (see step 1).

### Clinical Features:

Tourette's disorder is 3 times more common in boys than in girls. The motor tic usually emerges by the age of 7, and vocal tics typically appear by the age of 11 years. Examples of the motor component may include body gyrations, eye blinking, head shaking, kicking, grimacing, abdomen tensing, nasal exhalations, nasal flaring, echopraxia, or copropraxia. Examples of the vocal component may include coprolalia, palilalia, echolalia, grunting, sniffing, throat clearing, humming, or clucking.

### Next Step:

**Step 1)** Tourette's disorder is a clinical diagnosis based on the following features:

- Onset before the **age of 18 years**.
- **Both multiple motor and ≥1 vocal tics** are present during the course of the disorder, but they don't have to be present at the same time.
- Tics occur multiple times per day and almost every day for **>1 year** without a tic-free period greater than 3 consecutive months.

**Step 2)** An early part of management is to provide education to the patient, family, and those who interact with the patient.

**Step 3)** Patients that are doing well academically and socially may not require any treatment. On the other end of the spectrum, patients that are having a difficult time academically, professionally, or socially may require some type of intervention. The following therapies are available:

#### Nonpharmacologic Therapy

**Behavioral therapy**—Habit reversal training (HRT) may be effective in some patients.

#### Pharmacologic Therapy

**Antipsychotics**—Haloperidol, pimozide, and fluphenazine can reduce the effects of the tics.

**SSRIs**—SSRIs (eg, fluoxetine) are effective in treating comorbid OCD.

**Stimulants**—Stimulants (eg, methylphenidate, dextroamphetamine) are used in patients with comorbid ADHD.

### Follow-Up:

Patients that are on antipsychotics should be closely monitored for extrapyramidal symptoms (EPS).

### Pearls:

- Up to 30% to 40% of patients with Tourette's disorder will have OCD.
- Up to 50% to 60% of patients with Tourette's disorder will have ADHD.
- Patients with comorbid ADHD are treated with CNS stimulants, but caution is advised because the stimulants can potentially exacerbate preexisting tics.
- Tourette's disorder is a lifelong disease that can wax and wane throughout the course of the disorder.
- **Clinical snapshot:** A 12-year-old boy with a history of ADHD has rapid, recurrent shoulder shrugging and eye blinking that started by age 6. By age 10, he feels compelled to chirp in the classroom. After school, most of his peers tease him, calling him "birdman."

## ▌ PERSISTENT (CHRONIC) MOTOR OR VOCAL TIC DISORDER

Chronic motor or vocal tic disorder is characterized by the presence of a tic for a longer period of time compared to provisional tic disorder.

**DSM-5 Alert:** Chronic motor tic disorder can now synonymously be called persistent motor tic disorder. In addition, the DSM-5 criteria no longer require a tic-free period of more than 3 consecutive months (see step 1).

### Clinical Features:

Unlike Tourette's disorder, patients can only have a motor or vocal tic. In addition, patients cannot have a history of Tourette's disorder.

### Next Step:

**Step 1)** The diagnosis of chronic motor or vocal tic disorder is based on the following features:

- Onset before the **age of 18 years**.
- **Single or multiple motor or vocal tics** are present, not both.
- Tics occur multiple times per day and almost every day for **>1 year** without a tic-free period greater than 3 consecutive months.

**Step 2)** Depending on the severity of the tic and how debilitating it is socially or academically, psychotherapy may be helpful.

**Follow-Up:**

Patients that develop the disorder between 6 and 8 years of age usually do well. Symptoms may last 4 to 6 years and then resolve in early adolescence.

**Pearls:**

- Chronic motor or vocal tic disorder is more common than Tourette's disorder.
- **Clinical snapshot:** A 10-year-old boy has chronic throat clearing for the past 2 years. He does not have any comorbid conditions and he has never been diagnosed with Tourette's disorder.

## ▌ PROVISIONAL TIC DISORDER

Provisional tic disorder is characterized by the presence of tics for relatively short periods.

**DSM-5 Alert:** Transient tic order has been replaced with the name provisional tic disorder. In addition, the DSM-5 criteria no longer require a minimum of 4 weeks, but still require that tics are no longer than 1 year since tic onset (see step 1).

**Clinical Features:**

Similar to Tourette's disorder, patients can have both motor and vocal tics. However, patients cannot have a history of Tourette's disorder or chronic motor or vocal tic disorder.

**Next Step:**

**Step 1)** The diagnosis of transient tic disorder is based on the following features:

- Onset before the **age of 18 years**.
- **Single or multiple motor and/or vocal tics.**
- The time frame is for at least **4 weeks**, but **no longer than 12 consecutive months**.

**Step 2)** The initial step in management is to encourage the family to disregard the tic because focusing attention on the tic may exacerbate the problem. Psychopharmacology is not necessary unless it is causing severe impairment.

**Follow-Up:**

Patients may have complete resolution of their tics, or they may recur during periods of stress.

**Pearls:**

- A small subset of patients can progress to Tourette's disorder or chronic motor or vocal tic disorder.
- **Clinical snapshot:** An 8-year-old boy had echolalia for the past 6 weeks that seemed to abate.

# CLINICAL ATTENTION

The content in this section represents issues that can be seen in clinical practice, but do not represent true mental disorders.

## ▌ MALINGERING

Malingering can be characterized by the perpetrator's objective in achieving a recognizable goal through fabricating signs and symptoms of a medical condition.

**Clinical Features:**

The goal of the perpetrator is to reach external incentives through means of intentionally producing a false medical or mental disorder. External incentives may include avoiding responsibilities (eg, military duty), punishment (eg, criminal prosecution), danger (eg, gang/mobs), difficult times (eg, unemployment), or obtaining rewards (eg, workers' compensation, drugs, free room and board). Once the perpetrators have achieved their goals or realize that it is too dangerous to continue, they can usually stop producing their signs and symptoms.

**Next Step:**

**Step 1)** Suspicion should arise when there is a discrepancy between the history and physical examination, the patient is presented in a medicolegal context, or the patient is uncooperative with care.

**Step 2)** Avoid confronting or accusing the patient of malingering. By not discrediting the perpetrator, the doctor-patient relationship can be preserved and further positive intervention is still possible.

**Follow-Up:**

Care must be taken to avoid hostile behavior from the perpetrator if the malingerer's claims are continually challenged.

**Pearls:**

- Malingering and factitious disorders are voluntarily produced, but not somatoform disorders.
- The objective in malingering is to reach an external incentive through means of a medical problem, but external incentives are absent in factitious disorder.
- Antisocial personality disorder is associated with malingering.
- **Clinical snapshot:** A 32-year-old homeless person is in the emergency department complaining of upper back pain. He is requesting to have pain medication (ie, drug seeking) to alleviate his pain and hoping to stay in the hospital (ie, to get room and board).

# 17

# Pulmonary

## KEYWORDS REVIEW

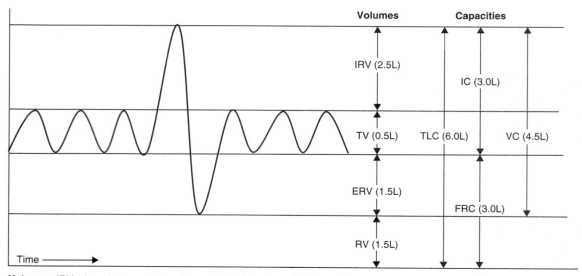

**Volumes:** IRV—inspiratory reserve volume; TV—tidal volume; ERV—expiratory reserve volume; RV—residual volume.
**Capacities:** TLC—total lung capacity; IC—inspiratory capacity; FRC—functional residual capacity; VC—vital capacity.
**Note:** Values are approximates for a 70-kg person.

**Bilevel positive airway pressure (BPAP)**—Also incorrectly referred to as BiPAP, since BiPAP is the name of a portable ventilator device. BPAP is a mode used to deliver a preset inspiratory positive airway pressure (IPAP) and an expiratory positive airway pressure (EPAP).

**Continuous positive airway pressure (CPAP)**—The continuous delivery of airflow throughout the respiratory cycle with no difference in the pressures delivered from inspiration to expiration.

**Expiratory reserve volume (ERV)**—The maximum volume of air that can be expired starting at the end of a normal tidal expiration.

**FEF$_{25\%-75\%}$**—Forced expiratory flow between 25% and 75% of the FVC, or in other words, the airflow halfway through a forced exhale after a maximal inspiration. The FEF$_{25\%-75\%}$ generally indicates the status of medium to small sized airways. Decreased flow rates are usually seen in the early stages of obstructive diseases. However, in restrictive diseases the FEF$_{25\%-75\%}$ values are usually normal. Although abnormal findings may suggest small airway changes, the FEF$_{25\%-75\%}$ should not be used to diagnose small airway disease because of poor reproducibility.

**FEV$_1$**—Forced expiratory volume in one second after a maximal inspiration.

**FEV$_6$**—Forced expiratory volume in 6 seconds, which is sometimes used as a surrogate for FVC.

**Forced vital capacity (FVC)**—The amount of air that can be forcibly expired after a maximal inspiration.

**Functional residual capacity (FRC)**—The volume of air remaining after the tidal volume is expired. FRC cannot be measured by spirometry because it includes the residual volume.

**Inspiratory capacity (IC)**—The volume of air inhaled during a maximal inspiratory effort starting at the end of a normal tidal expiration.

**Inspiratory reserve volume (IRV)**—The maximum volume of air that can be inspired starting at the end of a normal tidal inspiration.

**Peak expiratory flow rate (PEFR)**—The PEFR can be obtained by a handheld device that measures the greatest flow velocity during a forced exhalation starting from a maximal inhalation. PEFR is not sufficient to diagnose asthma, but it is useful for home monitoring in asthma patients because it can detect gross changes in airway function. PEFR is also useful for making bedside assessments in response to bronchodilators, given that there is a baseline PEFR.

**Positive end-expiratory pressure (PEEP)**—The positive airway pressure (alveolar pressure > atmospheric pressure) in the lungs at the end of expiration to help prevent atelectasis. PEEP can be applied by a mechanical ventilator (extrinsic PEEP) or caused by an incomplete exhalation (intrinsic PEEP). Extrinsic PEEP (applied PEEP) can range from 0 to 20 cm $H_2O$ and is usually adjusted in 2.5 to 5.0 cm $H_2O$ increments.

**Residual volume (RV)**—The volume of air that remains in the lungs after a maximal expiration. RV cannot be measured by spirometry.

**Tidal volume (TV)**—The volume of air that is inspired or expired with each normal breath.

Total lung capacity (TLC)—The sum of all 4 lung volumes. TLC cannot be measured by spirometry because it includes the residual volume.

Vital capacity (VC)—The volume of air expired after a maximal inspiration. VC usually decreases with diseases that decrease pulmonary compliance.

# OBSTRUCTIVE DISEASES

## ▌NONACUTE ASTHMA

Asthma is a chronic disorder of the airways that can be characterized by **reversible airway obstruction**, **bronchial hyperresponsiveness**, and an **underlying inflammation**. The cumulative effect of secretions in the airway, mucosal edema, and contraction of the smooth muscle within the bronchial walls result in a decrease in airway diameter with increased airway resistance.

### Asthma Triggers:

**Allergens**—Animal dander, house-dust mites, cockroaches, pollens, mold

**Climate changes**—Cool dry air, hot humid air, barometric pressure changes

**Inhaled irritants**—Smoke, odors, fumes, dust, pollutants, aerosol sprays

**Medical conditions**—Stress, depression, rhinitis, sinusitis, GERD

**Medications**—Nonselective beta-blockers, aspirin, NSAIDS

**Physical activity**—Exercise

**Respiratory infections**—Primarily viral infections

**Sulfite-containing foods**—Dried fruit, processed potatoes, shrimp, wine, beer, pickles, vinegar

### Clinical Features:

The presentation of asthma can vary among individuals from progression of the disease to signs and symptoms. The following are key elements to consider:

**Onset**
- Asthma can occur at any age.
- In the majority of cases, asthma is diagnosed in childhood or by adolescence.
- Asthma can occur in older people, but they will less frequently develop new-onset asthma.

**Pattern**
- Episodic—Patients can be asymptomatic between periods of recurrent symptoms.
- Continual—Patient can have chronic symptoms with intermittent worsening of their symptoms.

**History**
- Previous hospitalizations for asthma.
- Childhood diagnosis of "wheezy bronchitis" or "recurrent bronchitis."
- Inquire about a history of atopic diseases since there is an association between asthma and atopic diseases (eg, atopic dermatitis, allergic rhinitis, food allergy, allergic conjunctivitis).

**Severity**
- The severity of asthma can be classified as intermittent, mild persistent, moderate persistent, and severe persistent (see Table 17-1).

## Table 17-1 • Asthma Severity and Treatment for Youths ≥12 Years Old and Adults

| Normal FEV$_1$/FVC Reference Values | Severity | Lung Function | Symptoms | Nighttime Awakenings | Treatment Initiation |
|---|---|---|---|---|---|
| 8-19 yrs: 85%<br>20-39 yrs: 80%<br>40-59 yrs: 75%<br>60-80 yrs: 70% | **Intermittent** | • FEV$_1$/FVC normal<br>• FEV$_1$ >80% predicted | ≤2 dys/wk | ≤2x/mo | **PRN:** SABA |
| | **Mild persistent** | • FEV$_1$/FVC normal<br>• FEV$_1$ >80% predicted | >2 dys/wk, but not daily | 3-4x/mo | **Option 1:** Low-dose ICS<br>**PRN:** SABA |
| | **Moderate persistent** | • FEV$_1$/FVC reduced 5%<br>• FEV$_1$ 60%-80% predicted | Daily | >1x/wk, but not nightly | **Option 1:** Low-dose ICS + LABA<br>**Option 2:** Medium-dose ICS<br>**PRN:** SABA<br>**Note:** Consider short course of oral corticosteroids |
| | **Severe persistent** | • FEV$_1$/FVC reduced >5%<br>• FEV$_1$ <60% predicted | Throughout the day | Often 7x/wk | **Option 1:** Medium-dose ICS + LABA<br>**Option 2:** High-dose ICS + LABA<br>**PRN:** SABA<br>**Note:** Consider short course of oral corticosteroids, and for patients with allergies consider omalizumab. |

*ICS—inhaled corticosteroid; LABA—inhaled long-acting beta$_2$-agonist; SABA—inhaled short-acting beta$_2$-agonist; wk—week.*
*Note: Assign the severity of the asthma to the most severe category for which any of the three features are present.*

## Symptoms

- Patients may report some or all of the following symptoms:

    **Cough**—Nocturnal cough, recurrent cough during specific seasons, cough in the presence of triggers, or persistent cough (several weeks).

    **Wheeze**—A high-pitched whistling sound may be heard on expiration.

    **Difficulty breathing**—Patients may complain of chronic or acute episodes of shortness of breath (SOB).

    **Chest tightness**—A bandlike constriction will commonly be reported as opposed to a sharp pain.

## Physical Exam

- Physical exam findings may be unremarkable when the patient is asymptomatic, but the presence of abnormal findings becomes more prominent with increasing severity of asthma or during acute exacerbations.

    **Inspection**—An increase in anterior-posterior diameter of the chest due to air trapping; hunched shoulders; use of accessory muscles.

    **Percussion**—Hyperresonant.

    **Auscultation**—Prolong expiratory phase; wheezes typically heard on expiration; wheezes can be heard on both inspiration and expiration as the severity of the obstruction increases and then becomes potentially inaudible with no airflow.

    **Extrapulmonary findings**—Conjunctival congestion (allergic conjunctivitis), eczematous lesions (atopic dermatitis), or pale bluish nasal mucosa with turbinate edema (allergic rhinitis).

Next Step:

**Step 1**) Establishing a diagnosis of asthma involves a careful **clinical assessment** that should determine **(1) episodic symptoms of airflow obstruction are present**, **(2) airflow obstruction is reversible**, and **(3) exclusion of alternative diagnoses**. Pulmonary function testing (PFT) such as a **spirometry** is an objective tool that can establish airflow obstruction, severity, and reversibility. Spirometry can be performed in children ≥5 years of age, and spirometry measurements should be taken before and after administration of a short-acting bronchodilator to assess reversibility. Spirometry results may show the following:

## Airflow Limitation

- $FEV_1$ and $FEV_1/FVC$ (or $FEV_1/FEV_6$) values are typically reduced relative to the predicted or reference values that indicate an airflow obstruction (see Table 17-1).

- Reversibility is indicated by an increase in $FEV_1$ of ≥12% and >200 mL from baseline after inhalation of a short-acting bronchodilator.

## No Airflow Limitation

- Patients may have a normal spirometry test at the time of an evaluation.

- The next step in these patients is to either repeat the spirometry when they are symptomatic or challenge them with a **bronchoprovocation test** with methacholine, mannitol, or exercise to demonstrate reversible airflow obstruction.

**Step 2**) Once the diagnosis has been established, it is important to characterize the severity of the asthma, which will help guide decisions for initiating treatment (see Tables 17-1 and 17-2).

**Step 3**) Educate patients on asthma self-management, which can take the form of a written "asthma action plan" that will

| Table 17-2 • Asthma Medications | | |
|---|---|---|
| Medications | Drug Category | Net Effect |
| **Inhaled Short-acting β2-agonists (SABA)** | | |
| • Albuterol<br>• Levalbuterol<br>• Pirbuterol | Beta₂ agonist | Bronchodilates |
| **Inhaled Long-acting β2-agonists (LABA)** | | |
| • Salmeterol<br>• Formoterol | Beta₂ agonist | Bronchodilates |
| **Inhaled Corticosteroids (ICS)** | | |
| • Beclomethasone<br>• Budesonide<br>• Flunisolide<br>• Fluticasone<br>• Mometasone<br>• Triamcinolone acetonide | Corticosteroid | Anti-inflammatory |
| **Systemic Corticosteroids** | | |
| • Methylprednisolone<br>• Prednisolone<br>• Prednisone | Corticosteroid | Anti-inflammatory |
| **Immunomodulator** | | |
| • Omalizumab | Monoclonal antibody (Binds to IgE) | Mitigates an allergic response to an allergen |
| **Leukotriene Modifiers** | | |
| • Montelukast<br>• Zafirlukast<br>• Zileuton | LTRA<br>LTRA<br>5-Lipoxygenase inhibitor | ↓ bronchoconstriction + ↓ vascular permeability |
| **Methylxanthines** | | |
| • Theophylline | Theophylline derivative | Bronchodilates |
| **Mast Cell Stabilizers** | | |
| • Cromolyn<br>• Nedocromil | Mast cell stabilizer | Modulates mast cell mediator release |

*LTRA—Leukotriene Receptor Antagonist*

help guide patients to recognize and handle worsening asthma and daily management.

## Follow-Up:

Patients should be periodically evaluated for their asthma control. Well-controlled patients may be seen every 1 to 6 months, but uncontrolled asthma patients should be seen more frequently (eg, 2-6 weeks). In addition, patients that are on chronic high-dose inhaled glucocorticoids should be monitored for potential side effects such as thrush, dysphonia, cataracts, or growth velocity deceleration (in children).

## Pearls:

- Not every asthmatic patient will wheeze.
- Bronchoprovocation challenge testing is contraindicated in patients with known aortic aneurysm, myocardial infarction, or stroke in the last 3 months, uncontrolled hypertension, and severe airflow limitation (ie, $FEV_1$ <50% predicted).
- Children are more likely to have complete remission compared to adults; however, children with severe asthma are more likely to continue to have asthma as adults.
- Peak expiratory flow rate (PEFR) can be measured by a peak flow meter, which is a relatively inexpensive, portable device in which the patients draws in a maximal inhalation and then exhales forcefully into the device. PEFR is not particularly useful in detecting airflow limitation, and thus not a primary tool for the diagnosis of asthma, but rather it is used to monitor trends in the patient's lung function.
- The forced expiratory volume in 6 seconds ($FEV_6$) is sometimes used as an approximation for the FVC.
- The diffusing capacity for carbon monoxide (DCLO) is normal to elevated in patients with asthma, but decreased in patients with emphysema.
- The chest x-ray is usually normal or may demonstrate hyperinflation in patients with asthma, but ordering a chest x-ray may be useful for excluding other diagnoses.
- Allergy testing is not useful for the diagnosis of asthma but as a useful adjunct in determining contributing factors to asthma. Allergy testing may be useful in patients with a history of allergies, persistent asthma, and in patients with moderate-to-severe symptoms.
- A spacer or valved holding chamber is attached to the metered dose inhaler (MDI), which is typically recommended for children or any patient that has difficulty with the coordination between actuation and inhalation of the MDI or when inhaled glucocorticoid is being administered.
- By adding a spacer or holding chamber to the MDI, there is some evaporative loss of the propellant (chlorofluorocarbon [CFC] or hydrofluoroalkane [HFA]) that decreases the size of the medication droplets and thereby leads to an increase in smaller particles being inhaled and reduces the amount of medication being deposited in the back of the throat.
- Asthma patients should avoid nonselective beta-blockers (including eye preparations).

- Patients with asthma plus chronic rhinosinusitis with nasal polyposis may experience asthmatic symptoms, conjunctival congestion, nasal congestion, rhinorrhea, and facial flushing upon ingesting a cox-1 inhibitor (eg, aspirin, NSAIDs). This condition is referred to as aspirin exacerbated respiratory disease (AERD).
- Leukotriene modifiers, theophylline, and the mast cell stabilizers are not the preferred agents to treat asthma, but are considered alternative agents.
- Theophylline requires regular drug level monitoring to avoid toxicity, and zileuton requires liver function testing to monitor hepatotoxicity.
- Cromolyn and nedocromil can be used as preventive treatment for either exercise-induced bronchoconstriction or unavoidable exposure to known allergens.
- An inhaled short-acting β2-agonist (SABA) is the preferred prophylactic agent for exercise-induced bronchoconstriction and should be taken 10 minutes before exercise.
- **Foundational point**—Bronchi and bronchioles can be plugged up by mucous plugs. On microscopic findings of the plugs, Curschmann's spirals can be seen. Curschmann's spirals are coiled shed epithelium that can be seen in asthma, bronchitis, and other lung diseases.
- **Foundational point**—Charcot-Leyden crystals can also be found in sputum from patients with asthma or parasitic infections (eg, ascariasis). On microscopic findings of the sputum, Charcot-Leyden crystals appear as needlelike structures with pointed ends. These crystals consist of lysophospholipase, which is an eosinophil-derived enzyme, and their presence indicates an eosinophil response.
- **Foundational point**—Typical lung volume and capacities seen in asthma are normal or ↑ total lung capacity (TLC), ↑ functional residual capacity (FRC), and ↑ residual volume (RV).
- **On the CCS**, it is important to order "advise patient, asthma care" because education is a component of asthma management.
- **On the CCS**, "advise patient, side effects of medication."
- **On the CCS**, if you order "spirometry" to evaluate a patient for asthma, be careful not to order "incentive spirometry," which is used for a breathing exercise, especially after surgery.
- **On the CCS**, it is acceptable to order either "PFT" or "spirometry, flow" to evaluate for asthma, but be aware that the PFTs will provide a more inclusive set of lung function tests compared to the spirometry in the practice CCS.

## ▌ NONACUTE COPD

Chronic obstructive pulmonary disease (COPD) is characterized by a **progressive airflow limitation** that is **not fully reversible**. It is thought that the parenchymal tissue destruction that results in **emphysema** (↓ elastic recoil) and the structural changes of the small airways that result in **obstructive bronchiolitis** (↑ increased airway resistance) are due to a chronic inflammatory response to noxious particles or gases.

## Clinical Features:

### Symptoms

- The three most common symptoms in COPD are cough, sputum production, and exertional dyspnea.

  **Cough**—Chronic cough is usually the first symptom to develop in COPD, which may start as an intermittent cough that then becomes more noticeable throughout the day.

  **Sputum production**—Patients may have a pattern of chronic sputum production that is usually mucoid in appearance but can become purulent during exacerbations.

  **Dyspnea**—Patients may describe their dyspnea as "air hunger" or "heaviness." As COPD advances, the principal feature is dyspnea on exertion, which can then become noticeable even at rest.

### Physical Exam

- Physical exam findings may be unremarkable in the early stages of COPD but becomes more prominent in the presence of significant impairment of lung function.

  **Inspection**—An increase in anterior-posterior diameter due to hyperinflation ("barrel chest"); sitting in the characteristic "tripod" position to facilitate the accessory muscles.

  **Percussion**—Hyperresonant.

  **Auscultation**—Prolong expiratory phase; expiratory wheezes; diffusely decreased breath sounds; coarse crackles on inspiration.

## Next Step:

**Step 1)** A diagnosis of COPD should be considered in any patient who reports any combination of chronic cough, chronic sputum production, dyspnea, and a history of exposure to smoke, dust, or chemicals. Patients who have any of these indicators for COPD should have a PFT such as a **spirometry**. The diagnosis of COPD is confirmed when there is airflow limitation based on the spirometry (FEV1/FVC <0.70), symptoms compatible with COPD, and exclusion of other diagnoses.

**Step 2)** Managing patients with stable COPD involves multiple medical therapies, which include:

### Bronchodilators

- **Inhaled short-acting bronchodilators**—A **short-acting β2-agonists** (see Table 17-2) or a **short-acting anticholinergic** (eg, ipratropium) can be used for symptomatic relief when needed. Combination therapy with both beta agonist and anticholinergic (eg, albuterol/ipratropium) can provide a greater bronchodilator response compared to using a single agent, but monotherapy is still acceptable.
- **Inhaled long-acting bronchodilators**—Either a **long-acting β2-agonists** (see Table 17-2) or a **long-acting anticholinergic** (eg, tiotropium) should be regularly scheduled when the short-acting bronchodilators cannot control the symptoms.

### Pulmonary Rehabilitation

- Pulmonary rehabilitation should be considered in patients that have persistent pulmonary symptoms or have decreased functional status despite optimal medical therapy.

### Smoking Cessation

- Smoking cessation is important because it can reduce the rate of $FEV_1$ decline in smokers with COPD.
- A guideline to help patients quit smoking is: Ask → Advice → Assess → Assist → Arrange.

### Supplemental Oxygen

- Long-term oxygen therapy should be given to patients with a resting arterial oxygen tension ($PaO_2$) ≤55 mm Hg or a pulse arterial oxygen saturation ($SaO_2$) ≤88%.
- In the presence of cor pulmonale, long-term oxygen therapy should be given to patients with a $PaO_2$ ≤59 mm Hg or $SaO_2$ ≤89%.
- Long-term oxygen therapy reduces mortality rates in patients with severe resting hypoxemia.

### Vaccinations

- An annual influenza vaccine should be given to all COPD patients.
- A pneumococcal vaccine should be offered to all patients ≥65 years old or <65 years old with a $FEV_1$ <40%.

**Step 3)** Patient education is an important part of COPD management because it can help improve the patient's health status.

## Follow-Up:

Routine follow-up care is important in patients with COPD. Monitoring airflow (ie, spirometry), symptoms, and functional status can determine when to modify therapy or identify any complications.

## Pearls:

- DCLO is decreased in proportion to the severity of emphysema.
- The chest x-ray is not required to make the diagnosis of COPD, but is still commonly performed. Radiographic features of COPD may reveal hyperinflation of the lungs, increase in retrosternal airspace, and flattening of the diaphragm.
- Pulse oximetry can be used as a simple test to assess for hypoxemia by measuring the arterial oxygen saturation ($SaO_2$).
- An ABG can also assess for hypoxemia by measuring the arterial oxygen tension ($PaO_2$), but also the severity of the hypercapnia. For reference, a patient with mild COPD may only have mild to moderate hypoxemia with no hypercapnia.
- Chronic respiratory acidosis leads to compensatory metabolic alkalosis (ie, ↑ serum bicarbonate).
- Chronic hypoxemia can lead to polycythemia (ie, ↑ hematocrit level).
- When patients continue to have significant symptoms or repeated exacerbations even with the optimal use of a

long-acting bronchodilator, the next best step is to add an inhaled corticosteroid (see Table 17-2) as part of a combination therapy.

- Theophylline (oral or IV) is considered a second-line agent compared to the other bronchodilators.

- Roflumilast is an oral medication (phosphodiesterase-4 enzyme inhibitor) that is used to reduce the frequency of COPD exacerbations.

- Guaifenesin is an oral expectorant that offers little value to patients with COPD.

- Mucolytic agents (eg, acetylcysteine, dornase alfa) should not be used as routine care for patients with stable COPD because long-term studies have been controversial.

- Prophylactic antibiotics are not recommended in patients with stable COPD.

- The short-acting anticholinergic ipratropium can be remembered because of its "immediate" effect, and the long-acting anticholinergic, tiotropium can be remembered because it is "totally longer."

- Surgery may be considered when patients continue to have significant symptoms despite optimal medical therapy and pulmonary rehabilitation. Lung transplantation or a lung volume reduction surgery (for patients with emphysema) may be helpful.

- The definition of chronic bronchitis as a chronic productive cough for 3 months in each of 2 consecutive years with other causes of cough excluded is still used clinically, but is not included in the Global Initiative for Chronic Lung Disease (GOLD) reports.

- Since most COPD patients have a mixture of emphysema and small airway disease, the terms "pink puffer" and "blue bloater" are incorrectly applied because both terms represent pure forms of emphysema and bronchitis, respectively.

- Type A pathophysiology: "Pink puffer," predominantly emphysema, dyspnea, thin, wasted, not cyanotic, $\downarrow PO_2$, normal or $\downarrow PCO_2$, $\downarrow$ elastic recoil, $\downarrow$ DCLO, normal hematocrit, cor pulmonale is infrequent.

- Type B pathophysiology: "Blue bloater," predominantly bronchitis, cough and sputum, obese, cyanotic, $\downarrow\downarrow PO_2$, normal or $\uparrow PCO_2$, normal elastic recoil, normal DCLO, hematocrit is often elevated, cor pulmonale is common.

- **Foundational point**—PFT measurements that are indicative of hyperinflation include a $\uparrow$ TLC, $\uparrow$ FRC, $\uparrow$ RV, $\downarrow$ inspiratory capacity, and $\downarrow$ vital capacity.

- **Foundational point**—In restrictive lung disease, the lung volumes typically show a pattern of $\downarrow$ TLC, $\downarrow$ FRC, and $\downarrow$ RV.

- **Foundational point**—In restrictive lung disease, the $FEV_1$ and FVC are both typically reduced in proportion to decreased lung volumes, resulting in a FEV1/FVC ratio that is normal or increased. In obstructive lung disease, the $FEV_1$ is reduced more than FVC, therefore if the numerator is reduced more than the denominator, the resulting $FEV_1$/FVC ratio is reduced.

- **Foundational point**—Three morphologic forms of emphysema are centriacinar (associated with smoking), panacinar (associated with alpha 1-antitrypsin deficiency), and paraseptal/distal acinar (least common, associated with bullae formation which can lead to spontaneous pneumothorax).

- **Foundational point**—Ipratropium is a quaternary derivative of atropine and when inhaled, it competitively blocks muscarinic receptors in the airway and thereby, prevents vagally mediated bronchoconstriction.

- **On the CCS**, remember to "counsel family/patient" since education is a component of COPD management.

- **On the CCS**, remember to "advise patient, no smoking."

- **On the CCS**, "advise patient, side effects of medication."

# RESTRICTIVE DISEASE

## ASBESTOSIS

Asbestosis is a pneumoconiosis caused by inhaling asbestos fibers (ie, fibrous silicate). The asbestos fibers can be long and curly, which are referred to as serpentine fibers (eg, chrysotile), or fibers can be long and straight and are referred to as amphibole fibers (eg, crocidolite, amosite). Asbestos exposure has been associated with the following:

- Parenchymal interstitial fibrosis
- Pleural plaques
- Pleural thickening
- Pleural effusions
- Small-cell and non-small cell carcinoma of the lungs
- Mesothelioma

**Risk Factors:**

Individuals at risk of developing asbestosis are workers in asbestos mining and milling, textiles, shipyard workers, cement workers, plumbers, electricians, carpenters, insulators, welders, sheet metal workers, pipefitters, steamfitters, boilermakers, power plant workers, workers in brake linings and clutch pads, and individuals exposed to the soiled clothes brought home by an asbestos worker.

**Clinical Features:**

Patients are typically asymptomatic for 20 to 30 years from the time of the initial asbestos exposure. However, it is thought that the duration and intensity influences the latency period. Typically, short-term, high-intensity asbestos exposure is associated with a shorter latency compared to prolonged, lower intensity exposure. Patients may develop any of the following clinical manifestations:

- Dyspnea on exertion is a common symptom.
- End-inspiratory crackles can be fine or coarse, usually at the bases of the lungs.

- Dry, nonproductive cough.
- Clubbing.
- Cor pulmonale is usually seen in advanced disease and can present as jugular venous distention, hepatojugular reflux, and peripheral edema, and a loud $P_2$ heart sound may be heard if there is pulmonary hypertension.

## Next Step:

**Step 1)** Diagnosis of asbestosis is based on evidence of exposure, evidence of pathology consistent with asbestos-related disease, and exclusion of other causes. Diagnostic modalities include the following:

**PFT**—The classic finding is a **restrictive pattern**, although a mixed restrictive and obstructive pattern can sometimes be seen. Characteristic findings include ↓ vital capacity, ↓ TLC, ↓ DLCO, normal ratio of $FEV_1/FVC$.

**Chest X-ray**—Initially, irregular parenchymal opacities begin in the lower lobes bilaterally, and over time, the opacities can be seen in the middle and upper zones of the lung. Abnormal pleural findings on chest x-ray are good indicators of asbestos exposure since pleural findings in other interstitial lung diseases are uncommon.

**High resolution computed tomography (HRCT)**—HRCT is the next best step when PFTs or chest x-ray findings are indeterminate because HRCT is better at delineating pleural plaques, thickening, "rounded atelectasis" due to pleural adhesions, and parenchymal lesions.

**Bronchoalveolar lavage (BAL)**—BAL can detect asbestos fibers and asbestos bodies (ie, fibers coated with protein and iron, which appear as beaded rods with knobbed ends). When inorganic particulates become coated with protein and iron complexes, the generic term *ferruginous bodies* is used.

**Transbronchial biopsy**—Rarely performed to establish a diagnosis since BAL recovers more material and therefore offers a better indicator of tissue burden.

**Step 2)** There is no specific therapy for asbestosis. Managing patients with asbestosis includes the following:

- Withdraw from further asbestos exposure, and report to state or federal agencies
- Smoking cessation

- Prompt attention and treatment of respiratory infections
- Pneumococcal and influenza vaccinations
- Assess the degree of functional impairment because it will determine how closely they need to be monitored (ie, PFT's, chest films, office visits)

## Follow-Up:

Screening patients for lung cancer or mesothelioma with chest x-ray or CT is not recommended because it has not been shown to prevent mortality.

## Pearls:

- There is a higher risk of lung cancer in people who were exposed to asbestos and are smokers since there is a multiplicative effect.
- Asbestos exposure increases the risk of developing malignant mesothelioma.
- It appears that long, straight asbestos fibers (ie, amphibole fibers) are more toxic than long, curly asbestos fibers (ie, serpentine fibers) because they are deposited further into the distal lung tissue and therefore, the rate of clearance is reduced.
- It appears that exposure to amphibole fibers has a higher risk of lung cancer compared to the serpentine fibers.
- Asbestos bodies are not pathognomonic for asbestos since asbestos bodies can be seen in people without known exposure.
- Honeycombing is typically seen in advanced disease.
- When there is a good history of asbestos exposure and chest x-ray findings clearly demonstrate asbestos-related disease, no further imaging is necessary for diagnosis.
- The clinical exam findings in patients with interstitial lung disease are typically nonspecific.
- **Foundational point**—Asbestos bodies can be found inside macrophages in the process of phagocytosis. The iron component of the asbestos body is thought to arise from phagocyte ferritin.
- **On the CCS,** "pulmonary function tests" or "PFT" is available in the practice CCS.
- **On the CCS,** basic chest x-ray films should include both the PA and lateral views.
- **On the CCS,** "bronchoalveolar lavage" or "BAL" is not recognized in the practice CCS.

# VASCULAR DISEASE

## PULMONARY EMBOLISM

Pulmonary embolism (PE) refers to an obstruction of the pulmonary artery or one of its branches by any substance that can travel within the bloodstream such as air, fat, tumor cells, foreign bodies, amniotic fluid, septic emboli, or thrombus. For the remainder of the review, this topic will focus on pulmonary embolism secondary from a thrombus.

## Risk Factors:

Risk factors for pulmonary emboli can be remembered by Virchow's triad:

**Stasis**

Immobility, postoperative state, prolong inactivity during travel, obesity, stroke, paralysis, CHF

**Endothelial Injury**

Surgery, trauma, central venous instrumentation

## Hypercoagulable States

**Acquired conditions**—Medications (eg, OCP, HRT, tamoxifen), pregnancy, smokers, medical illness (eg, malignancy, multiple myeloma, polycythemia, nephrotic syndrome, antiphospholipid syndrome, history of venous thromboembolism, burns)

**Inherited conditions**—Factor V Leiden mutation, prothrombin gene mutation, protein C deficiency, protein S deficiency, antithrombin III deficiency, hyperhomocystinemia

## Clinical Features:

There is no single symptom or sign that is specific to pulmonary embolism. However, commonly reported signs and symptoms include acute onset of dyspnea, pleuritic chest pain, cough, hemoptysis, tachypnea, tachycardia, and rales. Keep in mind that patients can be completely asymptomatic to having clinical features suggestive of a massive PE, which may include any of the following:

- Hypotension
- Syncope
- Cyanosis
- JVD
- Right-sided $S_3$
- Parasternal lift

## Next Step:

**Step 1)** The initial steps to a patient suspected of having a PE is to **stabilize the patient**. Provide supplemental oxygen to patients with hypoxemia, and consider intubation if the patient is in respiratory failure. Intravenous fluids (eg, normal saline) can be carefully given to patients who present with hypotension and appropriate monitoring are important initial steps in caring for the patient.

**Step 2)** Administer empiric anticoagulation in patients for whom clinical suspicion of PE is high. Do not delay treatment in these patients while awaiting diagnostic confirmation for a PE. Patients that have low or moderate clinical suspicion for a PE may proceed with prompt diagnostic investigations for a PE.

**Step 3)** There are several different diagnostic modalities to evaluate a patient with suspected PE. Not every test should be ordered, but for board purposes, it is important to know the different features of each test.

**ABG**—ABG results are nonspecific for PE, but possible findings include hypoxemia, hypocapnia with respiratory alkalosis (due to hyperventilation), or hypercapnia with respiratory acidosis (due to a massive PE causing respiratory collapse). The alveolar-to-arterial $O_2$ partial pressure gradient (A-a gradient) is typically elevated in patients with PE, but a small subset of patients will have a normal A-a gradient.

**Chest x-ray**—Possible findings include a normal chest x-ray, atelectasis, pleural effusions, localized area of decreased vascular markings corresponding to vessel occlusion (Westermark's sign), or a wedge-shaped opacity near the pleural base which represents a pulmonary infarction

(Hampton's hump). Chest x-ray is an appropriate study to rule out other diseases, but it also allows interpretation of the V/Q scan if the scan is going to be ordered in the near future.

**EKG**—Possible abnormalities include sinus tachycardia, nonspecific ST-segment and T-wave changes, $S_1Q_3T_3$ pattern, new incomplete right bundle branch block, RVH, or right axis deviation.

**D-dimer**—D-dimer is a protein that represents a degradation product of cross-linked fibrin, which can be detected in the serum by using different assays (eg, ELISA). D-dimer is a good "rule-out" test because a PE can be excluded in patients with low or moderate clinical pretest probability for a PE with a normal D-dimer level. However, a D-dimer has rather poor specificity since an elevated D-dimer level is considered nonspecific. Elevated D-dimer can also be seen in patients with an MI, atrial fibrillation, stroke, DIC, sepsis, surgery, trauma, malignancy, severe liver disease, renal disease, and pregnancy. Therefore, ordering a D-dimer level in the hospital setting has a limited role.

**Duplex ultrasound**—Since DVT and PE are closely related, ultrasound of the lower extremities is sometimes performed in the evaluation of a PE. When a positive ultrasound confirms a DVT, no further testing is required and treatment can be initiated. However, a normal ultrasound of the lower extremities does not rule out a PE since a clot could be in the pelvic veins, iliac veins, or has already embolized to the lungs. Further diagnostic testing is often required in patients with a normal ultrasound but with suspicion for a PE.

**CT pulmonary angiography (CTPA)**—CTPA is rapidly becoming the initial diagnostic evaluation for suspected PE. CTPA involves the use of intravenous contrast to detect a clot as a filling defect in the pulmonary vasculature from a CT scan. Advantages of CTPA is the availability, relative quickness of the procedure, noninvasive, less costly than conventional pulmonary angiography, and the ability to diagnosis other diseases (especially if there is an underlying cardiac or lung disease). Disadvantages of CTPA is that it requires an experienced reader, is contraindicated in patients with renal insufficiency and contrast allergy, and finally, is not as sensitive at detecting thromboemboli in smaller vessels compared to conventional pulmonary angiography.

**V/Q scan**—The diagnostic evaluation for a PE is in a state of transition as CPTA is emerging as the imaging modality of choice. However, V/Q scans are still used, especially if there is a contraindication to CPTA such as contrast allergy or renal disease. The V/Q scan involves two parts that include injecting an isotope into the patient and observing for a perfusion defect, and secondly, having the patient inhale an isotope to observe for ventilation defects. Patients with a PE will typically have a perfusion defect, but a normal ventilation scan. Patients with airway disease will typically have both a perfusion and ventilation defects in the same corresponding areas. The probability of having a PE from the V/Q scan can be categorized as high, intermediate, low, and normal. V/Q scans that are high probability or normal are most helpful because there is sufficient evidence to initiate treatment for high probability scans and to exclude the diagnosis of PE in normal scans. Unfortunately, up to 75% of V/Q scans are nondiagnostic (ie, low or intermediate) and further testing is usually required.

**Pulmonary angiography**—Conventional pulmonary angiography is considered the "gold standard" in the diagnosis of PE. Pulmonary angiography is a safe, but invasive procedure that involves threading a catheter through the jugular or femoral vein into the pulmonary arteries and injecting contrast to detect a clot as a filling defect.

**Step 4)** The primary treatment for a PE is anticoagulation, but other therapies include thrombolysis, IVC filter, and embolectomy.

## Anticoagulation

Unfractionated heparin (UFH)

- UFH has a short half-life, which would be a good choice to treat a patient if they were to undergo an invasive procedure (eg, embolectomy), the patient has a risk of bleeding because it can be reversed with protamine sulfate, or allows for a smoother transition from UFH to thrombolytic therapy when thrombolysis is still considered during the evaluation process.
- When severe renal insufficiency exists (ie, CrCl <30 mL/min), UFH is the preferred agent over LMWH or subcutaneous fondaparinux.
- Disadvantages of UFH are monitoring the aPTT to achieve a target level, heparin dose adjustments, and risk of developing heparin-induced thrombocytopenia (HIT).
- The importance of achieving a therapeutic aPTT within 24 hours cannot be overstated because failure to do so has been associated with a higher risk of PE recurrence.

Low molecular weight heparin (LMWH)

- LMWH such as enoxaparin, dalteparin, tinzaparin exhibit a longer half-life, more predictable dose-response, requires no monitoring, less likely to cause a HIT, and ideal for home-based therapy.

Factor Xa inhibitor

- Fondaparinux can be given subcutaneously, requires no monitoring, but is contraindicated in patients with severe renal insufficiency.
- Consider fondaparinux in patients with a history of HIT because it has little to no antiplatelet effects.

Warfarin

- The effects of warfarin are monitored by the INR with a target of 2.5 for an acute PE.
- Warfarin can be initiated on the same day as UFH, LMWH, or fondaparinux.
- Overlap UFH, LMWH, or fondaparinux with warfarin for at least 5 days until the INR is in the therapeutic range of 2.0 to 3.0 for at least 24 hours.
- Duration of anticoagulation should be individualized to the patient's circumstances, but typically 3 months of treatment and then reassessed. Patients that have reversible risk factors (eg, surgery, trauma, immobilization) may only require a total

of 3 months, but patients that have recurrent disease or irreversible risk factors (eg, cancer, factor V Leiden mutation, protein C and S deficiency) usually require long-term anticoagulation.

## Thrombolytic Therapy

- Thrombolytic agents such as alteplase (rtPA), streptokinase, and urokinase increase plasmin levels, which cause lysis of the clot.
- The main indication for thrombolysis is in a patient with confirmed diagnosis of PE who is hemodynamically unstable (ie, hypotension) in which thrombolytic therapy may be lifesaving.
- Contraindications to thrombolytic therapy include: bleeding diathesis, internal bleeding within the past 6 months, recent surgery or trauma, intracranial disease (eg, neoplasm, aneurysm), stroke within past 2 months, and uncontrolled hypertension.

## IVC Filter

- The two main indications for an IVC filter placement is a contraindication to anticoagulation or failure of anticoagulation.

## Embolectomy

- Embolectomy can be performed surgically or using a catheter and is considered a last resort effort in patients who have failed thrombolytic therapy or a contraindication exists for thrombolytic therapy.

Disposition:

Patients diagnosed with acute PE are typically admitted to the hospital and patients with severe PE may require admission to the ICU.

Pearls:

- It can be easily remembered that warfarin is in "war" with the vitamin K-dependent clotting factors (II, VII, IX, and IX), which results in impaired production of the factors. Factor VII (extrinsic pathway) can be considered the first victim because any preexisting factor VII in the circulation will be cleared fairly quickly because it has a short half-life (4-6 hours) which will eventually result in a prolong PT in the first few days of therapy. However, it takes approximately 5 days for the full effect of anticoagulation with warfarin because the intrinsic and common pathways are still intact (ie, longer half-lives of the other clotting factors).
- UFH and LMWH are the preferred agents to use during pregnancy since warfarin is a category X drug and is generally contraindicated in pregnancy, but it is okay to give warfarin postpartum since it does not cross into breast milk.
- Serum troponins can be elevated in 50% of patients with moderate to large pulmonary embolism, which is thought to be due to an acute right ventricular myocardial stretch.
- Care should be taken when administering IV fluids to patients with hypotension because an increase in right

ventricular stress, especially in patients with right ventricular dysfunction, can result in worsening of their heart.

- **Foundational point**—Of the several different fibrin degradation products (FDP), one is called a D-dimer. The D stands for domains, hence, two identical domains that have been crosslinked by factor XIII.

- **Foundational point**—If there is complete airway obstruction, but perfusion is normal, then the V/Q is equal to zero and thus, referred to as intrapulmonary shunt. In contrast, if perfusion is completely obstructed (eg, pulmonary embolus), but ventilation is normal, then the V/Q approaches infinity and is referred to as alveolar dead space.

- **Foundational point**—Ventilation and perfusion are both greater in the bases (gravity-dependent regions) compared to the apices. Since the gradient between the apical and basilar perfusion is greater than the gradient between the apical and basilar ventilation, the V/Q ratio is higher in the apices compared to the bases. In an upright lung, the V/Q ratio in the apices is >1.0 resulting in $\uparrow$ $PO_2$ and $\downarrow$ $PCO_2$, but the V/Q ratio in the bases is <1.0 resulting in $\downarrow$ $PO_2$ and $\uparrow$ $PCO_2$.

- **CJ:** A 32-year-old businesswoman presents with an acute onset of dyspnea, cough, right-sided chest pain, but no reports of leg pain. She is a heavy smoker, on OCPs, with no previous history of DVT/PE, no history of malignancy, no recent surgeries or trauma, no contraindications to anticoagulation, but has an anaphylactic reaction (type I hypersensitivity) to contrast media. Her vitals are 37.0°, 95/62, HR-115, RR-32. What are your initial steps?

**First Order Sheet:**

1) IV access
2) NSS, 0.9% NaCl, IV, continuous
3) Pulse oximetry, stat      **Result:** 87%
4) Supplemental oxygen
5) Continuous cardiac monitor, stat
6) Continuous blood pressure cuff, stat

**Physical Examination:**

**General appearance:** In apparent respiratory distress

**Chest/Lungs:** Tachypnea. Clear breath sounds over left lung; rales over right lower lobe.

**Heart/Cardiovascular:** Tachycardia. No extra heart sounds. No JVD.

**Abdomen:** Normal bowel sounds. No bruits. No mass or tenderness.

**Extremities/Spine:** No edema. No clubbing or cyanosis.

**Second Order Sheet:**

1) ABG, stat — **Result:** pH-7.5, $pCO_2$-30, $pO_2$-60, $HCO_3$-22
2) CXR, portable, AP, stat — **Result:** Normal findings
3) EKG, 12 lead, stat — **Result:** Sinus tachycardia, T-wave inversion in aVR
4) CBC with diff, stat — **Result:** Leukocytosis
5) BMP, stat — **Result:** WNL
6) CK-MB, stat — **Result:** WNL
7) Troponin I, stat — **Result:** WNL
8) PT/INR, stat — **Result:** PT-13.0 seconds (nl: <12), INR-0.9
9) PTT, stat — **Result:** 30.0 seconds (nl: <28)

**Third Order Sheet:**

1) Heparin, IV, continuous
2) PTT, routine, q4 hours

**Fourth Order Sheet:**

1) V/Q scan, stat — **Result:** Perfusion scan—Diminished perfusion in right lower lobe, Ventilation scan—Normal findings
2) D-Dimer, stat — **Result:** 500 mcg/L (nl: <250)

**Pearl:**

- **On the CCS,** "V/Q scan" and "CTA, chest, with contrast" are both available in the practice CCS.

---

# INFECTIONS

## ▍ TUBERCULOSIS

Tuberculosis (TB) is caused by *Mycobacterium tuberculosis* and is transmitted from person to person through direct inhalation of aerosolized droplets of the organism. Upon establishing a focus infection in the lung, the infection can progress to clinically active disease (progressive primary disease), remain dormant with reactivation at a later time, or immediate clearance of the organism.

**Risk Factors:**

Close contact to a person with active TB, recent immigrant (≤5 years) where TB incidence is high, history of a positive test for *M tuberculosis*, health-care workers, homeless people, prisoners, nursing home residents, alcoholics, drug users, and patients with medical conditions that put them at risk for TB (eg, AIDS, HIV, transplant recipients, silicosis, renal failure requiring dialysis, head and neck cancer, lung cancer, lymphoma, leukemia, intestinal bypass surgery (eg, jejunoileal bypass), gastrectomy, diabetes, chronic glucocorticoid users, >10% below ideal body weight).

## Clinical Features:

**Latent TB**—Patients are asymptomatic.

**Active TB**—Patients may present with any of the systemic and pulmonary features:

> **Systemic**—Fever, night sweats, malaise, weight loss.
>
> **Pulmonary**—Productive cough, hemoptysis, pleuritic chest pain, rales, or bronchial breath sounds over involved lung (ie, indication of consolidation).

**Extrapulmonary TB**—Up to 20% of TB cases will be extrapulmonary. Extrapulmonary manifestations can occur at the same time as the primary infection or at the time of reactivation. The following are extrapulmonary sites with its manifestations listed from a relative head to toe fashion:

> **Neurologic**—Tuberculous meningitis, tuberculoma (round mass lesion).
>
> **Cardiac**—Pericarditis.
>
> **Pleura**—Pleural effusions.
>
> **GI**—Peritonitis, enteritis, liver disease.
>
> **Genitourinary**—Renal granulomas, ureteral strictures, genital TB.
>
> **Adrenals**—Adrenal insufficiency.
>
> **Bone**—Spinal TB (Pott's disease).
>
> **Lymphatics**—Painless cervical and supraclavicular lymphadenopathy. Mediastinal, hilar, and retroperitoneal lymph nodes are other sites.
>
> **Dermatologic**—Ulcers, abscesses, lupus vulgaris.
>
> **Disseminated**—Also referred to as miliary TB; results from hematogenous dissemination of *M tuberculosis* that can affect multiple organs. Clinical manifestations are usually nonspecific and can occur at the time of a primary infection or at the time of reactivation. The lesions within the organs typically resemble "millet seeds."

## Next Step:

**Step 1)** Patients suspected of having TB should be placed into a separate waiting room wearing a surgical mask, and health-care workers caring for the patient should also be masked.

**Step 2)** Evaluation for latent, active, and extrapulmonary TB is the following:

## Latent TB

- Evaluate for latent TB in individuals with contact to patients with active TB or individuals with an increased risk of reactivation (eg, silicosis, diabetes, renal failure requiring dialysis, head and neck cancer, lung cancer, lymphoma, leukemia, >10% below ideal body weight, transplant recipients, TNF-alpha inhibitors, chemotherapy, glucocorticoid users, CXR with fibrotic changes consistent with prior TB, HIV infection).

- Treatment for latent TB (see step 3) should only commence once active TB has been ruled out.

### Table 17-3 • Interpretation of the PPD

| PPD Size | Groups |
|---|---|
| ≥5 mm | • HIV-infected<br>• Close contact with someone with active TB<br>• CXR with fibrotic changes consistent with prior TB<br>• Immunosuppressed (transplant recipients, TNF-alpha inhibitors, chemotherapy, glucocorticoid users) |
| ≥10 mm | • Children <4 years<br>• Recent immigrants (≤5 years) where TB incidence is high<br>• Health care workers<br>• Prisoners, homeless, IV drug users<br>• Risk of reactivation (silicosis, diabetes, RF requiring dialysis, head and neck cancer, lung cancer, lymphoma, leukemia, >10% below ideal body weight) |
| ≥15 mm | • No known risk factors for TB |

*CXR—chest x-ray; IV—intravenous; RF—renal failure; TB—tuberculosis*

- The tuberculin skin test (TST) and the interferon gamma release assay (IGRA) are tests used to evaluate latent TB by assessing the cell-mediated immunity of the patient. Consider the two tests:

> **TST**—The Mantoux test involves the intradermal injection of purified protein derivative (PPD) to assess previous exposure to mycobacterial antigens by stimulating the type IV–delayed type hypersensitivity response. Only skin induration is assessed 48 to 72 hours after injection, and a positive test is interpreted as indicated in Table 17-3.

>> **PPD positive**—Proceed to evaluate for active TB, but keep in mind that false positive tests can occur in patients that received the Bacille Calmette-Guèrin (BCG) vaccination or have been exposed to nontuberculous mycobacteria (eg, *M avium* complex, *M kansasii*).

>> **PPD negative**—Repeat the PPD in 8 weeks for patients exposed to someone with active TB because it take as long as 8 weeks for the sensitization and development of the delayed hypersensitivity response in someone never exposed to the mycobacterial antigen. Keep in mind that false negative tests can result from improper administration, waning immunity, or someone who is immunosuppressed.

### IGRA

- IGRA is an in vitro blood test that can detect the production of IFN-gamma from T lymphocytes following stimulation with M. tuberculosis antigens.

- IGRA testing does not give false positive results because it is not affected by prior BCG vaccination or prior sensitization from nontuberculous mycobacteria.

- Routine testing with both IGRA and PPD is not recommended.

- The CDC recommends that IGRA testing is preferred in individuals with a history of a BCG vaccination and individuals from groups that have historically have poor rates of returning to have their PPD read (eg, homeless people, drug users).

## Active TB

- Evaluate for active TB in individuals where there is a suspicion for tuberculosis, which can be based on the presence of risk factors, history of prior TB infection (ie, positive PPD or IGRA), possible exposure to active TB, signs and symptoms of TB, or an incidental finding on CXR suggestive of TB.
- It may not always be possible to establish a definitive diagnosis of TB prior to the start of treatment, therefore, **empiric therapy** to treat active TB (refer to step 3) can be initiated when there is a high clinical suspicion for TB based on the patient's history including epidemiologic factors (ie, exposure to TB), physical findings, radiographic findings, and a preliminary AFB smear-positive result.

    **Chest X-ray**—The CXR is the initial diagnostic step in evaluating a patient with active TB. In primary active TB, nonspecific infiltrates may be found in any area of the lung. In reactivation TB, cavitation can sometimes be present, and infiltrates are typically found in the upper lobes (apical-posterior segments) or lower lobes (apical segment) of the lungs. Other features that may be present in active TB are hilar or mediastinal adenopathy, pleural effusions (ie, exudate), tuberculoma (mass lesion), and reticulonodular infiltrates (ie, miliary pattern).

    **Sputum samples**—Sputum samples should be collected in patients whose chest x-ray demonstrate infiltrates ± cavitation. Three samples should be collected for acid-fast bacilli (AFB) smear and culture, and at least one specimen should be reserved for nucleic acid amplification (NAA) testing in individuals with signs and symptoms of pulmonary TB for which a diagnosis of TB is still considered.

    **AFB smear**—AFB smear is rapid and inexpensive, but has relatively low sensitivity (40%-80%). The smears can be stained with the traditional Ziehl-Neelsen dye or with a more sensitive dye, auramine-O.

    **Culture**—Culture is important for identification of M. tuberculosis and drug susceptibility. Unfortunately, results can take a long time (3-8 weeks).

    **Nucleic acid amplification**—NAA testing is a useful adjunct in the early stages of patient evaluation because results can be obtained fairly quickly (24-48 hours) while the cultures are still pending. NAA testing provides a greater positive predictive value in AFB smear-positive results where nontuberculous mycobacteria is common, and NAA testing can rapidly confirm the presence of M. tuberculosis in 50%-80% of AFB smear-negative results, but culture-positive specimens.

## Extrapulmonary TB

- To establish a diagnosis of extrapulmonary TB, obtain fluid or tissue specimens for AFB smear, culture, and drug susceptibility testing (eg, synovial, pericardial, peritoneal, pleural fluid, CSF, bone, or lymph tissue).

**Step 3)** Treatment for tuberculosis typically consists of a combination of first-line antituberculosis agents which are isoniazid (INH), pyrazinamide (PZA), ethambutol (EMB), rifampin (RIF), and the newer rifamycins, rifabutin and rifapentine.

## Latent TB

- Treatment for latent TB includes INH therapy for 9 months in HIV-negative or HIV-infected patients.
- Regardless of the test result for latent TB infection, HIV-infected patients should still be treated in cases of recent contact with someone with active TB or in a HIV-infected patient with a history of untreated TB.

## Active TB

- For the first 2 months (initial phase) treat with **RIPE** (**R**ifampin + **I**soniazid + **P**yrazinamide + **E**thambutol), then obtain sputum cultures at the completion of the initial phase, followed by INH + RIF for the next 4 months (continuation phase) for a total of 6 months of treatment.
- Extend treatment in the continuation phase to 7 months (total of 9 months of treatment) in patients who did not receive PZA in the initial phase or patients that initially had a cavitation in the initial chest films + positive sputum cultures at the completion of the initial phase.

## Extrapulmonary TB

- The basic principles for the treatment of pulmonary TB applies to extrapulmonary TB with a standard 6-month course of treatment, except for TB meningitis (total of 9-12 months) and bone and joint TB (total of 6-9 months of at least including RIF).
- Adjunctive glucocorticoid therapy is recommended in patients with TB meningitis and TB pericarditis.

## Special Populations

### Pregnancy

- The same basic principles are used to treat latent TB and active TB with the exception of excluding PZA from the initial phase because of the uncertainty of causing adverse effects in pregnancy (Category C drug rating).
- Do not use streptomycin because it is a known teratogen that can cause congenital deafness (Category D drug rating).
- Breastfeeding is not a contraindication in mothers being treated only with first-line agents for active or latent TB.
- Mothers that are breastfeeding and receiving INH should be given supplemental pyridoxine (vitamin $B_6$) to both infants and mothers.

### Children

- Drug regimens for adults are generally the same regimens for children.

- Treatment should be started as soon as the diagnosis is suspected in children <4 years because of a high risk of TB to disseminate.

- Visual acuity monitoring is usually performed in patients receiving ethambutol (EMB) since the drug can cause optic neuritis.

### HIV-infected

- The general approach to TB treatment is the same as HIV-negative patients. However, HIV-infected patients should be treated with rifabutin instead of rifampin because there are drug interactions, particularly with protease inhibitors.

**Step 4)** TB is a reportable disease, and any suspected or confirmed cases of TB should be reported to the health department.

### Disposition:

In the majority of cases, patients with TB can be initially treated as an outpatient, but it is important for the ER physicians to contact public health services or physicians for the long-term management of the patient.

### Pearls:

- Individuals with latent TB are not considered contagious.

- Individuals with active, untreated pulmonary TB (especially in the presence of cavitary lesions) are considered contagious.

- Individuals with only extrapulmonary TB without pulmonary disease are *not* contagious.

- TB is not transmitted by fomites.

- IGRA or PPD should not be used to diagnosis active TB.

- Patients receiving INH can have neurologic side effects such as peripheral neuropathy, ataxia, or paresthesia, therefore, add vitamin $B_6$ (pyridoxine) in patients who are at risk for INH-induced neurotoxicity, which includes pregnant women, breastfeeding women, infants, children, elderly, HIV-infected, diabetics, alcoholics, chronic liver disease, renal failure, and nutritional deficiency.

- A two-step skin testing involves a second PPD testing 1 to 2 weeks after a negative PPD result. The idea behind a second testing is for individuals who were previously exposed to TB may have a waning response to the PPD over time that may give a false-negative result if only one PPD test is given. Performing the first PPD in the two-step testing may actually "boost" the immune system, which will allow a better reflection of the patient's status when given a second PPD. If the second test is negative, then the patient is truly negative. Two-step testing is useful for individuals that are tested periodically (eg, health-care workers, nursing home residents).

- Patients with continued positive cultures after 4 months of treatment are considered a failing course of treatment, and another single agent should never be added to a failing regimen because of concerns for resistance to the drug.

- Direct observation of therapy (DOT) is to assure that patients are ingesting anti-TB agents by having a health-care provider watch the patient swallow the medications. DOT should be instituted in children, individuals with memory impairment, psychiatric illness, drug users, homeless, HIV infection, pulmonary TB with positive sputum cultures, prior treatment with active or latent TB, drug resistance, relapse, and patients with treatment failure.

- Ghon focus refers to a granulomatous structure (tubercle) which represents the initial primary lesion in the lung from a TB infection.

- Ghon complex refers to the Ghon focus accompanied by perihilar lymph node involvement (ie, remember it's a complex of things together).

- Ranke complex refers to the evolution of the Ghon complex as a healed, calcified lesion.

- Formation of a cavity can occur when a caseous lesion erodes into a bronchiole allowing drainage of the necrotic material.

- Since *M tuberculosis* is an obligate aerobe, it has a predilection to settle in areas of high oxygen content after hematogenous spread. Therefore, upon reactivation, characteristic locations typically involve the apical segment of the upper lobe since there is a higher oxygen partial pressure.

- **Foundational point**—*Mycobacterium tuberculosis* is an obligate aerobic, acid-fast, non-spore-forming, rod-shaped bacterium. Although *M tuberculosis* is neutral on Gram's staining, it is still considered a gram-positive bacterium since it lacks a true outer membrane. However, the cell envelope distinguishes this organism. The constituents of the cell envelope include mycolic acids, peptidoglycan, arabinogalactan, lipopolysaccharide (but without a lipid A), and lipoarabinomannan (LAM).

- **Foundational point**—Two notable organisms that are acid-fast are *Mycobacteria* species and *Nocardia*. What makes acid-fast unique is the ability of the mycolic acids (large fatty acid) to resist destaining by acid alcohol after being stained and holding "fast" to the initial stain.

- **Foundational point**—Although *M tuberculosis* does not have exotoxins or endotoxins, what makes *M tuberculosis* virulent is the sulfatides, catalase-peroxidase, LAM, mycolic acid glycolipids, and trehalose dimycolate (also known as cord factor).

- **Foundational point**—One of the defense mechanisms to contain the bacteria is the presence of a caseous necrotic ("soft cheese") granuloma that has a low pH and low oxygen tension that inhibit the growth of the bacteria but keep them viable for dormancy.

- **Foundational point**—Within the caseating granulomas are Langhans giant cells, which have a characteristic "horseshoe" pattern of nuclei.

- **CJ:** A 45-year-old HIV-infected man started anti-TB medications 5 days ago and presents with fever, presence of new lymph nodes, inflamed and increased size of preexisting lymph nodes, and worsening of his respiratory symptoms along with worsening of his CXR. What is your next step? **Answer:** The patient is experiencing a paradoxical reaction or immune reconstitution syndrome, which is a temporary exacerbation of the infection after starting anti-TB medications. Although this reaction can occur in anybody, HIV-infected patients are commonly affected. The first step is to rule out other causes (eg, treatment failure, resistance), but the treatment for a paradoxical reaction is supportive as it is a self-limited condition.

- **CJ:** A 35-year-old woman is on RIF, INH, PZA, and EMB. Her AST is 5 times the upper limit of normal but she is asymptomatic. Do you want continue treatment? **Answer:** No. Hepatotoxicity can occur in RIF, INH, PZA, or EMB. Discontinue anti-TB agents if a patient's aminotransferase is 5 times the upper limits of normal ± symptoms or 3 times the upper limit of normal in the presence of symptoms.

- **Connecting point** (pg. 290)—Patients that are taking TNF-alpha inhibitors (eg, adalimumab, etanercept, infliximab) for their rheumatoid arthritis are at risk of reactivation of TB.

- **Connecting point** (pgs. 8, 9)—Know the other types of hypersensitivity reactions.

- **On the CCS,** "PPD" or "Tuberculin skin test" are available in the practice CCS.

- **On the CCS,** ordering "sputum" will allow you to select the AFB smear and C&S in the practice CCS.

- **On the CCS,** "NAA" is not recognized, but "Nucleic acid amplification, mycobacteria RNA" is available in the practice CCS.

- **On the CCS,** remember to order "Notify public health department" during the case.

- **On the CCS,** "Advise patient, side effects of medication" since anti-TB agents can cause the following:

  **Rifampin**—Red-orange discoloration of body fluids, flulike syndrome, hepatitis

  **Isoniazid**—CNS effects, lupus-like syndrome, hepatitis

**Pyrazinamide**—Hyperuricemia, GI upset, hepatitis

**Ethambutol**—Optic neuritis, decrease in red-green color discrimination, hepatitis

## ▌COMMUNITY-ACQUIRED PNEUMONIA—ADULTS

Community-acquired pneumonia (CAP) refers to a pneumonia that is acquired in the community as opposed to the hospital (ie, hospital-acquired pneumonia).

### Clinical Features:

The clinical presentation of CAP is usually nonspecific and no single sign or symptom is pathognomonic for CAP. However, classic findings for "typical" bacterial pneumonias include fever, dyspnea, pleuritic chest pain, and a productive cough. Although the patient's history and clinical features cannot always identify the etiologic pathogen, the clinical clues are listed in Table 17-4 for background knowledge.

### Next Step:

**Step 1)** The initial approach to a patient with CAP is the **clinical assessment** followed by a **chest x-ray.** Unfortunately, the radiographic findings cannot reliably distinguish bacterial from nonbacterial causes of pneumonia. However, it is still good to keep in the back of your mind that lobar consolidation, cavitation, and pleural effusions are suggestive of a bacterial etiology, while interstitial infiltrates are associated with viral causes.

**Step 2)** Once CAP is diagnosed or suspected, the decision has to be made to care for the patient either as an outpatient, inpatient, or in the ICU. There are several different prediction scores (eg, CURB-65, PSI) that can assess the severity of the illness;

### Table 17-4 • Clinical Clues to Pathogens in Community-acquired Pneumonia

| Pathogen | Associations | Clinical Features |
|---|---|---|
| Anaerobes (eg, Bacteroides spp, Fusobacterium) | • Aspiration<br>• Anesthesia<br>• Alcoholics | Gradual onset, "foul-smelling" sputum, poor dental hygiene, chills are uncommon |
| Chlamydophila pneumoniae | • Atypical bug<br>• Young adults<br>• Elderly people | Gradual onset, hoarseness, sore throat (pharyngitis), occasional sinusitis |
| Chlamydophila psittaci | • Atypical bug<br>• Exposure to infected birds | Abrupt onset of fever; dry cough, headache; other manifestations that may be present include chest pain, splenomegaly, maculopapular rash (Horder spots) |
| Coxiella burnetti (Q fever) | • Atypical bug<br>• Tick bite or inhalation of contaminated aerosols from birth products of infected animals (eg, goats, cattle, sheep, cats, dogs, rabbits) | **Acute:** Self-limited flulike illness, pneumonia, hepatitis<br>**Chronic (>6 months):** Endocarditis, vascular aneurysm |
| Haemophilus influenzae (nontypeable) | • COPD<br>• Cystic fibrosis<br>• Elderly | Gradual onset, fever, dyspnea, productive cough |
| Klebsiella pneumoniae | • Alcoholics<br>• Diabetics<br>• Nosocomial | Acute onset, fever, dyspnea, cough, "currant jelly" sputum |

(Continued)

**Table 17-4 • Clinical Clues to Pathogens in Community-acquired Pneumonia (Continued)**

| Pathogen | Associations | Clinical Features |
|---|---|---|
| *Legionella spp* | • Atypical bug<br>• Exposure to aerosolized water with the bug (eg, AC, whirlpool, showers)<br>• Causes legionellosis | Legionellosis is associated with two clinically distinct syndromes:<br>1) **Legionnaire's disease**—Fever, pneumonia, and any of the following may be present: nausea, vomiting, diarrhea, lethargy, confusion, chest pain, hyponatremia, hematuria<br>2) **Pontiac fever**—Fever, flulike illness, but self-limited condition |
| *Moraxella catarrhalis* | • COPD | Less commonly, *M catarrhalis* causes pneumonia, which presents similarly to *H influenzae* (gradual onset, fever, dyspnea, productive cough). More commonly, *M catarrhalis* causes COPD exacerbation (dyspnea increases, cough frequency increases, sputum production volume increases). |
| Mycoplasma pneumoniae | • Atypical bug<br>• Young adults | Gradual onset, fever, chills (rarely rigors), dry cough, headache, and sometimes extrapulmonary causes (eg, bullous myringitis, hemolytic anemia, skin rashes, CNS, cardiac, and GI involvement) |
| *Pseudomonas aeruginosa* | • COPD<br>• Cystic fibrosis<br>• Immunocompromised<br>• Recently hospitalized | Fever, chills, dyspnea, productive cough, confusion |
| *Staphylococcus aureus* | • Postinfluenza<br>• IV drug users<br>• Nosocomial | Fever, dyspnea, productive cough |
| *Streptococcus pneumoniae* | • Most common cause of CAP | Classic presentation includes acute onset, fever, chills, dyspnea, productive cough, "rust-colored" sputum, pleuritic chest pain |
| Viruses (eg, influenza, RSV, adenovirus) | • Influenza is a common viral cause of CAP seen in adults | Sudden onset of fever, chills, nonproductive cough, rhinorrhea, sore throat, myalgias, headache |

*A/C—air conditioner; RSV—respiratory syncytial virus; spp—species*

however, in clinical practice the prediction scores serves as an adjunct to the physician's overall clinical judgment. For board purposes, the following will serve as a general guideline for managing a patient with CAP:

>**Reasons to manage as an outpatient**—Relatively young (<50 years), healthy, active, compliant, no comorbidities, unremarkable physical exam

>**Reasons to admit to the inpatient**—Any combination of the following using your clinical judgment: elderly, presence of comorbid conditions, altered mental status, ↑ respiratory rate, ↑ heart rate, ↑ temperature, ↓ blood pressure, hypoxemia based on the pulse oximetry, inability to maintain oral intake, possible complications of the pneumonia itself (eg, development of pleural effusions, abscess, or respiratory failure)

>**Reasons to admit to the ICU**—Patient in septic shock requiring vasopressors, or patient requiring intubation and mechanical ventilation

**Step 3**) Initial treatment for adults with CAP is empiric antibiotics, which depends on the clinical setting. The following list is based on the guidelines from the Infectious Diseases Society of America/American Thoracic Society (IDSA/ATS):

**Outpatient treatment for the uncomplicated patient**

If the patient is previously healthy and no antibiotics within the previous 3 months, then:

>**Option 1:** Macrolide (eg, azithromycin, clarithromycin, or erythromycin)

>**Option 2:** Tetracycline (eg, doxycycline)

## Outpatient treatment for the more complicated patient

If the patient has comorbidities, use of immunosuppressive drugs, or use of antibiotics within the previous 3 months, then:

**Option 1:** Respiratory fluoroquinolone (eg, moxifloxacin, gemifloxacin, or levofloxacin)

**Option 2:** Beta-lactam (eg, amoxicillin) + macrolide

## Inpatient treatment

**Option 1:** Respiratory fluoroquinolone

**Option 2:** Antipneumococcal beta-lactam (eg, ceftriaxone, cefotaxime, or ampicillin-sulbactam) + macrolide

## ICU treatment

**Option 1:** Antipneumococcal beta-lactam + azithromycin

**Option 2:** Antipneumococcal beta-lactam + respiratory fluoroquinolone

**Option 3:** For penicillin-allergic patients use respiratory fluoroquinolone + aztreonam

## Treatment with Special Concerns

## Community-acquired MRSA

**Option 1:** Add vancomycin or linezolid to the inpatient or ICU regimens.

## Pseudomonas infection

**Option 1:** Antipseudomonal beta-lactam (eg, piperacillin-tazobactam, cefepime, imipenem, or meropenem) + ciprofloxacin or levofloxacin

**Option 2:** Antipseudomonal beta-lactam + aminoglycoside + azithromycin

**Option 3:** Antipseudomonal beta-lactam + aminoglycoside + respiratory fluoroquinolone

**Option 4:** For penicillin-allergic patients, substitute aztreonam for above beta-lactam

**Step 4)** Vaccinate for the influenza infection during the influenza season. Pneumococcal vaccination should also be given to:

- Persons ≥65 years old
- Younger people that are at risk of pneumococcal disease: immunocompromised, asplenia, alcoholics, smokers, nursing home residents, CSF leaks, DM, and chronic cardiac, pulmonary, renal, or liver disease

## Follow-Up:

Patients managed in the outpatient setting or discharged from the hospital should follow up in 1 week with their physician for a reassessment, but a repeat chest x-ray is unnecessary if the patient is clinically improving.

## Pearls:

- Routine diagnostic testing to establish an etiologic diagnosis in outpatients with CAP is usually unnecessary since empiric treatment is usually successful.

- Patients admitted to the inpatient ward usually require more diagnostic testing such as blood and sputum cultures.

- Patients in the ICU usually require extensive diagnostic testing such as blood cultures, sputum specimen for culture and Gram stain, urinary antigen testing (UAT) for *Legionella* and *Streptococcus pneumoniae*, and endotracheal aspirate if intubated.

- "Atypical" bugs are atypical because they cannot be detected on Gram's stain or cultivated on standard bacteria media.

- In approximately 50% of patients with CAP, no specific pathogen can be identified, and if identified, it is usually *Streptococcus pneumoniae.*

- The most common cause of pneumonias in children <5 years old are viral pathogens (RSV most common), but in older children ≥5 years old the most common causes of CAP are *Streptococcus pneumoniae, Mycoplasma pneumoniae,* and *Chlamydophila pneumoniae.*

- Both *Chlamydophila pneumoniae* and *Chlamydophila psittaci* are transmitted by respiratory route.

- Duration of antibiotic treatment for patients with CAP is a minimum of 5 days.

- Patients that are on intravenous antibiotics can be switched to oral therapy when they are hemodynamically stable, able to ingest orals, and are clinically improving.

- **Foundational point**—*Bacteroides melaninogenicus* and *Fusobacterium* are both anaerobic, gram-negative rods that can cause a necrotizing aspiration pneumonia. A key difference between the organisms is that *Bacteroides melaninogenicus* does not contain lipid A (ie, no endotoxin), but *Fusobacterium* does contain an endotoxic LPS.

- **Foundational point**—*Coxiella burnetii* is morphologically similar to *Rickettsia.* They are both obligate intracellular (use host ATP), gram-negative bacteria. What is unique to *Coxiella* is that it can exist in an endospore form, which can make it resistant to heat and drying conditions. In addition, it does not require an arthropod vector, unlike *Rickettsia.*

- **Foundational point**—*Haemophilus influenzae* is a gram-negative coccobacillus. *H influenzae* can be encapsulated ("typeable") or unencapsulated ("nontypeable"). The encapsulated has six serotypes (a, b, c, d, e, f), and type b is known for causing meningitis, epiglottitis, sepsis, and septic arthritis. The nontypeable *H influenzae* species are involved in upper and lower respiratory tract infections such as sinusitis, otitis media, pneumonia, and bronchitis. As with most gram-negative bacteria, the outer membrane has an endotoxic LPS. *H influenzae* can also produce IgA proteases, which makes sense since they are under attack from the humoral immunity. *H influenzae* can be grown on chocolate agar, but require factor V (NAD) and factor X (hemin), which are both found in blood, hence the term *Haemophilus* ("blood loving").

- **Foundational point**—*Klebsiella pneumoniae* is a gram-negative, nonmotile, lactose-fermenting, rod. *K pneumoniae* is encapsulated, and some strains can produce a mucoviscous capsule.

- **Foundational point**—*Legionella pneumophila* is a gram-negative, motile rod that is a facultative intracellular parasite to macrophages. What is unique about this organism is that it poorly stains with a Gram's stain, but can be stained using a silver stain. In addition, *L pneumophila* grows on specialized media of buffered charcoal yeast extract with L-cysteine, iron, antibiotics, and dyes. *L pneumophila* is not transmitted from person to person.

- **Foundational point**—*Moraxella catarrhalis* (also known as *Neisseria catarrhalis* and *Branhamella catarrhalis*) is a gram-negative, aerobic diplococcus. M catarrhalis resembles *Neisseria* species on gram stain, but what is unique to this organism is that when grown on agar (chocolate or blood); the colonies can be pushed across the surface like a hockey puck ("hockey puck sign").

- **Foundational point**—*Mycoplasma pneumoniae* is one of the smallest free-living bacteria. It lacks a cell wall (ie, no peptidoglycan layer) and therefore, you cannot gram stain it and certain antibiotics (eg, penicillins, cephalosporins) are ineffective. However, *M pneumoniae* does have a cell membrane that is composed of cholesterol, which allows for the various shapes of the organism. Antibodies (IgM) to M. pneumoniae can develop and cross react with RBC antigens (ie, I antigen) at cold temperature, hence cold agglutinins (ie, RBCs clumping together secondary to antibodies binding to antigen). Other causes of cold agglutinin include infectious mononucleosis, influenza, and *Rickettsia* infection. Warm agglutinins (IgG instead) can be caused by CLL, SLE, viral infections, blood transfusions, and drugs (eg, methyldopa, penicillin). Autoimmune hemolytic anemia can be due to the presence of warm or cold agglutinins.

- **Foundational point**—*Pseudomonas aeruginosa* is a gram-negative, obligate aerobe, non-lactose-fermenting, oxidase positive rod that can produce pyocyanin (blue pigment) and pyoverdin (fluorescent pigment) giving it a blue-green appearance. It also has a distinctive fruity, grapelike smell. Some of the key distinctive features include the presence of an endotoxin, produces exotoxin A, produces alginate (biofilm formation to protect against antibiotics), secretes phospholipase C (lyses RBCs), and secretes elastase (degrades IgG).

- **Foundational point**—*Staphylococcus aureus* is a gram-positive coccus that appears in grapelike clusters on Gram's stain and has a golden pigment, hence the word *aureus* (Latin for gold). *S aureus* is also catalase positive (converts $H_2O_2$ to $H_2O$ and $O_2$) and coagulase positive (fibrin formation for protection). Distinctive features of *S aureus* include protease A (binds Fc region of IgG thereby preventing opsonization and phagocytosis), leukocidins (kills leukocytes), hemolysins (lysis of RBCs), beta-lactamase (hydrolysis of the β-lactam ring), lipase (digests lipids), hyaluronidase (breaks down connective tissue), staphylokinase (dissolves fibrin), transpeptidase (cross-links peptidoglycan chains to form a cell wall), and releases exotoxins (eg, TSST-1, exfoliatin, enterotoxin).

- **Foundational point**—*Staphylococcus epidermidis* and *Staphylococcus saprophyticus* are both catalase positive but **coagulase negative**.

- **Foundational point**—Methicillin-resistant *Staphylococcus aureus* (MRSA) is defined by the presence of the mec gene, which encodes for penicillin binding protein 2a (PBP2a). Penicillin binding protein is a normal constituent of most bacteria and naturally binds to penicillins, hence the name. The function of these proteins is the biogenesis of the cell wall; however, PBP2a has a low affinity for the beta-lactam antibiotics, making these bugs resistant.

- **Foundational point**—Streptococci are gram-positive cocci that can exist in pairs or chains. They are also **catalase negative**. There are five major types of streptococci to consider based on their surface (Lancefield) antigens and simply by their species: Lancefield group A, Lancefield group B, Lancefield group D, *Streptococcus viridians* (no Lancefield), and *Streptococcus pneumoniae* (no Lancefield). The organisms can also be classified by their ability to lyse RBCs on blood agar. Beta-hemolytic organisms can completely lyse RBCs, alpha-hemolytic can partially lyse RBCs leaving a green color on culture, and gamma-hemolytic (ie, nonhemolytic) cannot lyse RBCs on blood agar. Examples of the streptococci include *Streptococcus pyogenes* (group A, beta-hemolytic, bacitracin sensitive), *Streptococcus agalactiae* (group B, beta-hemolytic, bacitracin resistant), and *Streptococcus bovis* (group D, nonhemolytic). It should be noted that Enterococci are gram-positive cocci that were formerly classified as group D streptococci.

- **Foundational point**—*Streptococcus pneumoniae* and *Streptococcus viridians* are both alpha-hemolytic. However, *Streptococcus pneumoniae* is optochin sensitive, bile soluble, and has a positive Quellung reaction (ie, indicates the presence of a capsule since it swells when antisera against the capsule is added). On the contrary, *Streptococcus viridians* is optochin resistant, bile insoluble, and lacks a capsule.

- **Foundational point**—Influenza virus is an orthomyxovirus that has a negative, segmented, single-stranded RNA that can replicate within the nucleus. There are three types of influenza (A, B, and C). Influenza A and B can cause seasonal epidemics in the United States, but influenza C does not appear to cause epidemics. Influenza A and B both have important antigenic glycoproteins studded along the surface membrane. First, **hemagglutinin (H)** is a protein that binds to host sialic acid receptors. Second, **neuraminidase (N)** is an enzyme that cleaves sialic acid allowing the virus to be released from the host cell. The hemagglutinin and neuraminidase is often used to describe the strain of the virus (eg, H1N1 influenza).

- **Foundational point**—Antigenic drift occurs when there is a relatively minor change in the antigenicity of the virus (eg, point mutation in the H or N) that can result in a localized outbreak with mild disease. Antigenic shifts can also occur in the influenza virus because it has a segmented genome that can result in high rates of reassortment leading to complete different antigenicity. The result can be more serious leading to epidemics and pandemics.

- **Foundational point**—RSV is a paramyxovirus that has a negative, unsegmented, single-stranded RNA that replicates in the cytoplasm. It does not have hemagglutinin or neuraminidase. As with most paramyxovirus (eg, mumps, measles, parainfluenza), it has an F protein on the surface of the virus that allows them to fuse with other cells resulting in multinucleated cells (ie, syncytial cells).

- **Foundational point**—Adenovirus is a lytic, nonenveloped virus that contains a double-stranded linear DNA. Host defense against adenovirus is through cell-mediated immunity.
- **Connecting point** (pg. 166)—Know the different serotypes of *Chlamydia trachomatis*. Also, know the microbiologic features and life cycle of *Chlamydophila* (formerly *Chlamydia*) *pneumoniae* and *Chlamydophila* (formerly *Chlamydia*) *psittaci*, which are both similar to *Chlamydia trachomatis*.
- **On the CCS,** "advise patient, no smoking."

- **On the CCS,** if you order "vaccine" you will be able to select influenza and pneumococcal vaccine in the practice CCS.
- **On the CCS,** "urinary antigen test" is not recognized in the order menu, but type in "antigen" and you will be able to locate "Antigen, bacterial, pneumococcus, urine" and "Antigen, Legionella, urine" in the practice CCS. If you cannot find your order in the CCS, there are three approaches to take. First, type the order in the most specific format (eg, urinary antigen test). Second, type in a very broad term (eg, antigen). Finally, if you cannot find your order then you can click on the "Broaden Search" tab under the "Order Verification" screen. The "Broaden Search" tab will provide you with a larger list of items from your original order input.

# NEOPLASM

## ▌LUNG CANCER

Lung cancer is the leading cause of cancer-related death in both men and women not only in the United States, but also worldwide. There are several different histologic types of lung cancer (see Table 17-5).

**Clinical Features:**

The clinical presentation of lung cancer can be best understood by the "on-site" or "off-site" effects of the lung cancer.

**On-site Effects (Direct Invasion)**

**Lung parenchyma invasion**—Cough, hemoptysis, dyspnea

**Tumor obstruction**—Pneumonia

**Esophageal invasion**—Dysphagia

**Chest wall invasion**—Chest pain

**Recurrent laryngeal nerve invasion**—Hoarseness

**Phrenic nerve invasion**—Diaphragm paralysis (ie, elevated hemidiaphragm, dyspnea)

**Pleural invasion**—Pleural effusion (ie, exudates)

**Pericardial invasion**—Pericarditis, tamponade

**Superior vena cava (SVC) obstruction**—SVC syndrome (ie, facial and arm swelling, dyspnea, cough)

**Sympathetic ganglia invasion**—Horner's syndrome (ie, miosis, ptosis, anhidrosis/no sweating)

**Superior sulcus tumors with invasion into adjacent tissues**—A constellation of symptoms referred to as Pancoast's syndrome: SVC syndrome, Horner's syndrome, brachial plexus invasion (shoulder pain, atrophy of hand and arm muscles), recurrent laryngeal nerve invasion (hoarseness), phrenic nerve invasion (diaphragm paralysis), supraclavicular lymph node enlargement, spinal cord compression

**Off-site Effects (Distant Effects)**

**Metastasis**—Frequent sites are **LABB** (**L**iver, **A**drenal, **B**one, **B**rain)

**Paraneoplastic syndromes**

**Cushing's syndrome**—"Moon facies," hirsutism, HTN, muscle weakness, glucose intolerance

**Dermatomyositis/Polymyositis**—Symmetrical proximal muscle weakness ± skin manifestations

**Hypercalcemia**—Nausea, vomiting, constipation, polyuria, polydipsia, lethargy

**Hypertrophic osteoarthropathy**—Clubbing, symmetrical painful arthropathy of the elbows, wrist, knees, and ankles

**Lambert-Eaton myasthenic syndrome**—Symmetrical proximal muscle weakness, extraocular muscles usually spared (unlike myasthenia gravis), muscle strength improves after brief muscle stimulation (myasthenia gravis), dry mouth, erectile dysfunction, ↓ DTR

**SIADH**—Symptoms related to hyponatremia that may include nausea, vomiting, irritability, malaise, anorexia, muscle cramps, or neurologic dysfunction

**Trousseau's syndrome**—Migratory or recurrent superficial thrombophlebitis

**Next Step:**

**Step 1**) The initial approach to a patient with suspected lung cancer is a thorough **clinical assessment** followed by a **chest x-ray (CXR)**. If a mass is identified on CXR, the location of the lesion may provide an indirect clue to the histology of the cancer (see Table 17-5).

**Step 2**) Further testing is usually performed if a mass is identified on CXR:

**CBC**—To check for anemia

**CMP**—To check for electrolytes, calcium level, alkaline phosphatase, and aminotransferases

**CT Chest with contrast**—Characterizes the primary tumor with possible pleural and mediastinal extension

**Step 3**) To establish a diagnosis and to differentiate small-cell lung cancer (SCLC) from non-small cell lung cancer (NSCLC), tissue sampling is required from any of the following modalities:

## Table 17-5 • Histologic Types of Lung Cancer

| Type | Location | High Yield Features |
|------|----------|---------------------|
| **Small Cell (Oat Cell)** | | |
| | Central | • Strongly related to smoking<br>• Highly malignant<br>• Commonly presents as a large hilar mass with mediastinal adenopathy<br>• Usually metastatic at the time of diagnosis<br>• Rarely amenable to surgery<br>• Median survival is 6-18 weeks if untreated<br>• Frequently associated with the paraneoplastic syndromes:<br><br>　1) SIADH<br>　2) Cushing's syndrome ($\uparrow$ ACTH)<br>　3) Hypercalcemia<br>　4) Lambert-Eaton myasthenic syndrome<br>　5) Dermatomyositis/polymyositis<br><br>**Foundational point**—Histologically, small "blue" malignant cells that can contain neurosecretory granules. |
| **Non-Small Cell** | | |
| Squamous cell | Central | • Related to smoking<br>• Cancer spread may be associated with hilar adenopathy and mediastinal widening on CXR<br>• Lesion can cavitate<br>• Frequently associated with the paraneoplastic syndrome:<br><br>　1) Hypercalcemia due to $\uparrow$ PTHrP<br><br>**Foundational point**—Histologically, the presence of keratin and/or desmosomes ("intracellular bridges"). |
| Adenocarcinoma | Peripheral | • Overall, most common type of lung cancer<br>• Commonly seen in women and nonsmokers<br>• Frequently associated with the paraneoplastic syndrome:<br><br>　1) Hypertrophic osteoarthropathy<br>　2) Trousseau's syndrome<br>　3) Dermatomyositis/polymyositis<br><br>**Foundational point**—Histologically, the presence of mucin or neoplastic gland formation. |
| Large cell | Peripheral | • Least common compared to the other types<br>• Undifferentiated tumor<br>• Typically, presents as a large peripheral mass<br>• Lesion can cavitate<br><br>**Foundational point**—Histologically, large pleomorphic cells with vesicular nuclei, prominent nucleoli, and abundant cytoplasm. |

ACTH—adrenocorticotropic hormone; CXR—chest x-ray; PTHrP—parathyroid hormone-related protein; SIADH—syndrome of inappropriate antidiuretic hormone secretion

- Transbronchial needle aspiration or biopsy
- Transthoracic needle aspiration or biopsy
- Thoracoscopic lung biopsy or pleural biopsy
- Thoracentesis of the pleural effusion
- Bronchoscopy with direct biopsy
- Mediastinoscopy with tissue sampling
- Fine-needle aspiration (FNA) of the lymph node
- Needle biopsy
- Sputum cytology

**Step 4)** Once the diagnosis of lung cancer is established, staging the disease will provide information on the extent of the cancer and management of the disease. Additional testing is usually required and may include a CT abdomen with contrast (to detect liver or adrenal metastasis), CT or MRI of the brain (to detect brain metastasis), bone scan, PET scan primarily for patients with NSCLC, or bone marrow biopsies primarily for patients with SCLC who have an abnormal CBC or peripheral blood smear. The staging system for SCLC and NSCLC differ in the following way:

## SCLC Staging Schema

**Limited disease**—Disease confined to one hemithorax and regional lymph nodes

**Extensive disease**—Disease outside of the hemithorax to distant sites

## NSCLC Simplified Staging Schema

**Stage I**—Cancer confined to lung with no lymph node involvement

**Stage II**—Cancer spread to adjacent structures or lymph nodes within the lung

**Stage IIIA**—Cancer spread to adjacent structures with mediastinal lymph node involvement

**Stage IIIB**—Cancer spread to adjacent structures with lymph node involvement of the mediastinum, supraclavicular, or scalene regions

**Stage IV**—Metastatic

**Step 5)** Treatment of lung cancer depends on the cell type, stage of the disease, and the functional capacity of the patient.

## SCLC Treatment

**Limited disease**—Chemotherapy (eg, cisplatin) + radiation

**Extensive disease**—Chemotherapy (eg, cisplatin)

## NSCLC Treatment

**Stage I**—Consider surgical resection

**Stage II**—Consider surgical resection

**Stage IIIA**—Chemotherapy (eg, cisplatin) + radiation, but surgical resection in select patients

**Stage IIIB**—Chemotherapy (eg, cisplatin) + radiation

**Stage IV**—Palliative systemic therapy that may include chemotherapy, radiation therapy, or molecular-targeted therapy

## Follow-Up:

Patients treated with a curative intent approach should have regular surveillance with a clinical assessment and imaging study (CXR or CT) every 6 months for 2 years, then annually.

Pearls:

- Patients with NSCLC in stages I-III are managed with a curative intent approach.
- Patients should have a PFT prior to having a surgical resection.
- Any of the histologic types of lung cancer can result in a paraneoplastic syndrome.
- It is not recommended to routinely screen for lung cancer with a CT, CXR, or sputum cytology.
- Hypercalcemia of malignancy can be due to an ectopic production of PTH, secretion of PTHrP, osteolysis from the tumor cells, or an increased production of 1,25-dihydroxyvitamin D.
- 5-year survival rate for SCLC-limited disease is 10% to 13% and for SCLC-extensive disease 1% to 2%.
- 5-year survival rate for NSCLC is Stage I >60%, Stage II 40% to 50%, Stage IIIA 10% to 35%, and Stage IIIB and IV <5%.
- Bronchoscopy is well suited for suspected central lesions since it allows for direct visualization of the tumor with biopsy, cytology brushing or lavage, or transbronchial biopsies.
- The sensitivity of sputum cytology varies by location of the lung cancer with the highest yield from large central tumors. Further diagnostic testing is recommended in patients with a negative or equivocal sputum cytology, but with clinical suspicion for lung cancer.
- The treatment approach to patients with small-cell lung cancer and SIADH should be focused on treating the malignancy since the hyponatremia will usually resolve once chemotherapy is started. However, patients with severe symptomatic hyponatremia should be treated with hypertonic (3%) saline infusion.
- **On the CCS**, "advise patient, no smoking."
- **On the CCS**, a "transthoracic needle biopsy" is equivalent to a "percutaneous biopsy, lung" in the practice CCS.
- **On the CCS**, a "transbronchial biopsy" will automatically be converted to a "bronchoscopy" in the practice CCS.
- **On the CCS**, remember that a thoracoscopic lung biopsy or lung resection will require a surgical consult. This would be the appropriate time and consultant for this type of procedure.
- **On the CCS**, remember to order an oncology consult if you're going to use chemotherapy.

# TRAUMA

## PNEUMOTHORAX

Pneumothorax (PTX) refers to an accumulation of air into the pleural space. The pressure in the intrapleural space is subatmospheric resulting in the tendency for air to readily flow into the pleural space if there is any communication with atmospheric pressure. There are several descriptions of pneumothorax that include the following:

**Primary spontaneous pneumothorax (PSP)**—A pneumothorax that occurs in the absence of a precipitating event and without an underlying history of lung disease. PSP is usually the result of a pleural bleb rupture and typically seen in tall, thin, young adults who are smokers.

**Secondary spontaneous pneumothorax (SSP)**—A pneumothorax that occurs as a complication from an underlying lung disease (eg, COPD, cystic fibrosis).

**Traumatic pneumothorax**—Blunt or penetrating trauma that disrupts the parietal or visceral pleura.

**Iatrogenic pneumothorax**—A pneumothorax that results from any diagnostic or therapeutic interventions.

**Tension pneumothorax**—A buildup of air in the pleural space without means of escape because of a check-valve mechanism.

**Open pneumothorax**—A chest wall defect that appears as a "sucking chest wound" upon inspiration and resulting in equilibration of atmospheric pressure within the intrapleural space.

**Hemopneumothorax**—An accumulation of blood and air in the pleural cavity.

**Catamenial pneumothorax**—A pneumothorax believed to be caused by endometriosis of the pleura. Onset of symptoms usually occurs within 24 to 48 hours of menstruation, and typically the pneumothorax is on the right side.

## Clinical Features:

Patients may be completely asymptomatic, especially if the pneumothorax is small. If the pneumothorax is large, then any of the following features may be present:

- Sudden onset of dyspnea
- Subcutaneous emphysema may be present
- Decreased tactile fremitus
- Decreased chest movement on the affected side
- Absent or decreased breath sounds on the affected side
- Hyperresonance to percussion on the affected side
- Acute pleuritic chest pain
- Hypoxemia

## Next Step:

**Step 1)** The patient's clinical condition determines the initial management in patients with a pneumothorax. Patients that are **clinically unstable** (eg, tension pneumothorax), require immediate intervention. Patients that are **clinically stable** based on the respiratory rate, pulse, blood pressure, and oxygen saturation can undergo a **chest x-ray** to establish the diagnosis of a pneumothorax. The expected finding on chest x-ray is a white visceral pleural line separated by a radiolucent area devoid of vascular markings. For board purposes, it may be helpful to estimate the size of a pneumothorax if the exam presents a radiograph. Based on the American College of Chest Physicians, a small pneumothorax is a measurement of <3 cm from the thoracic apex to the lung cupola and a large pneumothorax has a size ≥3 cm apex-to-cupola distance (see Figure 17-1).

**Step 2)** Patients should be provided **supplemental oxygen** while in the emergency room or in the inpatient unit. A summary of the different treatments for pneumothorax is as follows:

**Clinically unstable with any size PTX**—Chest tube + admit to hospital

**Clinically stable with large PTX**—Chest tube + admit to hospital

**Clinically stable with first small PSP**—Observe → repeat CXR → PTX does not progress → Discharge

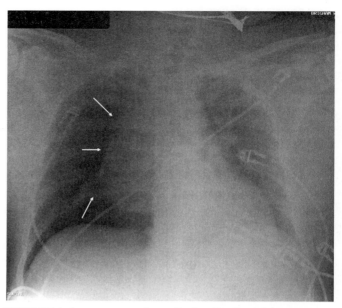

**FIGURE 17-1 • Large pneumothorax.** Depicted is a large right pneumothorax. Note the white visceral pleural line (arrows) that has a convex shape toward the chest wall. Beyond the visceral pleura is an increased lucency (air density) with avascular lung markings. (Reproduced with permission from Loscalzo, J. Harrison's *Pulmonary and Critical Care Medicine*. New York: McGraw-Hill; 2010:53.)

**Clinically stable with recurrent PSP**—Chest tube followed by thoracoscopy + admit to hospital

**Hemopneumothorax**—Chest tube followed by thoracoscopy + admit to hospital

**Clinically stable with small SSP**—Admit to hospital and either observe or simple aspiration

## Disposition:

Upon discharge from the hospital, patients should have close follow-up with their physician to assess the patient's condition.

## Pearls:

- Instilling a sclerosing agent through a chest tube (ie, chemical pleurodesis) to prevent a recurrent pneumothorax is an acceptable alternative if thoracoscopic pleurodesis (ie, surgically creating adhesions) is not available.

- Chest x-ray is the most common diagnostic tool for detecting a pneumothorax, but CT scanning is more accurate and is usually used in more complex or equivocal cases.

- A pneumothorax may be detected by CXR in the supine, lateral decubitus, or upright position. The lateral decubitus position is the most sensitive, while the supine position is the least sensitive.

- Providing supplemental oxygen is an important part of management because it can increase the rate of pleural air resorption three- to fourfold compared to room air.

- Patients with catamenial pneumothorax are acutely managed as other patients with a pneumothorax, but the underlying cause is eventually treated with either hormonal therapy (eg, oral contraceptives, progestins) or surgery.

- Caution is advised in patients with SSP because they have an underlying lung disease that compromises their pulmonary reserve volume.

- **CJ:** A 30-year-old man presents to the ED with an apparent chest wound. As the patient breathes, air can be seen bubbling through the blood surrounding the wound. What are your next steps? **Answer:** The diagnosis is an **open pneumothorax**, and the initial steps is to provide oxygen to the patient and then cover the wound with an impermeable dressing taped on three sides. Once the size of the hole is two-thirds the diameter of the trachea, air will preferentially enter the hole rather than the trachea because of lower airflow resistance. The dressing creates a one-way flap valve that prevents air into the chest on inspiration, but allows air to escape on the untaped side on expiration. Taping on all four sides of the dressing can create a tension pneumothorax. Definitive treatment is to close the wound and place a chest tube.

- **On the CCS**, "advise patient, no smoking" since smoking cessation will reduce the risk of a recurrent pneumothorax.

- **On the CCS**, both "chemical pleurodesis" and "thoracoscopic pleurodesis" are available in the practice CCS, but a surgical consult with a reason for the consult is required for the thoracoscopic pleurodesis.

- **On the CCS**, "video-assisted thoracoscopic surgery (VATS)" is not recognized in the practice CCS, but a "thoracoscopy" requiring a surgical consult is available.

- **On the CCS**, if a procedure is not warranted, the patient will let you know on a "Patient Update" screen that the "procedure is declined at this time."

- **On the CCS**, be aware that consultants are rarely helpful. Remember that the CCS is designed to assess your reasoning process and not to rely on the consultants. However, you are still evaluated on ordering the appropriate consultant at the appropriate time.

## TENSION PNEUMOTHORAX

A tension pneumothorax is a life-threatening condition that occurs when air is trapped in the pleural space. A one-way valve mechanism allows air to enter the pleural space on inspiration but prohibits outflow of air on expiration. Accumulation of gas within the pleural space can result in collapse of the ipsilateral lung and tracheal and mediastinal shift toward the contralateral side, which can compress the contralateral lung as well as impair venous return to the right atrium (see Figure 17-2).

### Clinical Features:

Patients with tension pneumothorax may present with any of the following features:

- Respiratory distress
- Hypotension
- Marked tachycardia
- Tracheal and mediastinal deviation away from the injured side
- Jugular venous distension (↑ central venous pressure)

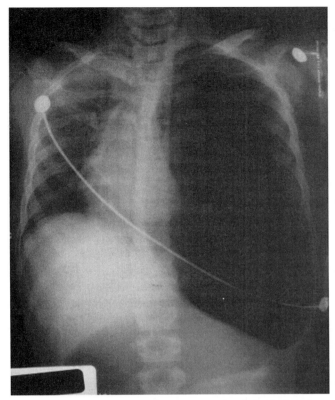

**FIGURE 17-2 • Tension pneumothorax.** Depicted is a left-sided tension pneumothorax. Note the "tense" pressure that results in tracheal deviation, mediastinal shift to the right, contralateral compressed lung, ipsilateral collapsed lung, and a marked depression of the left hemidiaphragm. Also, examine the striking left-sided "deep sulcus sign" that is seen in the supine position. In this position, air is able to collect anteriorly and basally, which accentuates the deepening of the left costophrenic angle. (Reproduced with permission from Knoop KJ, Stack LB, et al. *The Atlas of Emergency Medicine.* 3rd ed. New York: McGraw-Hill; 2010:161.)

- Absent or decreased breath sounds on injured side
- Hyperresonance to percussion on injured side
- Acute pleuritic chest pain
- Hypoxemia

### Next Step:

**Step 1)** Tension pneumothorax is a clinical diagnosis and a medical emergency that requires immediate decompression. Rapidly decompress with a **needle thoracostomy** performed on the injured side through the second or third intercostal space at the anterior, midclavicular line. A rush of air should be heard upon insertion of the needle and diagnosis of a tension pneumothorax is then confirmed. The tension pneumothorax has now been converted to a simple pneumothorax.

**Step 2)** Arrange for a **chest tube thoracostomy,** which is considered definitive treatment. Chest tube placement is typically placed through the fifth intercostal space at the midaxillary line.

**Step 3)** Connect the chest tube to a water seal device ± suction (ie, some physicians will only apply suction if the lungs fail to re-expand).

**Step 4)** Order a portable chest x-ray to confirm chest tube placement and assess lung re-expansion.

## Disposition:

Remember to treat and stabilize the patient in the emergency room before admitting the patient into the hospital for further observation.

## Pearls:

- Do not order a chest x-ray and wait for confirmation of the results before treating the patient because it may lead to the patient's death.

- Upon placing a needle into the intercostal space, remember to avoid the lower margin of the involved rib to prevent injury to the neurovascular bundle.

- Tension pneumothorax is commonly caused by trauma (blunt or penetrating) and iatrogenic (eg, medical procedures, barotrauma secondary to positive pressure ventilation), but 1% to 2% of PSP may develop a tension pneumothorax.

- A chest tube thoracostomy is preferable over a needle thoracostomy because of controlled placement of the chest tube compared to blindly inserting a needle. However, if the chest tube is not readily available or your clinical judgment (ie, respiratory distress, hemodynamically unstable) tells you

that the patient would not be able to withstand the few extra minutes to perform a tube thoracostomy, the best next step would be the needle thoracostomy, which would serve as a bridge until a chest tube can be placed.

- **On the CCS**, remember not to do a complete physical exam in acute cases, but rather a focused physical exam.

- **On the CCS**, remember to monitor patients closely during emergent cases. In this case, you want to measure the oxygen saturation with a pulse oximetry. Also, try typing in "continuous" in the order menu, and a list of monitoring devices will be available. In this particular case, you will want to order "continuous blood pressure cuff" and "continuous cardiac monitoring." For future blood pressure and cardiac readings, you will have to order "check blood pressure" and "check cardiac monitor," respectively.

- **On the CCS**, timing is critical in this type of case. Remember not to order anything that would delay treatment.

- **On the CCS**, you will be evaluated on your sequence of actions. Therefore, do not order a chest x-ray before treatment, but rather after treatment to assess lung re-expansion.

# CCS: COPD EXACERBATION CASE INTRODUCTION

Day 1 @ 17:00
Emergency Room

A 67-year-old white male comes to the emergency department because of worsening dyspnea, increased frequency of cough, increased volume of sputum production, and change in color of sputum from white to yellow.

**Initial Vital Signs:**
Temperature: 38.6°C (101.5°F)
Pulse: 110 beats/min, bounding
Respiratory: 28/min
Blood pressure: 140/90 mm Hg
Height: 177.8 cm (70.0 inches)
Weight: 68.2 kg (150 lb)
BMI: 21.6 kg/m$^2$

**Initial History:**
Reason(s) for visit: Dyspnea, productive cough, sputum changes

**HPI:**
The patient, a 67-year-old retired physician, has been experiencing increased dyspnea, increased frequency of cough, and increased sputum volume with purulence over the past 4 days, which has been beyond his normal day-to-day variation. He states that he

feels better when he is sitting up and in the forward position to alleviate his dyspnea. He admits to being a long time smoker and states "back in my day, we use to smoke inside the hospital." He has been admitted to the hospital 4 times over the past year for COPD exacerbation with his most recent admission 2.5 months ago.

| | |
|---|---|
| **Past Medical History:** | Four hospitalizations for COPD exacerbations that each required antibiotic therapy. Hypercholesterolemia. |
| **Past Surgical History:** | None |
| **Medications:** | Atorvastatin, tiotropium once daily, albuterol prn, supplemental home oxygen |
| **Allergies:** | None |
| **Vaccinations:** | Up to date |
| **Family History:** | Father died of lung cancer. Mother died of breast cancer. No siblings. |
| **Social History:** | Quit smoking 7 years ago, but previously smoked 1 ppd × 42 years; no longer drinks alcoholic beverages; denies use of illegal drugs; married; four children; retired physician; enjoys playing golf and going to operas. |

**Review of Systems:**

| | |
|---|---|
| General: | See HPI |
| Skin: | Negative |
| HEENT: | Negative |
| Musculoskeletal: | Negative |
| Cardiorespiratory: | See HPI |
| Gastrointestinal: | Negative |
| Genitourinary: | Negative |
| Neuropsychiatric: | Negative |

Day 1 @ 17:07

**Physical Examination:**

**General appearance:** Thin, undernourished; in respiratory distress, sitting in the tripod position.

**HEENT/Neck:** Normocephalic. EOMI, PERRLA. Copious oral secretions. No cyanosis of the lips. Full use of the accessory muscles of the neck. Trachea midline. Thyroid normal.

**Chest/Lungs:** Increase AP diameter of the chest. Hyperresonant to percussion. Expiration through pursed lips. Generalized expiratory wheezes, bilateral crackles at the lung bases. Inward retraction of the lower rib cage on inspiration.

**Heart/Cardiovascular:** Tachycardia. No murmurs, rubs, gallops, or extra sounds. No JVD.

**Abdomen:** Normal bowel sounds; no bruits. No tenderness. No masses. No hernias. No hepatosplenomegaly.

**Extremities/Spine:** Extremities symmetric. No cyanosis or clubbing. No edema. Peripheral pulses bounding. Full range of motion of the extremities. Spine examination normal.

**First Order Sheet:**
1) Sit upright
2) Suction upper airway, stat — **Result:** Difficult to clear all secretions
3) Pulse oximetry, stat — **Result:** 87% (nl: 94-100)
4) Supplemental oxygen, continuous
5) PEFR, stat — **Result:** The patient is unable to cooperate.
6) IV access
7) Continuous cardiac monitoring, stat — **Result:** Sinus tachycardia
8) Continuous blood pressure cuff, stat — **Result:** 140/90 mm Hg

**Second Order Sheet:**
1) Albuterol, inhalation, continuous
2) Ipratropium, inhalation, continuous
3) Methylprednisolone, IV, one time/bolus
4) Levofloxacin, IV, continuous

**Third Order Sheet:**
1) ABG, stat — **Result:** pH-7.35, pCO$_2$-50 mm Hg, pO$_2$-52 mm Hg, HCO$_3$-30 mEq/L, O$_2$ saturation-87%
2) EKG, 12-lead, stat — **Result:** Rhythm- sinus tachycardia, Axis- +30 degrees, P waves-wnl, QRS complexes-wnl, ST-T waves-wnl, Other findings-none, Interpretation-sinus tachycardia
3) Chest x-ray, PA/lateral, stat — **Result:** Increased radiolucency in both lung fields, flattened diaphragm, nodular infiltrate with tree-in-bud opacities in left lower lobe.
4) CBC with differential, stat — **Result:** WBC-14,000, H/H-16/55%, Plt-300,000, Differential: Neutrophils-65% (nl: 54%-62%) Band neutrophils-10% (nl: 3%-5%), Lymphs-25% (nl: 25%-33%)
5) BMP, stat — **Result:** Glu-100, Urea-16, Na-143, K-4.0, Cl-103, HCO3-30, Cr-0.8, Ca-9.5
6) Urinalysis, stat — **Result:** WNL

**Follow-Up History:**
The patient is feeling better.

**Physical Examination:**

**HEENT/Neck:** No straining of the accessory muscles of the neck.

**Chest/Lungs:** Improved breath sounds. Minimal wheezing.

**Heart/Cardiovascular:** S1 and S2 normal. No murmurs, rubs, gallops, or extra sounds. No JVD.

**Fourth Order Sheet:**
1) Pulse oximetry, stat — **Result:** 90% (nl: 94-100)
2) Check cardiac monitor, stat — **Result:** Regular sinus
3) Vital signs, stat — **Result:** 37.8°C (100.2°F), HR-96, RR-20, BP-138/88 mm Hg
4) ABG, stat — **Result:** pH-7.37, pCO$_2$-48 mm Hg, pO$_2$-58 mm Hg, HCO$_3$-29 mEq/L, O$_2$ saturation-90%

**Actions:**
1) Change location to inpatient unit

**Fifth Order Sheet:**
1) Ambulate at will
2) Urine output, routine
3) Low fat diet

**This case will end in the next few minutes of "real time."**
You may **add** or **delete** orders at this time,
then enter a diagnosis on the following screen.

**Sixth Order Sheet:**
1) Counsel family/patient
2) Advise patient, no smoking
3) Advise patient, side effects of medication
4) Vaccine, influenza, IM, one time
5) Vaccine, pneumococcal, IM, one time

**Please enter your primary diagnosis only:**
COPD Exacerbation

## DISCUSSION:

COPD exacerbation is typically triggered by a respiratory infection, but other precipitants that have been implicated are environmental pollutants, medications, and medical conditions (eg, pneumonia, pulmonary embolism, CHF). Common viral causes include influenza, rhinoviruses, adenoviruses, and coronaviruses. Common bacterial causes include nontypeable *Haemophilus influenzae*, *Streptococcus pneumoniae*, *Moraxella catarrhalis*, and *Pseudomonas aeruginosa* (particularly in patients with severe COPD).

## Clinical Features:

Patients with a COPD exacerbation will usually have acute changes from their baseline symptoms, which can include any of the following: ↑ dyspnea, ↑ cough, ↑ sputum production, and/or changes in the quality of sputum. Patients with worsening dyspnea will try to alleviate their symptom by leaning forward with outstretched arms, exhaling through pursed lips, and using their accessory muscles (scalene, sternocleidomastoid, and intercostal muscles). Patients with worsening hypoxemia (ie, $SaO_2$ <90%) will start to have changes in mental status, tachycardia, tachypnea, hypertension, and cyanosis.

## Next Step Summary:

**Step 1)** Perform a targeted physical exam as with most acute cases.

**Step 2)** Address the oxygen status and cardiovascular status with the appropriate monitoring equipment.

**Step 3)** Diagnosis of a COPD exacerbation is based on the clinical presentation (ie, acute changes from their baseline symptoms); therefore, no single test will confirm the diagnosis. Do not delay treatment in a patient that is in respiratory distress. Once treatment is given to the patient (see Step 4), initial evaluation should include:

**ABG**—To access the acid-base status.

**BMP**—To access the electrolytes and to have a baseline potassium since β2-agonists can lower potassium levels.

**CBC**—In this case, elevated white count with increase in bands suggest an infection. Also, the hematocrit is elevated, which suggest chronic hypoxemia.

**CXR**—To exclude other causes and to identify coexisting diseases.

**EKG**—To access for other coexisting cardiac disease since cardiac ischemia can also cause hypoxia.

**UA**—To identify potential sources of infection.

**Step 4)** Treatment for COPD exacerbation should strive for adequate oxygenation, "open up the airways," and treat the underlying cause. Consider the following interventions:

**Supplemental oxygen**—The target for adequate oxygenation is an arterial oxygen saturation ($SaO_2$) of 90% to 94% or an arterial oxygen tension ($PaO_2$) of 60 to 70 mm Hg.

**Bronchodilators**—The combination therapy of an inhaled short-acting β2-agonist (eg, albuterol) with an inhaled short acting anticholinergic (eg, ipratropium) is thought to have an additive effect than either agent alone.

**Systemic corticosteroids**—Adding systemic corticosteroids can improve symptoms, lung function, shorten the length of hospital stays, and decrease the rate of return of ED visits. Route of administration can be given orally (eg, po prednisone) or intravenously (eg, IV methylprednisolone). In this CCS case, if there is any concern for the patient to swallow, the intravenous route would be safer, and once the patient is able to tolerate orals, then you can switch to oral medication. Typical duration of corticosteroid therapy is 10 to 14 days.

**Antibiotics**—Antibiotic therapy is usually given to patients when there is evidence of infection. In this particular CCS case, the patient had an increase in sputum production, increase in sputum purulence, increase in dyspnea, and the CBC showed an elevated white count with bands, which cumulatively suggests a bacterial infection. In addition, this patient had risk factors for a pseudomonas infection because he was recently hospitalized within the past 90 days and he had multiple antibiotics over the past year (≥4 courses of antibiotics). In this particular CCS case, the choice of antibiotics was tailored towards a pseudomonas infection with levofloxacin, but other antipseudomonals can also be used such as ciprofloxacin, piperacillin-tazobactam, cefepime, or ceftazidime. Ideally, initial antibiotics should target the most likely bacteria (ie, *H influenzae*, *M catarrhalis*, *S pneumoniae*), and good empiric treatment can be started with trimethoprim-sulfamethoxazole (TMP-SMZ), doxycycline, or amoxicillin-clavulanate. Typical duration of antibiotic therapy is 3 to 7 days.

**Noninvasive positive pressure ventilation (NPPV)**—NPPV refers to positive pressure ventilation delivered by nasal mask, facemask, or mouthpiece. Positive pressure ventilation can be delivered by either one of two modes: continuous positive airway pressure (CPAP) or bilevel positive airway pressure (BPAP). Indications for NPPV include severe dyspnea with use of accessory muscles or pH ≤7.35 and/or $PaCO_2$ ≥45 mm Hg. Contraindications to NPPV include copious secretions, inability to clear secretions, high risk of aspiration, uncooperative patient, obtunded patient, hemodynamic instability, unstable cardiac arrhythmia, respiratory arrest, recent facial or gastroesophageal surgery, burns, extreme obesity, or craniofacial abnormalities.

**Step 4)** Reassess the patient by using the interval/follow-up, performing a focus physical exam, monitoring the vitals and oxygen saturation.

## Disposition:

Patients should be considered for admission when they fail to improve adequately despite treatment, significant comorbidities, change in mental status, older age, inability to care for themselves, or inadequate home support.

## Pearls:

- Oral or intravenous glucocorticoids are both equally effective in treating COPD exacerbations.
- The route of delivery of an inhaled short-acting bronchodilator can be given by a nebulizer or metered-dose inhaler (MDI) with proper technique since studies have shown no difference in $FEV_1$ when either device is given.
- The PEFR, which is also known as "peak flow," can be obtained by spirometry or a peak flow meter (inexpensive portable device). If the patient is able to cooperate during a COPD exacerbation, a value of <100 L/min usually indicates a severe exacerbation.
- Patients that are taking theophylline should have their theophylline levels checked because of concerns for toxicity.
- Sputum cultures and gram stain is usually not useful in patients with COPD exacerbations, however, the sputum cultures and antibiotic sensitivities should be considered when the patient is not responding to the initial antibiotic treatment.
- Patients with severe airway obstruction will have the characteristic hyperinflation of the lungs with a flattened diaphragm that can result in inward contraction of the diaphragm instead of downward, which will appear as a paradoxical retraction of the lower intercostal spaces on inspiration (Hoover's sign).
- **On the CCS,** both "CPAP" and "Continuous positive airway pressure" are available in the practice CCS.
- **On the CCS,** either "BiPAP" or "Bilevel positive airway pressure" is available in the practice CCS, but not "BPAP."
- **On the CCS,** delaying treatment would be considered suboptimal management.
- **On the CCS,** failure to monitor or follow up on the patient's oxygen status, vital signs, cardiac status, and physical condition would be considered suboptimal management.
- **On the CCS,** be cognizant about the simulated time because you want to complete your diagnostic and therapeutic interventions in a timely fashion in acute cases.

# 18

# Renal and Genitourinary

## KEY FINDINGS REVIEW

### URINE INSPECTION

#### Color

**White-cloudy**—Due to chyle, pus, or phosphate crystals.

**Red-brown**—Due to hematuria, hemoglobinuria, myoglobinuria, bile pigments, fava beans, or beets.

**Black-brown**—Due to methemoglobin, melanin, methyldopa, or levodopa.

**Green-blue**—Due to biliverdin, Pseudomonas infection, or propofol.

#### Odor

**Sweet or fruity**—Due to ketones.

**Fecal**—Due to GI-bladder fistula.

**Maple**—Due to maple syrup urine disease

**Mousy or musty**—Due to phenylketonuria (PKU).

**Pungent**—Think UTIs.

**Ammoniac**—Think urease-producing organisms or struvite stones.

### URINE DIPSTICK

**Urine pH**—Urine pH ranges from 4.5 to 8.0. Urine pH >7.0 suggests calcium phosphate or struvite stones. Urine pH <5.5 suggests uric acid stones. Urine pH <5.3 suggests type 4 RTA, urine pH >5.3 suggests type 1 (distal) RTA, and a variable urine pH suggests type 2 (proximal) RTA.

**Specific gravity (SG)**—SG can range from 1.003 to 1.030. SG can give you an idea of the kidney's ability to concentrate, patient's hydration status, or an estimate of the urine osmolality. A rough SG guideline includes SG <1.003 indicates a very dilute urine, SG <1.010 indicates hydration, SG >1.020 indicates dehydration, and SG = 1.009 correlates with a urine osmolality of approximately 280 mOsmol/kg.

**Ketones**—Can be found in DKA, fasting, carb-free diets, strenuous exercise, or pregnancy. A positive dipstick indicates the presence of acetoacetate or acetone (ie, only nitroprusside reacts with those 2 ketones), but not β-hydroxybutyrate.

Glucose—Glycosuria occurs if the kidneys cannot reabsorb filtered glucose (eg, Fanconi's syndrome) or urinary spillage of glucose because of high plasma glucose levels which is not seen until plasma glucose is >180 mg/dL.

Nitrites—Indicates bacteriuria because the bacteria (primarily Enterobacteriaceae species, which are gram-negatives) can convert nitrates to nitrites from the enzyme nitrate reductase. However, false negatives can occur if there is an infection with enterococcus (gram-positive), which expresses low levels of nitrate reductase.

Leukocyte esterase (LE)—Indicates the presence of white blood cells (ie, produces LE). A positive result is suggestive of a bacterial infection, but not diagnostic.

Bilirubin—No bilirubin should be detected on dipstick. A positive dipstick suggests an elevated conjugated bilirubin because it is water soluble, which allows it to pass through the glomerulus, but unconjugated bilirubin is water insoluble, which does not pass through the glomerulus.

Urobilinogen—Urobilinogen is an end product of conjugated bilirubin, and only small amounts are normally present in the urine. If elevated levels are seen, it may be due to hemolysis or liver disease, while a decreased level may be due to bile duct obstruction or antibiotics.

Blood—A positive dipstick can be the result of erythrocytes, hemoglobin, myoglobin, menstrual bleed, or semen (ie, false positive). If you centrifuge your sample and a red color is seen in the supernatant, then it suggests hemoglobin or myoglobin, but if the sediment appears red, then it suggests hematuria. Further microscopic studies are needed by taking the sediment and examining for red blood cells as the cause of hematuria.

Protein—Dipstick is sensitive for albumin, but not for other types of proteins (eg, globulins, Bence-Jones proteins). However, performing a follow-up test with sulfosalicylic acid (SSA) can detect all proteins in the urine. The dipstick is not sensitive enough to detect moderately increased albuminuria (formerly called microalbuminuria). The level of proteins (ie, trace, 1+, 2+, 3+) in the urine is not completely reliable because it depends on the urine concentration. If proteinuria is found, break it down to primary glomerular causes (eg, nephrotic syndrome), secondary glomerular causes (eg, SLE, DM), tubular causes (eg, tubulointerstitial nephritis, drugs), overflow causes (eg, multiple myeloma), or transient causes (eg, dehydration, exercise, orthostatic postural proteinuria).

## URINE SEDIMENT (MICROSCOPIC EXAM)

After centrifugation of the urine sample, the supernatant is poured off and the remaining pellet is agitated so that the sediment can be placed on a slide for evaluation.

### Cells

Transitional epithelial cells—Normal finding, but if found in clumps or large numbers then it suggests neoplasm.

Squamous epithelial cells—Suggests contamination.

Renal tubular cells—Larger than WBCs; their presence suggests tubular damage or inflammation.

Erythrocytes—Findings ≥2 RBCs on high-power field (HPF) is considered abnormal.

Leukocytes—Men generally have <2 WBCs on HPF, and women typically have <5 WBCs on HPF. Eosinophils detected with either Hansel's or Wright's stain suggests allergic interstitial nephritis.

Bugs—Bacteria can be further characterized by gram staining, yeast will show hyphae or budding forms, and Trichomonas will be swimming around with their motile flagellum.

### Casts

Casts have a cylindrical structure that are formed in the distal tubules and collecting ducts as result of the precipitation of a protein (ie, Tamm-Horsfall mucoprotein).

RBC casts—Suggests glomerulonephritis or vasculitis.

WBC casts—Suggests pyelonephritis, interstitial nephritis, or glomerulonephritis.

Fatty casts—Suggests heavy proteinuria or nephrotic syndrome. Under polarized light, a "Maltese cross" can be seen in the fat droplets.

Broad casts—Suggests advanced chronic kidney disease.

Waxy casts—Nonspecific finding, but can be seen in renal failure patients and in rapidly progressive glomerulonephritis.

Hyaline casts—Nonspecific finding, but can be seen in concentrated normal urine or in renal disease.

Granular casts—Nonspecific finding, but may suggest renal disease (ie, ATN, tubulointerstitial disease, glomerulonephritis) or the result of degeneration from other casts. Granular casts can be coarse ("muddy brown") or fine.

Epithelial casts—Renal tubular epithelial cell casts suggests acute tubular necrosis (ATN), acute interstitial nephritis, proliferative glomerulonephritis, or nephrotic syndrome.

## Crystals

See Nephrolithiasis section (see Table 18-1, Figure 18-1, and Color Plate 14).

| Table 18-1 • Nephrolithiasis Profile | | | |
|---|---|---|---|
| **Stones** | **Causes** | **Diagnostic Clues** | **Next Step Treatment Approach** |
| **Calcium oxalate (CaOx)** | **Hypercalciuria:** Idiopathic hypercalciuria, primary hyperparathyroidism<br>**Hyperoxaluria:** Diet high in oxalate (eg, spinach, rhubarb, kale, beets, berries, bean, nuts, wheat, chocolate), enteric causes (eg, fat malabsorption, bowel diversion or resection, IBD), or conversion to oxalate (eg, vitamin C)<br>**Hypocitraturia:** Distal (type 1) RTA, chronic diarrhea, carbonic anhydrase inhibitors | **Imaging:** Radiopaque<br>**Urine pH:** Crystal formation is independent on the urine pH<br>**Crystal shape:** Dumbbell-shaped or envelope-shaped (Note: Looks like squares with lines intersecting in the center. If the lines do not intersect in the middle, it may be mistaken for a triple phosphate crystal.)<br>**Color:** Colorless | **Step 1)** Initial treatment should begin with dietary changes (ie, ↑ fluid intake, ↑ phytate, ↑ $K^+$, ↑ diet $Ca^{2+}$, ↓ sucrose, ↓ fructose, ↓ animal protein, ↓ oxalate foods, ↓ $Na^+$, reduce excessive $Ca^{2+}$ and vitamin C supplements) for at least 3-6 months.<br>**Step 2)** If resistant to step 1, then consider meds:<br>**Hypercalciuria:** Thiazides<br>**Hyperoxaluria:** Cholestyramine<br>**Hypocitraturia:** Alkalinization (eg, $K^+$ citrate, $K^+$ bicarbonate) |
| **Calcium phosphate** | Same as calcium oxalate except for hyperoxaluria. Distal RTA usually causes an alkaline pH, which favors calcium phosphate crystals. | **Imaging:** Radiopaque<br>**Urine pH:** Alkaline (>7.0)<br>**Crystal shape:** Pleomorphic (needle, star, rosette, prism, flat plates)<br>**Color:** Colorless | **Step 1)** Same as CaOx, except for limiting oxalate foods or vitamin C.<br>**Step 2)** Meds can be attempted with thiazides to ↓ urine calcium, and alkalinization should be used with caution. |
| **Struvite ($MgNH_4PO_4$)** | Infection with urease-producing organisms such as:<br>• *Klebsiella species*<br>• *Proteus species*<br>• *Pseudomonas aerugionsa*<br>• *Providencia species*<br>• *Haemophilus influenzae*<br>• *Staphylococcus aureus*<br>• *Ureaplasma urealyticum* | **Clinically:** Look for a UTI (more common in women)<br>**Imaging:** Radiopaque, staghorn (branched) calculus<br>**Urine pH:** Alkaline (>7.0)<br>**Crystal shape:** Rectangular prisms or "coffin lids"<br>**Color:** Colorless | **Step 1)** Treat the acute infection (eg, UTI) with antibiotics.<br>**Step 2)** Definitive therapy is to remove the stone with PNL as the preferred surgical approach in most patients. Patients that cannot tolerate surgical intervention may be given a urease inhibitor (acetohydroxamic acid) instead. |
| **Uric acid** | ↑ Uric acid production<br>• Gout<br>• Alcohol<br>• High purine diet<br>• Lesch-Nyhan syndrome<br>Diabetes mellitus<br>Obesity<br>Metabolic syndrome<br>Chronic diarrhea (ie, ↓ $HCO_3^-$) | **Imaging:** Radiolucent<br>**Urine pH:** Acidic (<5.5)<br>**Crystal shape:** Pleomorphic (rosette, rhomboid prism, diamond, amorphous, needle)<br>**Color:** Colorless to yellow or red-brown | **Step 1)** Initial treatment may begin with ↑ fluid intake, ↓ alcohol intake, ↓ protein intake, and alkalinizing the urine with either potassium bicarbonate or potassium citrate.<br>**Step 2)** Allopurinol may be given in patients resistant to step 1. |
| **Cystine** | Cystinuria, which is an inherited disorder that results in a defective transport channel in the proximal convoluted tubule leading to excess cystine in the urine. | **Imaging:** Radiopaque<br>**Urine pH:** Presents primarily in acidic urine, but as the pH rises so does the solubility of cystine.<br>**Crystal shape:** Hexagonal<br>**Color:** Colorless | **Step 1)** Initial treatment may begin with ↑ fluid intake and alkalinizing the urine with either potassium bicarbonate or potassium citrate.<br>**Step2)** A thio-containing drug (penicillamine or tiopronin) can increase the solubility of cystine and may be given to patients resistant to step 1. |

*PNL—percutaneous nephrolithotomy*

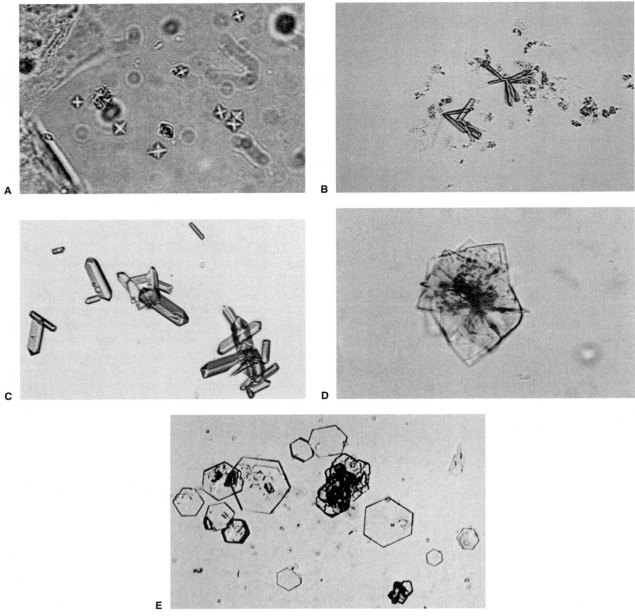

**FIGURE 18-1 • Urinary crystals. A. Calcium oxalate**—Envelope-shaped crystals with a prominent "X" crossing at the center. **B. Calcium phosphate**—Needle-shaped crystals. **C. Triple phosphate**—"Coffin lid" appearance. **D. Uric acid**—Rosette formation. **E. Cystine**—Hexagonal plates. (Reproduced with permission from Mundt LA, Shanahan K. Graff. *Textbook of Urinalysis and Body Fluids*. 2nd ed. Philadelphia, LWW; 2011: 66, 67, 76, 123, 133.)

# HEREDITARY DISORDERS

## ▌AUTOSOMAL DOMINANT POLYCYSTIC KIDNEY DISEASE

Autosomal dominant polycystic kidney disease (ADPKD), formerly called adult polycystic kidney disease, is the most common inherited kidney disease. The two genes that account for ADPKD include mutations in the PKD-1 (encodes polycystin-1) and PKD-2 (encodes polycystin-2) genes. PKD-1

mutations are more common, present earlier, and cause more severe disease compared to PKD-2 mutations. PKD-2 mutations have a later onset and slower progression.

**Clinical Features:**

Symptoms of ADPKD often do not appear until ages 30 to 40, but they can begin in childhood. The most common symptom is **pain in the abdomen, flank, or back**. The development of cysts is universally bilateral, and palpable bilateral flank masses felt on exam may suggest advanced ADPKD. Consider the following renal manifestations:

**Hypertension**—Hypertension is an early manifestation with a mean age of onset of 30 years. HTN occurs in approximately 60% of patients with normal kidney function before a reduction in GFR. Once kidney function is impaired, a progressive decline ensues with an average decline in the GFR of 4.0 to 5.0 mL/min/yr.

**Hematuria**—Hematuria is frequently a presenting manifestation and can be due to a cystic rupture into the collecting system, nephrolithiasis, or UTI.

**Stones**—Nephrolithiasis can occur in up to 20% to 25% of patients with 50% composed of uric acid stones and the remainder as calcium oxalate stones.

**Concentrating defect**—A decrease in the concentrating ability is usually an early manifestation that is initially mild, but worsens with increasing age and declining kidney function. Patients will often complain of polydipsia, polyuria, and nocturia. Plasma vasopressin is usually elevated with normal serum osmolarity.

**Proteinuria**—Patients may have mild proteinuria (ie, not a prominent feature in ADPKD).

**Pain**—An acute sharp pain may be due to a cystic rupture, hemorrhage into a cyst with expansion, cyst infection, parenchymal infection, or passage of a stone. A chronic, dull, nagging pain may be the result of an enlarged kidney with a mass effect. If the kidney enlarges such that there is an increase in abdominal girth, patients may complain of lower back pain secondary to lumbar lordosis.

ADPKD can also have extrarenal manifestations that include the following from a relative head to toe fashion:

**Cerebral aneurysms**—Approximately 5% to 20% of patients will have an aneurysm, which most often occurs in the anterior circulation. A ruptured aneurysm can result in either a subarachnoid or an intracerebral hemorrhage.

**Cardiac valve disease**—Valve disease include mitral valve prolapse, aortic regurgitation, or mitral regurgitation.

**Hepatic cysts**—Hepatic cysts are a common extrarenal manifestation with most patients that are asymptomatic with preserved hepatic function. However, hepatic enlargement secondary to hepatic cyst formation can result in pain, early satiety, or shortness of breath.

**Abdominal wall and inguinal hernias**—These hernias occur with a higher frequency than the general population.

**Colonic diverticula**—Colonic diverticula are common and can potentially result in colonic perforation.

**Cysts**—Other possible cysts seen in ADPKD include subarachnoid, thyroid, pancreatic, splenic, and seminal vesicle cysts.

### Next Step:

**Step 1)** Diagnosis of ADPKD is most often made by a positive family history (ie, every generation will be affected with an autosomal dominant inheritance) and imaging studies. The best initial imaging modality is with an **ultrasound**, which will typically show multiple bilateral kidney cysts with possible evidence of liver, splenic, or pancreatic cysts. In cases when ultrasound

findings are equivocal and disease status must be determined with greater certainty (eg, potential kidney donor), then the next best step is to consider genetic testing ± MRI or CT.

**Step 2)** Counseling should be offered once the diagnosis is established, and patients should be advised to avoid competitive contact sports.

**Step 3)** There is no specific treatment that will delay or prevent ADPKD. Treatment is mainly supportive. However, there may be concerns during the management of ADPKD. Consider the following:

**ESRD**—Approximately 60% of patients with ADPKD will have end-stage renal disease (ESRD) by the age of 70, and either dialysis or renal transplantation is required. Nephrectomy is typically avoided, but may be warranted prior to a transplant in cases of recurrent infection or very large kidneys.

**Hypertension**—Target blood pressure should be <130/80 mm Hg. Choice of agent can be with either an ACE inhibitor (eg, lisinopril) or an ARB (eg, losartan) for those intolerant of an ACE inhibitor (eg, cough, angioedema).

**Hematuria**—Hematuria secondary to a cystic rupture into the collecting system will typically resolve within 7 days, and supportive therapy is generally recommended.

**Infected cyst**—Most cysts are infected with gram-negative organisms. Antibiotics that have good lipid-soluble penetration into the cysts are with fluoroquinolones (eg, ciprofloxacin), trimethoprim sulfamethoxazole, or chloramphenicol. Unfortunately, cephalosporins and aminoglycosides do not adequately penetrate infected cysts.

**Cerebral aneurysms**—Routine screening for cerebral aneurysms is not recommended unless there is a family history of cerebral aneurysms, personal history of a rupture, high-risk occupation, or prior to surgery (eg, renal transplant).

### Follow-Up:

The most common cause of death from ADPKD is from **cardiovascular-related problems**. Therefore, periodic follow-ups for blood pressure management and lipid assessment are essential. If plasma creatinine or potassium levels are elevated secondary to an ACE inhibitor or ARB, consider another agent (eg, calcium channel blocker, beta-blocker).

### Pearls:

- ADPKD accounts for approximately 5% of ESRD in the United Sates and Europe.
- Risk factors for progressive kidney disease include PKD-1 mutation, early onset, HTN, male, black race, and large kidneys.
- There is an inverse relationship between the kidney size and GFR.
- ADPKD does not appear to increase the risk of renal cell carcinoma (RCC) compared to the general population.
- Perinephric abscess should be considered in patients who continue to have persistent symptoms (eg, fever, flank pain, dysuria) despite antibiotic therapy, and therefore drainage of the abscess may be indicated.

- **Caveat 1**—Avoid using gadolinium-containing contrast (eg, MRI) since it can cause nephrogenic systemic fibrosis in patients with kidney failure.

- **Caveat 2**—Avoid ACE inhibitors and ARBs during pregnancy (Category D) and consider alternative agents (eg, methyldopa, hydralazine, labetalol).

- **Caveat 3**—Infected cysts may not always communicate with the collecting system, and therefore your urinalysis and urine culture will be negative. Blood cultures may in fact identify the organism more often than the urine culture.

- An elevated hematocrit and hemoglobin concentration can sometimes be seen in ADPKD because of an increase in erythropoietin secretion from the cysts.

- GERD-like symptoms and early satiety can result from a mass effect of the enlarged kidneys onto the GI tract.

- ADPKD is predominantly seen in adults, although it can occur in childhood. Children may be asymptomatic until adulthood or they may present during childhood with renal manifestations similar to adults, but hepatic, splenic, and pancreatic cysts are uncommon manifestations. However, children may have a higher frequency in an increased left ventricular mass.

- Routine screening for ADPKD in patients <18 years of age is controversial.

- **Foundational point**—The PKD-1 gene is located on chromosome 16, and the PKD-2 gene is located on chromosome 4.

- **Connecting point** (pg. 156)—Know the management of subarachnoid hemorrhage.

- **Connecting point** (pgs. 30, 32, 35)—Be able to differentiate the murmur sounds of mitral regurgitation, mitral valve prolapse, and aortic regurgitation.

- **Connecting point** (pg. 271)—Know the management of calcium oxalate and uric acid stones.

- **Connecting point** (pg. 163)—Recognize the genetic pedigree chart of autosomal dominant genes and know that children have a 50% chance of acquiring ADPKD.

- **On the CCS**, "genetic counseling" is available in the practice CCS.

- **On the CCS**, if you're not sure which ultrasound to choose for ADPKD (abdomen vs transabdominal/pelvis), there is an option for "kidney ultrasound" on the practice CCS. The kidney ultrasound is essentially the same as the abdomen ultrasound and will provide you with the essential information for ADPKD (ie, findings of the kidney, liver, spleen, and pancreas).

# AUTOSOMAL RECESSIVE POLYCYSTIC KIDNEY DISEASE

Autosomal recessive polycystic kidney disease (ARPKD), formerly called infantile polycystic kidney disease, is less common than ADPKD. The gene that accounts for ARPKD is a mutation in the PKHD1 gene that codes for a protein called polyductin or fibrocystin. ARPKD is primarily a disease of infants and children with the **kidney** and **liver** as the primary affected organs.

## Clinical Features:

The clinical presentation of ARPKD can vary. There may be prominent features in different age settings. Consider the following:

**Neonates**—**Enlarged echogenic kidneys** is usually present in the neonatal period, and in fact, enlarged kidneys may be seen after 24 weeks gestation by ultrasound. **Hypertension, oliguria**, and **acute renal failure** may be seen in the neonatal period. Pregnancies may be complicated by oligohydramnios, which could result in **Potter syndrome** (ie, pulmonary hypoplasia, clubfeet, Potter's facies [flat nose, low-set ears, micrognathia, pseudoepicanthus]). **Feeding difficulties** may also may be present secondary to fatigue (eg, pulmonary insufficiency) or compression of the stomach by the enlarged kidneys. **Death** can occur in approximately 30% to 50% of neonates due to pulmonary insufficiency secondary to pulmonary hypoplasia.

**Infants**—Bilateral palpable **flank masses** may be appreciated on physical exam and may even be felt soon after birth. **Renal dysfunction** may become more noticeable during this time period and beyond such as hyponatremia, reduced concentrating ability, proteinuria, or metabolic acidosis. **Hypertension** continues to occur during the first few years of life and if inadequately controlled, then CHF or cardiac hypertrophy may develop. Infants may also present with pneumomediastinum or **pulmonary related-complications** (eg, pneumothorax secondary to poor lung development).

**Childhood and young adulthood**—Hepatic abnormalities are the prominent presenting features in this age group. Biliary ductal plate abnormalities can result in **congenital hepatic fibrosis**, and the fibrosis can lead to **portal hypertension** and its complication (eg, esophageal varices). In addition, patients have a higher risk of developing **bacterial cholangitis**. On exam, **hepatosplenomegaly** may be appreciated secondary to portal hypertension. Again, **hypertension** may be present and typically occurs in more than 60% of children. Interestingly, the kidney size does not continue to grow significantly anymore, but eventually there is a **progressive decline in kidney function** in most patients.

## Next Step:

**Step 1)** Diagnosis of ARPKD is most often made by the clinical evaluation, labs, and imaging. The best initial imaging modality is with an **ultrasound**, which will typically show bilateral enlarged echogenic kidneys with poor cortico-medullary differentiation. The ultrasound of the liver may reveal dilatation of the intrahepatic biliary ducts (ie, duct ectasia) and occasionally hepatic cysts. In cases when ultrasound findings are equivocal, an MRI or CT may be considered as adjunctive testing, but remember to limit the radiation exposure in children (ie, CT). Genetic testing is not routinely performed to make the diagnosis, but in cases of uncertainty, genetic testing can be used to confirm the diagnosis. The following labs may also support the diagnosis:

**CBC**—Low platelet levels may be seen secondary to splenic sequestration.

**CMP**—Hyponatremia may be seen; creatinine levels may be normal or elevated; low $HCO_3^-$ may be seen secondary to metabolic acidosis; LFTs are usually normal; check albumin level to assess hepatic synthetic function.

**Coags**—PT and PTT will also give you an idea of the hepatic synthetic function.

**Urine osmolality**—Assess for impaired urinary concentration (ie, ↓ urine osmolality)

**Step 2)** Counseling should be offered to families and individuals once the diagnosis is established.

**Step 3)** There is no specific treatment that will delay or prevent ARPKD. Treatment is mainly supportive. However, there may be concerns during the management of ARPKD. Consider the following:

**ESRD**—Dialysis or renal transplantation are options for ESRD.

**Hypertension**—Multiple agents may be required to control the hypertension, but ACE inhibitors may be initially attempted.

**Respiratory distress**—Neonates may require mechanical ventilation secondary to pulmonary hypoplasia.

**Feeding difficulties**—Patients may need a higher caloric formula or supplemental feedings with an NG or gastrostomy tube.

**Progressive portal hypertension**—A portacaval shunt may be necessary or liver transplantation is another viable option.

**Esophageal varices**—Nonselective beta-blocker, sclerotherapy, or endoscopic banding may be necessary.

**Immunizations**—Patients with severe portal hypertension and splenic dysfunction should be immunized against encapsulated bugs (eg, meningococcus, pneumococcus, *H influenza* type B).

**Nephrotoxic agent avoidance**—Patients should avoid aminoglycosides and NSAIDs.

### Follow-Up:

Patients need frequent monitoring for their blood pressure, renal function, liver assessment, weight gain, and linear growth.

### Pearls:

- Neonates that survive the neonatal period (ie, first month of life) have approximately an 80% chance of living >10 years of age.

- ARPKD patients that have findings of congenital hepatic fibrosis with bile duct dilatation have a syndrome referred to as Caroli syndrome.

- Patients that develop acute cholangitis may have the classic Charcot triad (ie, fever, RUQ pain, and jaundice).

- The absence of renal cysts in either parent on ultrasound helps to differentiate ARPKD from ADPKD (ie, ADPKD parents will typically demonstrate cysts, but if they are young parents without cysts then you might have to look at the grandparents for the cysts).

- **Foundational point**—The PKHD1 gene is located on chromosome 6.

- **Foundational point**—Macrocysts are more typical of ADPKD.

- **Foundational point**—Microcysts (ie, less than 3-4 mm) are seen in ARPKD and typically radiate from the medulla to the cortex, but macrocysts can be seen in older children with ARPKD, which could make it difficult to differentiate between ADPKD.

- **Foundational point**—Cystic dilatations can be seen in all parts of the nephron in ADPKD, but cystic dilatations in ARPKD are typically in the collecting tubules.

- **Connecting point** (pg. 184)—Oligohydramnios (ie, amniotic fluid index <5 cm) can also be the result of ruptured fetal membranes.

- **Connecting point** (pg. 161)—Prenatal genetic testing can be offered to patients affected with the mutation. Know what week of gestation to do either an amniocentesis or chorionic villus sampling (CVS).

- **Connecting point** (pg. 163)—Recognize the genetic pedigree chart of autosomal recessive genes. If the parents are heterozygotes (ie, carriers of one disease allele), then their child has a 25% chance (1 out of 4) of inheriting both disease alleles and developing the disease, 50% chance of inheriting one disease allele and being a carrier (1 out of 2), 25% chance of not inheriting any disease allele, and 75% chance (3 out of 4) of becoming asymptomatic (remember heterozygotes can be asymptomatic). Also, know that consanguinity is suggestive of autosomal recessive inheritance.

- **On the CCS**, both "peritoneal dialysis" and "hemodialysis" are available in the practice CCS.

- **On the CCS**, "renal transplant" is available in the practice CCS, but remember to get a pediatric nephrology consult.

- **On the CCS**, if you require mechanical ventilation during any CCS cases, the prerequisites are either an intubation or tracheostomy. You are not required to know the mechanical ventilator settings (eg, PEEP, tidal volume, respiratory rate, $FiO_2$, I:E ratio).

---

# URINARY TRACT DISORDER

## ▎NEPHROLITHIASIS

Nephrolithiasis involves the interplay between supersaturation of urinary solutes and the lack of inhibitors (eg, citrate) in the urine that prevent crystal formation. The majority of stones are calcium stones (75%), which are primarily composed of calcium oxalate and less often of calcium phosphate. Other stones include struvite stones (10%-15%), uric acid stones (5%-10%), and cystine stones (1%-2%).

### Clinical Features:

Patients with nephrolithiasis can sometimes be asymptomatic with stones that are discovered incidentally on radiologic imaging for an unrelated reason. However, the classic symptom is an acute onset of intermittent pain. The pain in acute renal colic can vary from mild to excruciating and typically waxes and wanes. The location of the stone usually correlates with the location of the pain in that an obstruction in the upper ureter will refer pain to the flank, mid-ureter will refer pain to the lower anterior quadrant, and lower ureter obstruction will refer pain to the ipsilateral testicle or labium. If the stone is lodged in the ureterovesical junction, patients will often complain of urinary urgency, frequency, and dysuria. Associated signs and symptoms that may or may not be present include nausea, vomiting, and hematuria. On physical examination, most patients will be unable to find a comfortable position or they may appear to wiggle on the stretcher or writhe in pain, which is unlike an acute abdomen where patients tend to be still. Ipsilateral costovertebral angle tenderness is also a common finding on exam.

### Next Step:

**Step 1)** Patients in severe pain should be given analgesics. NSAIDs provide pain relief and have a direct effect on the ureter by the inhibition of prostaglandin synthesis. Opiates do not have a direct effect on the ureter but are still used for pain relief. However, the combination of **NSAIDs** (eg, ketorolac) and **opioids** (eg, morphine) is effective in pain control and may be superior to either agent alone based on randomized trials. The route of administration can be IV for faster pain relief, but the oral form can be given if the patient is able to tolerate oral intake.

**Step 2) Antiemetics** (eg, metoclopramide) should be given to patients with nausea and vomiting, as these symptoms are often associated with acute renal colic. In addition to providing relief from nausea, metoclopramide has also been shown to provide pain relief that is equivalent to narcotic analgesics in 2 double-blinded studies.

**Step 3)** The initial workup in patients with nephrolithiasis should include labs and imaging. First, consider the following labs and use your clinical judgment on what tests are appropriate for that given patient.

   **β-HCG**—A qualitative β-HCG should be obtained in females of childbearing age due to a risk of radiation exposure if imaging is pursued and to differentiate from other possible diagnoses.

   **Urinalysis**—UA will determine the pH of the urine where a pH <5.5 would suggest a uric acid stone but more alkaline urine with a pH >7 would suggest a struvite or calcium phosphate stone. UA can also detect hematuria and possible infection. A positive leukocyte esterase (LE) plus a positive nitrite should prompt you to order a urine culture with sensitivities. Microscopic examination of the urine sediment can detect crystals that would provide information on the type of stone (see Figure 18-1 and Color Plate 14).

   **Urine culture**—Obtain a urine culture if an infection is found. In addition, a urine culture should be obtained in all pediatric patients suspected of having nephrolithiasis because a UTI may also be present.

   **BMP**—Assess for the BUN and creatinine since some stone formers will have a reduced creatinine clearance.

   **CBC**—Check to see if there is leukocytosis if the patient is febrile or you speculate a systemic infection. However, be aware that mild leukocytosis can accompany acute renal colic secondary to an adrenergic response.

Second, the initial evaluation should also include imaging studies. Consider the following imaging modalities and again using your clinical judgment on what tests are appropriate for that given patient.

   **Noncontrast CT**—The preferred imaging modality is with a noncontrast abdomen/pelvis CT because it has a very high sensitivity and specificity. However, a CT should be avoided in pregnant women to avoid radiation exposure. CT has the advantage of detecting radiolucent uric acid stones that are often missed on KUB. Unfortunately, nonopaque stones due to HIV protease inhibitors (eg, indinavir, atazanavir) are often missed with noncontrast CT scan, and in these patients, a contrast CT should be considered.

   **Ultrasound**—Ultrasound is the preferred imaging modality in pregnant women and in patients where you want to minimize radiation exposure (eg, children). Ultrasound has the advantage of detecting hydronephrosis and can detect radiolucent stones that are missed on KUB. The disadvantage of ultrasound is that it may miss small stones (<5 mm) and stones located in the mid-ureter region.

   **Abdominal plain film**—A flat plate or kidney-ureter-bladder film (KUB) can detect large radiopaque stones (eg, calcium, cystine, and struvite) but will often miss radiolucent stones (eg, uric acid). The KUB is not the best initial test because it has a fairly low sensitivity and specificity.

   **Intravenous pyelogram (IVP)**—IVP or urography was once considered the gold standard but has been largely replaced by noncontrast CT. IVP has the advantage of outlining the urinary system where a mild hydronephrosis could easily be detected or nonopaque stones could be identified as a filling defect. The disadvantage of IVP is that contrast material is required and patients are exposed to radiation.

**Step 4)** Most stones that are ≤4 mm (0.4 cm) will spontaneously pass, but as the stone becomes larger in diameter (≥5 mm), the passage rates decline and stones ≥10 mm (1.0 cm) are unlikely to pass. Patients who have well-controlled symptoms, adequate renal function, and stones <10 mm can initially be observed and offered medical expulsive therapy (MET) during the observation period. However, patients that have unrelenting symptoms or persistent obstruction should be seen by a urologist with possible intervention. Consider the following management approach:

### Acute Management

- **Hydration**—Patients should be encouraged to increase their fluid intake. However, forced IV hydration does not necessarily increase the rate of stone passage.

- **Pain control**—Provide adequate analgesics but be aware of the potential for drug abuse with opioids and avoid NSAIDs in patients with a history of GI bleeds or preexisting renal disease.

- **Stone passage facilitators**—MET with alpha-blockers (eg, tamsulosin, doxazosin) or calcium channel blockers (eg, nifedipine) can increase the rate of ureteral stone passage.

- **Straining**—Patients should be advised to strain their urine for the next several days to retrieve any stone for analysis, which will elucidate the type of stone and will help target preventative therapy.

- **Empiric antibiotics**—Patients can be given empiric antibiotics on an outpatient basis if there is an associated UTI, but without systemic infection or significant obstruction. The choice of antibiotics should cover gram-negative rods and reasonable options include ciprofloxacin for 10 to 14 days, levofloxacin for 10 to 14 days, or other antibiotics based on local sensitivities.

- **Urology consult**—An urgent urologic consult should be obtained in patients with intractable pain or vomiting, anuria, acute renal failure, obstruction (hydronephrosis), or urosepsis. An outpatient urologic referral should be obtained in patients with stones >10 mm (1.0 cm), stones that have not passed in more than 4 to 6 weeks despite fluid intake or with MET, or if significant discomfort develops.

- **Urologic procedures**—Shock wave lithotripsy and ureteroscopy are two common techniques used to remove ureteral stones, and both are considered first-line procedures.

  **Extracorporeal shock wave lithotripsy (ESWL):** ESWL is the procedure of choice for small proximal ureteral stones (<10 mm). However, ESWL is not the ideal modality for large stones, stones of harder composition (eg, calcium oxalate, cystine), or patients with complex renal anatomy.

  **Ureteroscopy (URS):** URS is the procedure of choice for middle and distal ureteral stones, although the procedure can still be performed for proximal ureteral stones. URS involves the passage of a small endoscope into the bladder and up the ureter with retrieval of the stone using a grasping forceps or stone basket.

  **Percutaneous nephrolithotomy (PNL):** PNL involves percutaneous access to the kidney that requires general anesthesia. The stones can be visualized with a nephroscope and the calculi can be fragmented using a device attached to the scope that delivers localized energy (eg, laser, ultrasonic, pneumatic) to a specific area (intracorporeal lithotripsy). The urologist can then retrieve the stones using grasping forceps. PNL is typically reserved for large stones (>20 mm or 2.0 cm) or complex renal stones.

**Chronic Management**

- **24-hour urine collection**—A 24-hour urine collection may be advisable in recurrent stone formers with an unknown stone composition or in patients with their first stone but with high risk features for a stone (eg, family history, obesity, diabetes, bowel surgery, malabsorption). The patient's interest to perform a urine study and willingness to make lifestyle changes after the study are important factors to proceed with a metabolic evaluation. The urine study has the benefit of targeting preventive therapy and detecting possible metabolic disorders. The test is usually performed twice on an outpatient basis and usually 1 to 2 months after the acute episode or after any intervention. The idea is to evaluate the urine composition while the patient is on his or her normal day-to-day diet. The variables that are usually measured include the urine volume, pH, calcium, oxalate, citrate, uric acid, sodium, potassium, phosphorus, and creatinine.

- **Preventative therapy**—Once the stone is analyzed and/or the urine collections are evaluated, then management can be tailored to the underlying stone (see Table 18-1).

Disposition:

Patients should be admitted to the hospital if they have urosepsis, acute renal failure, intractable pain or vomiting, medical comorbidities, or significant obstruction with infection.

Pearls:

- Approximately 25% to 40% of patients will have recurrence of another stone within 5 years.

- Open stone surgery has a limited role since the advent of other procedures (eg, ESWL, URS).

- A phlebolith (ie, a calculus in a vein) can be confused with a ureteral stone. On KUB, a lucent center can be seen in a phlebolith but not with a ureteral stone. On CT, a "rim" sign, which is a halo surrounding the stones (secondary to circumferential edema of the soft tissue), can be seen.

- Two common stones seen in ADPKD are calcium oxalate and uric acid stones.

- The predominant type of stones in pregnancy is calcium phosphate because of an increase in calcium excretion and a rise in pH during pregnancy.

- Transvaginal ultrasound can detect distal ureteral stones better than a transabdominal ultrasound.

- **Caveat 1**—Alkali therapy is the treatment for distal (type 1) RTA, but caution is advised in patients with calcium phosphate stones since alkalinization of the urine promotes this type of stone.

- **Caveat 2**—Acetohydroxamic acid (AHA) should be used with caution because it has many side effects such as nausea, vomiting, tremors, palpitations, and headaches. AHA is contraindicated in pregnancy (Category X).

- **Caveat 3**—ESWL is contraindicated in pregnancy.

- **Caveat 4**—Cholestyramine is an oxalate and bile acid resin that may cause unwanted side effects (eg, abdominal pain, bloating, nausea, constipation).

- **Caveat 5**—Sodium salts used in alkalinization (eg, sodium bicarbonate, sodium citrate) can actually increase urinary calcium excretion.

- **Caveat 6**—An expanding or ruptured AAA is often misdiagnosed as an acute renal colic.
- There is controversy in the role of hyperuricosuria in the formation of calcium oxalate stones.
- Low dietary calcium may actually increase the risk of calcium stone formation because calcium normally binds to oxalate in the gut forming an insoluble salt, thereby preventing free oxalate from absorption and eventual excretion into the urine.
- Patients with fat malabsorption will cause calcium to bind with fatty acids instead of oxalate in the gut resulting in free oxalate absorption and eventual excretion into the urine (referred to as enteric hyperoxaluria).
- The dietary risk factors that increase the risk of calcium stone formation include ↓ fluid intake, ↓ phytate (eg, seeds, grains, nuts), ↓ potassium (eg, fruits and vegetables), ↓ diet calcium, ↑ sucrose, ↑ fructose, ↑ animal protein, ↑ oxalate foods, ↑ sodium intake, ↑ vitamin C.
- Citrate is a principal inhibitor in the urine to prevent calcium stone formation. Excretion of citrate is enhanced by alkalinizing the plasma because it will decrease the uptake of citrate from the proximal tubular cells.
- Although there are many foods that contain oxalate, there is no need to have complete restriction of oxalate-containing foods because of the potential health and nutritional benefits from the foods.
- Thiazides cause reabsorption of calcium in the distal tubules resulting in a decrease in urinary calcium, unlike loop diuretics (eg, furosemide) which causes the calcium to "loop" through the tubules resulting in an increase in urinary calcium.
- The formation of calcium oxalate crystals does not depend on urine pH since the crystals can form in acidic, neutral, or alkaline urine.
- In the event of ethylene glycol (antifreeze) poisoning, an increased number of calcium oxalate crystals can be seen in the urine since ethylene glycol is an oxalate precursor that becomes oxidized by alcohol dehydrogenase and aldehyde dehydrogenase. Fomepizole or ethanol is used to treat ethylene glycol poisoning since both competitively inhibit alcohol dehydrogenase.
- Struvite stones are usually composed of magnesium-ammonium-phosphate crystals admixed with calcium carbonate apatite.
- Urease-producing organisms produce urease, which results in an increase in ammonium ($NH_4^+$) in the urine and causes the urine to become alkaline, which in turn favors the precipitation of struvite and apatite.
- Patients treated with medical management alone for struvite stones are rarely successful.
- Uric acid crystals are seen primarily in acidic urine (pH <5.5), but when the urine pH is >5.5 the uric acid is in its ionized form as urate salts (eg, amorphous urates).
- Alkalinizing the urine in patients with cystine stones increases the solubility of cystine.

- Cystine can be detected by the cyanide-nitroprusside test. A positive reaction turns the urine into a red-purple color and indicates a urine cystine concentration of at least >75 mg/L. A quantitative urinary cystine excretion test can be performed and most individuals with cystinuria will excrete >400 mg/dy.
- The defective cystine transporter is not only involved in cystine, but also other dibasic amino acids such as lysine, arginine, and ornithine. Although these dibasic amino acids are also lost in the urine, they are relatively soluble and thereby do not lead into stones.
- Indinavir crystals can appear as a starburst shape, fan-shaped, or platelike shape.
- **Foundational point**—Cystine is made up of two cysteine molecules linked by a disulfide bond.
- **Connecting point** (pg. 24)—Know the drug profile for bile acid sequestrants.
- **Connecting point** (pg. 73)—If the clinical picture presents as "bones, stone, abdominal and psychic moans" think primary hyperparathyroidism and order a serum calcium level along with an intact PTH.
- **Connecting point** (pg. 162)—Know the other types of autosomal recessive disorders.
- **CJ:** A 52-year-old man was found to have urosepsis with an obstructing stone in the ED. What is your next step? **Answer:** The patient needs an emergent decompression with either percutaneous drainage (ie, nephrostomy tube) or a ureteral stent in combination with appropriate antibiotics. An emergency decompression is also warranted in patients with a solitary kidney with complete obstruction and in patients with bilateral obstruction with acute kidney injury.
- **On the CCS,** "percutaneous nephrostomy" and "ureteral stent" are available in the practice CCS.
- **On the CCS,** "lithotripsy" is available in the practice CCS, but remember to order a consult for the procedure.
- **On the CCS,** "strain urine for stone" is available in the practice CCS.
- **On the CCS,** if a stone is retrieved during the CCS, there is an option for "ureteral calculi analysis" in the practice CCS.
- **On the CCS,** a "24-hour urine collection" is not available in the practice CCS. Instead, you are required to order the specific components of the urine collection and only urine calcium, oxalate, uric acid, phosphorus, and creatinine will give you the results based on a 24-hour time period in the practice CCS.
- **On the CCS,** remember to use the "Interval/follow up" to see how the patient is doing, especially after giving analgesics.
- **On the CCS,** remember to "bridge" your therapy by addressing the acute stages of your therapy (eg, analgesics) with the chronic stages of therapy (eg, prevention).
- **On the CCS,** this a type of case that will require you to become comfortable in moving patients to different locations and advancing the time. Therefore, start practicing with each chapter review!

# NEOPLASM

## ▌WILMS' TUMOR

Wilms' tumor is the most common renal malignancy in children younger than 15 years of age. Wilms' tumor is associated with a number of gene alterations (eg, deletions, mutations), but the exact pathogenesis to the development of Wilms' tumor is still unknown. Interestingly, the genetic abnormalities in Wilms' tumor are mapped to the same general vicinity (chromosome 11) as 3 recognizable malformation syndromes: WAGR, Denys-Drash, and Beckwith-Wiedemann.

### Clinical Features:

Wilms' tumor is more common in blacks compared to whites with even a lower risk in the Asian population. In the majority of cases, children will present with an asymptomatic abdominal mass that is usually discovered incidentally by the parents. Wilms' tumor can be bilateral or unilateral with usually an earlier diagnosis or later diagnosis, respectively. The mass is usually smooth and nontender and typically does not cross the midline unless the mass is very large. Other possible signs and symptoms to be aware of include abdominal pain, vomiting, hematuria, hypertension, fever, anemia, anorexia, weight loss, intestinal obstruction, or venous obstruction (eg, edema, varicocele, engorged veins). In advanced disease, children may have respiratory problems secondary to metastases to the lungs. Consider the associated syndromes of Wilms' tumor:

WAGR—**W**ilms' tumor, **A**niridia, **G**enitourinary anomalies, **R**etardation (intellectual disability)

**Deny-Drash syndrome**—Wilms' tumor, male pseudohermaphroditism, early onset nephrotic syndrome that progresses to renal failure

**Beckwith-Wiedemann syndrome**—Wilms' tumor (5%-20% of cases), macrosomia, macroglossia, gigantism, omphalocele/exomphalos, enlarged organs (visceromegaly), earlobe creases, hyperinsulinemia, hypoglycemia

### Next Step:

**Step 1)** The best initial test in patients suspected of having Wilms' tumor is an **abdominal ultrasound** because it is relatively inexpensive and it does not give off harmful radiation. Doppler ultrasound can detect the patency of blood flow in the event that the tumor has infiltrated the IVC. Further evaluation with a **contrast abdominal CT** is recommended to assess if there is bilateral renal involvement, lymph node involvement, or metastases to the liver. Imaging should also be performed on the chest to evaluate for lung metastases, but the preferred modality (chest x-ray vs chest CT) is still under debate.

**Step 2)** Laboratory testing should include the following:

**CBC**—Look for signs of anemia (ie, ↓ Hb).

**CMP**—Assess LFTs to check for possible liver metastases; calcium levels for hypercalcemia; and serum creatinine levels to detect a decrease in GFR.

**Coags**—PT and PTT should be checked since approximately 5%-10% of patients will have acquired von Willebrand's disease at the time of diagnosis.

**Urinalysis**—Assess for hematuria; check proteinuria which would suggest Deny-Drash syndrome.

**Step 3)** Definitive diagnosis of Wilms' tumor requires a tissue sample usually at the time of surgical excision. At the time of surgical excision, staging is performed based on the anatomic extent of the malignancy. In the United States, attempts are made to obtain a unilateral nephrectomy prior to the initiation of chemotherapy unless there is bilateral renal involvement (in which case preoperative chemotherapy followed by surgery is considered). In Europe, attempts are made to give preoperative chemotherapy (ie, shrink the tumor) prior to resection. Therefore, there are two different staging systems and the major system used in the United States is the National Wilms' Tumor Study (NWTS). For board purposes, the following is a simplified staging schema for Wilms' tumor:

**Stage I**—Tumor limited to the kidney.

**Stage II**—Tumor extends beyond the kidney, but is completely resected without evidence of tumor at or beyond the margins of resection.

**Stage III**—Residual tumor confined to the abdomen after surgery.

**Stage IV**—Hematogenous metastases or metastases to distant lymph nodes (beyond abdomen/pelvis).

**Stage V**—Bilateral renal involvement.

**Step 4)** Treatment is typically based on staging and tumor histology. In patients with stage I-IV and a favorable histology, the common approach is first with a unilateral nephrectomy followed by chemotherapy with radiation reserved for stages III and IV. Treatment in stage V is more challenging, and treatment approach is usually individualized with the oncologist (eg, preoperative chemo followed by surgery or initial surgical resection).

### Follow-Up:

Follow-up care is important for treatment-related complications and ongoing surveillance with the lungs as the most common site for recurrence.

### Pearls:

- The 5-year overall survival rate is approximately 90% with either the US or European treatment approach.
- The mean age at diagnosis is approximately 3.5 years of age.
- **Caveat 1**—Avoid vigorous abdominal palpation on exam because the tumor can rupture and result in spillage into the peritoneal cavity leading to a higher tumor stage.
- **Caveat 2**—Avoid transcutaneous biopsy because tumor spillage can occur in the peritoneal cavity.
- **Caveat 3**—Patients treated for Wilms' tumor can develop secondary malignancies (eg, leukemias, solid tumors).

- **Caveat 4**—Common chemotherapeutic agents used to treat Wilms' tumor can cause cardiotoxicity (ie, doxorubicin), or hepatotoxicity (ie, vincristine and dactinomycin).

- Aniridia is the congenital absence of the iris seen in WAGR syndrome.

- Wilms' tumor is a nephroblastoma not a neuroblastoma. A neuroblastoma is a tumor that arises from primitive sympathetic ganglion cells.

- **Foundational point**—Patients with the WAGR syndrome have a chromosomal deletion of the WT1 gene located on chromosome 11.

- **Foundational point**—Patients with the Denys-Drash syndrome have a mutation in the WT1 gene located on chromosome 11.

- **Foundational point**—Patients with the Beckwith-Wiedemann syndrome have a mutation in the WT2 gene located on chromosome 11.

- **Foundational point**—Favorable histology seen in Wilms' tumor includes epithelial cells, stromal cells, and blastemal cells. An unfavorable histology includes anaplastic features (eg, enlarged hyperchromatic nuclei, abnormal mitoses), which have a poorer outcome.

- **Foundational point**—On pathological exam of a Wilms' tumor, the mass is typically a well-circumscribed mass with a tan to gray color appearance on cut section.

- **Connecting point** (pg. 132)—Know the other types of acquired von Willebrand disease (vWD).

- **On the CCS**, if you decide to order a pediatric nephrology consult, remember to implement a course of action before the consultant is able to see your patient (eg, preordering ultrasound, CT, and labs).

# Rheumatology

## KEYWORDS REVIEW

**Bouchard's nodes**—Hard, bony enlargements at the PIP joints, which are characteristic of OA.

**Boutonnière deformity**—Flexion at the PIP joint with hyperextension of the DIP joint, which is characteristic of rheumatoid arthritis.

**Chondrocalcinosis**—Calcification of cartilage. In pseudo-gout, the calcification is due to CPPD crystals depositing into fibrocartilage (eg, menisci of the knee) or articular cartilage that will appear as punctate or linear densities on x-ray. Chondrocalcinosis is not pathognomonic for pseudogout.

**Heberden's nodes**—Prominent osteophytes in the DIP joints, which are characteristically seen in OA (women > men).

**Mononeuritis multiplex**—Nerve damage that occurs in two or more separate areas of the body and can be due to

infections, vasculitis, tumor involvement, autoimmune-mediated diseases, or diabetes.

**Pannus**—An inflammatory exudate that overlies the synovial membrane in rheumatoid arthritis. In Latin, *pannus* means "a piece of cloth."

**Peak bone mass**—The maximum amount of bone mass accumulated during early adult life.

**Podagra**—A painful condition at the base of the great toe usually caused by gout.

**Swan-neck deformity**—Hyperextension at the PIP joint with flexion at the DIP joint, which is characteristic of rheumatoid arthritis.

**Tophus**—Deposits of monosodium urate crystals into soft tissue with a surrounding inflammatory response. Tophi (plural) are pathognomonic for gout.

# METABOLIC DISORDER

## ▌ OSTEOPOROSIS

Osteoporosis is the most common metabolic bone disease in the United States. Osteoporosis ("porous bone") can be characterized by low bone mass and microarchitectural deterioration, which can lead to fractures.

### Risk Factors:

Advanced age, white or Asian race, female gender, postmenopause, low body weight (<127 lbs [58 kg]), personal history of fracture, family history of osteoporotic fracture, excessive alcohol intake (>3 drinks/dy), tobacco use, low calcium or vitamin D intake, excess vitamin A intake, **medications** (glucocorticoids ≥5 mg/dy for ≥3 months, phenytoin, phenobarbital, heparin, lithium, proton pump inhibitors, cyclosporine), **endocrine disorders** (Cushing's syndrome, adrenal insufficiency, diabetes mellitus, hyperparathyroidism, thyrotoxicosis, hypogonadism, estrogen deficiency, androgen deficiency), **genetic disorders** (osteogenesis imperfecta, Marfan's syndrome), **GI disorders** (celiac disease, chronic liver disease, gastric bypass), **heme disorders** (leukemia, lymphoma, multiple myeloma), **renal disorders** (renal failure, dialysis patients), **respiratory disorder** (COPD), **rheumatoid disorders** (rheumatoid arthritis, ankylosing spondylitis, SLE), **organ transplantation**.

### Clinical Features:

Osteoporosis is usually an asymptomatic condition. Patients can have fragility fractures, which are fractures that would normally not occur due to minimal force or low trauma. Common sites for fractures include the hip, humerus, distal radius (Colles fracture), and vertebrae. Patients with vertebral fractures will typically show progressive kyphosis ("dowager's hump") or a loss of height. Approximately two-thirds of patients with vertebral fractures will be asymptomatic. Patients that are symptomatic from a vertebral fracture will usually complain of acute back pain after bending, lifting, or coughing.

### Next Step:

**Step 1)** Based on the National Osteoporosis Foundation (NOF) guidelines, perform a dual-energy x-ray absorptiometry (DEXA) of the hip and spine in all women ≥65 years old and all men ≥70 years old, regardless of risk factors. Also, perform a DEXA in younger postmenopausal women and men 50 to 69 years of age who have risk factors for a fracture.

**Step 2)** The World Health Organization (WHO) has established diagnostic categories based on the bone mineral density (BMD):

> **Normal:** T-score ≥−1.0
>
> **Osteopenia:** T-score between −1.0 and −2.5
>
> **Osteoporosis:** T-score ≤−2.5
>
> **Severe osteoporosis:** T-score ≤−2.5 and in the presence of one or more fragility fractures

**Step 3)** Any postmenopausal women or men with a T-score ≤−2.5 or has a fragility fracture should have baseline labs to help exclude secondary causes of osteoporosis (see list of medications and medical conditions in "Risk Factors" section). The labs should include a CBC, CMP (to look at calcium, alkaline phosphatase, LFTs, electrolytes, creatinine, albumin, protein), serum phosphorus, 24-hour urinary calcium level, 25-hydroxyvitamin D, and serum testosterone (only men).

**Step 4)** Encourage nonpharmacologic treatment to postmenopausal women and all men >50 years of age that includes:

> **Lifestyle modification**—Reduce alcohol consumption to <3 drinks/dy, smoking cessation, weight-bearing and muscle-strengthening exercise.
>
> **Calcium and vitamin D intake**—Calcium intake of at least 1200 mg/dy and vitamin D intake of 800 IU.
>
> **Fall prevention**—Identify risk factors for falls, check hearing and vision, review medications.

**Step 5)** In general, patients that are at risk of developing fractures should be treated with pharmacologic therapy. The NOF recommends treatment in patients with hip or vertebral fractures, T-score ≤−2.5 at the femoral neck or spine by DEXA, or those with osteopenia (T-score between −1.0 and −2.5) who have a 10-year hip fracture probability of ≥3% or a 10-year major osteoporosis-related fracture probability ≥20% based on the US-adapted WHO absolute fracture risk model. The following are the approved FDA pharmacologic modalities for the prevention and/or treatment of osteoporosis:

### Bisphosphonates

- Bisphosphonates are considered first-line agents.
- Bisphosphonates inhibit osteoclastic activity.
- Alendronate, risedronate, and zoledronic acid reduce vertebral and hip fractures. Only zoledronic acid is available in the IV route of administration.
- Ibandronate is only effective at reducing vertebral fractures.
- Oral bisphosphonates can cause GI problems such as difficulty swallowing, esophagitis, gastric ulcers, or GERD.
- IV zoledronic acid can cause an acute phase reaction (eg, flu-like symptoms, fever, myalgia) and rare reports of osteonecrosis of the jaw.

### Selective Estrogen Receptor Modulator (SERMs)

- Raloxifene can increase BMD.
- Raloxifene is only effective at reducing vertebral fractures.
- Raloxifene has estrogen agonist activity on the bones and lipids, but has estrogen antagonistic activity on the breast and uterus.
- Raloxifene can increase vasomotor symptoms (hot flashes), increase the risk of venous thromboembolism, and although it can decrease total cholesterol and LDL, it does *not* reduce the risk of coronary heart disease.
- Raloxifene can decrease the risk of invasive breast cancer in postmenopausal women with osteoporosis.
- Ideally, raloxifene would be best suited for a patient who does not have hot flashes, and has no risk of thromboembolism but a high risk of breast cancer.

- Tamoxifen is another SERM, but it is not prescribed for the treatment of osteoporosis.
- Tamoxifen has estrogen agonist activity on the bones (preserves bone density) and on the endometrium (↑ risk of endometrial cancers), but it has estrogen antagonistic activity on the breast.

### Estrogen-Progestin Therapy

- Estrogen-progestin therapy is not considered a first-line agent because the benefits do not outweigh the risk of a stroke, venous thromboembolism, coronary heart disease, and breast cancer.
- Consider other medical treatment if estrogen-progestin therapy is used only for the treatment of osteoporosis.
- If estrogen-progestin therapy is used, it should be in the lowest effective dose and for the shortest period of time that attains treatment goals.

### Calcitonin

- Salmon calcitonin is not considered first-line treatment.
- Salmon calcitonin can be used in women who are at least 5 years postmenopausal.
- Salmon calcitonin is only effective at reducing vertebral fractures.

### Parathyroid Hormone

- Teriparatide is a recombinant human parathyroid hormone that is typically reserved for patients with severe osteoporosis, high risk for fractures, or failed other treatments.
- Teriparatide reduces vertebral and hip fractures.

### Follow-Up:

Monitor the response to osteoporosis therapy every 2 years with DEXA testing and then less frequently thereafter if the BMD assessments show signs of improvement or are stable.

### Pearls:

- Be vigilant about patients that have a history of an osteoporotic fracture because they are prone to have another fracture in the future.

- Although men have a lower lifetime risk of a hip fracture compared to women, men have twice the mortality from hip fractures compared to women.
- Peak bone mass most likely occurs by the third decade of life, and age-related bone loss occurs soon thereafter with most of the bone loss occurring at >65 years of age.
- A T-score is a comparison of the BMD (BMD) of a patient to that of a young healthy adult of the same sex and is expressed in terms of standard deviations (SD) above or below the mean.
- A Z-score is a comparison of the BMD of a patient to that of the patient's age and sex (age-matched population). A Z-score ≤−2.0 is considered a low BMD for that chronological age, but a Z-score >−2.0 would be considered within the expected range for that age.
- Osteoporosis will typically have a reduction in both bone matrix and mineralization, but osteomalacia will have an intact bone matrix but reduced bone mineralization.
- Common lab findings for nutritional osteomalacia include ↓ calcium, ↓ phosphorus, ↓ 25-hydroxyvitamin D level, ↑ PTH, ↑ alkaline phosphatase.
- Although patients can be asymptomatic with osteomalacia, bone pain is a common symptom.
- Bisphosphonates that are not FDA approved for osteoporosis include pamidronate, etidronate, and tiludronate.
- **On the CCS**, "DEXA scan" or "bone densitometry" are available in the practice CCS.
- **On the CCS**, the practice CCS does not recognize "zoledronic acid."
- **On the CCS**, if you order a medication during the case, remember to "advise patient, side effects of medication."
- **On the CCS**, be sure to also order "advise patient, limit alcohol intake," "advise patient, no smoking," and "advise patient, exercise program."

# CRYSTAL-INDUCED ARTHROPATHIES

## ❙ GOUT

Gout is a disease that is associated with hyperuricemia due to an overproduction or underexcretion of uric acid (see Table 19-1). When uric acid levels reach the point of supersaturation or exceed the solubility limits, urate salts can precipitate out into monosodium urate (MSU) crystals and deposit into joints, soft tissues, and kidneys. The resulting clinical manifestations include gouty arthritis, tophi, uric acid nephrolithiasis, and urate nephropathy.

### Clinical Features:

Gout commonly affects adult men and postmenopausal women. Gout occurs in three progressive stages: acute gouty arthritis, intercritical (interval) gout, and chronic (tophaceous) gout.

**Acute gouty arthritis**—The majority of initial gout attacks are monoarticular, especially the first metatarsophalangeal joint (**podagra**). In addition to the great toe, other sites include the insteps, heels, ankles, knees, wrists, fingers, or bursae. Patients will often present with signs of inflammation, which include a sudden onset of pain, erythema, edema, and warmth, and sometimes with fever. In some cases, the inflammation can extend beyond the joint mimicking a cellulitis or tenosynovitis. In elderly people who have concomitant osteoarthritis, inflamed Heberden's or Bouchard's node may

## Table 19-1 • Causes of Hyperuricemia

| Overproducers | Underexcretors |
|---|---|
| • Conditions<br>  • Lymphoproliferative disorders<br>  • Myeloproliferative disorders<br>  • Malignancies<br>  • Hemolytic disorders<br>  • Polycythemia vera<br>  • Psoriasis<br>  • Obesity<br>  • Purine-rich diet<br>  • Vitamin B$_{12}$ deficiency<br>• Agents<br>  • Alcohol<br>  • Fructose<br>  • Nicotinic acid<br>  • Warfarin | • Conditions<br>  • Renal insufficiency<br>  • Volume depletion<br>  • DKA<br>  • Lactic acidosis<br>  • Sarcoidosis<br>  • Berylliosis<br>  • Obesity<br>  • Hypothyroidism<br>  • Hyperparathyroidism<br>• Agents<br>  • Alcohal<br>  • Loop and thiazide diuretics<br>  • Low-dose aspirin<br>  • Levodopa<br>  • Pyrazinamide<br>  • Ethambutol |

be the sole or initial manifestation of a gout attack. Untreated gout attacks typically resolve within 7 to 10 days.

**Intercritical gout**—After an acute gout attack resolves, the patient enters an **asymptomatic** period. Most untreated patients will have another gout attack within 2 years of the initial attack, and over time the asymptomatic intervals will shorten between the attacks.

**Chronic gout**—This stage can be characterized by the presence of **tophi** and is typically seen 10 years after the initial attack. Tophi are usually nontender, but the tophi are surrounded by an intense inflammatory response that can cause symptoms similar to an acute gouty attack. Tophi can deposit into the helix of the ear, olecranon bursae, prepatellar bursae, Achilles tendon, toes, and over the Heberden's or Bouchard's node. Often the presence of subcutaneous nodules is mistaken for the diagnosis of rheumatoid arthritis. Over time, tophi can lead to nerve compression, joint destruction, or soft tissue damage.

Next Step:

**Step 1)** Definitive diagnosis should be made with a needle aspiration of the joint fluid or tophi, which will reveal the **needle-shaped**, **negatively birefringent** urate crystals when examined under a compensated polarized light microscope. See Table 19-2 for synovial fluid analysis.

**Step 2)** Gout is managed with anti-inflammatory therapy, antihyperuricemic therapy, and lifestyle modifications. Treatment of gout is as follows:

**Acute Gout Therapy**

- **NSAIDs** (eg, indomethacin, naproxen) are considered first-line therapy at the first sign of an attack, but it should be avoided in patients with renal insufficiency or those intolerant to the GI side effects.
- **COX-2 inhibitors** (eg, celecoxib) is an alternative for patients that have GI side effects associated with NSAIDs and do not have known cardiovascular disease.

## Table 19-2 • Synovial Fluid Analysis

| Parameters | Normal | Noninflammatory | Inflammatory | Septic | Hemorrhagic |
|---|---|---|---|---|---|
| Volume (mL) at the knee | <3.5 mL | Usually >3.5 mL | Usually >3.5 mL | Usually >3.5 mL | Usually >3.5 mL |
| Color | Clear | Yellow | Yellow | Yellow-green | Red |
| Clarity | Transparent | Transparent | Cloudy | Cloudy | Bloody |
| Viscosity | High/thick | High/thick | Low/thin | Variable | Variable |
| Glucose (mg/dL) | Close to serum glucose | Close to serum glucose | Low, but >25 mg/dL | Very low, <25 mg/dL | Close to serum glucose |
| WBC per mm$^3$ | <200 | 200-2000 | 2000-100,000 | 15,000-200,000 | 200-2000 |
| PMN cells (%) | <25% | <25% | >50% | >75% | 50%-75% |
| Culture | Negative | Negative | Negative | Usually positive | Negative |
| Other features | - | Osteoarthritis and trauma are examples. | **Gout**—MSU crystals; needle shaped, negatively birefringent.<br><br>**Pseudogout**—CPPD crystals; rhomboid shaped, weakly positively birefringent. | Usually presents with a single swollen, painful joint. | Look for a history of trauma or bleeding disorders. |

CPPD—calcium pyrophosphate dihydrate; MSU—monosodium urate; PMN—polymorphonuclear

- **Colchicine** is an alternative agent that would be an appropriate therapy for patients who cannot take NSAIDs or steroid therapy. Low-dose oral colchicine is most effective if it is given within the first 24 hours of an attack. Oral colchicine does have GI side effects (ie, nausea, vomiting, diarrhea, abdominal cramping), and intravenous colchicine is no longer produced or shipped to the United States because of the risk of bone marrow suppression, hepatic necrosis, and death.
- **Intra-articular glucocorticoid** (eg, triamcinolone) injection can be used in patients who cannot take NSAIDs or colchicine (eg, both NSAIDs and colchicine have GI side effects) and present with only one or two inflamed joints.
- **Systemic glucocorticoid** (eg, prednisone) therapy would be appropriate in patients who cannot take NSAIDs or colchicine but present with polyarticular joint involvement.

### Prophylactic Gout Therapy

- The goal of prophylactic gout therapy is to prevent another gout attack.
- Low-dose colchicine can be given for a period of time (eg, 3-6 months) to help serve as a bridge from an acute attack to preventive therapy (ie, lowering uric acid levels) since colchicine only decreases the frequency of gout flares without lowering uric acid levels.

### Preventive Gout Therapy

- The goal of preventive gout therapy is to lower uric acid levels by dietary changes, adjusting medications (see Table 19-1), and antihyperuricemic medications.
- **Weight reduction**—Patients that are obese can reduce their risk of gout by reducing their weight.
- **Dietary changes**—Reduce red meat, seafood, alcohol (particularly beer and hard alcohol), high-fructose corn syrup based drinks, but encourage low-fat dairy products.
- **Medication changes**—Consider alternatives to medications when appropriate. For example, both thiazide and loop diuretics can elevate urate levels, but the antihypertensive medication losartan, might be a preferable choice because it can actually lower the urate levels.

### Antihyperuricemic Medications

- Antihyperuricemic medication should be encouraged in patients with frequent painful gout, recurrent kidney stones, presence of tophi, joint damage seen on x-ray, or those with disabling gout.
- Underexcretors as determined by excreting <800 mg of uric acid in a 24-hour urine sample on a standard diet can be treated with the uricosuric agent **probenecid**. Probenecid is contraindicated in patients with uric acid kidney stones or those taking aspirin concomitantly.
- Overexcretors (ie, >800 mg of uric acid in 24-hour urine sample on a standard diet) can be treated with **allopurinol**.
- Both probenecid and allopurinol should not commence until after the acute gout attack resolves because it can precipitate another attack.

- Patients that have a gout attack while on antihyperuricemic medications should continue to take their antihyperuricemics, but also treat the acute gout with NSAIDs, colchicine, or steroids.

### Follow-Up:

Patients should initially be seen every 1 to 2 months when starting antihyperuricemic medication to achieve a target serum uric acid level of ≤6 mg/dL, because this is below the level of its saturation point (ie, 6.7 mg/dL).

### Pearls:

- Although hyperuricemia is a risk factor for the development of gout, not all people with hyperuricemia will develop gout and therefore they should not be treated if there are no symptoms.
- Although serum uric acid levels can be elevated during an acute gout attack, some people may have normal or even low serum uric acid levels at the time of an attack.
- An elevated serum uric acid level does not confirm the diagnosis of acute gout, and a normal serum uric acid level does not rule out the diagnosis of acute gout.
- Less than 20% of initial gout attacks will be polyarticular, but over time, the gout attacks will be polyarticular later in the course of untreated gout.
- Although aspirin is considered an NSAID, it is not recommended to treat an acute gout attack because it can alter the uric acid levels either (high or low) depending on the dose.
- **Foundational point**—Colchicine is an inhibitor of microtubule assembly by binding to tubulin. The end result is reduced leukocyte migration, chemotaxis, and phagocytosis.
- **Foundational point**—Probenecid competes with uric acid for reabsorption at the proximal convoluted tubule, thereby promoting net renal excretion of uric acid.
- **Foundational point**—The sequential steps to uric acid synthesis includes nucleic acids → hypoxanthine → xanthine → uric acid. Xanthine oxidase is an enzyme that catalyzes the oxidation of hypoxanthine to xanthine and again catalyzes the oxidation of xanthine to uric acid. Allopurinol is an inhibitor of xanthine oxidase, thereby reducing the production of uric acid, but without disrupting the biosynthesis of vital purines.
- **On the CCS**, "arthrocentesis" and "joint fluid tap" are the same procedure and are both available in the practice CCS. The results will provide you with the amount (mL) of fluid withdrawn from the joint and the color of the fluid.
- **On the CCS**, either arthrocentesis or joint fluid tap are prerequisites to obtaining specific joint fluid tests (eg, joint fluid culture).
- **On the CCS**, when you type in "joint fluid" in the order menu, a list of joint fluid items can be selected.
- **On the CCS**, manage gout by selecting "join fluid analysis" which will give you the glucose, cell count, crystals, mucin, and viscosity. However, you will have to order the "joint fluid culture" and the "joint fluid Gram stain" individually.
- **On the CCS**, in addition to ordering a CBC, BMP, PT, PTT, and UA, other ancillary testing would include an ESR, serum

uric acid level, 24-hour urine uric acid, and an x-ray of the involved joint (radiographic findings may reveal either soft tissue swelling [early phase], punched-out lesion [intermediate phase], or tophi [late phase]).

- **On the CCS**, by the end of the case, be sure to order "advise patient, medication compliance," "advise patient, no alcohol," "advise patient, no aspirin," "advise patient, side effects of medication," and "diet, low protein."

- **On the CCS**, remember to "bridge" your therapy by treating the acute stages of the disease (eg, gout attack) with the long-term care (eg, prevention).

## ▌ PSEUDOGOUT

Pseudogout is a calcium pyrophosphate dihydrate (CPPD) crystal deposition disease that can be characterized by acute gout-like attacks. The attacks are elicited from CPPD crystals that can deposit into articular cartilage, synovium, tendons, ligaments, and soft tissues.

### Risk Factors:

Although the cause of CPPD crystal deposition is unknown, the following conditions increase the risk of accumulating CPPD crystals: old age, joint trauma, join surgery, familial chondrocalcinosis, hemochromatosis, hyperparathyroidism, hypothyroidism, hypophosphatasia, hypomagnesemia, Gitleman's syndrome (inherited renal tubular disorder).

### Clinical Features:

Pseudogout attacks usually affect one or a few joints at a time (ie, monoarticular > oligoarticular). The **knees** and **wrists** are common affected sites, but other places include the shoulders, elbows, hands, and ankles. Similarly to gout, signs of inflammation can occur that include pain, erythema, edema, and warmth. The attacks are usually self-limiting, lasting days to weeks. Interestingly, attacks commonly occur following a parathyroidectomy.

### Next Step:

**Step 1)** Definitive diagnosis should be made with a needle aspiration of the joint fluid or articular tissue, which will reveal the **rhomboid-shaped, weakly positively birefringent** crystals when examined under a compensated polarized light microscope. See Table 19-2 for synovial fluid analysis.

**Step 2)** Pseudogout is primarily managed with anti-inflammatory therapy since there is no effective treatment for preventing the deposition of CPPD crystals or removing CPPD crystals that are already deposited. Treatment of pseudogout is as follows:

### Acute Pseudogout Therapy

- **Joint aspiration** can serve as both diagnosis and treatment.
- **Joint immobilization** should be temporarily advised until the pain and swelling reduce.
- **NSAIDs** (eg, indomethacin, naproxen) can be used if there is no contraindication.
- **Colchicine** is an alternative agent that can be used to treat acute inflammation.
- **Steroids** can be used if there is a contraindication to NSAIDs or colchicine. Either intra-articular glucocorticoid (eg, triamcinolone) injection for 1 or 2 involved joints, or systemic (oral) glucocorticoids for multiple joints may be attempted.

### Prophylactic Pseudogout Therapy

- **Low-dose colchicine** can be given to patients that have recurrent attacks (ie, ≥3 attacks/yr).

### Follow-Up:

Patients treated for an acute attack may return to baseline in less than 10 days. If patients continue to have symptoms, consider the worst-case scenario (ie, septic arthritis) that may require prompt reassessment.

### Pearls:

- Pseudogout is associated with normal serum urate levels.
- CPPD crystal deposition disease can present similarly to rheumatoid arthritis and is notably termed pseudorheumatoid arthritis. Patients can present with multiple joint involvement with symmetric distribution, morning stiffness, fatigue, synovial thickening, elevated ESR, and 10% of patients will have a positive rheumatoid factor (RF).
- CPPD crystal deposition disease can present similarly to osteoarthritis and is notably termed pseudo-osteoarthritis. Patients can have progressive joint degeneration involving the shoulders, elbows, wrists, metacarpophalangeal (MCP) joints, hips, knees, and spine.
- **On the CCS**, other testing that might be helpful (refer to the risk factor section) include serum calcium, phosphorus, magnesium, iron, ferritin, transferrin, TSH, and an x-ray of the involved joint (radiographic findings may reveal chondrocalcinosis).

# INFLAMMATORY MYOPATHIES

## ▌ DERMATOMYOSITIS AND POLYMYOSITIS

Dermatomyositis (DM) and polymyositis (PM) are both idiopathic inflammatory myopathies that are thought to be mediated by an immunologic mechanism.

### Clinical Features:

Females are twice as likely as males to have both DM and PM. Peak age of onset for DM is 5 to 10 years old and 40 to 50 years old. Peak age of onset for PM is also 40 to 50 years old, but children are rarely affected with juvenile PM. Both DM and PM are multisystem disorders whose principal clinical feature is **proximal muscle weakness**. The following are other affected organ systems in a relative head to toe fashion:

**Esophagus**—Involvement of the oropharyngeal muscles or upper esophagus can result in dysphagia, nasal regurgitation, or aspiration.

**Cardiac**—Arrhythmias, conduction disturbances, myocarditis, pericarditis, or CHF.

**Respiratory**—Interstitial lung disease (ILD) or thoracic muscle weakness that can lead to pulmonary dysfunction.

**Musculoskeletal**—A symmetric, proximal weakness that progresses over a period of weeks to months. Patients will have difficulty combing their hair, climbing steps, or getting up from a chair. Both facial and ocular muscles are spared (unlike myasthenia gravis), but neck muscles can be affected resulting in a head drop. Fine-motor movements are usually affected late in the disease. Myalgias and muscle tenderness can occur in a subset of patients.

**Systemic**—Fever, weight loss, malaise, nondestructive arthritis, or Raynaud's phenomenon.

**Skin**—Cutaneous manifestations are usually associated only with DM. However, PM has been associated with mechanic's hands. The following are rashes that can precede or accompany the muscle weakness:

**Heliotrope rash**: A violaceous erythematous rash over the upper eyelids ± periorbital edema (see Figure 19-1 and Color Plate 15).

**Gottron papules**: Violaceous erythematous papules over the dorsal aspects of the MCP and interphalangeal (IP) joints (see Figure 19-2 and Color Plate 16). Note that Gottron "sign" may be referred to as erythematous lesions at sites other than the hands (eg, elbows, knees, or ankles).

**Shawl sign**: An erythematous rash over the chest, shoulders, and upper back.

**V sign**: An erythematous rash over the anterior neck and chest.

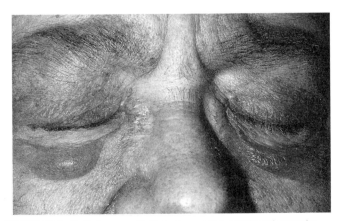

**FIGURE 19-1 • Heliotrope rash.** Note the reddish-purple rash over the upper eyelid with edema over the lower lids. The purplish hue is likened to the flower *Heliotropium peruvianum*. This patient developed severe muscle weakness of the shoulder girdle and presented with a lump in the breast that proved to be carcinoma. (Reproduced with permission from Wolff K, Johnson RA. *Fitzpatrick's Color Atlas of Synopsis of Clinical Dermatology*. 6th ed. New York: McGraw-Hill; 2009:371.)

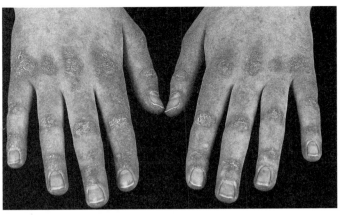

**FIGURE 19-2 • Gottron papules.** A raised, erythematous, scaly eruption can be seen over the dorsa of the hands and fingers, especially over the metacarpophalangeal and interphalangeal joints. (Reproduced with permission from Wolff K, Johnson RA. *Fitzpatrick's Color Atlas of Synopsis of Clinical Dermatology*. 6th ed. New York: McGraw-Hill; 2009:372.)

**Mechanic's hands**: Rough, scaly, cracked, fissured hands seen in both DM and PM.

**Erythema**: Erythema can be seen over the forehead and malar region (resembles SLE). Violaceous linear streaks on the trunk can also be observed (flagellate erythema).

**Periungual changes**: Periungual erythema and telangiectasias can be observed.

**Calcinosis cutis**: Deposition of calcium in the skin that commonly occurs in juvenile DM.

**Next Step:**

**Step 1)** Initial diagnostic testing may include the following with the expected results:

**Muscle enzymes**—↑ creatine kinase, ↑ aldolase, ↑ LDH, ↑ ALT, ↑ AST

**Autoantibodies**—ANA elevated 80% of the time, anti-Jo-1 elevated 20% to 30% of the time

**RF**—Elevated only 20% to 30% of the time

**ESR**—Elevated only 50% of the time

**EMG**—Myopathic pattern

**Step 2)** Definitive diagnosis is made by muscle biopsy. In PM, there is direct injury to the myofibers, but without vacuoles. Inflammatory cells (CD8+ T cells) are found primarily within the muscle fiber and the fibrous sheath that surrounds an individual muscle fiber (**endomysium**). In DM, the inflammatory cells (CD4+ T cells) are located around capillaries (**perivascular**), around a bundle of muscle fibers (**perifascicular**), fibrous sheath that surrounds the muscle fascicles (**perimysium**), and will demonstrate atrophy around the fascicle (**perifascicular atrophy**). Often the presence of perifascicular atrophy is sufficient to diagnosis DM, even in the absence of inflammation.

**Step 3)** Initial treatment for both DM and PM involves systemic steroids (eg, prednisone) for 4 to 6 weeks, followed by tapering doses until the lowest effective dose is reached. Unfortunately, about 75% of patients will ultimately require other adjuvant immunosuppressive therapy (eg, azathioprine, methotrexate).

**Step 4)** Initiate gender and age-appropriate cancer screening. Although both DM and PM are at risk of cancer, it appears that there is a higher risk of cancer with DM. The most common tumors include breast cancer, ovarian cancer, cervical cancer, lung cancer, gastric cancer, colon cancer, melanoma, and non-Hodgkin's lymphoma.

**Follow-Up:**

Once therapy has started, patients should be seen every few weeks to objectively assess their muscle strength. Obtaining serum creatine kinase (CK) does not reliably assess the response to treatment.

**Pearls:**

- Patients with SLE will also have an erythematous rash over the dorsal aspect of the hand, but will spare the skin over the IP joints, which is opposite to the Gottron sign.

- It is not uncommon to have an elevated CK-MB, but order a troponin I if there is suspicion for cardiac damage.

- The anti-Jo-1 antibody is associated with the antisynthetase syndrome, which includes mechanic's hand, ILD, arthritis, and Raynaud's phenomenon.

- **On the CCS**, remember to order "sun block" and "advise patient, avoid sun" in patients with DM because the rash is often related to photosensitivity.

## ▌INCLUSION BODY MYOSITIS

Inclusion body myositis (IBM) is considered the most common acquired idiopathic inflammatory myopathy after the age of 50.

**Clinical Features:**

Men are more likely to be affected than women, with the mean age of onset of 60 years old. IBM follows an insidious course, occurring over a period of years rather than weeks or months. Muscular weakness can affect both **proximal** and **distal** muscles groups. An index of suspicion should occur when there is involvement of the quadriceps, foot extensors, and wrist/finger flexors. Patients may have a history of falls (ie, quadriceps weakness), difficulty with ankle dorsiflexion, or difficulty with grip strength (eg, holding objects). The muscular weakness can sometimes be accompanied with muscular atrophy or myalgias. The distribution of the symptoms can be **symmetric** or **asymmetric**. IBM can also affect facial muscles, but the ocular muscles are usually spared. The cricopharyngeal muscles can be affected resulting in dysphagia, which occurs in approximately 60% of patients with IBM. On exam, sensory evaluation is usually normal, but deep tendon reflexes can be normal or decreased.

**Next Step:**

**Step 1)** Initial diagnostic testing may include the following with the expected results:

> **Muscle enzyme**—Serum CK may be normal or moderately elevated.
>
> **Autoantibodies**—ANA is usually not elevated.
>
> **ESR**—ESR is usually not elevated.
>
> **EMG**—Myopathic pattern or mixed pattern showing both myopathic and neurogenic changes.
>
> **Nerve conduction studies**—Normal.

**Step 2)** Definitive diagnosis is made by muscle biopsy. Similar to PM, inflammatory cells (CD8+ T cells) are found within the endomysium. Characteristic findings include **rimmed vacuoles** within the muscle fiber, **beta-amyloid deposits**, and **tubular filamentous inclusions** seen on electron microscopy.

**Step 3)** IBM is resistant to immunosuppressive therapies. Often, prednisone is combined with azathioprine or methotrexate for several months, but then ultimately discontinued because of minimal benefit from the therapy.

**Follow-Up:**

An evaluation for an assistive device (eg, walker) may be necessary for patients with an older age of onset (>60 years old), since there is a rapid decline compared to an earlier age of onset.

**Pearls:**

- IBM has the least favorable prognosis compared to DM and PM.

- **On the CCS**, remember that medications cannot be ordered as PRN.

# INFLAMMATORY DISORDERS

## ▌RHEUMATOID ARTHRITIS

Rheumatoid arthritis (RA) is a chronic systemic inflammatory condition that can affect many tissues and organs, but principally affects the synovial membranes of multiple joints. Over time, there is proliferation and hyperplasia of the synovial linings that can lead to the development of **pannus**. The pannus contains proteinases that can ultimately lead to cartilage destruction and bony erosions. The etiology of rheumatoid arthritis is unknown.

**Clinical Features:**

Rheumatoid arthritis affects women 3 times more than men. The peak age of onset is 30 to 50 years of age. The onset of RA is usually insidious, but approximately 10% of patients can have an acute onset of polyarthritis along with constitutional symptoms. **Prodromal symptoms** of weight loss, fever, malaise, weakness, and vague arthralgias can occur before joint pain or articular inflammation is apparent. Patients will typically present with **joint pain**, **swelling**, and **stiffness**. Stiffness is frequently seen after a period of prolonged inactivity or morning stiffness >1 hour that eventually subsides during the day. The pattern of joint involvement is usually **symmetric**, but a subset of patients can have asymmetry. Patients may initially have polyarthritis or they may have monoarthritis for a period of time before polyarthritis develops. In other cases, patients may only have monoarthritis usually of the large joints (eg, shoulder, hip, knee). Patients can have episodic attacks of one or more joints before abating to a symptom-free period that is referred to as **palindromic rheumatism**. There are a number of joints involved in RA, which include, from head to toe:

1) Temporomandibular joint can result in jaw pain.

2) Cricoarytenoid joint can result in hoarseness or stridor.

3) Cervical spine can result in cervical subluxation.

4) Shoulders are usually involved late in the disease.

5) Elbows are very common sites for subcutaneous rheumatoid nodules.

6) Wrists are common sites that can result in carpal tunnel syndrome.

7) Hands—MCP and PIP joints are commonly affected (DIP joints are rarely affected, instead think of OA or psoriatic arthritis), swan-neck deformities, Boutonnière deformities, ulnar deviation of the digits with radial deviation at the wrist, and tenosynovitis can be seen.

8) Hips are usually involved late in the disease.

9) Knees—Baker's cyst can develop behind the knees secondary to an extended inflamed synovium.

10) Ankles can develop arthritis.

11) Feet—Especially the MTP joints are involved early in the disease.

Rheumatoid arthritis can also have extra-articular involvement, which includes the following in a relative head to toe fashion:

**Neurologic**—Nerve entrapments, mononeuritis multiplex (eg, foot-drop and wrist-drop), CNS rheumatoid nodules

**Eye**—Episcleritis, scleritis

**Cardiac**—Atherosclerotic coronary artery disease, pericarditis, cardiac rheumatoid nodules

**Respiratory**—Pleural effusions, interstitial fibrosis, BOOP, pulmonary rheumatoid nodules

**Hematologic**—Anemia (ie, normochromic-normocytic), Felty's syndrome (ie, RA, neutropenia, splenomegaly), lymphoma

**Dermatologic**—Subcutaneous rheumatoid nodules, skin ulcers, digital necrosis

**Autoimmune**—Sjögren's syndrome (dry eyes, dry mouth) has been associated with RA

## Next Step:

**Step 1)** There is no single clinical feature or test used to make the diagnosis of RA. Instead, the diagnosis is based on a combination of clinical features, laboratory studies, and imaging features. Based on the American College of Rheumatology (ACR) 1987 revised classification criteria for RA, the presence of 4 or more criteria must be present in order for the patient to be classified as having RA. The classification criteria were intended for investigational purposes, but they have been useful as a guideline for making a diagnosis of RA.

1) Morning stiffness lasting 1 hour for >6 weeks

2) Arthritis involving ≥3 joint areas for >6 weeks

3) Arthritis of hand joints (wrist, MCP, or PIP joint) for >6 weeks

4) Symmetric arthritis for >6 weeks

5) Presence of subcutaneous rheumatoid nodules

6) Positive RF

7) Bony erosions on x-ray

**Step 2)** Pharmacotherapy is the primary treatment for patients with rheumatoid arthritis. No single medication can cure rheumatoid arthritis, but the goal is to provide pain relief, control inflammation, and maintain structure and function. Five classes of drugs to consider are nonbiologic disease-modifying antirheumatic drugs (DMARDs), biologic DMARDs, steroids, NSAIDs, and analgesics.

### Nonbiologic DMARDs

- Improvement in symptoms can take weeks to months with nonbiologic DMARDs.

- Nonbiologic DMARDs can be given alone or in combination with other medication.

**Methotrexate**—Considered first-line, but contraindicated in pregnancy, chronic liver disease, and blood dyscrasias.

**Leflunomide**—Commonly used in RA patients who do not respond to methotrexate. Contraindicated in pregnancy and patients with preexisting liver disease.

**Sulfasalazine**—Considered a second-line agent; can cause hemolysis in G6PD-deficient patients.

**Hydroxychloroquine**—An antimalarial drug that necessitates periodic eye exams because of the feared adverse effect of ophthalmologic toxicity.

### Biologic DMARDs

- The basis of biologic DMARDs therapy is to target cytokines or molecules on the cell surface.

- Biologic DMARDs tend to work rapidly compared to nonbiologic DMARDs.

- Biologic DMARDs are typically started after an unsuccessful attempt with a nonbiologic DMARD.

- Patients taking biologic DMARDs are at risk of opportunistic infections.

- TB screening with a PPD should be given to RA patients being considered for biologic DMARDs.

- Biologic DMARDs are not recommended in patients with untreated chronic hepatitis B, or treated chronic hepatitis B with Child-Pugh class B and higher.

- Biologic DMARDs can be given alone or in combination with other medication.

## Anti-TNF Agents

- Anti-TNF agents include adalimumab, infliximab, and etanercept.

- Anti-TNF agents are not recommended in patients with CHF (NYHA class III/IV with EF ≤50%).

## Non-TNF Agents

- Non-TNF agents include anakinra (IL-1 receptor antagonist), tocilizumab (IL-6 receptor antagonist), abatacept (T-cell co-stimulator blocker), and rituximab (B-cell depleting monoclonal antibody).

## Steroids

- Glucocorticoids are commonly used to treat flares or to bridge the time until DMARDs become effective.

- Glucocorticoids (eg, prednisolone) can be given by oral, intravenous, or intra-articular routes.

## NSAIDs

- NSAIDs have both analgesic and anti-inflammatory properties and are ideally used for short-term management.

## Analgesics

- Analgesics such as acetaminophen, tramadol, or topicals (eg, capsaicin) can be used for pain control.

## Follow-Up:

Regular follow-ups are necessary to monitor side effects from the medications and to assess disease activity, most often by clinical evaluation, imaging, and laboratory studies. It should be noted that RF titers are not useful for following disease activity.

## Pearls:

- **Anti-cyclic citrullinated peptides (CCP)** are often used to evaluate patients with RA since they have similar sensitivity to RF, but much **better specificity**.

- **ESR** and **CRP** are often elevated in patients with active RA. Both ESR and CRP are used to follow disease activity and to assess the response to medications.

- RF is not specific for rheumatoid arthritis as it is found in 5% of healthy people and it is also associated with other diseases including SLE, sarcoidosis, Sjögren's, scleroderma, syphilis, schistosomiasis, subacute bacterial endocarditis, TB, hepatitis B, chronic liver disease, DM, and PM.

- Subcutaneous rheumatoid nodules are firm or rubbery lesions that are typically seen over pressure points (eg, olecranon process), but also on tendon sheaths (eg, Achilles tendon, palmar tendon). The lesions are usually not painful, but in a subset of patients they can be painful, especially if the overlying skin breaks down.

- Morning stiffness is not pathognomonic for RA as it is seen in other inflammatory disorders.

- When you think of OA, think of Heberden's nodes, Bouchard's nodes, involvement at the carpometacarpal joint of the thumb, affected joints are hard and bony, "evening stiffness," stiffness after effort, normal ESR and CRP, negative RF and CCP, noninflammatory synovial fluid (WBC <2000 cells/mm³, see Table 19-2).

- Prior and current cigarette smoking increases the risk of RA.

- The life expectancy of patients with RA is shortened by approximately 3 to 7 years.

- Pregnant women with RA often have improvement during pregnancy, but approximately 90% of patients will have postpartum flares.

- Thrombocytosis is associated with very active disease.

- RA patients that have not started anti-TNF or non-TNF agents can receive live attenuated vaccines (eg, herpes zoster), killed vaccines (eg, influenza, pneumococcal, hepatitis B), and recombinant vaccines (eg, HPV vaccine for cervical cancer). However, once the patient starts an anti-TNF or non-TNF agent, the patient should not receive any live vaccines, but it is acceptable to receive killed and recombinant vaccines.

- Patients with RA have an increase in mortality due to accelerated cardiovascular disease.

- **Foundational point**—Adalimumab and infliximab can bind to TNF-alpha molecules and thereby block their action to the cell surface TNF receptors. Etanercept can bind both TNF-alpha and TNF-beta molecules and thereby block their action to the cell surface TNF receptors. The end result of anti-TNF agents is neutralizing the biological activity of TNF-alpha, which is normally involved in induction of proinflammatory cytokines (ie, interleukins), leukocyte migration, leukocyte activation, induction of tissue degrading enzymes, and induction of acute phase reactants.

- **Foundational point**—TNF-alpha and interleukin-1 (IL-1) are two important cytokines that are involved in inducing an inflammatory response. Once these cytokines bind to their cell surface receptors, they activate NF-κB proteins, which are normally sequestered in the cytosol in the inactive form. Once activated, they can translocate into the nucleus and turn on the transcription of genes that are involved in the inflammatory response. Unfortunately, when the actions of NF-κB proteins are excessive, the overdrive of the inflammatory response can damage healthy tissue and cause pain as seen in rheumatoid arthritis.

- **CJ:** An RA patient is about to start a biologic agent, but the PPD is positive. What is your next step? **Answer:** The patient should be followed up with a chest x-ray, and if suggestive of TB (ie, infiltrates ± cavitation), then obtain sputum cultures for acid-fast bacilli (AFB). Patients that have active TB should be treated completely for the active TB before starting a biologic agent. Patients that have latent TB should be treated for at least 1 month for the latent TB before starting a biologic agent.

- **On the CCS,** patients with RA have an increased risk of coronary atherosclerosis, and it is important to "advise patient, no smoking," "diet, low cholesterol," and "advise patient, exercise program."

- **On the CCS**, remember to "refer patient, physical therapy" and "refer patient, occupational therapy."

- **On the CCS**, consider an arthrocentesis to rule out other causes (see Table 19-2).

- **On the CCS**, remember to bridge the early stage of treatment (ie, pain relief) with NSAIDs or glucocorticoids with the later stages of treatment (ie, slowing joint damage) with the DMARDs.

- **On the CCS**, in office-based cases, you will need to advance the clock (sometimes in weeks) to see if there is a response to the medications you ordered.

# CCS: POLYMYALGIA RHEUMATICA CASE INTRODUCTION

Day 1 @ 15:00
Office

A 70-year-old white female comes to the office because of pain and stiffness in the shoulders and hips.

**Initial Vital Signs:**
Temperature: 37.3°C (99.14°F)
Pulse: 70 beats/min, regular rhythm
Respiratory: 16/min
Blood pressure: 130/86 mm Hg
Height: 152.4 cm (60.0 inches)
Weight: 57.6 kg (127 lb)
BMI: 24.8 kg/m$^2$

**Initial History:**
Reason(s) for visit: Shoulder and hip pain; stiffness

**HPI:**
A 70-year-old white female has experienced "achiness" and stiffness in the shoulders and hips for the past 5 weeks. Initially, the pain and stiffness started in her left shoulder, but now it has progressed to the right shoulder and both hips. Her pain is worse with movement, which has caused many sleepless nights. Acetaminophen provides minimal pain relief. She also reports having stiffness after periods of prolonged inactivity and morning stiffness lasting at least 30 to 60 minutes, but eventually "loosens up" by the midafternoon. She has difficulty combing her hair, brushing her teeth, putting on a coat or jacket, getting up from a chair or bed, and turning over in bed. There is also diffuse swelling and pitting edema over her hands and feet. She reports having fatigue, low-grade fever, and weight loss accompanying her musculoskeletal symptoms.

| | |
|---|---|
| **Past Medical History:** | Hypercholesterolemia, hypertension, history of breast cancer, osteopenia (T-score: −1.5) |
| **Past Surgical History:** | Left-sided mastectomy 15 years ago; childbirth at ages 25 and 27 |

| | |
|---|---|
| **Medications:** | Atorvastatin, amlodipine, alendronate |
| **Allergies:** | None |
| **Vaccinations:** | Up to date |
| **Family History:** | Mother died of myocardial infarction, age 60. Father died of prostate cancer, age 70. One younger sister is still alive, age 65, and has hypertension. |
| **Social History:** | Never smoked; no longer drinks alcoholic beverages; denies use of illegal drugs; widowed; two children; retired; college education; enjoys reading and playing bridge. |

**Review of Systems:**

| | |
|---|---|
| General: | See HPI |
| Skin: | See HPI |
| HEENT: | Negative |
| Musculoskeletal: | See HPI |
| Cardiorespiratory: | Negative |
| Gastrointestinal: | Negative |
| Genitourinary: | Negative |
| Neuropsychiatric: | Negative |

Day 1 @ 15:11

**Physical Examination:**

| | |
|---|---|
| **General appearance:** | Well nourished, well developed; in no apparent distress. |
| **Skin:** | Normal turgor. No nodules. Scar noted over left breast area. Hair and nails normal. |
| **Breasts:** | Left breast removed without any abnormal mass. Right breast exam normal. |
| **Lymph nodes:** | No lymphadenopathy. |
| **HEENT/Neck:** | Normocephalic. EOMI, PERRLA. Hearing normal. Ears, nose, mouth normal. Pharynx normal. Neck supple; trachea midline; no masses or bruits; thyroid normal. |

**Chest/Lungs:** Chest wall normal. Diaphragm moving equally and symmetrically with respiration. Auscultation and percussion normal.

**Heart/Cardiovascular:** S1, S2 normal. No murmurs, rubs, gallops, or extra sounds. No JVD.

**Abdomen:** Normal bowel sounds; no bruits. No tenderness. No masses. No hernias. No hepatosplenomegaly.

**Extremities/Spine:** Bilateral swelling and pitting edema over the hands, wrists, ankles, and feet. Decrease range of motion, most notably over the shoulders, neck, and hips. Muscle tenderness to palpation, but no pain along the tender point areas. No muscle atrophy. Mild kyphosis on spine exam

**Neuro/Psych:** Mental status normal. Cranial nerve and sensory exam normal. Motor strength 5/5 throughout. Cerebellar function normal. Deep tendon reflexes normal. Gait normal.

**First Order Sheet:**

1) CBC with differential, routine — **Result:** WBC-7000, H/H-11/37%, Plt-450,000, Differential- WNL, MCV-85, MCHC-33% (nl: 31%-36%), RDW-12% (nl: 11.5-13.6).

2) Peripheral smear, routine — **Result:** Normochromic normocytic erythrocytes; leukocytes normal in number and morphology; platelets elevated in number.

3) CMP, routine — **Result:** Ca-9.5, Glu-100, Urea-15, Cr-1, Prot.-7.2, Alb.-4.5, T.Bil.-0.7, AlkP-130, AST-30, ALT-30, Na-141, K-4.2, Cl-103, $HCO_3$-24

4) ESR, routine — **Result:** 87 mm/hr (nl: 0-20)

5) Creatine kinase, serum, routine — **Result:** 50 U/L (nl: 10-70)

6) Aldolase, serum, routine — **Result:** 8.3 U/L (nl: 1.5-12.0)

7) TSH, serum, routine — **Result:** 4.0 mU/L (nl: 0.5-5.0)

8) ANA, serum, routine — **Result:** Negative

9) Rheumatoid factor, routine — **Result:** 1:20 (normal <1:40)

10) Anti-CCP, routine — **Result:** Negative

11) Urinalysis, routine — **Result:** WNL

**Second Order Sheet:**
1) Prednisone, oral, continuous
2) Calcium-enriched diet
3) Calcium carbonate, oral, continuous
4) Vitamin D3 (cholecalciferol), oral, continuous

**Actions:**
1) Change location to home
2) Schedule appointment: In 3 days

**Day 3**
The patient has arrived for the appointment.

**Recorded Vital Signs:**
Temperature: 37.0°C (98.6°F)
Pulse: 70 beats/min, regular rhythm
Respiratory: 16/min
Blood pressure: 130/86 mm Hg

**Follow-Up History:**
The patient's pain and stiffness has improved significantly.

**Physical Examination:**
**Extremities/Spine:** Reduced swelling of the hands, wrists, ankles, and feet. Improved range of motion over the shoulders, neck, and hips. Decrease muscle tenderness. Normal peripheral pulses. Mild kyphosis on spine exam.

**Neuro/Psych:** Mental status normal. Normal motor, sensory, and cranial nerve exam. Cerebellar function normal. Deep tendon reflexes normal. Gait normal.

**Actions:**
1) Reevaluate case: In 14 days

**This case will end in the next few minutes of "real time."**
You may **add** or **delete** orders at this time, then enter a diagnosis on the following screen.

**Third Order Sheet:**
1) ESR, routine
   Future date: In 60 days — **Result:** 15 mm/hr (nl: 0-20)

2) CBC with differential, routine
   Future date: In 60 days — **Result:** WBC-7000, H/H-14/37%, Plt-300,000, Differential- WNL, MCV-85, MCHC-33% (nl: 31%-36%), RDW-12% (nl: 11.5-13.6).

3) Peripheral smear, routine
   Future date: In 60 days — **Result:** Normochromic normocytic erythrocytes; leukocytes and platelets normal in number and morphology.

4) Advise patient, side effects of medication

5) Advise patient, medication compliance

6) Advise patient, exercise program

**Please enter your diagnosis:**

Polymyalgia Rheumatica

## DISCUSSION:

Polymyalgia rheumatica (PMR) is an inflammatory condition of unknown etiology. PMR is closely associated with giant cell arteritis (GCA), which is also known as temporal arteritis. It is still not clear if PMR and GCA represent two separate diseases or part of a spectrum from a single disease process. Approximately 30% of patients with PMR will develop GCA, while 50% of patients with GCA will develop PMR. It should be noted that the clinical course of PMR and GCA may not be synchronous (ie, one condition may be completely inactive while the other condition starts to flare, and vice-versa).

## Clinical Features:

The average age at diagnosis for PMR is 70 years, and symptoms are generally present for more than 1 month before patients seek help. Symptoms of PMR may develop abruptly or insidiously. The classic presentation is **pain** and **stiffness** in the shoulders, hips, neck, and upper body. Pain is usually worse with movement. Early in the course of the disease, shoulder pain may be the initial presentation while sparing the lower extremities. However, in a subset of patients the neck and hip are involved at onset. Symptoms may initially begin unilaterally, but eventually they become bilateral after a few weeks. Morning stiffness lasting 30 minutes and stiffness after periods of rest (gel phenomenon) are characteristic of PMR. Synovitis, tenosynovitis, and bursitis can occur around the joints. As a result, the local inflammation is thought to contribute to the swelling and pitting edema seen over the hands, wrists, ankles, and feet. In some cases, patients can develop carpal tunnel syndrome from the tenosynovitis. Despite the term *polymyalgia* ("pain in many muscles"), patients may exhibit muscle tenderness, but the tenderness is most likely due to the synovial and bursal inflammation. On examination, patients will have **normal muscle strength** and decrease range of motion of the involved areas secondary from the pain. Constitutional symptoms such as fever, fatigue, and weight loss may be associated with the PMR symptoms as they are thought to represent the systemic effects of the cytokines that are released from the inflammatory process.

## Next Step Summary:

**Step 1)** PMR is a clinical diagnosis. Although there are no validated diagnostic criteria, the presence of the following can help with the diagnosis of PMR:

- Age of onset ≥50 years
- ESR ≥40 mm/hr
- Morning stiffness lasting ≥30 minutes
- Pain persisting for ≥1 month involving at least two areas including the neck, shoulders, or pelvic girdle
- A response to low-dose steroids

**Step 2)** As you approach this case, think about the labs or tests that you would order. The characteristic laboratory finding for PMR is an elevated ESR that can exceed 100 mm/hr. Nonspecific laboratory findings that may be present in patients with PMR include thrombocytosis (reflects an inflammatory response), normocytic anemia, and elevated liver enzymes, particularly the alkaline phosphatase. Also, as you go through the case, consider the differential diagnosis and the tests that you would order. The following are the differentials to consider:

**Polymyositis (PM)**—Patients with PM will have proximal muscle weakness and will have elevated muscle enzymes (ie, creatine kinase (CK), aldolase).

**Fibromyalgia**—The patient in this case had no abnormalities on tender point examination, and the ESR is usually normal in patients with fibromyalgia.

**Malignancy**—Patients can have a paraneoplastic syndrome that can result in myalgias or joint pain. In this case, the patient did have a history of breast cancer and presented with weight loss, but the breast and lymph node exam appeared normal, calcium levels were within normal limits, and she responded well to low-dose steroids.

**Drug-induced myalgia**—The patient in this case was on a statin, but the CK was within normal limits.

**Pseudogout**—Patients with pseudogout can present with pain and edema of the shoulders and lower extremities, but they will have the characteristic rhomboid-shaped, weakly positively birefringent crystals on synovial fluid analysis and chondrocalcinosis may be present on x-ray.

**Hypothyroidism**—Patients with hypothyroidism can present with stiffness and arthralgias. However, the thyroid exam appeared normal and the TSH was within normal limits in this case.

**Rheumatoid arthritis**—Patients with rheumatoid arthritis can also present with joint pain, swelling, stiffness, and constitutional symptoms. However, in this case the patient did have a rheumatoid factor (RF) level within normal limits, a negative anti-cyclic citrullinated peptide (CCP), which has a better specificity than RF at detecting rheumatoid arthritis, and the patient responded well to low-dose steroids.

**Step 3)** Patients with PMR typically respond well to low-dose oral steroids (eg, prednisone), typically within 3 days of starting the medication. Although there are no evidence-based guidelines for the dosing and duration of treatment, most patients are maintained on steroids until they are asymptomatic and then eventually tapered off. If patients do not respond to low-dose steroids, then you can try to incrementally increase the dose of the steroids to see if there is a response. However, there is no option to increase the dose on the CCS, and therefore, you have to reconsider the differential diagnosis and pursue further workup (eg, imaging, muscle biopsy, EMG, joint fluid analysis). In this particular case, the patient responded well to low-dose steroids, and thereby, we did not have to subject the patient to unnecessary radiation or painful procedures.

**Step 4)** Most patients with PMR will be on steroids for several months and it is important to prevent glucocorticoid-induced osteoporosis. In this case, the patient is already on a bisphosphonate (alendronate) for her osteopenia, but we also added calcium and vitamin D supplementation.

### Follow-Up:

Patients on steroid treatment should have monthly follow-ups to monitor the response to therapy and to assess the side effects of steroids including hypertension, glucose intolerance, and osteoporosis. Lab testing for ESR is often obtained every 2 to 3 months while on steroid therapy as normalization of the acute-phase reactant is expected with remission of the symptoms.

### Pearls:

- PMR can affect not only the shoulder and hip girdle, but also the proximal aspects of the upper arms and thighs, respectively.

- Muscle atrophy is not typically seen early in the course of the disease, but can be seen later if there is disuse of the proximal muscles.

- EMG and muscle biopsy findings are normal in patients with PMR.

- Inflammation is not at the level of the muscle, but rather the synovium and bursae.

- One of the side effects of amlodipine is peripheral swelling, which might have thrown you off in this case.

- Most patients with GCA will typically respond to high-dose steroids rather than low-dose steroids.

- PMR is a self-limited disorder with a duration of approximately 2 to 3 years.

- Patients can relapse from the steroid therapy, especially if the steroid dose is tapered too quickly.

- **CJ:** A 75-year-old woman has pain and stiffness in the shoulder and also complains of jaw pain, headaches, visual disturbances, and tenderness over the right temporal area. What is your next step? **Answer:** When GCA is suspected, initiate high-dose steroids (eg, prednisone). Do not delay treatment because the patient can potentially lose her vision.

- **Connecting point** (pg. 296)—Know the clinical features of GCA.

- **On the CCS**, it is acceptable to pick either "vitamin $D_3$" (ie, cholecalciferol) or "vitamin D, therapy" (ie, ergocalciferol) for prevention of glucocorticoid-induced osteoporosis, but some studies have suggested that cholecalciferol increases 25-hydroxyvitamin D (ie, 25OHD) more efficiently than ergocalciferol (ie, vitamin $D_2$).

- **On the CCS**, once you advance the clock forward, you cannot go backward in simulated time.

- **On the CCS**, after you treat a patient, be sure to monitor the patient's condition. As in this case, a follow-up office visit with the appropriate physical exam was performed with labs ordered for a future date.

# 20

# Vascular

## KEYWORDS REVIEW

**Desquamation**—Shedding or peeling of the epidermis.

**Livedo reticularis**—A mottled reticulated or lacelike (netlike) vascular pattern that appears purplish or bluish (livedo) in color that typically does not blanch upon active pressure. Livedo reticularis can be seen during a cold response in patients with Raynaud's phenomenon and can be reversible upon rewarming. Livedo reticularis can also be seen in other vasculitis disease (eg, PAN), vascular occlusive disease (eg, PAD), or autoimmune disease (eg, antiphospholipid syndrome).

**Phlegmasia alba dolens**—A clinical manifestation as a result of a massive venous thrombosis obstruction of the venous vasculature. It is commonly the result from precipitants of thrombosis (eg, DVT, malignancy, hypercoagulability). The thrombosis typically obstructs the major deep venous channels of the extremity, but sparing the collateral veins and thereby preserving some venous flow. Clinical features include edema, pain, and blanching or white (alba)

appearance of the affected extremity, but without ischemia. Phlegmasia alba dolens can potentially progress to phlegmasia cerulea dolens.

**Phlegmasia cerulea dolens**—Phlegmasia cerulea dolens occurs by the same mechanism as phlegmasia alba dolens, but both major deep venous channels and collateral veins are affected resulting in complete venous outflow obstruction. The result is significant edema (ie, ↑ venous congestion), pain, cyanosis (ie, cerulea means blue), and with ischemia. In addition, gangrene can develop as a sequela of the disease. Approximately 50% to 60% of cases of phlegmasia cerulea dolens is preceded by phlegmasia alba dolens.

**Sclerotherapy**—A type of medical procedure that involves injecting a sclerosing agent into a target vein with the goal of shrinking the vessel over a period of time. Sclerotherapy is primarily used to treat telangiectasias, reticular veins, or small varicose veins.

# ARTERIAL

## ▌ GIANT CELL ARTERITIS

Giant cell arteritis (GCA), also referred to as temporal arteritis, is a chronic vasculitis that affects **medium** and **large**-sized arteries. GCA has a predilection for the extracranial branches of the carotid artery, most notably the temporal artery. The etiology of GCA is unknown.

### Clinical Features:

GCA is typically seen in patients ≥50 years of age, female > male, and in individuals of European descent. Onset of symptoms is usually gradual, but abrupt presentations can occur. Clinical manifestations can vary, and it may be helpful to consider the features from a relative head to toe fashion:

**Neurologic**—New onset headache in any location (frontal, temporal, parietal, occipital)

**Eyes**—Diplopia or visual loss in one or both eyes that can be due to amaurosis fugax, anterior ischemic optic neuropathy (AION), posterior ischemic optic neuropathy (PION), central retinal artery occlusion, branch retinal artery occlusion, or homonymous hemianopsia

**Lower face**—Jaw claudication, tongue pain

**Neck**—Throat pain

**Respiratory**—Nonproductive cough

**Aorta**—Aortic aneurysms (ascending > descending), arm claudication, aortic dissection

**Musculoskeletal**—Polymyalgia rheumatic (PMR)

**Systemic**—Fever, fatigue, or anorexia

On physical exam, several key elements should be inspected. The **temporal artery** may be tender, thickened, or cordlike. Early in the disease, the temporal artery may be pulsatile, but it may diminish over time. Individuals may also have **scalp pain** upon palpation. On **funduscopic exam**, a pale swollen optic disc may be seen if AION has developed. In addition, if the optic nerve circulation is compromised, patients can develop a relative afferent pupillary defect (ie, Marcus-Gunn pupil). Finally, **bruits** may be heard over the carotids, axillary, brachial, abdomen, or femorals, which may be an indication of a partial occlusion.

### Next Step:

**Step 1)** Clinical suspicion for GCA (eg, age ≥50, new onset headache, temporal artery tenderness, jaw claudication, Hx or symptoms of PMR, visual disturbances, constitutional symptoms) should prompt you to initiate treatment with **glucocorticoids** before the diagnosis is confirmed! Either oral prednisone or IV methylprednisolone is an acceptable choice. Patients will typically report clinical improvement within 48 hours of initiating steroids, which would also support the diagnosis of GCA. In addition to giving steroids, **low-dose aspirin** should be given to reduce ischemic complications.

**Step 2)** Schedule the patient for a temporal artery biopsy to confirm the diagnosis. Other adjunctive testing to support the diagnosis includes:

**ESR**—Elevated ESR can reach ≥100 mm/hr.

**C-reactive protein (CRP)**—CRP levels may also be elevated. In some patients, the CRP shows a better reflection of disease activity compared to the ESR. In other cases, the CRP may be a better indicator of disease activity, therefore, order both CRP and ESR.

**CBC**—Normocytic normochromic anemia and thrombocytosis can sometimes be present.

**CMP**—Alkaline phosphatase and aminotransferases can sometimes be elevated; albumin levels can sometimes be decreased.

**Step 3)** Counsel patients about the anticipated side effects of steroids (eg, emotional instability, insomnia, impaired wound healing, osteoporosis) since the duration of glucocorticoid treatment is typically for one month followed by a gradual taper. Supplemental calcium and vitamin D may be recommended, and if there is concern for osteoporosis, your next best step is to order a DEXA scan and possibly treat with bisphosphonates if the T-score is ≤−2.5.

### Disposition:

GCA usually runs a self-limited course that can take several months to years. The ESR or CRP are useful indicators of disease activity and may be used as adjuncts to the clinical decision making for a steroid tapering schedule.

### Pearls:

- Takayasu arteritis is also a chronic vasculitis with an unknown etiology that can affect medium and large-sized arteries, primarily the aortic arch and its primary branches. The presentation to look for includes Asian descent, **age ≤40 years**, female > male, constitutional symptoms, claudication of the extremities, skin lesions, marked weakening of the arterial pulses in the upper and lower extremity that may be asymmetric (**pulseless disease**), >10 mm Hg systolic BP difference between the arms, bruits (ie, carotids, subclavian, brachial, or abdomen), renovascular hypertension, ↑ ESR, ↑ CRP. Unlike GCA, do not take a biopsy (ie, Do you really want take a biopsy of the aorta or its primary branches?); rather, imaging is usually used to confirm the diagnosis (eg, arteriography, MRI/MRA). Like GCA, treatment is with glucocorticoids.

- **Foundational point**—Histopathologically, GCA has predilection for the internal elastic lamina, which is usually fragmented. In addition, granulomatous inflammation is seen with variable numbers of multinucleated giant cells in close proximity to the fragmented elastic lamina. It should be noted that the morphologic changes seen in Takayasu arteritis may be indistinguishable from GCA (ie, presence of a granulomatous inflammation with giant cells).

- **Connecting point** (pg. 19)—Know the clinical clues of renovascular hypertension that can be seen in Takayasu arteritis.

- **Connecting point** (pg. 140)—Know the meaning of homonymous hemianopsia.

- **Connecting point** (pg. 142)—Know the meaning of a Marcus Gunn pupil.

- **Connecting point** (pg. 144)—Recognize the clinical features of amaurosis fugax.

- **Connecting point** (pg. 293)—Recognize the clinical features of polymyalgia rheumatica.

- **Connecting point** (pg. 282)—Know the management of osteoporosiss.

- **On the CCS,** timing is important in the management of GCA, and poor management would include delaying treatment (eg, waiting for the results of the ESR or temporal artery biopsy) since withholding glucocorticoid treatment can potentially result in irreversible vision loss.

- **On the CCS,** remember to order oral prednisone in the continuous mode of frequency. Once you decide to taper the prednisone, then you can discontinue the medication since it will be understood by the CCS and the examiner.

- **On the CCS,** "temporal artery biopsy" is available in the practice CCS.

- **On the CCS,** when the case is about to end, you will receive a 2-minute warning. If you feel that you managed GCA appropriately, you can order an ESR and/or CRP to follow disease activity at a later date.

- **On the CCS,** remember to "advise patient, side effects of medication."

## KAWASAKI DISEASE

Kawasaki disease (KD), also referred to as mucocutaneous lymph node syndrome, is a vasculitis that affects **small, medium,** and **large**-sized arteries. KD has a predilection for medium-sized arteries, especially the coronary arteries, which can lead to its most notable complication of a **coronary artery aneurysm (CAA).** Therefore, early diagnosis is essential to achieve the best possible treatment result. The etiology of KD is unknown.

### Clinical Features:

KD is a common vasculitis seen in children. Boys are affected more than girls, and in the majority of cases, KD is seen in children <5 years old and uncommonly seen in children <6 months. A higher incidence of KD is seen in children of Asian descent. The clinical features of KD will be reviewed in step 1 (see Next Step) since the diagnostic criteria are based on the clinical manifestations of KD. For the remainder of this section, the disease stages will be discussed with important highlights in each stage.

Acute stage—The acute phase is approximately the first 2 weeks. The hallmark of this stage is **fever.** Clinical manifestations of KD are likely to be present in this stage such as a rash or edema and induration of the hands or feet. Inflammation during this phase can also affect the myocardium, pericardium, AV node, and coronary artery, which can lead to myocarditis, pericarditis, arrhythmias, and coronary arteritis (without aneurysms), respectively. Do not be surprised if you observe tachycardia, a gallop, hyperdynamic precordium, or an innocent flow murmur in this stage of the disease.

Subacute stage—The subacute phase is approximately the next 2 to 4 weeks. The hallmark of this stage is a decrease or abatement of the fever, thrombocytosis (usually peaks in the third week), periungual desquamation (usually of the hands or feet) within 2 to 3 weeks after fever onset, and the development of coronary artery aneurysms.

Convalescent stage—The convalescent phase is approximately the next 4 to 6 weeks. CAA may still be apparent in this stage.

### Next Step:

**Step 1)** Early recognition of KD is important because you want to provide timely and appropriate treatment, which could potentially mitigate the morbidity and mortality associated with KD. Diagnosis of KD includes the presence of unexplained **FEVER FOR ≥ FIVE DAYS** and at least **FOUR of the FIVE** physical findings. Think of the physical findings in a relative head to toe fashion:

1) **Eyes**—Bilateral bulbar nonexudative conjunctivitis

2) **Oral**—Lips and oral mucous membrane changes that can include a strawberry tongue, injected oral or pharyngeal mucosae, or injected, cracked, or fissured lips

3) **Neck**—Cervical lymphadenopathy (at least one lymph node >1.5 cm in diameter)

4) **Extremities**—Peripheral extremity changes that can include erythema of the palms or soles, edema of the hands or feet, or periungual desquamation

5) **Dermatologic**—Polymorphous (ie, many forms or stages) rash

**Step 2)** Treatment should be initiated if patients fulfill the diagnostic criteria seen in step 1. **IVIG** should be administered as an infusion over 8 to 12 hours and is typically effective in reducing the prevalence of CAA if given within the first 7 to 10 days of the illness. Oral administration of **high-dose aspirin** should also be given to achieve an anti-inflammatory effect.

**Step 3)** Echocardiography should also be performed expeditiously and definitely within the acute phase to establish a baseline study (ie, keep in mind that you may not find a CAA in the acute stage but rather after the acute phase subsides).

**Step 4)** Once the patient is afebrile for at least 48 to 72 hours, you can switch high-dose aspirin to **low-dose aspirin** for its antiplatelet effect.

**Step 5)** Counsel patients and families about discontinuing aspirin therapy upon signs and symptoms of a varicella or influenza infection since aspirin is a risk factor for the development of Reyes syndrome. However, patients deemed to be on long-term aspirin therapy after being discharged from the hospital should receive an inactivated influenza (≥6 months of age) and varicella (≥12 months of age) vaccination to prevent the possibility of developing Reyes syndrome.

### Disposition/Follow-Up:

Patients seen in the ED and who fulfill the diagnostic criteria for KD should be admitted to the hospital for IVIG infusion and an echo. After hospital discharge, patients should have a repeat echo in the subacute stage, convalescent stage, and beyond.

### Pearls:

- KD is usually a self-limited condition.
- The use of glucocorticoids is controversial in the initial therapy of KD.
- Aspirin does not appear to affect the formation of CAA.
- Low-dose aspirin can usually be discontinued once the patient has a total of 6 to 8 weeks of aspirin therapy and there is no evidence of coronary artery abnormalities via echocardiography. Patients with coronary artery abnormalities should continue with low-dose aspirin until it resolves or indefinitely.
- CAA can lead to myocardial ischemia, MI, or sudden death.
- Not every child will develop a CAA, and in fact, approximately 25% of untreated children will develop CAA.
- Valvular dysfunction (eg, mitral regurgitation) can occur if inflammation affects the heart valves.
- Other possible features to be aware of in KD include anterior uveitis, sensorineural hearing loss, arthritis, Raynaud's phenomenon, gallbladder hydrops, or an induration of a BCG inoculation site.
- Reyes syndrome typically develops several days after recovery from a viral illness (usually varicella or influenza, but other viruses can also precipitate the disease), and salicylates (particularly aspirin) have been implicated as a risk factor. Reyes syndrome can also develop after vaccination with live viral vaccines. Features to look for in Reyes syndrome include vomiting, altered consciousness, seizures, coma, hepatomegaly, ↓ DTRs, ↑ AST, ↑ ALT, ↑ PT and PTT time, ↑ ammonia levels, hypoglycemia, or metabolic acidosis.
- **CJ:** A 3-year-old Asian boy presents with fever for the last 5 days, diffuse maculopapular eruption, dry red lips, and edematous feet. What is your next step? **Answer:** The patient does not fulfill the criteria for classic KD but rather **incomplete KD**. Incomplete KD is considered in patients with fever ≥5 days but associated with only 2 or 3 of the classic features of KD. In our patient, the patient had fever for 5 days and only had 3 of the diagnostic criteria, and therefore, the next best step is to order an ESR and CRP. Based on the recommendation of the American Heart Association (AHA)/American Academy of Pediatrics (AAP), an ESR and CRP should be obtained in patients suspected of having incomplete KD. Treatment with IVIG plus high-dose aspirin should be initiated (echo can be obtained afterward) if the ESR is ≥40 mm/hr **and/or** CRP is ≥3 mg/dL **plus** the presence of ≥3 supplemental labs that include either an al-

bumin ≤3 g/dL, anemia for age, ↑ ALT, platelets ≥450,000/mm³ (after 7 days of fever onset), WBC >15,000/mm³, or the presence of pyuria (urine ≥10 WBCs/high power field). However, if the ESR is ≥40 mm/hr and/or CRP is ≥3 mg/dL, but the laboratory criteria is not met (ie, <3 supplemental labs), then the next best step is to order an echo, and if the echo is abnormal then treat.

- **On the CCS,** "IVIG" is available in the practice CCS.
- **On the CCS,** "counsel family/patient" since the development of a CAA puts a patient at risk for early atherosclerotic disease.
- **On the CCS,** a pediatric cardiologist should be consulted because patients should have regular follow-ups with the cardiologist if they developed any cardiovascular complications during the course of the disease.
- **On the CCS,** if the patient fulfills the diagnostic criteria for classic KD, it should prompt you to initiate treatment without delay. Suboptimal management includes ordering unnecessary tests that would waste time because you have to keep in mind that there is no single definitive diagnostic test for classic KD.
- **On the CCS,** poor management includes failure to order an echo to possibly detect a CAA (remember not everybody will develop a CAA but the presence of a CAA is still a major complication that you need to potentially identify).

## ▌ PERIPHERAL ARTERIAL DISEASE

Peripheral arterial disease (PAD) is characterized by stenosis of the aorta and its branch arteries. The most common disease process affecting the arterial vasculature is **atherosclerosis**. The lower extremity vessels are affected more commonly than the upper extremity vessels, and therefore the remainder of the discussion will be based on the lower extremities.

### Risk Factors:

Risk factors for PAD are similar to those of coronary artery disease, which include smoking, diabetes, hypertension, hyperlipidemia, homocysteinemia, and metabolic syndrome. It should be noted that **smoking** (current and past) or **diabetes** are both very strong risk factors that have a two- to fourfold increase in the development of lower extremity PAD.

### Clinical Features:

Approximately 20% to 50% of patients with PAD are asymptomatic. The classic symptom that is seen in approximately 10% to 35% of patients with PAD is **intermittent claudication**. Claudication literally means "to limp" in Latin, however patients will often describe the symptom as cramping, aching, painful, numbness, weakness, or fatigue in the muscles (not joints) upon sustained exercise, but relieved by rest. The symptoms can be reproducible, and unlike neurogenic claudication (pseudoclaudication), there is no effect (ie, relief, exacerbation) with body positions seen in PAD (eg, relief with flexion or extension). Symptoms of claudication are typically distal to the site of the occlusion. For example, claudication in the lower calf may be the result of arterial disease in the popliteal artery, and discomfort in the butt or hips is usually the result of aortoiliac disease. In men, aortoiliac occlusive disease can give rise to **Leriche syndrome**, which is a triad of erectile dysfunction (impotence), claudication, and absent or decreased femoral pulses. On physical exam, possible findings in PAD include diminished pulses, bruits, hair loss, smooth and shiny skin, pallor, livedo reticularis, reduced skin temperature, or muscle atrophy. Approximately 1% to 2% of patients will have severe compromise of blood flow to an affected extremity, which is referred to as **critical limb ischemia**. Critical limb ischemia is characterized by rest pain and the development of ulcers or gangrene.

### Next Step:

**Step 1**) The best initial test to establish lower extremity PAD in patients with the classic symptoms of claudication is a calculation of the **ankle-brachial index (ABI)** (ie, compares the systolic BP in the arm to the ankle). The following is an interpretation of the ABI:

**ABI >1.3** (suggests calcified vessels)

**ABI between 0.91–1.3** (normal)

**ABI ≤0.90** (PAD)

**ABI ≤0.40** (severe PAD)

**Step 2**) Several different therapeutic strategies are recommended in the initial treatment approach with patients that have lifestyle-limiting claudication and an ABI ≤0.90. Consider the following:

### Risk Factor Reduction

1) **Smoking cessation** cannot be overstated. Help patients with either behavior modification or pharmacologic therapy (eg, nicotine patch, bupropion).

2) Appropriately treat diabetes mellitus.

3) Appropriately treat hypertension.

4) Appropriately treat hyperlipidemia.

### Lifestyle Changes

1) Implement a **supervised exercise program** in patients with a lifestyle-limiting claudication for at least a 3-month period.

2) Pharmacologic therapy with **cilostazol** may be used in conjunction with a supervised exercise program since it is effective in increasing walking distance. Once the drug is discontinued, the effect of increased distance is lost.

### Vascular Complication Prevention

1) **Aspirin** (75-325 mg) is given to reduce the risk of strokes or MI. Clopidogrel can be given as an alternative if aspirin cannot be given.

2) Do not give warfarin since it has not been shown to improve outcomes in patients with PAD.

### Follow-Up:

Patients should be seen regularly to assess the efficacy of treatment, and physicians should be aware that it may take up to 4 to 12 weeks for the benefits of cilostazol to be apparent. In addition, patients may need to be seen more frequently if being treated for coexistent diabetes, hypertension, or hyperlipidemia.

### Pearls:

- Cilostazol is a phosphodiesterase type 3 inhibitor that increases cAMP, which eventually results in arterial vasodilation and platelet aggregation suppression. **Cilostazol is contraindicated in patients with heart failure**.

- Pentoxifylline reduces blood viscosity and is considered a second-line agent compared to cilostazol. The efficacy of pentoxifylline in improving walking distances is still questionable.

- Beta-blockers are not contraindicated in patients with PAD who have coexistent hypertension or coronary artery disease.

- Conventional contrast angiography is considered the gold standard in assessing vascular anatomy, but neither conventional contrast angiography, MRA, nor CTA is routinely performed in the initial assessment of PAD unless revascularization intervention is considered.

- The diagnosis of PAD should serve as a marker for coexistent cardiovascular disease (eg, coronary artery disease).

- Buerger's disease (thromboangiitis obliterans) is a segmental, thrombosing vasculitis that affects small and medium-sized arteries and veins. There is minimal to absent atherosclerosis in the vessels. Patients are typically young (≤45 years) and there is a strong association with smoking or using tobacco products. Patients can present with claudication, Raynaud phenomenon, pain at rest, ulcers, or gangrene.

- **CJ:** A 62-year-old man with a history of smoking and coronary artery disease presents to the ED with an **acute onset** of the following signs and symptoms of his right leg: 1. Pain 2. Pallor 3. Pulselessness 4. Paralysis 5. Paresthesias 6. Polar (ie, cold). What is your next step? **Answer:** The patient has the hallmark signs and symptoms of an acute limb ischemia, which requires an emergent evaluation (eg, ABI or duplex ultrasound) and possibly immediate revascularization in consultation with a vascular specialist. The signs and symptoms of an acute limb ischemia can be easily remembered by the "Triple P's × 2." Be aware that an acute limb ischemia is not the same as critical limb ischemia (ie, chronic rest pain). However, critical limb ischemia needs to be evaluated and treated expeditiously as well.

- **Connecting point** (pgs. 142, 143)—Know the difference between neurogenic and vascular claudication.

- **Connecting point** (pgs. 79, 82)—Know the management of diabetes mellitus.

- **Connecting point** (pg. 19)—Know the management of hypertension.

- **Connecting point** (pg. 23)—Know the management of hyperlipidemia.

- **On the CCS**, "ABI" is available in the practice CCS.

- **On the CCS**, "cilostazol" is available in the practice CCS.
- **On the CCS**, remember to "advise patient, no smoking."
- **On the CCS**, remember to "advise patient, exercise program."

# POLYARTERITIS NODOSA

Polyarteritis nodosa (PAN) is a transmural necrotizing vasculitis that affects **small** and **medium**-sized muscular arteries and has multiorgan involvement. The etiology of PAN is unknown, but it has been associated with hepatitis B, hepatitis C, and hairy cell leukemia. Two unique features of PAN are that it is not associated with antineutrophil cytoplasmic antibodies (ANCA) and the lungs are usually spared (although the bronchial arteries have been involved on occasion).

## Clinical Features:

PAN is predominantly seen between the fourth and sixth decades of life, although it can still be seen in children. PAN is a "PAN-systemic" or multisystem disease that commonly affects the CNS (ie, neuropathy), renal, GI, derm, and musculoskeletal systems. However, it is good to see the whole clinical picture, and therefore, consider the following possible clinical manifestations from a relative head to toe fashion:

**Psychiatric**—Depression, psychosis

**Neurologic**—Strokes, AMS, seizure, confusion, or mononeuritis multiplex (ie, isolated damage in ≥2 separate nerves in different parts of the body, which can affect both sensory and motor function). Examples include a "wrist drop" (ie, radial nerve), "foot drop" (ie, sciatic or peroneal nerve), or an abnormal sensation along the little finger (ie, ulnar nerve). Mononeuropathy is usually asymmetric in the beginning, but over time, it can lead to distal symmetric polyneuropathy.

**Eyes**—Visual disturbances (eg, ischemic optic neuropathy)

**Cardiovascular**—CHF, myocardial infarction, or pericarditis

**Renal**—HTN, new onset diastolic BP >90 mm Hg, renal insufficiency/failure, or hematuria

**GI**—Abdominal pain (ie, mesenteric arteritis), GI bleed, nausea, or vomiting

**Genitourinary**—Testicular pain (ie, orchitis)

**Dermatologic**—Tender nodules, livedo reticularis, gangrene, ulcers, or purpura

**Musculoskeletal**—Arthralgias, myalgias, or muscle weakness

**Systemic**—Fever, fatigue, or weight loss

## Next Step:

**Step 1)** The clinical manifestation of PAN is nonspecific, and the initial diagnosis may not be readily apparent. In addition, there is no single diagnostic lab test to confirm the diagnosis of PAN. The following adjunctive tests may be used in the initial approach, and you should use your clinical judgment on what test would be appropriate for that given patient (ie, What symptoms is the patient complaining about?). Consider the possible findings of each test:

**CBC**—Normochromic anemia, leukocytosis, or thrombocytosis.

**CMP**—↑ BUN, ↑ Cr, or ↑ LFTs.

**ESR** or **CRP**—May be elevated.

**ANCA**—Usually negative, but if positive p-ANCA > c-ANCA. Also, the presence of antibodies against proteinase-3 and myeloperoxidase suggests a different vascular (ANCA) disease.

**Cryoglobulins and complements**—The presence of cryoglobulins and a fall in complements (↓ C3, ↓ C4) suggests mixed cryoglobulinemia, which is associated with hepatitis C and less often with hepatitis B and HIV.

**Hepatitis B and hepatitis C serologies**—May be positive.

**Rheumatoid factor**—If elevated levels are observed, you have to consider either rheumatoid vasculitis or mixed cryoglobulinemia (now you also have to consider hepatitis B and C).

**Creatinine kinase**—May be elevated.

**EMG**—In patients with mononeuritis multiplex, an EMG may help characterize the disease as myopathic or neurogenic.

**CXR**—Used to exclude other diseases since PAN usually spares the lungs.

**Occult blood, stool**—If positive, may suggest mesenteric arteritis.

**Urinalysis**—May show hematuria, may show mild proteinuria, but usually **no** red blood cell casts (ie, no glomerulonephritis).

**Step 2)** Diagnosis is confirmed with a **biopsy** of the affected organ (eg, skin, GI, renal) and preferably the most accessible site. It should be noted that a punch biopsy of the affected skin may not do the job since it may only reach the superficial dermis. Instead, you may need a deeper biopsy (eg, elliptical surgical biopsy) to reach a medium muscular artery. In the absence of an accessible tissue site, the alternative to a biopsy is an **arteriography** of the renal, hepatic, or mesenteric vasculature. Findings may reveal aneurysms of the vessels, but this is not a pathognomonic feature.

**Step 3)** Treatment in patients with PAN is with **glucocorticoids** (eg, prednisone). Oral prednisone is typically given for one month followed by a gradual taper. Patients that present with serious manifestations (eg, mesenteric ischemia, renal insufficiency) or are refractory to initial steroids should be given prednisone in conjunction with oral cyclophosphamide.

## Follow-Up:

Patients given cyclophosphamide should be monitored for **hemorrhagic cystitis**, and their blood counts should be checked regularly while on therapy.

## Pearls:

- When PAN is left untreated, the 5-year survival rate is approximately 13%. Major causes of mortality include strokes, MI, renal failure, and GI complications (eg, infarction, perforation).

- Keep in mind that IV drug users are predisposed to contracting hepatitis B or C, which would also predispose them to developing PAN.
- Patients with PAN-associated hepatitis B should also be treated with antivirals (eg, interferon alfa).
- High levels of eosinophilia suggest the diagnosis of Churg-Strauss syndrome.
- PAN is not associated with veins.
- PAN is not associated with granulomatous inflammation on histopathology.
- **Foundational point**—Histologically, PAN is characterized by a transmural inflammation of the muscular arterial wall with infiltration of neutrophils, eosinophils, and mononuclear cells. Necrosis of the arterial wall may be observed and is often referred to as fibrinoid necrosis.
- **Connecting point** (pg. 98)—Where else did we see ANCA? Crohn's disease is usually p-ANCA negative, and ulcerative colitis is usually p-ANCA positive.

- **On the CCS**, if you decide to treat with cyclophosphamide, you can give it orally (typically given everyday for one year) or it can be given intravenously (typically on a monthly basis for one year).
- **On the CCS**, remember to "advise patient, side effects of medication."
- **On the CCS,** remember to always use your clinical judgment when admitting a patient to the hospital. For example, if a PAN patient has a life-threatening GI bleed or you suspect a mesenteric arterial thrombosis (eg, sudden severe abdominal pain, abdominal tenderness, nausea, vomiting, guarding) and your clinical assessment coincides with your clinical diagnosis, be sure to work up your patient and treat the patient appropriately in the hospital. Do not send the patient home, or most likely the CCS case will end early.

# VENOUS

## VARICOSE VEINS

Varicose veins are characterized as dilated, tortuous subcutaneous veins. Most **primary varicosities** are due to hereditary causes, while **secondary varicosities** are due to the sequelae of trauma, prior DVT, pregnancy, prolonged standing, congenital lesions, perforator vein incompetence, or AV fistulas. However, the common feature of both primary and secondary varicosities is venous reflux caused by valvular incompetence. The venous anatomy of the lower extremity involves the deep and superficial veins. The two major superficial veins are the great and small (lesser) saphenous veins. The superficial venous system is interconnected to the deep venous system through perforator veins (which also have valves), the saphenofemoral junction, and the saphenopopliteal junction.

### Clinical Features:

Patients may complain for purely aesthetic reasons of the unsightly appearance of the veins. Others may complain of an "aching," "burning," "throbbing," "heaviness," or "soreness" in their legs. Symptoms may worsen with pregnancy, menstrual cycle, or from prolonged standing. Leg elevation usually relieves the symptoms, but if it worsens, then it is unlikely a varicosity. Keep in mind that the severity of the patient's symptoms does not necessarily correlate with the appearance of the visible varicosities or with the volume of the reflux. On exam, varicose veins may be visibly apparent, but if they are not visibly apparent then palpation of the lower extremity may reveal a dilated vein.

### Next Step:

**Step 1)** The diagnosis of varicose veins may be apparent on clinical evaluation. A duplex ultrasound is a useful adjunct in identifying varicose veins that are not visibly apparent, identifying a DVT, and useful in treatment planning.

**Step 2)** The initial treatment approach in patients with symptomatic complaints is with conservative management, which includes avoiding prolonged standing, elevating legs periodically, walking, exercise (eg, flexion and extension of the feet), and wearing elastic compression stockings for external support.

**Step 3)** Patients that are refractory to conservative management or who have cosmetic reasons may require a more invasive management approach to remove the varicose veins. Consider the following approaches:

- Sclerotherapy
- Endovenous laser ablation
- Endovenous radiofrequency ablation
- Ambulatory phlebectomy
- Surgical ligation and stripping

### Follow-Up:

When patients continue to have persistent symptoms despite conservative management, be sure to always rule out a DVT.

### Pearls:

- Varicosities should not be ablated or removed if there is a deep venous outflow obstruction because the enlarged superficial veins are serving as collaterals that bypass the obstruction.
- The Perthes maneuver involves placing a tourniquet over the proximal part of the leg to compress the superficial varicose veins, but without affecting the deep venous system. The patient is asked to walk or pump the calf muscle, which would normally empty or drain the varicose vein. If the varicose vein becomes paradoxically congested, that suggests a deep venous obstruction.

- When considering a DVT, think about the risk factors for DVT (eg, immobilization, travel, malignancy) and the signs and symptoms of DVT (eg, leg tenderness along the venous system, pitting edema, warmth, palpable cord, swelling, erythema, pain).

- Chronic venous insufficiency is usually associated with chronic venous reflux. Chronic venous insufficiency can typically be identified by the presence of skin changes (eg, discoloration of the skin), skin ulcer, or edema.

- Telangiectasias (also referred to as spider veins, thread veins, or hyphen webs) are a confluence of dilated intradermal venules.

- Reticular veins are dilated bluish subdermal veins that are larger than telangiectasias in diameter, but smaller than varicose veins.

- Both telangiectasias and reticular veins may also indicate the presence of chronic venous insufficiency.

- Superficial thrombophlebitis (STP) is the result of a thrombosis in the superficial vein that leads to inflammation, hence "thrombophlebitis." There may be tenderness, induration, erythema, and pain along the course of the superficial vein. Upon palpation, the vein may feel "cordlike." STP is often associated with varicose veins, IV injections, or indwelling catheters. Diagnosis of STP is mainly clinical, but if a DVT is suspected, then a duplex ultrasound should be ordered. STP is typically a self-limited condition, but treatment may include supportive measures such as NSAIDs, warm or cold compress, compression stockings, extremity elevation, and continuation of daily activities. Antibiotics are not routinely ordered unless there are signs of an infection (eg, purulent discharge, fever).

- **On the CCS**, in nonemergent CCS cases, you may be required to advance the clock in weeks to months. Prior to your Step 3 exam, select your own system of advancing the clock so that on exam day, you become more comfortable throughout your cases. Be aware that as you advance the clock, the patient's condition may change and a "Patient Update" will appear. At that point, you have to decide to either change the course of management or stay the course.

# APPENDIX A

# Pattern Recognition

The basis of pattern recognition is for you to "feel" or "recognize" the pattern of the disorder with both typical and atypical presentations. Pattern recognition is not meant for you to memorize every feature of the disorder, but rather to develop your gut instinct about a disease. Once you review this section several times, you should be able to quickly draw a clinical impression of the disorder on longer-type questions and answer the questions with more confidence. As you read through the pattern recognition, keep in mind that not every patient will present the same way, and some patients may only present with a partial list of the disease.

**Acute myelogenous leukemia (AML)**—Fatigue, anemia, thrombocytopenia, varied WBC count (low, normal, or high), hepatosplenomegaly, petechiae, ecchymoses, gingival bleeding, sternal tenderness, arthralgias, myeloid sarcoma (ie, extramedullary disease), fever secondary to infection, lymphadenopathy is uncommon, men > women, implicated risk factors (eg, radiation, chemotherapy, chemical exposures, familial syndromes, myelodysplastic syndrome), leukemic blasts in the peripheral blood and bone marrow, Auer rods (ie, indicates myeloid origin), myeloperoxidase positive, DIC, proliferation of myeloid precursors, maturational arrest of myeloid precursors, >20% of blasts in bone marrow as defined by the World Health Organization, most common in adults, infrequently seen in children (<10% of cases), pallor, cardiac flow murmur, hypokalemia, lactic acidosis, Sudan black B positive, leukemia cutis, ↑ LDH, ↑ uric acid, poor prognosis associated with advancing age.

**Acute promyelocytic leukemia (APL)**—Previously called AML-M3, is a distinct variant of AML, APL defined by the translocation of chromosome 15 and 17, which can be written as t(15;17) or defined by the product of the translocation PML/RARα, APL associated with bleeding secondary to DIC,

medical emergency, atypical promyelocytes in peripheral blood and bone marrow, dumbbell-shaped or kidney-shaped nuclei, granular cytoplasm obscuring the nucleus, common in adults, pancytopenia, menorrhagia, epistaxis, Auer rods in the cytoplasm, early mortality if untreated.

**Acute lymphoblastic leukemia (ALL)**—Bleeding, fever, bone pain, headache, lymphadenopathy, painless testicular enlargement, mediastinal mass, anemia, thrombocytopenia, varied WBC count (low, normal, or high), neutropenia, ↑ LDH, >25% lymphoblasts on bone marrow, most common in children, increased risk in Down syndrome, increased risk in neurofibromatosis type 1, negative myeloperoxidase, positive TdT, precursor B cell or precursor T cell ALL exists, precursor B cell ALL associated with poorer prognosis, Philadelphia chromosome in a minority of patients, ↑ uric acid secondary to high tumor burden, splenomegaly, petechiae, ecchymoses, pallor, cardiac flow murmur, infection, fatigue, dyspnea, infrequently DIC.

**Chronic myeloid leukemia (CML)**—Fatigue, weight loss, bleeding, abdominal fullness, hepatosplenomegaly, lower sternal tenderness, ↑ uric acid, asymptomatic, normochromic normocytic anemia, leukocytosis, normal or elevated platelets, ↓ leukocyte alkaline phosphatase (LAP) which is also called neutrophil alkaline phosphatase (NAP), elevated neutrophils, basophilia, eosinophilia, early satiety secondary to splenomegaly, triphasic course (accelerated phase, chronic phase, blast crisis), majority of patients have the Philadelphia chromosome that results from t(9;22) giving rise to a fusion protein product Bcr-Abl, constitutive kinase activity of Bcr-Abl, bone pain in blast crisis, peripheral smear demonstrates immature and mature granulocytes, most common in adults.

**Chronic lymphocytic leukemia (CLL)**—Lymphocytosis, absolute B-lymphocytes ≥5000/microL in the peripheral blood, painless lymphadenopathy (usually in the cervical area but can occur in the supraclavicular or axillary regions), hepatosplenomegaly, leukemia cutis, fevers, fatigue, weight loss, night sweats, common in the elderly, smudge cells on peripheral smear (ie, represents the fragility of the lymphocyte during slide preparation), expression of B cell antigens (CD19, CD20, and CD23), expression of T cell antigen (CD5), predominance of mature-appearing small lymphocytes, Richter's transformation (ie, CLL transformation to an aggressive diffuse large B cell lymphoma).

**Sickle cell disease (SCD)**—Recurrent painful episodes (previously called sickle cell crisis), bone pain, anemia, aplastic crisis due to parvovirus B19, growth retardation, avascular necrosis, stroke, ptosis, mutation in the β-globin gene that leads to a change in the sixth amino acid position from glutamic acid to valine (Glu → Val), cholelithiasis secondary to pigmented gallstones, leg ulcers, splenic sequestration, infection due to encapsulated bugs (ie, *Streptococcus pneumoniae* and *Haemophilus influenzae*), dactylitis/hand-foot syndrome (painful swelling of the hands and/or feet secondary to bone infarction of those small bones), delayed puberty, rapidly enlarging spleen, bone infarction, osteomyelitis secondary to *Salmonella* or *Staphylococcus aureus*, sensory hearing loss, vestibular dysfunction, cardiac involvement (chamber enlargement), priapism, pulmonary hypertension, acute chest syndrome, unconjugated hyperbilirubinemia, renal failure, retinopathy, reticulocytosis, ↑ LDH, ↓ haptoglobin, Howell-Jolly bodies, reduced splenic function (functional asplenia or hyposplenism), pneumonia, target cells and sickle cells on peripheral smear, HbSS or homozygous sickle cell anemia electrophoresis (zero percentage of HbA, ↑↑ HbS, ↑ HbF), structure of HbS (2 normal alpha chains/2 sickle beta chains).

**Systemic lupus erythematosus (SLE)**—Malar rash, fever, fatigue, weight loss, arthralgia, weight gain, discoid rash, Raynaud phenomenon, minimal mesangial lupus nephritis, mesangial proliferative lupus nephritis, alopecia, photosensitivity, purpura, urticaria, joint effusions, subcutaneous nodules, avascular necrosis, muscle weakness, fibromyalgia, annular plaques, erythematous papules, periungual erythema, telangiectasias, livedo reticularis, hypoalbuminemia, leukopenia, hemolytic anemia with reticulocytosis, thrombocytopenia, lymphadenopathy, splenomegaly, ↑ ESR, false-positive VDRL, focal lupus nephritis, diffuse lupus nephritis, membranous lupus nephritis, advanced sclerosing lupus nephritis, abnormal levels of IgG or IgM anticardiolipin antibodies, hepatomegaly, liver enzyme abnormalities, mesenteric vasculitis, pancreatitis, dysphagia, dyspepsia, pleural effusion, pulmonary hypertension, pericarditis, Libman-Sacks verrucous endocarditis, myocarditis, congenital heart block, delirium, psychosis, seizures, peripheral neuropathies, keratoconjunctivitis sicca, thromboembolic events, oral ulcers, ± HTN, creatinine levels (normal or elevated), ± hematuria, nasal ulcers, pleurisy, erythematous rash over dorsa of the hands sparing the interphalangeal joints, interstitial lung disease, ± subendothelial deposits on immunofluorescence, increased risk of coronary artery disease, persistent proteinuria >0.5 g/dy, headaches, arthritis, lymphopenia, anti-double stranded DNA (dsDNA), anti-Smith (SM) antibodies, cellular casts (granular, RBC, hemoglobin, tubular, mixed), pneumonitis, valvular disease, low C3, low C4, serositis, abdominal pain, nausea, vomiting, bullous skin lesions, >3+ proteinuria, thrombophilia, recurrent miscarriage, nephrotic syndrome, neonatal lupus (cardiac and cutaneous manifestations) from mothers that are positive for anti-Ro/SSA and/or anti-La/SSB antibodies, peritonitis, positive ANA, positive for lupus anticoagulant, anti-U1 RNP antibodies, early mortality due to disease activity (eg, CNS, cardiac, renal involvement, infection secondary to immunosuppression), late mortality due to strokes, MI, cancer, and treatment complications.

**Neurofibromatosis type 1 (NF1)**—Café au lait macules, freckling in the axillary or inguinal regions, learning disabilities, Lisch nodules (iris hamartomas), neurofibromas (cutaneous, subcutaneous, nodular plexiform, diffuse plexiform), long bone dysplasia, optic glioma, von Recklinghausen disease, familial disorder, autosomal dominant, hypertension, cognitive deficits, sporadic mutations, NF1 gene mutation on chromosome 17, decreased production of the protein product neurofibromin, increased risk for brainstem gliomas, astrocytomas, and soft tissue sarcomas, bony lesion, short stature, scoliosis, ↓ bone density, macrocephaly, pseudoarthrosis, seizures, speech delay, shortened life span compared to the general population.

**Neurofibromatosis type 2 (NF2)**—Bilateral vestibular schwannomas (ie, fairly common), meningiomas, dumbbell-shaped spinal cord schwannomas, neuropathies, cataracts, retinal hamartomas, absence of Lisch nodules, optic nerve meningiomas, skin plaques, unilateral vestibular schwannomas can occur, absence of cognitive impairment, posterior subcapsular lenticular opacities, autosomal dominant, sporadic mutations, NF2 gene mutation on chromosome 22, decreased production of the protein product merlin (also known as schwannomin) that acts as a tumor suppressor, ependymomas, epiretinal membranes, schwannomas rarely undergo malignant transformation, shortened survival.

**Parkinson's disease**—Resting tremor ("pill-rolling"), cogwheel rigidity (oscillating pattern of resistance and relaxation), bradykinesia, postural instability, positive "pull" test (ie, patient takes multiple steps backwards when pulled from behind), blurred vision, hallucinations, masked facial expression, decreased eye blinking, impaired upward gaze and convergence, positive glabellar tap sign (ie, persistent blinking with repetitive tapping over the glabella area), speech impairment, lead-pipe rigidity (smooth resistance), dysphagia, dystonia, stooped posture, rapid repetition of a word or phrase, Lewy bodies, excessive saliva, REM sleep behavior disorder, scoliosis, lid apraxia, impaired vestibulo-ocular reflex, myoclonus, shuffling gait, short strides, flexed posture, sensory abnormalities and pain, dementia, hyposmia, abulia, constipation, forgetfulness, urinary urgency, kyphosis, reduced pulmonary capacity secondary to kyphosis, depigmented cells in the substantia nigra and locus ceruleus, sleep disturbances, autonomic dysfunction, sexual dysfunction, seborrheic dermatitis, decreased arm swing, depression, slow thinking, weakness, excessive daytime somnolence, micrographia (small handwriting), soft speech, cognitive dysfunction, psychosis, fatigue, difficulty turning in bed, apathy, freezing (transient inability to walk), poor articulation, festination (acceleration of gait), orthostasis.

**Cystic fibrosis (CF)**—Thick secretions, meconium ileus, bronchiectasis, pancreatic insufficiency, chronic productive cough, PFTs consistent with obstructive disease ($\downarrow$ FEV$_1$, $\downarrow$ FEV$_1$/FVC ratio, $\uparrow$ RV/TLC ratio, $\downarrow$ FEF$_{25\%-75\%}$), male infertility secondary to absent vas deferens, normal spermatogenesis, obstructive azoospermia, females can become pregnant, $\downarrow$ fertility in females secondary to thick cervical mucus, osteoporosis, digital clubbing, sinusitis, wheezing, recurrent pancreatitis, rectal prolapse, amenorrhea, autosomal recessive, high prevalence in whites, sweat chloride $\geq$60 mmol/L (ie, abnormally high result), normal or intermediate sweat chloride result, mutation in the cystic fibrosis transmembrane conductance regulator (CFTR) gene located on chromosome 7, delta 508 mutation (most common mutation in the CFTR gene), nephrolithiasis, hypochloremic hyponatremic alkalosis, bronchiolitis, vomiting, jaundice, failure to thrive, diabetes mellitus, dermatitis, hyperinflated lungs on CXR (ie, $\uparrow$ TLC, $\uparrow$ residual volume), susceptible to colonization in the respiratory tract (ie, *Pseudomonas aeruginosa*, *Staphylococcus aureus*, *Haemophilus influenzae*, *Aspergillus*), allergic bronchopulmonary aspergillosis (ABPA), undescended testicles, fat malabsorption, GERD, intussusception, constipation, $\uparrow$ frequency of stools, vitamin deficiencies (A, D, E, K), nasal polyps, affected sibling, biliary cirrhosis, periportal fibrosis, portal hypertension, hypertrophic osteoarthropathy, cholelithiasis, foul-smelling stools, nephrocalcinosis, weight loss, abdominal distension, hyperresonant chest percussions, small intestine bacterial overgrowth, hydrocele, volvulus, abnormal nasal potential difference, airway hyperreactivity, peribronchial cuffing and "tram tracks" on CXR, steatorrhea, poor appetite, distal intestinal obstructive syndrome (DIOS), cause of death is typically due to respiratory failure and cor pulmonale, shortened survival.

**HIV**—Fever, sore throat, rash, myalgia, headache, nontender lymphadenopathy (occipital, cervical, axillary), arthralgia, fatigue, night sweats, diarrhea, hepatosplenomegaly, mucocutaneous ulcerations, rash, nausea, weight loss, anorexia, aseptic meningitis, asymptomatic (clinical latent period), STDs, contaminated blood products, high viral load >100,000 copies/mL, increased risk for opportunistic infections (*Pneumocystis jirovecii*, toxoplasma, Mycobacterium avium complex, histoplasma, candida, coccidioides, cryptococcus, cryptosporidium, CMV), positive p24 antigen (viral core protein), toxoplasmosis (fever, headache, seizure, focal neurologic deficits, aphasia, IgG anti-toxoplasma, hemiparesis, pneumonitis, altered mental status, single or multiple ring enhancing lesions with surrounding edema, posterior uveitis), $\downarrow$ CD4 T cell count after seroconversion (usually 1-6 months after exposure), CD4 count <200 mm$^3$ is considered AIDS, shared IV drug users, primary CNS lymphoma (aphasia, hemiparesis, seizures, confusion, lethargy, fever, memory loss, night sweats, focal neurologic deficits, headaches, ring enhancement lesions on MRI, multiple solitary enhancing lesions on MRI, ring and solitary lesions can occur concomitantly, systemic lymphoma), sexual intercourse transmission, mother-to-child transmission, progressive multifocal leukoencephalopathy (white matter demyelination secondary to JC virus, ataxia, hemiparesis, no mass effect, hemianopia, aphasia, cognitive impairment, visual field defects, no contrast enhancement on MRI), retroviruses, HIV-1 is responsible for the majority of infections, HIV encephalopathy (dementia, forgetfulness, depression, apathy, abnormal gait, poor balance, changes in the Mini-Mental Status Examination score, cerebral atrophy on MRI), HIV-2 infection is seen in endemic areas (eg, West Africa), HIV-2 is a slower progressing disease and does not transmit the infection as efficiently as HIV-1, CMV (polyradiculopathy, urinary retention, areflexia, hyperactive reflexes, difficulty walking, delirium, confusion, lower extremity weakness, peripheral neuropathy, altered mental status, encephalitis, periventricular enhancement on MRI, myelitis, CMV retinitis, painless progressive vision loss).

**Sarcoidosis**—Noncaseating granulomas (lung, heart, brain, kidneys, eyes, GI tract, lymph nodes, joints, skin), common in blacks, $\uparrow$ ESR, $\uparrow$ ACE, frequently affects the lungs, PFTs may or may not demonstrate a restrictive pattern ($\downarrow$ FVC, $\downarrow$ FEV$_1$, normal or $\uparrow$ FEV$_1$/FVC ratio, $\downarrow$ TLC, $\downarrow$ FRC, normal FEF$_{25\%-75\%}$), cough, chest pain, dyspnea, bilateral hilar adenopathy and reticular opacities on CXR, uveitis, fatigue, wheezing, weight loss, crackles, peripheral neuropathies, valvular dysfunction, keratoconjunctivitis, xerostomia, proximal muscle weakness, normal or elevated creatine kinase, nephrolithiasis, maculopapular eruptions, systemic inflammation, anemia of chronic disease, violaceous plaque (lupus pernio), unexplained hoarseness, splenomegaly, Bell's palsy, positive RF, hypercalcemia, $\uparrow$ alkaline phosphatase, $\uparrow$ GGT, tachyarrhythmias, sudden death, glomerulonephritis, cystic bone lesions, Löfgren syndrome (fever, polyarthralgias, hilar adenopathy, erythema nodosum), anorexia, hypercalciuria, nephrocalcinosis, heart block, sudden death, pulmonary hypertension, heart failure, hepatomegaly, presence of histiocytes in the granulomas on histology, interstitial nephritis, optic neuritis, cor pulmonale, carpal tunnel syndrome, central diabetes insipidus, pituitary or hypothalamic involvement disrupting the endocrine axis, cranial nerve palsies, hydrocephalus, lymphocytic meningitis, hypergammaglobulinemia, parotid gland enlargement, rhinosinusitis, goiter, leukopenia, eosinophilia, $\downarrow$ diffusing capacity for carbon monoxide (DLCO), nasal polyps, lacrimal gland swelling, $\uparrow$ CD4/CD8 ratio on bronchoalveolar lavage.

**Hepatitis B serologies**—The components include hepatitis B surface antigen (HBsAg), hepatitis B surface antibody (anti-HBs), hepatitis B core antibody (IgM or IgG), hepatitis B e antigen (HBeAg) ,which reflects HBV replication and infectivity, hepatitis B e antibody (anti-HBe), HBV DNA, and ALT. **Acute infection (early phase):** HBsAg (+), anti-HBs (−), IgM anti-HBc (+), HBeAg (+), anti-HBe (−), $\uparrow$ HBV DNA, $\uparrow$ ALT. **Acute infection (window phase):** Only IgM anti-HBc (+). **Acute infection (recovery phase):** IgG anti-HBc (+), anti-HBs (+), anti-HBe (+), ALT normalization. **Chronic infection (replicative phase):** HBsAg (+) for >6 months, anti-HBs (−), IgG anti-HBc (+), HBeAg (+), anti-HBe (−), ↑ HBV DNA. **Chronic infection (nonreplicative phase/inactive carrier state):** HBsAg (+) for >6 months, anti-HBs (−), IgG anti-HBc (+), HBeAg (−), anti-HBe (+). **Prior HBV infection:** IgG anti-HBc (+), anti-HBs (+), anti-HBe (+). **Vaccination:** Only anti-HBs (+).

**Celiac disease**—Also known as celiac (nontropical) sprue or gluten-sensitive enteropathy, malabsorption, flatulence, diarrhea, steatorrhea, weight loss, water- and fat-soluble vitamin deficiencies, bleeding diathesis secondary to vitamin K deficiency, fatigue, headaches, cheilosis, Down syndrome, Turner syndrome, histology on small bowel biopsy (crypt hyperplasia, villous atrophy, ↑ intraepithelial lymphocytes), minor GI complaints, recurrent abdominal pain, stunted growth/short stature, delayed puberty, learning disorders, first degree relatives, female infertility, common in whites, hypocalcemia, selective IgA deficiency, T-cell response, osteoporosis, osteopenia, hypothyroidism > hyperthyroidism, abdominal bloating, anemia, arthritis, GERD, anxiety, genetic predisposition (HLA-DQ2, HLA-DQ8), enamel defects, male infertility, motor weakness, ↑ aminotransferases, autoimmune thyroiditis, silent disease (asymptomatic but positive for serologies and intestinal mucosa consistent with celiac disease), latent disease (asymptomatic with normal intestinal mucosa), seizures, atrophic glossitis, type 1 diabetes, depression, delayed menarche, secondary amenorrhea, osteomalacia, tympanic abdomen, ataxia, peripheral neuropathy, iron deficiency, folate deficiency, dermatitis herpetiformis, IBD, triggering gluten-containing grains (wheat, barley, rye), resolution of symptoms and mucosal lesions upon withdrawal of gluten-containing foods, increased risk for lymphoma and GI cancers, positive antibodies (IgA or IgG) to the following: gliadin, endomysium, and tissue transglutaminase.

**Hemochromatosis**—Skin bronzing, hepatomegaly, hyperpigmentation, hypogonadism, cirrhosis, iron deposition (pituitary, heart, liver, pancreas), dilated cardiomyopathy, restrictive cardiomyopathy, ↑ plasma iron, ↑ plasma ferritin (in the absence of inflammation), ↑ transferrin saturation (ie, ratio of iron to TIBC with normal ranges expressed between 20% and 50%), weakness, heart failure, hypothyroidism, conduction defects, hepatocyte iron accumulation on Perls Prussian blue stain, amenorrhea, diabetes mellitus, asymptomatic, arthralgia, ↑ LFTs, impotence, supraventricular arrhythmias, homozygous C282Y mutation of the HFE gene (common), mutation in the transferrin receptor 2 gene (uncommon), increased risk of hepatocellular carcinoma (HCC), ↓ libido, hooklike osteophytes on x-ray, autosomal recessive, sick sinus syndrome, hair loss, chondrocalcinosis secondary to calcium pyrophosphate dihydrate (CPPD), ↓ bone density, koilonychia, ventricular arrhythmias, juvenile hemochromatosis (earlier onset, cardiomyopathy, hypogonadism, autosomal recessive, hemojuvelin gene mutation, liver disease not as prominent), absence or presence of cirrhosis is a major prognostic factor.

**Hypokalemia**—Muscle weakness, cardiac arrhythmias, muscle cramps, palpitations, fatigue, ↑ blood pressure, rhabdomyolysis, ↑ ammonia production, myoglobinuria, ileus, paroxysmal atrial tachycardia, sinus bradycardia, abdominal distension, asymptomatic, causes (↑ GI loss, ↑ urinary loss, hypothermia, ↓ potassium intake, ↑ sweat loss, ↑ insulin, dialysis), diaphragmatic weakness, AV blocks, premature atrial beat, ventricular fibrillation, constipation, premature ventricular beats, impaired renal concentrating ability, ↑ U wave amplitude, ↓ T wave amplitude, prolonged QT, ST segment depression, ↓ insulin secretion, worsening diabetes control.

**Hyperkalemia**—Muscle weakness, cardiac arrhythmias, palpitations, flaccid paralysis, ↓ deep tendon reflexes (DTRs), ↓ renal ammoniagenesis, LBBB, RBBB, AV blocks, sinus bradycardia, peaked T waves, widen QRS, shortened QT, prolonged PR, absent P wave, asymptomatic, causes (↓ insulin, ↓ urinary K+ loss, ↓ aldosterone secretion, renal failure, nonselective beta-blockers, succinylcholine, metabolic acidosis, acute digitalis toxicity, hyperosmolality), ventricular tachycardia, ventricular fibrillation, paresthesias, asystole.

**Hyponatremia**—Nausea, malaise, headache, lethargy, obtundation, dizziness, gait disturbances, seizures, coma, confusion, ileus, respiratory arrest, central pontine myelinolysis secondary to rapid sodium correction, hypotonic (<275 mOsmol/kg $H_2O$), normotonic (275-295 mOsmol/kg $H_2O$), hypertonic (>295 mOsmol/kg $H_2O$), hypertonic hyponatremia (eg, mannitol, maltose, hyperglycemia), normotonic hyponatremia (eg, hyperlipidemia, hyperproteinemia, bladder irrigation), hypovolemic hypotonic hyponatremia plus urine sodium <10 mmol/L (eg, extrarenal sodium losses), hypovolemic hypotonic hyponatremia plus urine sodium >20 mmol/L (eg, renal sodium loss, hypoaldosteronism, vomiting, diuretics), euvolemic hypotonic hyponatremia plus urine osmolality >100 mOsmol/kg $H_2O$ (eg, SIADH), hypotonic hyponatremia plus urine osmolality <100 mOsmol/kg $H_2O$ (eg, primary polydipsia), hypervolemic hypotonic hyponatremia (eg, CHF, cirrhosis, nephrotic syndrome, renal insufficiency).

**Hypernatremia**—Irritability, lethargy, weakness, subarachnoid hemorrhages, cognitive dysfunction, twitching, coma, seizures, confusion, intracerebral hemorrhage, focal neurologic deficits, causes (diuretics, central diabetes insipidus, nephrogenic diabetes insipidus, osmotic diuresis, mannitol, hyperglycemia, vomiting, diarrhea, NG suction, sweating, burns, impaired thirst/primary hypodipsia, sodium overload).

**Hypomagnesemia**—Neuromuscular hyperexcitability, hyperreflexia, hypocalcemia, hypokalemia, weakness, muscle cramps, ileus, apathy, cardiac arrhythmias, delirium, paresthesias, muscular fibrillation, coma, tremor, ventricular tachycardia, tetany, seizures, ↑ DTRs, muscle spasms, causes (vomiting, diarrhea, NG suction, malabsorption, laxatives, surgical bowel resection, diuretics, alcohol, hypercalcemia, aminoglycosides, amphotericin B, pentamidine, cisplatin, cyclosporine, acute pancreatitis, chronic metabolic acidosis, inherited disorders, hungry bone syndrome, proton pump inhibitors), ventricular premature contractions, positive Chvostek and Trousseau signs, vertical nystagmus, widen QRS, prolonged PR, prolonged QT, peaked T waves, depressed T waves, Na-K-ATPase inhibition, potentiates digitalis toxicity, ↓ PTH secretion, skeletal resistance to PTH, ↓ 1,25-dihydroxyvitamin D (calcitriol), common in ICU patients, respiratory muscle failure, torsades de pointes.

**Hypermagnesemia**—Lethargy, ↓ DTRs, hypocalcemia, hypotension, headache, nausea, vomiting, flushing, muscle weakness, drowsiness, bradycardia, somnolence, respiratory paralysis, cardiac arrest, muscle paralysis, prolonged PR, ↑ QT interval, ↑ QRS duration, complete heart block, respiratory failure, ↓ PTH secretion, causes (renal insufficiency, magnesium infusion, Epsom salts, lithium therapy, milk-alkali syndrome, tumor lysis syndrome, hypothyroidism, adrenal insufficiency, primary hyperparathyroidism, familial hypocalciuric hypercalcemia, magnesium-containing laxatives, enemas and antacids).

**Hypophosphatemia**—Muscle weakness, irritability, confusion, delirium, paresthesias, coma, seizures, dysphagia, ileus, asymptomatic, hemolysis, thrombocytopenia, impaired WBC function, ATP depletion, rhabdomyolysis, bone pain, ↓ myocardial contraction, heart failure, causes (↓ intestinal absorption, chronic diarrhea, vitamin D deficiency, malabsorption, inadequate intake, aluminum or magnesium-containing antacids, alcoholism, ↑ urinary loss, inherited disorders, Fanconi syndrome, primary and secondary hyperparathyroidism, acetazolamide, intracellular shift of phosphate, ↑ insulin, hungry bone syndrome, acute respiratory alkalosis), respiratory failure secondary to diaphragmatic weakness, ↑ CPK, impaired platelet function, ↓ 2,3-DPG shifting hemoglobin-O$_2$ dissociation curve to the left, ↑ affinity of hemoglobin for O$_2$.

**Hyperphosphatemia**—Asymptomatic, signs and symptoms of hypocalcemia, signs and symptoms related to the underlying cause, causes (extracellular shift of phosphate, tumor lysis syndrome, rhabdomyolysis, hemolysis, DKA, lactic acidosis, ↓ renal excretion, renal failure, ↑ absorption, vitamin D toxicity, bisphosphonates, leukemia, acromegaly, thyrotoxicosis, hypoparathyroidism, pseudohypoparathyroidism, phosphate-containing laxatives).

**Acute rheumatic fever**—Sydenham chorea, erythema marginatum, carditis, valvulitis, migratory arthritis (common sites include elbows, wrists, knees, and ankles), subcutaneous nodules, fever, ↑ ESR, ↑ CRP, arthralgia, prolonged PR, sequela of group A streptococcus pharyngitis, positive rapid antigen test or throat culture for Group A beta-hemolytic streptococci, involuntary movements, common in children 5 to 15 years of age, transient joint pain, muscle weakness, mitral valve prolapse, "milkmaid's grip" (unable to maintain a grip when asked to squeeze examiner's hand), hypotonia, crying outbursts, personality changes, ↑ antistreptolysin O (ASO) titers, synovial fluid analysis revealing sterile inflammatory fluid, mitral regurgitation, heart block, annular skin lesions with pale centers, heart failure, jerking of the face and feet, facial grimacing, ballismus, loss of fine-motor skills, pericarditis, cardiomegaly on CXR, pericardial effusion, motor symptoms improvement during sleep, emotional lability, tongue fasciculations, speech dysarthria, evanescent nonpruritic rash, pericardial friction rub, erythematous serpiginous skin lesions, pancarditis (pericardium, epicardium, myocardium, endocardium), painless nodules (bony surfaces, prominences, tendon sheaths), short-lived (1-2 weeks) subcutaneous nodules, rheumatic heart disease (mitral valve > aortic valve), erythema marginatum typically spares the face, cardiovascular disease is leading cause of death.

**Tetralogy of Fallot**—PROVe (pulmonary stenosis, right ventricular hypertrophy, overriding aorta, VSD, extracardiac anomalies: patent foramen ovale, atrioventricular septal defects, PDA, ASD, multiple ventricular defects, persistent left-sided superior vena cava, aortic valve regurgitation, right-sided aortic arch, LAD arising from the right coronary artery instead of the left coronary artery, collateral vessels arising from the aorta to the lungs, absent ductus arteriosus, bilateral ductus arteriosus, scoliosis), Down syndrome, Di George syndrome, left-to-right shunt (acyanotic), single S$_2$ (ie, inaudible P$_2$), right-to-left shunt (cyanosis), hypercyanotic ("tet") spells, right axis deviation, prominent R waves in lead V$_1$, small size for expected age, right ventricular predominance on palpation, failure to thrive, systolic thrill on palpation along the left sternal border, feeding difficulty, clubbing of the fingers and toes, early systolic click along the left sternal border, exertional dyspnea, asymptomatic/acyanotic ("pink tetralogy"), "boot-shaped" heart on CXR, absent murmur during tet spells, pulmonary valve (bicuspid or unicuspid), harsh systolic ejection murmur along the left sternal border and pulmonic area, decrease in pulmonary vascularity on CXR, continuous murmurs in patients with aorticopulmonary collateral vessels or PDA, anterior and cephalad displacement of the infundibular septum, right atrial enlargement, ↑ P wave amplitude in lead V$_1$, pulmonary valve atresia (uncommon), murmurs not related to VSD but rather right ventricular outflow obstruction (common cause), squatting improve symptoms (↑ peripheral vascular resistance and thereby ↓ right-to-left shunt).

**Henoch-Schönlein purpura**—Also known as IgA vasculitis, rash (face, upper extremities, trunk, buttocks, lower extremities), arthralgia, abdominal pain, nonthrombocytopenic palpable purpura, renal disease, arthritis (lower extremity > upper extremity), pruritic petechiae, fever, ecchymoses, common in children, intussusception, subcutaneous edema, hematuria, nausea, orchitis, vomiting, proteinuria, normal or ↑ platelet count, nonambulatory, diarrhea, normal coagulation studies, constipation, IgA deposition (arterioles, capillaries, and venules), nephritis, 50% of cases preceded by upper respiratory infection (usually streptococcus), ↑ ESR and leukocytosis secondary to infection, joint swelling without effusion, GI bleed, anemia secondary to GI bleed, urticarial wheals, normal hemoglobin levels, acute pancreatitis (uncommon), scrotal pain and swelling, absence of purpura as the initial presentation, unknown etiology, ± red cell casts, ± guaiac-positive stool, triggering event (infection, food, drugs, insect bites, vaccinations), mesangium deposits (IgA, C3, IgG, fibrin, IgM), transient arthritis, bowel perforation, ambulating with a limp, scalp edema, skin lesion biopsy revealing leukocytoclastic vasculitis, can still occur in adults but less common, male > female, self-limited condition, nephrotic syndrome uncommon, immune-mediated vasculitis, recurrence.

**Cor pulmonale**—Altered structure and/or function of the right ventricle secondary to disease of the lung parenchyma and/or pulmonary vasculature, right-sided heart failure *not* due to left-sided heart failure or congenital heart disease, shortness of breath, lethargy, dyspnea on exertion, dizziness, lower extremity edema, accentuated $P_2$ upon inspiration, chronic cor pulmonale (slow progressive course with development of RVH $\rightarrow$ RV dilatation $\rightarrow$ right-sided heart failure), pulmonary arterial hypertension, fatigue, palpitations, chest pain, acute cor pulmonale secondary to massive PE (RV dilatation $\rightarrow$ heart failure without RVH seen during the entire process), RBBB in PE, cardiomegaly on CXR, mean pulmonary artery pressure $\geq 25$ mmHg at rest, exertional syncope, systolic pulmonary ejection click over the pulmonic area, RVH, prominent "a wave" on jugular venous pulsations secondary to RVH, right-sided $S_4$, left parasternal heave, RVH on EKG (prominent R wave in lead $V_1$, right axis deviation), signs and symptoms of the underlying lung disease (eg, COPD, CF, sarcoidosis), prominent pulmonary arteries on CXR, $\uparrow$ BNP, pulmonary capillary wedge pressure <15 mmHg, right atrial enlargement on EKG ($\uparrow$ P wave amplitude in lead $V_1$ and/or lead II), tricuspid regurgitation secondary to right ventricular dilatation, holosystolic murmur along the left sternal border (tricuspid regurgitation), prominent "v wave" on jugular venous pulsations secondary to right ventricular dilatation, loss of retrosternal space on lateral view CXR, signs of RV failure ($\uparrow$ JVP, hepatomegaly, hepatojugular reflux, pulsatile liver, right-sided $S_3$, peripheral edema, $\pm$ ascites), end-stage cor pulmonale (cyanosis, low cardiac output, cool extremities, hypotension, cool extremities, pulmonary edema).

**Stevens-Johnson syndrome (SJS)**—Prodromal symptoms (fever, arthralgias, photophobia, skin tenderness, conjunctival itching or burning, malaise), milder form of toxic epidermal necrolysis (TEN), risk factors for SJS and TEN (HIV infection, genetics, SLE), drug exposure followed by 1 to 3 weeks before symptoms appear, diffuse erythema, targetlike erythematous macules, rash may initially start on the face and upper torso, vesicles and bullae form which then slough off, denuded skin, secondary infection, 80% of cases of TEN are triggered by medications, positive Nikolsky sign (ie, elicitation of a blister upon lateral pressure on the skin), 50% of cases of SJS are triggered by medications, mucosal involvement (conjunctiva, lips, buccal mucosa, esophagus, trachea, urethra, vagina, anus), SJS (skin sloughing <10%), TEN (skin sloughing >30%), SJS/TEN overlap syndrome (skin sloughing >10% but <30%), keratitis, triggering drugs for SJS and TEN (allopurinol, lamotrigine, sulfamethoxazole, sulfasalazine, sulfadiazine, sulfapyridine, ampicillin, amoxicillin, carbamazepine, phenobarbital, phenytoin, piroxicam, cephalosporins, NSAIDs), corneal erosions, urethritis, hyperemia, tracheobronchitis, mucous membranes (erosions, crusts, ulcerations, necrosis, blistering), 15% of cases of SJS are triggered by infections (eg, *Mycoplasma pneumonia*, herpes virus), full-thickness epidermal necrosis and detachment on histology.

**Alport syndrome**—Bilateral sensorineural hearing loss (high frequency initially), ocular abnormalities, renal abnormalities, X-linked (80% of cases), autosomal recessive (10%-15% of cases), autosomal dominant (5% of cases), early childhood hematuria, hereditary nephritis, multiple leiomyomas (found in the respiratory, GI, and female reproductive tracts), microscopic hematuria, anterior lenticonus (ie, conical protrusion of the anterior surface of the lens), gross hematuria, abnormalities in the alpha chains of type IV collagen (seen in the cochlea, eye, and kidney), progressive hearing loss to low frequencies, family history, glomerulosclerosis, primary dysfunction is type IV collagen, not an autoimmune disease, post–renal transplant anti-glomerular basement membrane antibody disease (3%-5% of transplanted males), hypertension, predominantly males in X-linked Alport syndrome (no male-to-male transmission), thinning of the glomerular basement membrane (early stage), X-linked female carriers (varied presentation secondary to lyonization), thickening of the glomerular basement membrane (over time), proteinuria, gene mutation (COL4A3, COL4A4, or COL4A5), corneal changes (posterior polymorphous dystrophy), end-stage renal disease, laminated GBM (ie, splitting of the lamina densa of the GBM over time), retinal changes (perimacular dot-and-fleck retinopathy).

**Hydrocele**—Painless scrotal mass, fluid between the parietal and visceral layers of the tunica vaginalis, communicating hydrocele (patent processus vaginalis, $\uparrow$ peritoneal fluid during Valsalva, reducible, associated indirect inguinal hernia), noncommunicating hydrocele (closed processus vaginalis, no affect during Valsalva, nonreducible, fluid arises from the mesothelial lining of the tunica vaginalis), positive scrotum transillumination, superior and anterior to the testis, unilateral or bilateral.

**Varicocele**—Painless scrotal mass, "bag of worms" texture upon standing or Valsalva, scrotal pain, dilated pampiniform plexus of the spermatic cord veins, left > right, diminished varicocele upon supine position, scrotal heaviness, negative scrotum transillumination, $\downarrow$ fertility, unilateral or bilateral, postpubertal males, rule out obstruction or thrombosis of the IVC (for right-sided varicocele, acute onset, or nonreducible varicocele in the supine position), "nutcracker effect" (ie, increased pressure in left testicular vein secondary to compression of the left renal vein by the superior mesenteric artery and aorta), testicular atrophy.

**Spermatocele**—Painless scrotal mass, arises at the head (caput) of the epididymis, positive scrotum transillumination, epididymal cyst, benign, no affect during Valsalva, fluid may contain sperm, located superior and/or posterior to the testicle, no effect on fertility, unknown etiology, incidental finding.

**Primary sclerosing cholangitis (PSC)**—Pruritus, jaundice, hepatomegaly, fatigue, excoriations, progressive disease, splenomegaly, right upper quadrant pain, asymptomatic, $\uparrow\uparrow$ alkaline phosphatase, unknown etiology, normal albumin levels (early stage), $\uparrow$ serum aminotransferases (usually $\leq 300$ IU/L), chronic cholestasis, men > women, inflammation and fibrosis of medium to large intrahepatic and/or extrahepatic biliary ducts, $\uparrow$ GGT, intrahepatic and extrahepatic biliary duct strictures and dilatations on cholangiography, $\pm \uparrow$ direct (conjugated) bilirubin (ie, bilirubin levels can fluctuate but an increase suggests biliary obstruction), mean age of diagnosis is 40 years old, steatorrhea, stricturing and beading on cholangiography, increased risk for cholangiocarcinoma, fat-soluble vitamin deficiencies (A, D, E, K), recurrent febrile bacterial cholangitis secondary to biliary obstruction (Charcot's triad—fever, RUQ pain, jaundice), positive P-ANCA, hypergammaglobulinemia, patients with PSC have a fairly high likelihood (75%-90% of cases) of IBD (ulcerative colitis > Crohn's disease), increased risk for colon cancer (in the presence of PSC + UC), patients with IBD have a fairly low likelihood of PSC (1%-5% of cases), hypoalbuminemia (seen with concomitant active IBD), concentric periductal fibrosis on histology ("onion skin" pattern), cholelithiasis, increased risk for gallbladder cancer, secondary biliary cirrhosis, portal hypertension, end-stage liver disease, small duct PSC or "pericholangitis" (ie, variant of PSC with histology consistent with PSC but normal cholangiography), increased risk for hepatocellular carcinoma in patients with cirrhosis, metabolic bone disease (ie, osteoporosis), histology may be similar to PBC (eg, bridging fibrosis), $\uparrow$ serum IgM, PSC-autoimmune hepatitis overlap syndrome (ie, cholangiographic abnormalities characteristic of PSC but serologic features of autoimmune hepatitis such as $\uparrow$ ANA or $\uparrow$ smooth muscle antibodies), median survival without liver transplantation from time of diagnosis is 9 to 12 years.

**Pelvic inflammatory disease (PID)**—Lower abdominal pain (dull, crampy, or constant), cervical motion tenderness, fever, uterine tenderness, infection of the upper genital tract (uterus, oviducts, ovaries) and nearby pelvic organs, adnexal tenderness, sexually active young women, abdominal pain <7 days (unlikely if >3 weeks), multiple partners, cervical or vaginal mucopurulent discharge, pelvic pain developing a few days after the onset of a menstrual period or at the end of menses, diffuse bilateral lower abdominal pain exacerbated by sexual activity or movement, palpable adnexal mass, tubo-ovarian abscess, history of STDs, bacterial vaginosis, nonbarrier contraception, Fitz-Hugh-Curtis syndrome (perihepatitis, pleuritic RUQ pain ± radiation to shoulder, "violin string" adhesions on the surface of the liver, $\pm \uparrow$ aminotransferases, jaundice), salpingitis, periappendicitis secondary to salpingitis, ectopic pregnancy, tubal edema and erythema, controversial role or lack of a clear consensus of OCPs on PID risk, decreased bowel sounds, Gram's stain positive for gram-negative intracellular diplococci, abnormal uterine bleeding, *Neisseria gonorrhoeae* infection, menorrhagia, urethritis, *Chlamydia trachomatis* infection, unknown etiology, polymicrobial, plasma cell endometritis, $\uparrow$ ESR, $\uparrow$ CRP, nausea, vomiting, leukocytosis, oophoritis, abnormal fimbriae, $\uparrow$ WBCs on saline microscopy of vaginal secretions, chills, $\uparrow$ CA-125, new vaginal discharge, postcoital bleeding, urinary symptoms, malaise, peritonitis, rebound tenderness, cul-de-sac fluid, involuntary guarding, previous history of PID, parametritis, young age at first intercourse, vaginal douching, fluid-filled oviduct (hydrosalpinx), myometritis, infertility, vaginal spotting, IUD increases risk only in the first 3 weeks after insertion, uncommon during pregnancy (except the first 12 weeks of gestation before mucus plug seals off the uterus), chronic pelvic pain (ie, sequela of PID).

**Irritable bowel syndrome (IBS)**—Chronic abdominal pain, absence of organic pathology, altered bowel habits, abdominal distention, diarrhea and/or constipation, absence of weight loss, flatulence, women > men, GERD, absence of anemia, dyspareunia, abdominal pain with variable locations (upper, lower, right-sided, left-sided), improvement with defecation, nausea, vomiting, unclear pathophysiology, absence of fever, abdominal discomfort (ie, not pain), pellet-shaped stools, postprandial stool urgency, dysmenorrhea, absence of rectal bleeding, subjective feeling of incomplete evacuation, abdominal pain without radiation, belching, hard narrow-caliber stools, constant abdominal pain, episodic abdominal pain superimposed on constant ache, stool straining, recurrent abdominal pain in the last 3 months, dysphagia, normal labs (CBC, BMP, ESR), absence of painless diarrhea, altered stool appearance and/or frequency at onset of symptoms, urinary frequency, abdominal pain precipitated by meals or stress, onset in young patients (<45 years old), absence of steatorrhea, comorbid fibromyalgia, crampy pain, dyspepsia, sexual dysfunction, absence of progressive abdominal pain, stool accompanied by mucus, small volumes of loose stools, stool urgency prior to defecation, work absenteeism, noncardiac chest pain, absence of nocturnal abdominal pain.

**Psoriasis**—Skin lesions, pruritus, asymptomatic, uveitis, conjunctivitis, genetic predisposition (HLA-Cw6), blepharitis, $\uparrow$ T cell activity, triggering factors (trauma, infection, stress, cold, alcohol, lithium, beta blockers, antimalarial drugs), corneal lesions, dry eye, plaque psoriasis (silvery scales, common type, affects the scalp, trunk, and extensor surfaces of the elbows and knees), inverse psoriasis (smooth red lesions without scales, inverse of extensor surfaces such as the flexural areas of the armpit, under the breast, groin, creases of the butt), guttate psoriasis ("droplike" lesions, small erythematous papules or plaques, preceded by streptococcal infection, primarily affects the trunk, spontaneously remits or progresses to chronic plaque psoriasis), pustular psoriasis (pustules affecting the palms, soles, distal digit, or anywhere on the body), nail psoriasis (nail pitting, nail bed hyperkeratosis, splinter hemorrhages, onycholysis, visually indistinguishable from onychomycosis, brown "oil spot" sign, occurs as a solo condition or commonly with psoriatic arthritis), psoriatic arthritis (DIP joint arthritis, symmetric polyarthritis, asymmetric oligoarthritis, sacroiliitis, spondylitis, arthritis mutilans/deforming arthritis, nail involvement, tenosynovitis, ± rheumatoid factor, enthesitis/inflammation at the ligament insertion into bone, dactylitis ("sausage digit"), psoriatic skin lesions, family history of psoriasis, ocular involvement, "pencil-in-cup" appearance on hand x-ray), erythrodermic psoriasis (uncommon type, generalized erythema and scaling of the entire body, constitutional symptoms, high risk for complications), worsening psoriasis in HIV patients, improvement in warm sunny weather.

**Hodgkin's lymphoma**—B symptoms (fever, night sweats, weight loss), mediastinal mass, painless lymphadenopathy (occipital, preauricular, cervical, Waldeyer's tonsillar ring, supraclavicular, infraclavicular, mediastinal, hilar, axillary, epitrochlear/upper inner elbow, spleen, liver, paraaortic, mesenteric, iliac, inguinal, femoral, popliteal), pruritus, hepatomegaly, supradiaphragmatic lymphadenopathy > subdiaphragmatic lymphadenopathy, contiguous spread via lymphatic system (early stage), splenomegaly, noncontiguous spread via lymphatic system (later in the course of disease), bimodal age distribution (15-30 years old and >50 years old), intermittent fever (ie, Pel-Ebstein fever), fatigue, hematogenous dissemination (later in the course of disease), mediastinal related problems (retrosternal chest pain, dysphagia, shortness of breath, cough, superior vena cava syndrome), rubbery consistency of the lymph node, anemia, ± EBV infection, extranodal involvement (eg, bone marrow, pulmonary, skeletal), hypercalcemia, pain over involved bone or nodal sites upon drinking alcohol, neoplastic Reed-Sternberg cells ("owl's eyes" appearance) in the setting of mixed inflammatory cells seen in classical Hodgkin's lymphoma, neoplastic cells derived from germinal center B cells, Reed-Sternberg cell positive for CD15 and CD30, 5 types of Hodgkin's lymphoma (4 subtypes of the classical Hodgkin's lymphoma and 1 type referred to as nodular lymphocyte predominant Hodgkin's lymphoma), 4 subtypes of classical Hodgkin's lymphoma: nodular sclerosis (70%-80% of cases) > mixed cellularity (20%-25% of cases) > lymphocyte rich (5% of cases) > lymphocyte depleted (<1% of cases), paraneoplastic syndrome (eg, CNS abnormalities, hypertrophic osteoarthropathy, nephrotic syndrome, cutaneous manifestations), nodular lymphocyte predominant Hodgkin's lymphoma ("nonclassical," 5% of cases of Hodgkin's lymphoma, L&H cell that is a variant of a Reed-Sternberg cell, L&H cell negative for CD15 and CD30), eosinophilia, neutropenia, leukocytosis, lymphopenia, thrombocytosis, thrombocytopenia, autoimmune hemolytic anemia, early stage large mediastinal mass (greater than one-third of the intrathoracic diameter of the chest wall) is an unfavorable prognostic factor.

**Amyotrophic lateral sclerosis (ALS)**—Also known as Lou Gehrig's disease or motor neuron disease, mixed upper and lower motor neuron deficit, anterior horn cell degeneration, corticospinal tract degeneration, loss of Betz cells in the motor cortex, asymmetric limb weakness, upper motor neuron findings (spasticity, stiffness, hyperreflexia, ↑ DTRs, poor dexterity, Babinski/extensor plantar response, Hoffman's sign), lower motor neuron findings (fasciculations, fibrillations on EMG, twitching, cramping, muscle weakness, reduced reflexes, amyotrophy/muscular atrophy, respiratory difficulties, tripping secondary to a foot drop), progressive neurodegenerative disorder, sporadic (90% of cases) > familial (5%-10% of cases), autosomal dominant pattern (superoxide dismutase 1 mutation) in familial cases, unknown etiology in sporadic cases, normal sensory exam, motor nuclei degeneration in the brainstem (trigeminal motor nucleus, hypoglossal nucleus, nucleus ambiguus), bulbar findings (dysarthria, dysphagia, drooling, aspiration, choking, tongue weakness, slurred speech, hoarseness, vocal cord weakness, trismus, chewing difficulty, laryngospasm, incomplete eye closure, reduced volume of speech, jaw stiffness/clenching, poor lip seal, pseudobulbar affect/involuntary crying or laughing), cervical findings (head drop, intrinsic hand muscle weakness, shoulder girdle muscle weakness, wrist drop, difficulty eating, grooming, bathing, or writing secondary to upper extremity weakness), thoracic findings (abdominal protuberance, truncal

weakness, difficulty maintaining an erect posture, hand walking on their thighs to support their trunk, diaphragmatic weakness, dyspnea, respiratory muscle weakness, weak cough, orthopnea, tachypnea, sleep disordered breathing), lumbosacral findings (lower extremity weakness, imbalance, foot drop secondary to foot/ankle weakness, gait dysfunction, difficulty rising from chairs or climbing stairs, lumbar lordosis), fibrillations and fasciculations on EMG, extraocular motility is typically spared but dysfunction can present in late stages, incontinence is uncommon, gliosis of the corticospinal tract, sphincter control of the bowel and bladder is typically spared, urinary and fecal urgency without incontinence (ie, preserved sphincter function) can occur in late stages, thinning of the ventral roots, sensory function is typically preserved, frontotemporal dementia (personality changes, ritualized behaviors, impaired judgment, unusual eating patterns), evidence of muscle denervation and reinnervation, normal sensory nerve conduction study, sometimes abnormal sensory nerve conduction study, sometimes abnormal sensory evoked potentials, signs of parkinsonism, reduced amplitudes of the compound motor action potential on nerve conduction studies, most common cause of death is respiratory failure, median survival from time of diagnosis is 3 to 5 years.

**Granulomatosis with polyangiitis (Wegener's)**—Also known as GPA, systemic vasculitis, systemic features (eg, fever, weight loss, malaise, migratory arthralgias, night sweats), necrotizing granulomatous inflammation, renal and respiratory tract manifestations predominate, whites > blacks, unknown etiology, multiorgan involvement (CNS, parotids, thyroid, lungs, heart, breast, GI, liver, prostate, ureters, skin), nasal crusting, epistaxis, sinusitis, tracheal stenosis, stridor, wheezing, proteinase 3-ANCA > myeloperoxidase-ANCA (Note: P-ANCA correlates with myeloperoxidase and C-ANCA correlates with proteinase 3), conjunctivitis, negative ANCA (<10% of cases), ↑ ESR, ↑ CRP, episcleritis, otitis media, ± ↑ creatinine levels, purulent nasal discharge, uveitis, corneal ulceration, few or absent immune deposits in the glomeruli (ie, pauci-immune glomerulonephritis), leukocytosis, thrombocytosis, ear pain, hemoptysis, DVT, acute kidney injury, urticaria, ± rheumatoid factor, dyspnea, nasal ulcers, chest discomfort, coronary vasculitis, normochromic-normocytic anemia, pericarditis, ↑ or ↓ DLCO, subglottic stenosis, strawberry gingival hyperplasia, pulmonary effusion, pulmonary consolidation, CNS granulomatous mass, visual loss, abnormal findings on CXR (cavitary pulmonary nodules, noncavitating pulmonary nodules, opacities, or hilar adenopathy), atelectasis, proteinuria, eye pain, oral ulcers, persistent rhinorrhea, dacryocystitis, hematuria, livida reticularis, hearing loss (conductive and sensorineural), absence of nasal polyps, diffuse alveolar hemorrhage (DAH) secondary to pulmonary capillaritis, cough, vesicles, papules, petechiae, mastoiditis, optic neuropathy, cranial nerve palsies, otorrhea, proptosis, focal and segmental glomerulonephritis that can evolve into a necrotizing crescentic glomerulonephritis, hyperthyroidism, bronchial stenosis, retinal vasculitis, renal failure, abdominal pain secondary to splanchnic vasculitis, myalgias, cardiac conduction defects, saddle nose deformity secondary to nasal septal perforation (ie, loss of nasal support), purpura ± ulceration, peripheral neuropathy, myocarditis,

± hypergammaglobulinemia (IgA), hoarseness, pleuritic pain, airflow obstruction, subcutaneous nodules, bronchial ulceration, leukocytoclastic vasculitis on skin biopsy, mononeuritis multiplex, ± red cell casts, limited GPA (ie, isolated respiratory tract manifestations with the possibility of renal manifestations later in the course of disease), biopsy of the involved organ may show some or all of the findings: granulomatous inflammation, necrosis, vasculitis.

**Anti-GBM antibody (Goodpasture's) disease**—Autoimmune disorder, rapidly progressive glomerulonephritis (RPGN), hematuria, hemoptysis, proteinuria, acute renal failure, red cell casts, granular casts, cough, shortness of breath, ↑ DLCO secondary to hemoglobin in the alveoli, pulmonary hemorrhage, hemoptysis precipitated by lung injury (eg, cocaine, smoking, inhaled hydrocarbons), hypertension, renal plus lung disease (most common presentation), bimodal age distribution (30s and 60s), isolated renal disease (20%-40% of cases), tachypnea, crackles, isolated lung disease (<10% of cases), ± ↑ creatinine, systemic features are usually absent (eg, fever, weight loss, malaise), myeloperoxidase-ANCA > proteinase 3-ANCA, absence of vasculitis, up to 30% of patients are double positive (ie, positive anti-GBM antibodies + positive myeloperoxidase ANCA), immunofluorescence demonstrating linear deposition of IgG (sometimes IgA or IgM) along the basement membranes (glomerular basement membrane > alveolar basement membrane), light microscopy from a renal biopsy demonstrating crescentic glomerulonephritis, cyanosis, nonspecific pulmonary infiltrates on CXR, edema, anti-GBM antibodies (mainly IgG but sometimes IgA or IgM) against the alpha chains of type IV collagen, oliguria, iron deficiency anemia secondary to prolonged pulmonary hemorrhage, genetic predisposition (HLA-DR15 previously known as HLA-DR2), pulmonary fibrosis secondary to recurrent episodes of pulmonary bleeding, type II hypersensitivity.

**Vitamin A (retinol)**—**Deficiency:** Night blindness, xerophthalmia (dry eye), poor bone development, Bitot's spots (abnormal squamous proliferation and keratinization of the conjunctiva), follicular hyperkeratosis, keratomalacia (ulceration of the cornea), dry skin, hyperkeratosis of the skin, impaired immune system. **Acute toxicity:** Nausea, vomiting, vertigo, blurry vision, drowsiness, irritability, teratogenic. **Chronic toxicity:** Dry skin, pruritus, yellow-orange skin discoloration (ie, excess β-carotene), alopecia, anorexia, ↑ CSF pressure, pseudotumor cerebri, papilledema, visual impairments, headache, hepatotoxicity, hepatomegaly, hyperostosis, bone pain, bone fractures, ataxia, teratogenic.

**Vitamin D (ergocalciferol/D$_2$, cholecalciferol/D$_3$)**—**Deficiency:** Rickets (children), osteomalacia (adults), hypocalcemia, secondary hyperparathyroidism, severe deficiency (↓ serum Ca, ↓ serum PO$_4$, ↓ 25 (OHD), ↑ PTH, ↑ alkaline phosphatase). **Toxicity:** Hypercalcemia, bone pain, backache, nausea, vomiting, polydipsia, polyuria, anorexia, abdominal pain, constipation, confusion, muscle weakness, shortened QT.

**Vitamin E (α-tocopherol)**—**Deficiency:** Hemolytic anemia, neurologic abnormalities (ataxia, hyporeflexia, ↓ proprioception, ↓ vibratory sensation, retinopathy, skeletal muscle atrophy. **Toxicity:** Nausea, fatigue, blurred vision, muscle weakness.

**Vitamin K (phylloquinone/K$_1$, menaquinone/K$_2$, menadione/K$_3$)**—**Deficiency:** Bleeding, easy bruisability, hematuria, melena, prolonged PT. **Toxicity:** Menadione formulation (vitamin K$_3$) can cause hyperbilirubinemia, hemolytic anemia, jaundice, kernicterus, and blocks the effects of oral anticoagulants.

**Vitamin C (ascorbic acid)**—**Deficiency:** Scurvy (poor wound healing, petechiae, ecchymosis, bleeding gums, coiled hairs, joint swelling, perifollicular hyperkeratotic papules, fatigue). **Toxicity:** Diarrhea, abdominal cramps, false-negative stool guaiac results.

**Vitamin B$_1$ (thiamine)**—**Deficiency:** Wernicke-Korsakoff syndrome (ataxia, confusion, nystagmus, ophthalmoplegia, memory impairment, confabulation), infantile beriberi (cyanosis, dyspnea, vomiting, tachycardia, cardiomegaly, heart failure), adult wet beriberi (high-output CHF, cardiomegaly, tachycardia, peripheral edema, peripheral neuritis), adult dry beriberi (↓ reflexes, motor and sensory peripheral neuropathy primarily affecting the legs).

**Vitamin B$_2$ (riboflavin)**—**Deficiency:** Angular stomatitis (inflammation at the corner of the mouth), smooth tongue secondary to glossitis (ie, loss of papillae), seborrheic dermatitis, corneal vascularization, anemia.

**Vitamin B$_3$ (niacin)**—**Deficiency:** Pellagra (dermatitis, diarrhea, dementia, death). **Acute toxicity:** Flushing can be seen with nicotinic acid but not with nicotinamide. **Chronic toxicity:** Nicotinic acid can cause elevated aminotransferases, elevated uric acid, and peptic ulcers.

**Vitamin B$_5$ (pantothenic acid)**—**Deficiency:** GI disturbances, paresthesias, dysesthesias ("burning feet" syndrome).

**Vitamin B$_6$ (pyridoxine)**—**Deficiency:** Stomatitis, glossitis, seborrheic dermatitis, peripheral neuropathy, depression, confusion, irritability, seizures, anemia, elevated homocysteine levels. **Toxicity:** Photosensitivity, dermatitis, unstable gait secondary to sensory neuropathy.

**Vitamin B$_{12}$ (cobalamin)**—**Deficiency:** Megaloblastic anemia (pernicious anemia), subacute combined degeneration of the dorsal and lateral columns, loss of vibration and position sense, positive Romberg test, ataxia, paresthesias, urinary and fecal incontinence, dementia, glossitis, optic neuropathy, elevated homocysteine levels, elevated methylmalonic acid, hypersegmented neutrophils.

**Folate**—**Deficiency:** Megaloblastic anemia, absence of neurologic disturbances, elevated homocysteine levels, hypersegmented neutrophils, neural tube defects, earlier disease onset compared to vitamin B$_{12}$ deficiency secondary to a smaller storage capacity for folate.

**Biotin**—**Deficiency:** Anorexia, nausea, paresthesia, psychological disturbances (depression, hallucinations, apathy), myalgia, rash, fine hair, alopecia, seborrheic dermatitis. (Note: Eating large amounts of raw egg whites can lead to biotin deficiency secondary to the protein avidin in egg whites that binds strongly to biotin.)

# APPENDIX B

# Rapid-fire Clinical Judgments

The rapid-fire clinical judgment section focuses on patient management with the intention to "keep you on your toes" during your preparation. Initially, try to answer the questions without looking at the answer. By your final review, you should be able to confidently answer all the questions without hesitation.

1) **45 y.o. man presents to the ED with cyanosis, dyspnea, headache, and weakness. Pulse oximetry reading demonstrates 86% on room air. The patient was given 100% oxygen with no improvement. Blood was drawn for further evaluation, and it was noted that his blood appeared "chocolate brown." He later tells the resident physician that earlier in the day he was given a topical mucosal anesthetic for an in-office biopsy procedure. The resident orders a co-oximeter, which reveals an elevated level of methemoglobin (>25%). What is the primary medical treatment?**

The treatment of choice for methemoglobinemia is an IV infusion of methylene blue given over 5 to 10 minutes. Methemoglobinemia can be due to congenital or acquired causes. Acquired causes include topical anesthetic agents (benzocaine, lidocaine, prilocaine), dapsone, nitrites/nitrates, nitroglycerin, metoclopramide, menadione, sulfonamides, primaquine, naphthalene, phenazopyridine, benzene derivatives, and aniline dyes. Pulse oximetry readings are unreliable because they only measure two wavelengths of light and the partial pressure of oxygen ($PO_2$) on ABG will be typically be normal. Co-oximetry can measure at least four wavelengths of light and is capable of detecting methemoglobinemia. Methylene blue should not be given to patients with G6PD deficiency because it is ineffective and it can potentially trigger an acute hemolytic anemia.

2) **62 y.o. woman presents to the office with a nonproductive cough, nasal congestion, facial edema, dyspnea on exertion, dilated right jugular vein, and a prominent venous pattern on her chest. A CXR reveals a widened mediastinum and a right-sided mass in her chest. A chest CT with contrast demonstrates a narrowed superior vena cava (SVC), presence of collateral vessels, and the absence of thrombosis. Sputum cytology results are pending, and a bronchoscopy is scheduled. The patient expresses significant discomfort and feels that she cannot wait until the scheduled bronchoscopy. What is the best treatment option in this patient?**

In this patient that presents with SVC syndrome, a percutaneous endovascular stent can be performed for rapid relief while the histologic diagnosis is being pursued. Upon histologic diagnosis of the malignancy, initiation of chemotherapy or radiotherapy can be performed for chemosensitive or radiosensitive tumors, respectively. Endovascular stenting is also a viable option in patients with SVC syndrome that have failed chemotherapy or radiotherapy.

3) **65 y.o. man presents with blood oozing from his IV lines in the inpatient ward. Lab workup demonstrates a low platelet count, prolonged PT/PTT, decreased plasma fibrinogen, increased fibrin degradation products, and an**

elevated D-dimer level. Peripheral smear demonstrates Auer rods in the cytoplasm and bilobed nuclei of abnormal promyelocytes. Your clinical suspicion suggests DIC with an underlying acute promyelocytic leukemia (previously called AML-M3). What is the primary medical treatment?

Treat the underlying disorder in DIC, which is the acute promyelocytic leukemia (APL). APL is considered a medical emergency, and when APL is suspected, treatment should be initiated with induction therapy of all-trans retinoic acid (ATRA) and chemotherapy.

4) **65 y.o. woman presents to the ED with clinical suspicion for diverticulitis. What is the imaging of choice to confirm the diagnosis of acute diverticulitis?**

A CT scan of the abdomen is the best imaging method. Institutions will vary on the use of oral plus IV contrast in the evaluation of acute diverticulitis, but typically, the oral contrast does not reach the sigmoid colon. However, the use of oral and IV contrast can reach sensitivities of 97% and specificities of 100%. Barium enema and colonoscopy are contraindicated in the acute stages due to a risk of peritonitis and perforation.

5) **What are the treatment options for acute diverticulitis?**

Uncomplicated diverticulitis can be treated with outpatient antibiotics that cover gram-negative rods and anaerobes. Oral metronidazole plus ciprofloxacin can be given 10 to 14 days. An alternative is oral amoxicillin-clavulanate monotherapy for 10 to 14 days. Patients with poor oral intake and patients who are elderly, have comorbidities, or are immunosuppressed usually require inpatient management, which include NPO, IV fluids, and IV antibiotics. Several options for IV antibiotics include IV ampicillin-sulbactam, IV piperacillin-tazobactam, or IV metronidazole plus IV ceftriaxone. Patients with a bowel perforation, obstruction, fistula, ruptured abscess, failed percutaneous drainage of the abscess, peritonitis, recurrent attacks, or failed medical response typically require surgical intervention, IV antibiotics, IV fluids, and NPO status.

6) **60 y.o. man on digoxin therapy for his heart failure presents to the ED with nausea, vomiting, weakness, abdominal pain, dizziness, and visualizing yellow-green halos for the past 10 hours. Vitals are HR- 55, BP- 105/70, RR- 16. Recently, the patient started taking clarithromycin for his community-acquired pneumonia. The treating resident physician orders IV access, pulse oximetry (result = 95%), continuous blood pressure monitoring, continuous cardiac monitor, EKG (result = sinus bradycardia), finger-stick glucose (result = 115 mg/dL), labs (potassium result = 6.0 mEq/L), and digoxin level (result = wnl). The resident orders IV atropine x 1 dose and the patient responds from the symptomatic bradycardia. What is the primary medical treatment in this patient?**

The treatment of choice for digoxin toxicity is digoxin-specific antibody (Fab) fragments given as a slow IV push (for unstable patients) or IV infusion. Atropine can be given as a temporizing measure prior to giving digoxin-specific antibody (Fab) fragments. Activated charcoal may be given as an adjunctive therapy and is effective if given within 1 to 2 hours of ingestion, but in this case, the patient is beyond that time period and is experiencing symptomatic bradycardia. Drugs that can increase digoxin serum levels include amiodarone, clarithromycin, cyclosporine, diltiazem, erythromycin, itraconazole, ketoconazole, quinidine, and verapamil. Digoxin toxicity can result in neurologic, cardiac, and GI manifestations. Digoxin toxicity can cause almost any arrhythmias (eg, sinus bradycardia, AV blocks, PVCs, ventricular tachycardia, ventricular fibrillation, junctional rhythms, ventricular bigeminy, supraventricular tachyarrhythmias). Remember that once you obtain the potassium level, toxicity will correlate with hyperkalemia rather than the serum digoxin level. The hyperkalemia will correct itself once digoxin-specific antibody (Fab) fragments are given, and therefore, caution is advised of aggressive correction of the hyperkalemia prior to digoxin-specific antibody (Fab) fragments since it can lead to hypokalemia.

7) **34 y.o. woman has been in the inpatient ward for the past 7 days. On day 1, she received a double lumen central catheter that is being flushed with heparin to maintain patency. Her platelet count has dropped to 75,000/mm³, which has been more than a 50% drop from her baseline platelet count on day 1. Skin necrosis can be observed near the heparin flush site. What is your next best step?**

The patient is presenting with heparin-induced thrombocytopenia (HIT). The next best step is to discontinue heparin flushes and stop any further heparin products including unfractionated and low molecular weight heparin. The patient needs anticoagulation because the risk for thrombosis is highest in the first 1 to 2 weeks. Acceptable nonheparin anticoagulation includes SubQ fondaparinux, IV argatroban, or IV bivalirudin. It should be noted that lepirudin and danaparoid are not available in the United States. The transition to warfarin should not occur until the platelet count is above 150,000/mm³ and the patient has been stably anticoagulated with the nonheparin agent. There are two types of HIT, type 1 (nonimmune) and type 2 (immune-mediated). In HIT 1, which occurs in approximately 10% of patients, a transient thrombocytopenia is usually observed 1 to 2 days after heparin administration and the platelet count returns to normal levels even in the presence of continued heparin therapy. In this case, HIT 2, which occurs in less than 5% of patients, the thrombocytopenia is usually seen 5 to 10 days after heparin administration, but it can occur earlier (ie, hours to <1 day) if previously exposed to heparin. The risk of thrombosis (arterial and venous) is seen with HIT 2, but not with HIT 1, which is more of a benign self-limited condition. When HIT is suspected, always remember the "4 T's": thrombocytopenia, timing of the platelet drop, thrombosis, and thrombocytopenia due to other causes. There are several different assays to diagnosis HIT 2, but the 14C-serotonin release assay is considered the gold standard.

8) **52 y.o. man presents to the ED with crampy abdominal pain and at least 10 episodes of watery diarrhea per day for the past 2 days. The patient is afebrile, and physical exam reveals decreased skin turgor and lower abdominal tenderness without guarding or rebound tenderness. Recently, the patient finished a course of levofloxacin for an upper respiratory infection. A workup of the patient revealed a WBC of 12,000/mm³, positive enzyme immunoassay (EIA) detection for *C difficile* glutamate dehydrogenase (GDH), and positive EIA detection for *C difficile* toxin A and B. What is the clinical management in patients with *Clostridium difficile* infection (CDI)?**

The general management is to discontinue the offending antibiotic, IV fluids for dehydration, avoid antimotility agents (eg, loperamide, opiates), place the patient on contact precautions, and good hand hygiene. Symptoms of CDI can occur during or after the antibiotic is discontinued. Almost any antibiotic can cause CDI, but common culprits include fluoroquinolones, cephalosporins, clindamycin, and ampicillin/amoxicillin. Patients that are asymptomatic but test positive for CDI do not require antibiotics. However, in this case, the patient has mild to moderate CDI and can be treated with oral metronidazole for 10 to 14 days. IV metronidazole is an alternative to oral therapy if the patient cannot tolerate oral intake. Patients with severe CDI (eg, marked leukocytosis, fever, ill appearance) are usually given oral vancomycin for 10 to 14 days in the inpatient unit. Unlike IV metronidazole, IV vancomycin is ineffective at the colonic level, and it is not recommended for CDI. The management in patients with their first recurrence depends on the severity as it did for the initial episode. Unfortunately, there is no standard treatment for patients that continue to have multiple recurrences.

9) **21 y.o. man presents to the ED after sustaining a bite to the hand from a raccoon. The patient states that he was opening the lid of his garbage can and saw a raccoon scavenging through his garbage. At that time, the raccoon bit the patient's hand and ran off. The patient is asymptomatic, and the physical exam revealed a deep bite wound on the dorsum of his right hand. The patient's history reveals that he is an avid spelunker, and 6 months ago he was bitten by a bat during one of his expeditions. At the time of the bat bite, the treating resident physician gave the patient a rabies postexposure prophylaxis (PEP) that included rabies immunoglobulin plus a rabies vaccine. (1) What is the treatment management in this patient? (2) The patient tells you that he completed the tetanus immunization series as a child and received his last booster Tdap at age 12. Would you still give him a tetanus prophylaxis? If yes, what would you give him? (Please see the discussion in question 10 for the answer in part 2.)**

The patient's wound should be cleansed with a virucidal agent (eg, povidone-iodine solution). At the time of his earlier bat bite, the patient was not previously immunized to rabies, and so it was acceptable to administer both immunoglobulin ("passive immunization") and vaccine ("active immunization") as a PEP. Recall that passive immunization refers to an immediate antibody neutralization from an already pooled source (eg, immunized humans), but active immunization requires time (7-10 days) for the human body to actively produce antibodies against a target antigen. In this case, the PEP should only include the rabies vaccine and not the rabies immunoglobulin because the patient is technically immunized and there should be an anamnestic immune response from the previous vaccine. When considering PEP, the type of animal is taken into account. Bats, raccoons, skunks, foxes, coyote, bobcats, and other carnivores are generally regarded as rabid unless proven negative. If these types of animals are not caught and unavailable to be euthanized for further testing, PEP should begin immediately. Keep in mind that capture and observation for signs of rabies is not recommended for these types of animals. Patients bitten by a dog, cat, or ferret may be given PEP if the bite was on the head or neck, the animal appeared rabid, the animal was available for observation for at least 10 days and showed signs of rabies, or the animal is unavailable for observation and there is uncertainty. In this area of medicine where there can be a great deal of uncertainty it is best to err on the side of safety because you can always discontinue PEP if testing is negative, but if treatment is delayed and clinical signs of rabies develop it is too late since it usually leads to a fatality. It should be noted that in most unprovoked attacks, the animal is most likely rabid. In this case, we are not sure if the raccoon was rabid or simply startled from the opening of the garbage can lid. As mentioned, symptomatic rabies virtually always leads to death, and unfortunately, there is no proven medical treatment. The goal of rabies management is prevention. Once rabies is confirmed in the patient, the rabies immunoglobulin and rabies vaccine no longer provide a pivotal role in management and should be avoided at this point.

10) **28 y.o. woman presents to the ED after sustaining a cut to her finger while slicing vegetables with a knife. The laceration is not deep, and it measures less than 1 cm long. There are no motor or sensory deficits of the finger, and there is no foreign body in the wound. The patient's tetanus immunization status is unknown. How do you manage tetanus prophylaxis in this patient?**

Recall that tetanus prophylaxis consists of a tetanus toxoid vaccine ("active immunization") ± tetanus immune globulin ("passive immunization"). In this case, the patient does not need the tetanus immune globulin (TIG) because it is a clean and minor wound. However, she does need the vaccine because we do not know her tetanus immunization history. The woman should receive her first dose of Td today in a 3-dose primary tetanus vaccination series.

The 3-dose primary series in adults consists of 3 doses of Td with the first 2 doses separated by 4 weeks and the third dose separated 6 to 12 months from the second dose. Tdap should be substituted for Td at least one time in the 3-dose primary series. If this patient had <3 doses of the tetanus toxoid vaccine, then she can continue to finish her vaccine series. If this patient had ≥3 doses of the tetanus toxoid vaccine and it has been ≥10 years since her last dose, then she can be given a single dose of Td or Tdap (if she never received Tdap before).

The 21-year-old patient in question 9 sustained a wound that would be considered risky because he was exposed to the saliva of a raccoon when he was bitten. Examples of riskier wounds would include puncture wounds, dirty wounds (eg, soil, saliva, or stool, which can be remembered by the "Triple S"), avulsions, burns, frostbite, crushing wounds, and shrapnel wounds. Since the patient completed his tetanus series as a child, which normally consists of a 5-dose primary series and a onetime booster, he does not require the tetanus immune globulin (TIG) because he received ≥3 doses of the tetanus toxoid vaccine. If his tetanus status was unknown or he received <3 doses of the tetanus toxoid vaccine, then the patient would require the tetanus immune globulin (TIG). The next part we have to consider in the tetanus prophylaxis is the tetanus toxoid vaccine for this young man. If a patient received ≥3 doses of the tetanus toxoid vaccine and his last dose of the tetanus toxoid vaccine was ≥5 years ago, the patient would require a dose of the tetanus toxoid vaccine. In this case, the 21-year-old man had ≥3 doses of the tetanus toxoid vaccine and his last vaccine dose was at age 12, which is ≥5 years ago, and so he should receive the Td vaccine. Note that he is due for his 10-year booster Td vaccine until age 22, but it is acceptable to give the Td now. If his tetanus immunization status were unknown or he had <3 doses of the tetanus toxoid vaccine, then you would administer the 3-dose primary tetanus vaccination series or continue to finish the vaccine series, respectively. To refresh your memory of the tetanus immunization schedule for children, the DTaP vaccine is given as a 5-dose series at ages 2, 4, 6, and 15 to 18 months and 4 to 6 years old. Then, the child receives a booster vaccine called the Tdap vaccine at age 11 or 12. Subsequently, at ages ≥19 years old the patient receives a booster called the Td vaccine every 10 years with a onetime substitution of Tdap for Td in those who have never had Tdap before or whose tetanus immunization status is unknown. It should be noted that Tdap vaccine is recommended to pregnant women with each pregnancy regardless of their last Td/Tdap vaccination. The major players in tetanus prophylaxis include tetanus immune globulin (TIG), which binds to unbound toxin for neutralization; diphtheria-tetanus-acellular pertussis (DTaP) vaccine, which is part of the routine immunization schedule in children; diphtheria-tetanus (DT) vaccine if pertussis antigen is contraindicated; and tetanus toxoid (TT) vaccine if pertussis and diphtheria antigens are contraindicated. Tetanus-reduced diphtheria-acellular pertussis (Tdap) and tetanus-reduced diphtheria (Td) vaccines are typically used as booster vaccines, but they can also serve as primary immunization as seen in the 28-year-old woman above.

11) **32 y.o. man was started on fluphenazine for his schizophrenia. Three days later the patient presents to the ED with lead pipe rigidity, agitation, profuse sweating, and a temperature of 38.3°C (100.94°F). Workup of the patient demonstrates a negative head CT scan, leukocytosis, elevated creatine kinase, elevated LDH, elevated alkaline phosphatase, elevated ALT and AST, hyperkalemia, hyponatremia, hypocalcemia, hypomagnesemia, and a decreased serum iron concentration. What is the diagnosis, management, and disposition for this patient?**

The patient is presenting with neuroleptic malignant syndrome (NMS). Triggering factors include typical antipsychotics, atypical antipsychotics, and antiemetics. NMS is characterized by a tetrad of hyperthermia, muscular rigidity (eg, cogwheel, tremor, dystonia, dyskinesia), altered mental status (eg, agitation, mutism, confusion, delirium), and autonomic dysfunction (eg, labile blood pressure, diaphoresis, tachycardia, tachypnea, urinary incontinence). Laboratory abnormalities can occur (eg, hyponatremia, hypernatremia, myoglobinuria, metabolic acidosis), but no single test is specific for NMS. In this case, the inciting agent is fluphenazine, and this medication should be discontinued along with any other psychotropic medications (eg, lithium, anticholinergics). The patient should be transferred to the ICU for further monitoring and supportive care. Supportive care may include mechanical ventilation, IV fluids for insensible fluid loss, IV fluids with urine alkalinization to prevent acute renal failure secondary to rhabdomyolysis, cooling blankets for fever, or IV lorazepam for agitation. Dantrolene, bromocriptine, amantadine, and electroconvulsive therapy have been used to treat NMS, but there are no controlled studies to support their efficacy. Reported mortality rates can be as high as 20%.

12) **20 y.o. man is in the operating room for an elective surgical procedure. This is the patient's first surgery, and no family perioperative problems could be obtained since he was adopted as a young boy. The anesthesiology resident premedicates the patient with IV midazolam. Subsequently, an induction sequence of propofol and a onetime dose of succinylcholine (to facilitate tracheal intubation) is administered. The patient is intubated, and inhalational sevoflurane is administered for maintenance anesthesia. Fifteen minutes into the case the patient develops sinus tachycardia, masseter muscle rigidity, and hypercarbia. Pulse oximetry demonstrates 98% oxygen saturation, capnography shows an end-tidal carbon dioxide ($ETCO_2$) of 70 mmHg, and the patient has a core temperature of 37°C (98.6°C). The concerned resident decides to increase the patient's minute ventilation to control the hypercarbia, but the $ETCO_2$ remains at 70 mmHg. The soda lime carbon dioxide absorbent canister is warm to touch (exothermic reaction), and there is a change in color from white to purple (indication of $CO_2$ exhaustion). The anesthesiology resident makes**

a presumptive diagnosis, tells the surgeon to abort the case, and calls for anesthesiology backup. Inhalational sevoflurane and succinylcholine are discontinued, IV propofol is administered to complete the case, and high-flow 100% oxygen is administered to hasten the removal of residual sevoflurane. What is the diagnosis and the next most important step?

The patient is presenting with malignant hyperthermia (MH). The next best step is to administer IV dantrolene, which will interfere with calcium release from the sarcoplasmic reticulum. Cooling measures should be instituted if there is hyperthermia, but be aware that hyperthermia is usually a late finding. Labs and venous blood gas should be sent out. Acidosis can be treated with bicarbonate. Hyperkalemia can be treated with insulin (drives $K^+$ into the cell), D50 (prevents hypoglycemia from the insulin), and bicarbonate. Dysrhythmias usually respond by correcting the hyperkalemia and acidosis. It is important not to administer a calcium channel blocker when using dantrolene because it can potentially exacerbate the hyperkalemia and enhance the negative inotropic effect on the heart. MH is caused by mutations in the RYR1 receptor gene that are inherited as an autosomal dominant trait. The receptor is involved in the regulation of calcium into the intracellular space. It should be noted that an elevated $ETCO_2$ level that is resistant to increasing the patient's minute ventilation is one of the most sensitive and early signs of MH. Triggering agents include anesthetic agents (eg, sevoflurane, desflurane, enflurane, isoflurane, halothane) and a depolarizing neuromuscular blocker (succinylcholine). Abnormal findings include elevated creatine kinase, myoglobinuria, elevated serum myoglobin, hyperkalemia, peaked T waves on EKG, and a mixed respiratory acidosis and metabolic acidosis ($\downarrow$ pH, $\uparrow$ $pCO_2$, $\downarrow$ $HCO_3^-$).

13) **12 y.o. boy presents to the ED with nausea, vomiting, and acute scrotal pain. The exact duration of pain is unknown, but the patient believes that is has been for at least 3 hours. The patient denies fever, chills, dysuria, or trauma. On exam, the right testicle is tender to touch and there is no scrotal edema. There is a high-riding right testicle in the horizontal position. Scrotal elevation does not alleviate the pain, and stroking the upper right thigh does not elicit the cremasteric reflex. What is the best treatment option in this patient?**

The patient is presenting with testicular torsion. The best treatment option in this patient is immediate surgical exploration with detorsion and fixation (orchipexy) because you want to preserve the viability of the affected testicle. It should be noted that testicular salvage rates are usually very good if detorsion occurs in less than 6 hours of symptoms, but salvage rates decline precipitously thereafter. In this case, we are not sure about the exact duration of symptoms, and therefore, time is of the essence. This patient is presenting with classic signs and symptoms of testicular torsion, so there is no need to do imaging. Color Doppler ultrasound (which would show decreased or absent testicu-

lar blood flow) or radionuclide scintigraphy (which would show decreased blood flow) can be used for equivocal presentations, but they should not delay treatment. If there is a delay in surgical intervention, manual detorsion is an option, but the procedure should not be performed if there is significant scrotal swelling. In the technique, with appropriate analgesia, the testicle is detorsed by rotating it in a medial to lateral motion since most testicular torsions twist in a lateral to medial rotation. An easy way to remember this is to rotate the "nut out" (take the testicle and laterally rotate the nut out toward the thigh). However, it should be noted that upon successful manual detorsion, the patient should still undergo surgical fixation (orchipexy) to prevent a recurrence. Testicular torsion is usually the result of abnormal fixation of the testicle within the tunica vaginalis. The tunica vaginalis is a closed peritoneal sac that covers the anterior portion of the testis and epididymis. If the tunica vaginalis is inappropriately high (covers the distal spermatic cord), the testis can lie horizontally ("bell clapper deformity") and the spermatic cord can twist. The absence of the cremasteric reflex can help differentiate other causes of scrotal pain, but the Prehn sign (relief with scrotal elevation) is unreliable for a clinical diagnosis. Scrotal swelling can occur early or late (>12 hours) in the course of disease.

14) **10 y.o. boy with a past medical history of 21-hydroxylase deficiency has recovered from a cough, sore throat, and runny nose 2 weeks ago. Subsequently, the patient develops palpable purpura over the buttocks and lower extremities and develops periarticular swelling and tenderness over the knees and ankles. One week after the skin and joint manifestations, the patient develops colicky abdominal pain and now presents to the office accompanied by his mother, who happens to be a nurse. The medical resident makes the diagnosis of Henoch-Schönlein purpura (HSP) and decides to order a urinalysis, stool guaiac, platelet count, and coagulation studies, which all turn out to be normal. The resident recommends supportive care, which included hydration and NSAIDs for abdominal and joint pain. The mother inquires if there is an increased risk of developing renal disease even though the patient is taking long-term glucocorticoid for his congenital adrenal hyperplasia. The resident finds a retrospective study that examined the relationship of developing renal disease in patients with HSP and the use of long-term glucocorticoids for other comorbid conditions (p = 0.004, odds ratio 0.65, 95% CI 0.63-0.67). What do you tell the mother, and what would be your next best step?**

Based on the article, it is less likely that the patient will develop renal disease when using long-term glucocorticoid. Since the odds ratio is less than one, the estimated risk of developing renal disease is decreased. The confidence intervals (CI) are narrow, which indicates a large sample size that will give a larger number of observations and more precise estimates. In addition, the CI may serve as a proxy for the presence of statistical significance if it does not overlap the null value (in this case it would be OR = 1), but we already see that the p-value is less than 0.05, which indicates statistical significance. In this case, the patient has not developed any signs of renal abnormalities such as hematuria or proteinuria. The next best step is to monitor the patient's blood pressure and urinalysis. In the event of elevated blood pressures, hematuria, or proteinuria, the patient should have his renal function assessed with a serum creatinine level. The classic tetrad of HSP includes a rash (95%-100%), arthralgias (60%-80%), abdominal pain (60%-80%), and renal disease (20%-60%) that can be preceded by an upper respiratory infection in approximately 50% of cases. In the majority of cases, HSP is a self-limited condition and treatment is aimed at supportive care and pain management. The use of glucocorticoids is controversial, but it has been used for severe GI, joint, or scrotal disease. There is no definitive evidence to support the use of glucocorticoids to prevent renal disease, and it is not recommended. However, in this case, the patient is using glucocorticoids for another purpose, and it is important to learn how to apply biostatistical concepts into patient management. In the majority of patients with mild nephropathy secondary to HSP, a renal biopsy is usually unnecessary unless there is severe renal disease or the diagnosis is in question. However, a skin biopsy, which is less invasive than a renal biopsy, is an alternative in confirming the diagnosis of HSP. Patients with mild nephropathy should be monitored closely for impaired renal function and elevated blood pressures (keep in mind that patients with 21-hydroxylase deficiency are usually hypotensive).

15) **65 y.o. man presents to the office with headache, amaurosis fugax, and vertigo. The patient states that he has intense itching after taking a shower, particularly with warm water. On exam, there is a ruddy complexion of the face, hepatomegaly, splenomegaly, and the patient is hypertensive. The medical resident performs a workup of the patient and significant findings include WBC (15,000/mm³), Hb (20 g/dL), Hct (60%), platelets (550,000/mm³), SaO$_2$ (98%), red cell distribution width (RDW) of 18% (normal: 11.5-13.5), red cell mass of 50 mL/kg (normal in males: 20-36 mL/kg), normal RBC morphology, and erythropoietin (EPO) level of 1 mU/mL (normal: 0-20). What is (1) the most likely diagnosis (2) the cornerstone of therapy, and (3) what would you recommend for his pruritus-related shower concerns?**

The diagnosis is polycythemia vera (PV). The cornerstone of therapy is serial phlebotomy to reduce the blood viscosity and maintaining a hematocrit below 45% in men and 42% in women. Although phlebotomy induces a relative state of iron deficiency, it is not recommended to give patients iron supplements because it can accelerate red cell mass production (ie, "adding fuel to the fire"). Adjunctive therapies may include hydroxyurea (for myelosuppression), anagrelide (to reduce platelet counts), and allopurinol (for gout). In addition, low-dose aspirin (if no contraindications exist)

is typically given to all patients to reduce the risk of blood clots, and aspirin is particularly helpful in patients with erythromelalgia. The intense itching after showering or bathing without visible skin changes is referred to as aquagenic pruritus. Initially, treatment of aquagenic pruritus may consist of reducing the temperature of the water and afterward gently patting the skin dry with a towel rather than rubbing the skin. In addition, patients may attempt to use an antihistamine to relieve their symptoms. PV involves the clonal proliferation of myeloid cells, which can affect the red blood cells, granulocytes, and platelets. Because there can be such a high turnover of hematopoietic cells, there may be an increase in uric acid, which can cause secondary gout or uric acid stones. One of the hallmark features of PV is the hyperviscosity of the blood, which can be deleterious to the body, and it makes sense that the EPO levels would be low to avoid further erythropoiesis. Clinical manifestations may relate to the involved vessels of the body (eg, neurologic, cardiac, mesenteric), and other findings that may be seen include systolic hypertension, thrombosis, bleeding, acquired von Willebrand disease, and erythromelalgia (ie, burning pain, erythema, and warmth in the hands or feet). Abnormal lab findings (other than described above) include an elevated leukocyte alkaline phosphatase, elevated serum B$_{12}$, elevated uric acid, iron deficiency secondary to bleeding, and the presence of JAK2 mutations. In this case, it should be mentioned that the elevated RDW is due to iron deficiency secondary to an occult bleeding and that the SaO$_2$ demonstrates the absence of hypoxia that could have been a possible cause of erythrocytosis.

16) **65 y.o. white woman presents to the office for a routine checkup. The patient is asymptomatic, and the physical examination is completely normal. The patient is a smoker and is trying to quit with the help of the resident physician. The patient relays her concerns about a family history of abdominal aortic aneurysms (AAA). The patient turned 65 years old last week and is now covered under the Medicare program, which allows a onetime ultrasound for patients with a family history of AAA. The ultrasound reveals a 3.2 cm abdominal aneurysm. What is the next best step, and what is the single most important modifiable risk factor for AAA?**

The next best step is for the patient to come back in 6 months for another ultrasound to assess for aortic expansion. The most important modifiable risk factor for AAA is smoking cessation, which the patient is already doing with her treating physician. In most adults, the abdominal aorta is approximately 2.0 cm, and AAA is diagnosed when the aorta is ≥3.0 cm. Risk factors for AAA include smoking, advancing age, atherosclerosis, white race, family history, presence of peripheral aneurysms, hypertension, and male gender. It should be noted that AAA is more prevalent in men, but the risk of rupture is higher in women compared to men of the same aortic diameter. The USPSTF recommends a one-time screening for AAA by ultrasound in men aged 65 to 75 who have ever smoked and actually recommends against routine screening for AAA in women. However, other organizations include women that are at risk (eg, smoker, family history, >65 years old) and, in fact, Medicare Part B actually covers a onetime ultrasound for women and men who have a family history of AAA. Clinical features of AAA may include any of the following: asymptomatic, pain (back, flank, abdominal, pelvic, or groin), nausea, vomiting, pulsatile abdominal mass, flank ecchymosis (Grey Turner sign), periumbilical ecchymosis (Cullen sign), limb ischemia, AMS, hypotension, tachycardia, cyanosis, mottling. Asymptomatic patients with AAA diameter <5.5 cm can be managed with risk modification, periodic clinical exams, and AAA surveillance. It should be noted that there is no standardized AAA surveillance schedule, but patients typically have annual imaging for aneurysms <4.5 cm or at more frequent intervals (eg, every 6 months) for those at higher risk (eg, rapid expansion, women, aneurysms ≥4.5 cm). In this case, the patient is a woman, which places her at a higher risk for rupture, and because it is her first ultrasound, we want to assess the expansion rate in 6 months or even in 3 months rather than a year. The decision to pursue elective AAA repair for asymptomatic AAA is based on the risk of the aneurysm to rupture, which is typically an AAA diameter of >5.5 cm and a rapidly expanding AAA. However, elective repair is also based on advanced comorbidities, advanced age, presence of PAD, and gender. An immediate surgical repair (emergent AAA repair) is performed on patients with a ruptured AAA. Features to look for are any combination of hemodynamically unstable (eg, hypotensive, tachycardic), back/flank pain, pulsatile mass, AMS, skin mottling, Cullen sign, or Grey Turner sign. The decision to pursue an urgent repair (within 24 hours) in a patient that is symptomatic (attributable to the AAA), hemodynamically stable, has an unruptured AAA, and irrespective of the aneurysm size presents more of a challenge. There is no clear-cut answer, and the clinical management is usually individualized. In one circumstance, the patient may benefit from an urgent AAA repair, but in another circumstance, the patient may benefit from preoperative optimization (eg, beta-blockers in the setting of hypertension). Notable figures who have died from AAA include Albert Einstein, Lucille Ball, and George C. Scott.

17) **35 y.o. woman presents to the office with nausea, vomiting, visual disturbances, and headaches. The headache is located over the right parietal region and is described as "throbbing" throughout the day. The headaches are aggravated by bending forward, and there is minimal relief with NSAIDs. The headaches do not seem to bother her at night, and there are no early morning awakenings secondary to the headache. The patient states that she hears a "rush of water" in her right ear intermittently during the daytime and says that she is not sure if it is associated with her headaches. The visual changes include double vision, sees "flashes of light," bilateral dimness in vision for approximately 20 seconds after standing up, and has pain behind the right eye. Initial** vital signs include a temperature of 37°C (98.6°F), pulse 78 bpm, respiration 16/min, blood pressure 138/88, height 152.4 cm (60.0 inches), weight 79.4 kg (175 lb), and BMI 34.2 kg/m². On exam, the right eye is turned medially (esotropia) and the left eye is in the normal position on forward gaze. Upon horizontal gaze to the patient's right side, there is limited abduction of the right eye and normal adduction of the left eye. Visual field loss is noted in both eyes, and the visual acuity testing demonstrates 20/70 OD (right eye) and 20/50 OS (left eye). On funduscopic exam, bilateral papilledema is seen. The medical resident orders labs (eg, CBC, BMP, ESR, ANA, anti-dsDNA, PT/INR, PTT, Lyme disease serology, and serum iron) and a head MRI with gadolinium. No significant findings are seen on imaging or lab workup. The resident decides to order a lumbar puncture (LP) with CSF studies, and the findings demonstrate a glucose of 50 mg/dL (nl: 40-70), protein of 20 mg/dL (nl: < 40), chloride of 120 mEq/L (nl: 118-132), opening pressure of 285 mm H₂O (nl: 70-180), zero cell count (nl: 0-5/mm³), no atypical cells on cytology, negative VDRL, and no growth on bacterial culture. What is the most likely diagnosis, and what is the best initial treatment management for this patient?

The diagnosis is idiopathic intracranial hypertension (IIH), also known as pseudotumor cerebri or benign intracranial hypertension. The initial treatment management should include weight reduction and the carbonic anhydrase inhibitor acetazolamide to lower the CSF pressure. In this case, the patient is obese (BMI 34.2 kg/m²), and weight loss would serve 3 purposes: (1) it may alleviate the symptoms of IIH; (2) the patient has prehypertension; and (3) the health benefits of losing weight. Patients that continue to have persistent headaches or progressive visual loss despite maximum medical treatment may consider surgical intervention. Optic nerve sheath fenestration and CSF shunting (eg, ventriculoperitoneal or lumboperitoneal shunt) are the main surgical procedures for IIH. Although IIH is idiopathic in nature, the strongest associations with this disease are the use of retinoids, tetracycline derivatives, growth hormone, and being an obese woman of childbearing age. The clinical features of IIH include visual abnormalities (eg, photopsia, papilledema, sixth cranial nerve palsy secondary to ↑ ICP on the abducens nerve, diplopia secondary to sixth cranial nerve palsy, transient visual obscurations, visual field loss, reduced visual acuity secondary to papilledema, retrobulbar pain), pulsatile tinnitus ("rush of water" sound), and headaches. The headaches in IIH are usually nonspecific and can vary from patient to patient. However, increasing intrathoracic pressure such as bending forward, Valsalva maneuver, coughing, or sneezing can sometimes worsen the headache by increasing the intracranial pressure (ICP). In this case, the patient has a unilateral abducens nerve palsy of the right eye. The inward deviation of the right eye is due to the loss of normal resting tone in the right lateral rectus muscle, and this condition might have contributed to the worsening of her visual acuity on the right eye compared to her left eye. Also, there is limited abduction of the right eye on horizontal gaze secondary to paresis of the right lateral rectus muscle. IIH is a diagnosis of exclusion, and in this case, all labs and neuroimaging were normal. To avoid a cerebral herniation, an intracranial mass was ruled out on neuroimaging prior to an LP. IIH will typically present with an elevated opening pressure on LP with normal CSF composition. Keep in mind that the opening pressure should be read with the patient in the lateral decubitus position to prevent a falsely elevated pressure reading that can occur if the patient is in the sitting position.

18) **20 y.o. man presents to the office complaining of a sore throat, rash, fatigue, fever, and nausea for the past 5 days. The medical resident performs a good physical examination and reveals bilateral upper eyelid edema, pharyngeal inflammation with tonsillar exudates, palatal petechiae, bilateral posterior cervical lymphadenopathy, generalized maculopapular rash, and splenomegaly. The resident orders labs, and significant findings reveal a WBC of 15,000/mm³ (nl: 4500-11,000), platelets of 145,000/mm³ (nl: 150,000-400,000), lymphocytes of 75% (nl: 25%-33%), ALT of 60 U/L (nl: 10-40), AST of 70 U/L (nl: 15-40), presence of atypical lymphocytes on peripheral blood smear, and a negative result on the heterophile antibody screen ("Monospot" test). The resident makes a diagnosis of infectious mononucleosis (IM) and recommends supportive care that includes rest and analgesia (eg, NSAIDs, acetaminophen). A follow-up appointment is scheduled in 2 weeks to reassess the patient and repeat the Monospot test. The patient is concerned because he is a college wrestler and he is competing in the Division 1 Collegiate Wrestling Championships next week. The medical resident strongly recommends against competing in the tournament and any other contact sports for 4 weeks. The patient ignores the resident's advice and competes the following week. During the tournament, the patient is injured. He is rushed to a nearby university hospital and is complaining of severe left shoulder pain that is worse upon inspiration in the ambulance. Vital signs include blood pressure 98/63, pulse 106, and respiration 14/min. No external hemorrhage is observed, and the patient continues to be tachycardic despite a fluid challenge. The bedside ultrasound or Focused Assessment with Sonography for Trauma (FAST exam) demonstrates intraperitoneal fluid in the splenorenal and splenodiaphragmatic recess. What is the most likely diagnosis, and what is the primary treatment option in this patient?**

The diagnosis is a splenic rupture as a complication from IM. Since the patient is hemodynamically unstable and intraperitoneal fluid is seen on the FAST exam, the patient needs an emergent exploratory laparotomy. If findings on the FAST exam were equivocal, a diagnostic peritoneal aspiration/lavage (DPA/DPL) could be performed to detect intraperitoneal blood. If the patient were hemodynamically stable, then there would be time for an abdominal CT scan with contrast. The CT scan can aid in the grading of the

splenic injury, and it may identify extravasation of the contrast. Once the splenic injury is graded, the patient may be observed, undergo splenic angiographic embolization, or go straight to surgery. Note that in this case the patient's left shoulder pain is a referred pain (Kehr's signs) secondary to the irritation of the phrenic nerve from blood that is located under the left hemidiaphragm. The patient's IM is due to the Epstein-Barr virus (EBV), which is part of the herpes virus family. The primary mode of transmission of EBV is through saliva ("kissing disease"). Clinical features of IM (other than described above) include hepatomegaly, hepatitis, myocarditis, cranial nerve palsies, enlarged tonsils ("kissing tonsils"), pharyngitis (exudative or nonexudative), Guillain-Barré syndrome, meningoencephalitis, aplastic anemia, hemolytic anemia, tender lymphadenopathy (posterior cervical chains > anterior cervical chains), transverse myelitis, optic neuritis, peripheral neuritis, and aseptic meningitis. Note that the viral rash of EBV in this case is not the same as the drug-induced rash (ie, from administration of ampicillin or amoxicillin) during an IM infection. However, both types of rashes are clues to an EBV infection, and it should be mentioned that the drug-induced rash of IM does not represent a true drug allergy. If this patient had waited until at least the third week of illness, the splenic rupture probably would not have occurred since the spleen usually returns to near normal size within 3 weeks of the illness. Expected abnormal lab findings include leukocytosis, lymphocytosis, >10% atypical lymphocytes on peripheral smear, mild thrombocytopenia, mild elevation of transaminases, and positive for heterophile antibodies. Keep in mind that the false negative rates for heterophile antibody test (Monospot test) is highest early in the course of the disease, and it may take until the second or third week of the illness for the heterophile antibody response to become positive or reactive to the Monospot test. In this case, a repeat Monospot test was recommended for the patient in 2 weeks, and it is very acceptable to repeat the test in a patient who has the clinical manifestations of IM but a negative Monospot test. Treatment of IM is mainly supportive, and it is recommended to avoid contact sports for 4 weeks, which is when the spleen should have receded. The routine use of corticosteroids is not recommended but can be given to patients with impending airway obstruction secondary to enlarged tonsils, persistent severe disease, severe thrombocytopenia, autoimmune hemolytic anemia, and aplastic anemia.

19) **22 y.o. woman presents to the office with lower abdominal pain and fishy vaginal odor, particularly after sexual intercourse, for the past week. The patient rates her abdominal pain as 6/10 in severity. The patient denies fevers, chills, nausea, vomiting, or diarrhea. On pelvic examination, there is cervical motion tenderness and adnexal tenderness on the right side without a palpable mass. On speculum exam, there is gray-white discharge on the vaginal walls. The ob-gyn resident orders labs that include a qualitative urine β-HCG (negative result), WBC of 9,000/mm³ (nl: 4500-11,000), ESR of**

82 mm/h (nl: 0-20), urinalysis (within normal limits), vaginal pH of 6.2 (nl: 3.8-4.5), wet mount of vaginal secretions (presence of clue cells detected and >10 WBC/high-power field), positive whiff test (aminelike odor upon KOH), VDRL (nonreactive), HIV rapid antibody test (none detected), Gram stain of the cervix (no gram-negative intracellular diplococci detected), Chlamydia culture of the cervix (pending), and Gonococcal culture of the cervix (pending). The ob-gyn resident prescribes IM ceftriaxone (single dose) + PO doxycycline (14-day course) + PO metronidazole (14-day course) and a follow-up visit to the office in 3 days. The patient returns to the office with minimal improvement, rating her abdominal pain as 5/10 in severity. The ob-gyn resident performs a transvaginal ultrasound that demonstrates a fluid-filled tube along with a complex adnexal mass on the right side. Further delineation of the mass reveals a thickened wall, fluid-containing mass, multiple internal echoes, and a size of 2.6 cm in diameter. What is the (1) diagnosis, (2) disposition of the patient, and (3) treatment management?

The diagnosis is a tubo-ovarian abscess (TOA) as a complication from pelvic inflammatory disease (PID). The disposition of the patient is to admit her to the hospital for further treatment. The majority of small TOAs (<9 cm in diameter) will resolve with antibiotics alone, but the initial antibiotic regimen should have broad coverage since TOAs are typically polymicrobial. There are 3 first-line inpatient antibiotic options that could be used to treat PID with TOAs and PID alone. The following options are based on the CDC recommendations, which include (1) IV cefoxitin + IV doxycycline; (2) IV cefotetan + IV doxycycline; or (3) IV clindamycin + IV gentamicin. Direct inpatient observation is recommended to see if the patient is clinically improving or worsening and to assess if the mass is enlarging (via imaging) or there are signs of a rupture TOA (eg, sepsis, acute abdomen). Patients with TOAs that do not respond to parenteral antibiotics after 48 to 72 hours require percutaneous drainage or surgery (laparoscopic or open). However, patients with TOAs that do respond to parenteral antibiotics can transition to oral therapy after 24 hours of sustained clinical improvement. Oral therapy should include PO clindamycin or PO metronidazole for anaerobic coverage plus PO doxycycline for a total of 14 days of antibiotic therapy. In addition to treating the patient, male sexual partners of women with PID should be evaluated and treated if they had sexual contact with the patient during the 60 days prior to the patient's onset of symptoms. In this case, there were several deviations from the classic presentation. First, the patient presented with bacterial vaginosis, which can be associated with PID. Second, the patient did not present with fever, which may only be seen in approximately 50% of patients with PID. Third, most patients with TOA will have leukocytosis, but not all patients. Finally, the patient did not present with an acute onset (eg, 2-day history of symptoms) that is typically seen in acute PID alone, but it may not be an unusual

presentation in PID with a complicating TOA. Also, note that the ob-gyn resident was unable to palpate an adnexal mass on the right side, which is not uncommon if the TOA is small. When you work up a patient with suspected PID, always remember to obtain a pregnancy test. Keep in mind that there is no single test that is highly sensitive or specific for PID. However, abnormal findings of PID may include ↑ ESR, ↑ CRP, ↑ WBCs on wet mount (vaginal secretions), ± leukocytosis, ↑ CA-125, leukocytes on urinalysis (secondary to pelvic inflammation). The decision to treat PID is based on the principle of having a high index of suspicion for PID with a low threshold to initiate treatment in order to minimize the long-term sequelae of untreated or delayed treatment. The CDC recommends that empiric therapy of PID should begin in sexually active women and those at risk of STDs in the presence of lower abdominal or pelvic pain plus ≥1 of the following: cervical motion tenderness, adnexal tenderness, or uterine tenderness. There are 3 first-line outpatient antibiotic options for PID. The following options are based on the CDC recommendations, which include (1) IM ceftriaxone (single dose) + PO doxycycline (14 days) ± PO metronidazole (14 days); (2) IM cefoxitin (single dose) + PO probenecid (single dose; probenecid prolongs cephalosporin serum levels) + PO doxycycline (14 days) ± PO metronidazole (14 days); or (3) IM cefotaxime or ceftizoxime (single dose) + PO doxycycline (14 days) ± PO metronidazole (14 days). Note that metronidazole can be added to any of the regimens if anaerobic organisms or bacterial vaginosis is suspected, as in this case. Once antibiotic therapy (oral or parenteral) is initiated, the patient should have significant clinical improvement within 72 hours. If a patient with PID does not respond to outpatient therapy, the patient should be admitted to the hospital for further management. The CDC recommends that admission to the hospital should be considered in pregnancy, TOAs, failure to respond to outpatient therapy, poor oral intake, noncompliance, severe illness (high fever, nausea, vomiting, intractable abdominal pain), or surgical emergencies that cannot be excluded (eg, appendicitis). If a patient with PID does not respond to inpatient therapy, additional diagnostic tests (eg, CT with contrast, diagnostic laparoscopy) and surgical intervention may be required. It should be noted that patients with PID may also be intrauterine device (IUD) users. Although IUD insertion poses a PID risk within the first 3 weeks of insertion, the CDC advises that there is insufficient evidence to recommend removal of IUDs in women diagnosed with acute PID, but close follow-up is mandatory if an IUD is left in place.

20) **62 y.o. white man presents to the ED with palpitations, dizziness, and fatigue. The patient is not sure when the symptoms started, but he believes that it has been 2 or 3 days. The patient states that he has never had palpitations before and is concerned about his heart. Past medical history includes asthma that is controlled with albuterol and hypertension that is controlled with benazepril. The patient denies any history of prior stroke. Vital signs include a temperature of 37°C (98.6°F), pulse 145 bpm,**

blood pressure 140/82, and respiration 18/min. Physical exam reveals an irregularly irregular pulse, and auscultation of the heart demonstrates an irregular rhythm with a rapid heartbeat. There is no JVD, carotid bruits, thyromegaly, wheezes, diminished breath sounds, hepatomegaly, cyanosis, clubbing, or edema on exam. The resident physician orders the following STAT items: IV access, pulse oximetry (96% oxygen saturation), continuous blood pressure (140/82), continuous cardiac monitor (irregular irregular rhythm, ventricular rate of 145 bpm), 12-lead EKG (no discrete P waves, chaotic f waves, irregular R-R intervals, atrial rate of 352 bpm, rapid ventricular response of 145 bpm, interpretation as atrial fibrillation). The resident orders a onetime bolus of IV diltiazem and waits 15 minutes to see if there is an adequate response. In the meantime the resident orders a CBC, electrolytes, BUN/creatinine, troponin-I, TSH, free T4, BNP, D-dimer, PT/INR, PTT, CXR, transthoracic echocardiography (TTE), and a toxicology screen. Fifteen minutes have passed, and the resident checks the cardiac monitor and reads an irregular irregular rhythm with a ventricular rate of 128 bpm. The resident decides to give one more bolus of IV diltiazem. Fifteen minutes later the cardiac monitor reads an irregular irregular rhythm with a ventricular rate of 98 bpm. The patient tells the resident physician, "I feel much better, doc." Results of the labs and imaging are all within normal limits. What is your next step management in this patient with atrial fibrillation (AF)?

The patient is presenting with new-onset AF. The resident made the correct decision by initially controlling the ventricular rate to less than 110 bpm without necessarily converting to normal sinus rhythm. Conversion to sinus rhythm will eventually be addressed with cardioversion ± anticoagulation (depending on duration of AF). Acute rate control can be achieved by intravenous metoprolol, esmolol, diltiazem, or verapamil, which are all effective in slowing the AV nodal conduction. Note that we used a calcium channel blocker (diltiazem) in this case instead of a beta-blocker because of his history of bronchospastic disease (asthma). In general, beta-blockers and calcium channel blockers should be avoided in patients with AV blocks and decompensated heart failure. Digoxin can also slow the AV nodal conduction, but it is not considered a first-line agent because it takes a longer time to achieve rate control. However, IV digoxin can be considered as the initial therapy for rate control in patients with significant hypotension or advanced heart failure. It should be noted that beta-blockers, calcium channel blockers, and digoxin should be avoided in patients with preexcited AF (eg, WPW syndrome) because these AV nodal blocking agents can actually encourage the conduction of impulses through the accessory pathway resulting in an increased ventricular rate and potentially ventricular fibrillation. Preexcited AF can be treated with IV procainamide in stable patients and synchronized direct-current (DC) cardioversion in unstable patients. The next question that the resident has to consider

is the duration of the AF because there is an increased risk of embolization the longer the duration of AF. In this case, the patient was symptomatic for the past 48 to 72 hours, but there is no documented AF on EKG until he arrives in the ED, so he fits into the category of unknown duration. If AF is known to be greater than 48 hours or the AF is of unknown duration, then there are two options. The options include (1) TEE (look for atrial thrombus) + IV heparin (anticoagulation before cardioversion) + cardioversion (if no thrombus seen) + oral warfarin after cardioversion; (2) oral warfarin for 4 weeks (target INR of 2.5) + cardioversion + oral warfarin after cardioversion for 4 weeks (target INR of 2.5). If AF is less than 48 hours, then there is a lower risk of embolization and it is acceptable to consider cardioversion by pharmacologic (eg, flecainide, propafenone, dofetilide, ibutilide) or electrical (direct-current) means. It should be noted that it can be difficult to determine the actual onset and duration of AF. However, keep in mind that if a patient is on the telemetry floor, the onset and duration of AF can easily be documented, but AF in the outpatient setting may prove to be more difficult to document unless a Holter monitor is used. The ACC/AHA/ESC guidelines recommend immediate synchronized DC cardioversion in patients with AF who do not respond promptly to a rapid ventricular response (RVR) with pharmacologic therapy and there is evidence of ongoing myocardial ischemia (eg, EKG evidence), chest pain (angina), heart failure, or symptomatic hypotension. In addition, immediate DC cardioversion can be performed in patients with preexcited AF who are hemodynamically unstable or in the presence of an extremely rapid ventricular rate secondary to an accessory bypass tract. DC cardioversion delivers electrical current in monophasic or biphasic waveforms that is synchronized to the QRS complex. An initial shock energy of 200 joules for monophasic devices or 120 to 200 joules for biphasic devices are recommended for AF. AF is characterized by rapid, disorganized electrical activity in the atria with uncoordinated atrial contraction. The ventricular response is always irregular, but the ventricular rate can be slow or rapid. A slow ventricular rate may be due to AV nodal disease, AV nodal blocking agents, or a long refractory period of the AV node (eg, aging, enhanced vagal parasympathetic tone, athlete). A rapid ventricular rate may be due to an accessory bypass tract (preexcitation syndrome) or a shortened refractory period of the AV node (eg, sympathetic stimulation, catecholamine excess). An easy way to estimate the ventricular rate is to count the number of QRS complexes in a 6-second EKG strip (ie, 30 big squares) and multiply by 10. AF is commonly associated with hypertension and coronary artery disease. Other associated conditions include heart failure, rheumatic valvular disease, congenital heart disease, hyperthyroidism, heavy alcohol use, and cardiac surgery. There are several terms used to describe AF which include new onset (first detection of AF), paroxysmal (≥2 episodes of AF that terminate within 7 days, typically <24 hours), persistent (AF >7 days that usually requires cardioversion), permanent (AF refractory to cardioversion), and lone AF (absence of structural heart disease, typically <60 years old). The 3 essential elements to consider in AF management are **(1)** rate control, **(2)** rhythm control, and **(3)** anticoagulation to prevent a stroke. Once the patient reverts to sinus rhythm, the decision to undergo rate control or rhythm control for long-term management is addressed. It should be noted that either strategy (rate or rhythm control) results in similar overall mortality and morbidity. However, anticoagulation is still recommended with either strategy in patients at high risk for stroke. To determine the risk of stroke, the CHADS$_2$ is a validated scoring system that has gained favor. Each letter in the **CHADS$_2$** (CHF,

HTN, **A**ge >75 years old, **D**iabetes, **S**troke) carries a single point except for stroke or TIA, which carries 2 points (ie, it is the strongest predictor of stroke). Patients with nonvalvular AF with a score of zero are considered low risk (no antithrombotic therapy necessary), those with a score of 1 are at intermediate risk (aspirin or oral anticoagulant therapy recommended), and those with a score ≥2 are at relatively high risk (oral anticoagulant therapy recommended).

Once you have read and understood the essence of each question in Appendix B, then you have sharpened your clinical judgment another sliver.

# Factoids

Factoids are another part of your armamentarium in conquering the Step 3 exam. The facts presented in this section will serve as building blocks to strengthen your knowledge base. Factoids should be viewed as another arsenal in your preparation because they will provide (1) "silver bullet" knowledge (ie, ability to answer the question with 100% conviction based on a fact); (2) improved deductive reasoning (ie, ability to eliminate wrong answers and make good educated choices based on facts); and (3) sharper analytical thinking on inference-type questions. The design of the following formation is so that you will be able to absorb as many facts as possible without turning a page.

- **Mini-Mental Status Exam** (MMSE) has a total of 30 points. Cognitive impairment is based on a score with ≤9 (severe), 10-20 (moderate), and ≥21 (mild). A score ≥24 is generally considered normal.

- Anion gap = Na − (Cl + HCO$_3$).

- High anion gap metabolic acidosis is **MUDPILES** (Methanol, Uremia, DKA, Propylene glycol, Isoniazid, Lactic acidosis, Ethylene glycol, Salicylates).

- Major depressive episode is ≥5 of the following symptoms (**SIGECAPS + D**) for 2 weeks that must include either depressed mood or loss of interest: **S**-sleep changes, **I**-interest loss, **G**-guilt, **E**-energy loss, **C**-concentration loss, **A**-appetite/weight changes, **P**-psychomotor agitation or retardation, **S**-suicide ideation + **D**-depressed mood most of the day.

- The following is the CDC recommended immunization schedule (2014) for aged 0-18 years.

- **Hepatitis A (2 doses):** 12-23 months of age (2nd dose separated by 6-18 months).

- **Hepatitis B (3 doses):** Birth, 1-2 months, 6-18 months of age.

- **MMR (2 doses):** 12-15 months, 4-6 years of age.

- **Varicella (2 doses):** 12-15 months, 4-6 years of age.

- **DTaP (5 doses):** 2, 4, 6, 15-18 months, 4-6 years of age.

- **Tdap (1 dose):** 11-12 years of age.

- **PCV (4 doses):** 2, 4, 6, 12-15 months of age.

- **Hib (3 or 4 doses depending on brand):** 2, 4, ±6, 12-15 months of age.

- **Phase 0 Clinical Trials:** Designed to evaluate the pharmacodynamics (drug does to body) and pharmacokinetics (body does to drug). Information is then used to refine the researchers' study in the traditional phase 1 testing. Phase 0 studies usually recruit a small number of patients, has a short testing period, and low dosages of the drug are given.

- **Phase 1 Clinical Trials:** Evaluate the safety of the drug. Researchers learn how the drug should be given, determine a safe dosage range, and identify any side effects. Only a small number of patients are recruited.

- **Phase 2 Clinical Trials:** Evaluate the effectiveness of the drug. Researchers continue to monitor side effects. A larger group of patients are recruited to the study.

- Apgar score performed at 1 and 5 minutes of age and a score ≥7 points is generally considered normal, 4-6 is fairly low and requires close attention, and a score 0-3 indicates a serious problem.

- **Apgar** stands for **A**-appearance/color, **p**-pulse, **g**-grimace/reflex response, **a**-activity/muscle tone, **r**-respiration/lung maturity.

- Median survival is <1 month in untreated acute promyelocytic leukemia (APL).

- **Hypovolemic shock:** ↓ CO, ↑ SVR, ↓ PCWP.

- **Cardiogenic shock:** ↓ CO, ↑ SVR, ↑ PCWP.

- **Distributive (vasodilatory) shock:** ↑ CO, ↓ SVR, ↓ or nl PCWP.

- **Uncompensated metabolic acidosis:** ↓ pH, ↓$HCO_3^-$ (primary process), nl $pCO_2$.

- **Compensated metabolic acidosis:** nl pH (ie, compensated), ↓ $HCO_3^-$, ↓ $pCO_2$ (ie, blowing off $CO_2$ through hyperventilation during compensation).

- **Uncompensated respiratory acidosis:** ↓ pH, ↑ $pCO_2$ (primary process), nl $HCO_3^-$.

- **Compensated respiratory acidosis:** nl pH (ie, compensated), ↑ $pCO_2$, ↑ $HCO_3^-$ (ie, kidneys are reabsorbing more base during compensation).

- **Uncompensated metabolic alkalosis:** ↑ pH, ↑ $HCO_3^-$ (primary process), nl $pCO_2$.

- **Compensated metabolic alkalosis:** nl pH (ie, compensated), ↑ $HCO_3^-$, ↑ $pCO_2$ (ie, $CO_2$ is retained during compensation).

- **Uncompensated respiratory alkalosis:** ↑pH, ↓$pCO_2$ (primary process), nl $HCO_3^-$.

- **Compensated respiratory alkalosis:** nl pH (ie, compensated), ↓$pCO_2$, ↓$HCO_3^-$ (ie, kidneys excreting more base during compensation).

- In simple acid-base disorders, $pCO_2$ and $HCO_3^-$ will move in the same direction during compensation to return the pH to normal range.

- **Mixed metabolic and respiratory acidosis:** ↓ pH, ↑ $pCO_2$, ↓ $HCO_3^-$.

- **Rotavirus (2 or 3 doses depending on brand):** 2, 4, ±6 months of age.

- **IPV (4 doses):** 2, 4, 6-18 months, 4-6 years of age.

- **Meningococcal (1 dose + booster):** Start at ages 11-12 years followed by a booster at age 16.

- **HPV (3 doses):** Start at ages 11-12 years. Second dose given 1-2 months after the first dose. Third dose given after 6 months from the first dose. Note that HPV2 vaccine protects from HPV types 16 and 18 and should be given to females only. The HPV4 vaccine protects from HPV types 6, 11, 16, and 18 and can be given to females and males.

- **Influenza (annual):** Ages 6-23 months use only inactivated vaccine. Ages 2-18 years old can use inactivated or live attenuated vaccine.

- CDC recommends against the use of inactivated influenza vaccine (IIV) in patients with severe allergic reactions to egg.

- CDC recommends against the use of live attenuated influenza vaccine (LAIV) in patients with severe allergic reactions to egg protein, gentamicin, gelatin, and arginine.

- LAIV should not be used concomitantly with aspirin in children and adolescents.

- LAIV should not be used in pregnant women, children <2 years, adults ≥50 years, asthmatic patients, children 2-4 years who had wheezing in the past 12 months, immunosuppressed patients, and underlying medical conditions that would predispose patients to complications.

- **Tanner Stage 1 (girls):** Prepubertal; elevation of the papilla; no pubic hair.

- **Tanner Stage 2 (girls):** Breast bud stage; sparse pubic hair.

- **Tanner Stage 3 (girls):** Further enlargement of breast and areola; pubic hair is darker, coarser, and curlier.

- **Tanner Stage 4 (girls):** Secondary mound formed above the level of the breast; adult hair covering most of the pubic region.

- **Phase 3 Clinical Trials:** Compare the efficacy and safety of the new treatment with the current standard treatment for that disease. Phase 3 studies usually include a large group of patients.

- **Phase 4 Clinical Trials:** Also referred to as postmarketing surveillance trials. After the drug is approved and marketed, researchers will learn the effectiveness of the drug in various populations and identify unanticipated side effects that were not seen earlier in the clinical trials.

- **Patient Safety**—A "time out" should occur prior to any surgical procedure. During the time out, verification of the correct patient, procedure, and site must be confirmed.

- **Glasgow coma scale (GCS)**—Three domains that include eye opening (4 points is the best possible score reflecting spontaneous eye opening), verbal response (5 points is the best possible score reflecting oriented), and motor response (6 points is the best possible score reflecting obeys command).

- **GCS**—The highest total score is 15 points and the lowest possible score is 3 points. A score ≥13 points reflects mild brain injury, a score 9 to 12 points reflects moderate brain injury, and a score ≤8 points reflects severe brain injury (ie, "less than 8 may be too late, so you better intubate").

- **Tanner Stage 1 (boys):** Prepubertal; no pubic hair.

- **Tanner Stage 2 (boys):** Enlargement of the scrotum and testes; scrotal skin reddens; sparse pubic hair.

- **Tanner Stage 3 (boys):** Enlargement of the penis in length; further growth of the testes and scrotum; pubic hair is darker, coarser, and curlier.

- **Tanner Stage 4 (boys):** The breadth of the penis enlarges; further growth of the testes and scrotum; scrotal skin becomes darker; adult hair covering most of the pubic region.

- **Mixed metabolic and respiratory alkalosis:** $\uparrow$ pH, $\downarrow$ pCO$_2$, $\uparrow$HCO$_3^-$.

- **Patient Safety**—A sentinel event is an unanticipated outcome that may result in death or serious physical or psychological injury. Keep in mind that not all sentinel events are due to error because some diseases have a natural course of terminal illness that may not be the physician's fault.

- **American mistletoe toxicity**—Gastroenteritis.

- **Ginseng toxicity**—Diarrhea, hypertension, headache, nausea, insomnia.

- **Gingko toxicity**—Headache, bleeding, emesis.

- Short stature is defined as a height that is $\geq$2 standard deviations (SD) below the mean for children of the same sex and age. The equivalent would be less than the third percentile for height on the growth curve.

- **Constitutional delay of growth:** Variant of normal growth, normal size at birth, delay in height and weight velocity, resumes normal height and weight growth but may be at the lower growth percentiles or parallel to the third percentile, normal final height, normal TSH and T$_4$, delayed skeletal age, delayed puberty, timing of puberty dependent on bone age and not chronologic age, normal average height of the parents, family history of delayed growth or puberty is frequently present.

- **Familial short stature:** Variant of normal growth, normal size at birth, low-normal growth velocity throughout life, short final height, normal TSH and T$_4$, bone age consistent with chronological age, normal puberty, normal onset of puberty since bone age is normal, short height of the parent(s).

- **Normal CSF:** Clear fluid, opening pressure 70-180 mmH$_2$O, glucose 40-70 mg/dL, protein <40 mg/dL, cells 0-5/mm$^3$ (lymphs).

- **Bacterial meningitis CSF:** Cloudy fluid, opening pressure >180 mm H$_2$O, glucose <40 mg/dL, protein >45 mg/dL, WBCs 10 µL-10,000 µL ($\uparrow$ neutrophils), Grams stain positive >60% of the time, culture positive >80% of the time.

- **Tanner Stage 5 (girls):** Mature appearing breast with recession of the areola; adult hair with extension onto thighs.

- **Sequence of pubertal events in girls:** thelarche $\rightarrow$ pubarche $\rightarrow$ peak height velocity $\rightarrow$ menarche.

- In a minority of girls, pubarche will be the first manifestation in pubertal maturation.

- The mean interval between the breast bud stage (Tanner Stage 2) and menarche is approximately 2.5 years.

- The mean age of onset of puberty is approximately 10.5 years of age in girls and 11.5 years of age in boys.

- Newborns will lose up to **10%** of their birth weight in the first few days and then regain their weight in approximately **10** days.

- **Approximate weight gain in babies is as follows:** 30 g/dy (for first 3 months of life) $\rightarrow$ 20 g/dy (3 to 6 months of life) $\rightarrow$ 10 g/dy (6 to 12 months of life).

- Average weight gain from 2 years old to puberty is 2 kg/yr or 4.4 lbs/yr.

- To convert pounds (lbs.) to kilogram (kg), take the number in pounds and divide by 2.2.

- Birth weight should have **doubled** by 4 months of age and **tripled** by age 1.

- **Cryptococcal meningitis CSF:** $\uparrow$ opening pressure, normal to $\downarrow$ glucose, normal to $\uparrow$ protein, $\uparrow$ cell count (10-200 cells/mm$^3$), mononuclear cell predominance ($\uparrow$ lymphs), India ink preparation of CSF demonstrates a halo surrounding the encapsulated yeast, CSF cryptococcal antigen positive, *Cryptococcus neoformans* is a fungus and may present similarly to other fungal meningitides.

- **Spina bifida occulta**—Also referred to as closed spinal dysraphism; "occulta" in Latin means hidden; mildest form of spina bifida; one or more vertebrae are malformed; meninges and spinal cord are normal and not exposed; dimpling of the skin or hairy patch may be seen at the site of the lesion.

- **Tanner Stage 5 (boys):** Adult size and shape of the genitalia; adult hair with extension onto thighs.

- **Sequence of pubertal events in boys:** testicular enlargement $\rightarrow$ penile enlargement $\rightarrow$ pubarche $\rightarrow$ peak height velocity.

- The peak height velocity (growth spurt) typically occurs 2 years earlier in girls than in boys.

- Nocturnal sperm emissions (wet dreams) are considered the male counterpart of menarche and typically occur shortly after peak height velocity.

- Precocious puberty occurs before the age of 8 in girls and 9 in boys.

- Delayed puberty is considered by age 13 in girls and 14 in boys.

- **Drug Schedule I**—Considered the most dangerous class of drugs, high abuse potential, no acceptable medical use, examples: heroin, LSD, ecstasy (MDMA), mescaline, methaqualone, peyote, marijuana (certain states such as Colorado and Washington state allows for medical marijuana use).

- **Drug Schedule II**—High abuse potential but less abuse potential compared to schedule I, accepted medical indications with severe restrictions, examples: morphine, hydromorphone, oxycodone, codeine, fentanyl, methadone, meperidine, methamphetamine, methylphenidate, amphetamine, cocaine, pentobarbital.

- **Drug Schedule III**—Abuse potential less than schedule I and II, low to moderate potential for physical and psychological dependence, accepted medical indications, examples: anabolic steroids, acetaminophen with codeine, acetaminophen with hydrocodone, ketamine, buprenorphine, dronabinol.

- **Drug Schedule IV**—Low potential for abuse, low risk for dependence, accepted medical indications, examples: benzodiazepines, phenobarbital, zolpidem, modafinil, pentazocine, carisoprodol.

- **Viral meningitis CSF:** Clear fluid, normal to slightly elevated opening pressure, normal to slightly reduced glucose, normal to slightly elevated protein, WBC <500 cells/μL (mononuclear cell predominance), sometimes polymorphonuclear (PMN) predominance within the first 48 hours, negative Gram's stain, negative acid-fast, negative India ink.

- **TB meningitis CSF:** Cloudy fluid, opening pressure 180-300 mm $H_2O$, ↓ glucose (usually <45 mg/dL), ↑ protein (usually 100-500 mg/dL), mononuclear cell predominance (↑ lymphs), but early in infection polymorphonuclear predominance (↑ neutrophils), CSF acid-fast stain positive.

- **Neoplastic CSF:** Positive CSF cytology, ↓ glucose, ↑ protein, presence of mononuclear cells (<500 cells/mm$^3$), negative Gram's stain.

- **Milestone—gross motor (2 months):** Head up and chest up when lying prone.

- **Milestone—gross motor (4 months):** Holds head steady when held upright.

- **Milestone—gross motor (6 months):** Rolls over, sits with little to no support.

- **Milestone—gross motor (9 months):** Pulls to stand, crawls, gets into sitting position.

- **Milestone—gross motor (12 months):** Holds onto furniture when walking ("cruising").

- **Milestone—gross motor (18 months):** Walks alone, may run well.

- **Milestone—gross motor (2 years):** Runs, dances, walks up and down stairs holding on, throws ball overhand.

- **Milestone—gross motor (3 years):** Pedals a tricycle, climbs well.

- **Milestone—gross motor (4 years):** Hops on one foot, stands on one foot for 2 seconds, catches a bounced ball.

- **Primary prevention**—Prevents the disease from occurring (eg, immunizations).

- **Secondary prevention**—Early detection of disease and treatment to stop progression of the disease (eg, routine Pap smears).

- **Aseptic meningitis** refers to meningeal inflammation not caused by pyogenic bacteria. The most common cause of aseptic meningitis is the enterovirus (eg, echovirus, coxsackievirus, poliovirus). However, other viruses can still cause aseptic meningitis (eg, HSV, HIV, EBV, CMV, VZV, mumps, measles, rubella) and other etiologic agents include bacteria (eg, *Borrelia burgdorferi*, *Mycobacterium tuberculosis*, *Treponema pallidum*), fungi (eg, *Cryptococcus neoformans*, *Coccidioides immitis*, *Histoplasma capsulatum*), parasite (eg, *Toxoplasma gondii*), malignancy (eg, leukemia, lymphoma, leptomeningeal cancer), systemic diseases (eg, SLE, sarcoid, Behcet's disease), and drugs (eg, NSAIDs, TMP-SMX, IVIG, azathioprine, vaccines).

- **Milestone—fine motor (2 months):** Holds hands together.

- **Milestone—fine motor (4 months):** Grasps rattle and brings to mouth.

- **Milestone—fine motor (6 months):** Transfers object from hand to hand.

- **Milestone—fine motor (9 months):** Pokes with forefinger, uses immature pincer grasp.

- **Milestone—fine motor (12 months):** Neatly picks up small objects with thumb and index finger (mature pincer grasp).

- **Milestone—fine motor (18 months):** Makes 4 cube tower.

- **Milestone—fine motor (2 years):** Makes 6 cube tower, makes a "train" of cubes.

- **Milestone—fine motor (3 years):** Copies a circle.

- **Milestone—fine motor (4 years):** Copies a cross and square.

- **Milestone—social (2 months):** Smiles.

- **Milestone—social (4 months):** Vocalizes.

- **Milestone—social (6 months):** Stranger anxiety.

- **Milestone—social (9 months):** Separation anxiety.

- **Drug Schedule V**—Least potential for abuse, preparations contain limited amounts of narcotics and stimulants, accepted medical indications, examples: antitussives (<200 mg of codeine), antidiarrheals (eg, diphenoxylate + atropine, difenoxin + atropine), pregabalin, decongestant (eg, propylhexedrine).

- **Neurosyphilis CSF:** Reactive CSF-VDRL, ↑ protein, lymphocytic CSF pleocytosis, ± CSF HIV genotype positive for the virus (keep in mind that patients at risk for syphilis are also at risk for HIV infection).

- **Milestone—language (2 months):** Coos.

- **Milestone—language (4 months):** Laughs.

- **Milestone—language (6 months):** Babbles.

- **Milestone—language (9 months):** Says mamma/dada (nonspecifically).

- **Milestone—language (12 months):** Says mamma/dada (specifically), uses 1-2 true words.

- **Milestone—language (18 months):** Says "no" a lot, names common objects.

- **Milestone—language (2 years):** Uses 2-word sentences, follows 2-step commands.

- **Milestone—language (3 years):** Uses 3-word sentences, plurals, and pronouns correctly (eg, *I, me, you*).

- **Milestone—language (4 years):** Tells stories, follows 3-step commands.

- **Milestone—cognitive (2 months):** Recognizes parent.

- **Milestone—cognitive (4 months):** Enjoys looking around.

- **Milestone—cognitive (6 months):** Shows curiosity.

- **Milestone—cognitive (9 months):** Waves bye-bye, plays pat-a-cake, plays peek-a-boo.

- **Root reflex**—Stroking the baby's cheek causes the baby to turn toward the stimulus and opens the mouth. Present at birth, and disappears by 3-6 months.

- **Sutures**—Basic concepts in sutures include: **(1) Absorbable vs. Nonabsorbable**: Absorbable sutures typically lose their tensile strength in <60 days, but nonabsorbable sutures retain their tensile strength for at least 60 days. **(2) Diameter** of the sutures is graded by the number of zeros (eg, 1-0, 2-0, 3-0, 4-0, 5-0, 6-0, 7-0, 8-0, 9-0, 10-0). There is an inverse relationship between the number of zeros and suture diameter plus suture strength. For example, a 10-0 suture has a high number of zeros, but a smaller diameter and low suture strength, while a 1-0 suture has a low number of zeros, but a large diameter and high suture strength (think of the Golden Gate Bridge with an increase in the number of parallel wires in each of the main cables that increases the cable diameter). **(3) Monofilament vs. Multifilament** (eg, braided, twisted). Monofilament is more resistant to harboring bacteria and therefore less prone to infection. Multifilament is susceptible to harboring bacteria between the strands and therefore are more prone to infection. Multifilament sutures are easier to handle and provide greater knot security compared to monofilament sutures. **(4) Tissue reactivity** to the sutures is commonly seen in chromic gut, plain gut, and silk sutures. However, suture materials made of polydioxanone, polyglyconate, and polypropylene have the least tissue reactivity. **(5) Location of the sutures**: Absorbable sutures are typically used for deeper structures such as the fascia. Nonabsorbable sutures are typically used for the outermost layer in which the sutures can be removed. Smaller caliber sutures (eg, 5-0, 6-0) are used for delicate tissues (eg, face, digits), larger caliber sutures (eg, 2-0, 3-0) are used for closure of deeper tissues, and tissues on the scalp, extremity, and torso are typically sutured with a 3-0 or 4-0 suture.

- **Milestone—social (12 months)**: Imitates actions or sounds to get attention.

- **Milestone—social (18 months)**: Plays in company with other children.

- **Milestone—social (2 years)**: Parallel play.

- **Milestone—social (3 years)**: Imaginative play, shares toys.

- **Milestone—social (4 years)**: Cooperative or group play.

- **Tertiary prevention**—Reduce complications of disease (eg, diabetic patients require glycemic control, foot and eye checkups, urine microalbumin test, lipid control, HTN control, ↓ smoking, aspirin, vaccinations).

- **Plantar grasp**—Placing a finger in the baby's palms causes the baby to grip the finger. Present at birth, and disappears by 9 months.

- **Nonabsorbable sutures**—Nylon, silk, polypropylene (Prolene), polyester (Mersilene), polybutester (Novafil).

- **Absorbable sutures**—Plain gut, chromic gut, polydioxanone (PDS), polyglyconate (Maxon), polyglactin (Vicryl), polyglycolic acid (Dexon), poliglecaprone (Monocryl).

- **Lead time bias** is the bias that survival rates may be increased by a screening test when in fact the disease course is not altered by earlier detection. Patients do not necessarily live longer, but rather the perception of increased survival from the time of diagnosis. Researchers should avoid lead-time bias by comparing age-specific mortality rates instead of survival rates.

- **Length time bias** is the bias that outcomes appear better than the actual prognosis and is often discussed in the context of screening. For example, most slow-growing tumors will be detected by screening, and those slow-growing tumors inherently have a better prognosis. However, faster-growing tumors may prompt patients to seek medical care because of symptoms and be diagnosed without screening. As a result, screening appears to be more effective compared to no screening.

- **Milestone—cognitive (12 months)**: Copies gestures.

- **Milestone—cognitive (18 months)**: Points to at least one body part.

- **Milestone—cognitive (2 years)**: Sorts objects by color and shape.

- **Milestone—cognitive (3 years)**: Knows own gender, age, and name; dresses and undresses self.

- **Milestone—cognitive (4 years)**: Sings a song from memory, draws a 4-part person, starting to count.

- **Moro reflex (startle reflex)**—A sudden, slight dropping of the head from a slightly raised supine position causes the baby to open the palms of the hand and extension and abduction of the arms, followed by flexion and sometimes crying. Present at birth, and disappears by 3-6 months.

- **Receiver operating characteristic (ROC)** curve is a graphical illustration of the relationship between the sensitivity (ie, true positive rate) along the vertical axis ($y$-axis) and 1-specificity (ie, false positive rate) along the horizontal axis ($x$-axis). The ROC curve allows you to identify a cutoff value that would minimize the false negatives and false positives. As you move from left to right on the ROC curve, the sensitivity increases while the specificity decreases. Ideally, you would want a test that would give a near 100% sensitivity and 100% specificity, which would reflect a curve closest to the far upper-left corner. On the board exam, there may be 2 or 3 curves on the graph that reflect 2 or 3 tests (eg, screening test). The curve that lies near the far upper-left corner will usually prove to be the superior test of them all. The area under the ROC curve represents the accuracy of the test. A near perfect test is seen when the area under the curve approaches one.

- **Placenta accreta**—Placenta attaches to the myometrium; think of **Ac-creta**-**Attachment**; prior C-sections increases the risk of placenta accreta; placenta previa after a prior C-section increase the risk of placenta accreta; consider placenta accreta in the setting of overt hemorrhage at the time of manual placental separation.

- **Placenta increta**—Placenta invades into the myometrium; think of Increta-Invades Internally.

- **Placenta percreta**—Placenta penetrates through the myometrium to the uterine serosa; think of **Percreta**-**Penetrates Powerfully**; placenta accreta (most common) > placenta increta > placenta percreta (least common).

- **Placenta previa**—Placenta is implanted over or very near to the internal cervical os; think of **Previa**-**Previous** (in other words, the placenta is lying previous or in front of the internal cervical os, which is the gateway to the outside world); painless vaginal bleeding usually beyond 20 weeks gestation; risk factors include prior C-sections, multifetal gestations, multiparity, advanced maternal age, prior placenta previa, prior abortions, prior uterine surgery, infertility treatment, smoking, and cocaine; complete placenta previa (placenta completely covers the internal os); partial placenta previa (placenta partially covers the internal os); marginal placenta previa (placenta is at the margin of the internal os, but does not cover it); low-lying placenta (placenta is in close proximity to the internal os).

- Normal sequential primary tooth eruption: lower (mandibular) central incisors → upper (maxillary) central incisors → lateral incisors → first molars → canines → second molars.

- **Patient Safety**—Use appropriate antibiotic prophylaxis to reduce surgical site infections.

- **Ultraviolet B (UVB) radiation** (280 to 320 nm) has a shorter wavelength compared to UVA radiation. UVB radiation damages the skin's superficial epidermal layers. UVB radiation has a principal role in skin cancer but a contributory role in photoaging.

- **Enuresis**—Repeated voiding of urine in an individual ≥5 years of age that may be involuntary or intentional and can occur during the night, day, or both. Enuresis occurs at least 2 times/wk for at least 3 consecutive months or in the presence of significant distress or the disturbance impairs functioning in important areas (eg, work, school, relationships). Enuresis is usually a self-limiting condition and children will typically be continent by adolescence. There are no significant changes from DSM-IV to DSM-5.

- **Velamentous umbilical cord insertion**—Umbilical cord inserts into the fetal membranes (chorioamniotic membranes) rather than the placenta mass. Remember that the umbilical cord has vessels and these vessels will continue to travel haphazardly through the chorioamniotic membranes to the placenta. The reason why the vessels are running haphazardly is that they are vulnerable to rupture since they are unprotected from Wharton's jelly. Wharton's jelly is a gelatinous substance that is normally found in the umbilical cord, and it serves to protect the umbilical vessels. Think of velamentous umbilical cord insertion as a defective insertion (ie, the umbilical cord should normally extend to the chorionic plate) with exposed umbilical vessels running from the end of the umbilical cord to eventually the placenta. The length of exposed umbilical vessels can be highly variable.

- **Vasa previa**—Fetal vessels crossing over the internal cervical os; think of **Vasa Previa**–**Vessel Previous** (in other words, *vasa*, which means vessel in Latin, lies previous or in front of the internal cervical os, which is the gateway to the outside world); vasa previa may be associated with velamentous umbilical cord insertion or vessels that cross between lobes of the placenta (eg, bilobate placenta, succenturiate placenta); consider rupture of the vessels secondary to digital manipulation, artificial rupture, or descent of the fetal head compressing the vessels during labor.

- **Encopresis**—Repeated fecal incontinence in an individual ≥4 years of age that may be involuntary or intentional and may occur with constipation and overflow incontinence or without constipation and overflow incontinence. Encopresis occurs at least 1 time/mo for at least 3 months. In the majority of cases, encopresis is usually a self-limiting condition, but intermittent exacerbations may persist for years. There are no significant changes from DSM-IV to DSM-5.

- **Asymmetric tonic neck reflex**—Rotating the baby's head to one side causes extension of the arm and leg on the side to which the head is turned and at the same time flexion of the arm on the opposite side, which gives the baby a fencing posture. Present at birth, and disappears by 4-9 months.

- **Placenta abruption (abruptio placentae)**—An abruption at the decidual-placental interface; consider placenta abruption in patients beyond 20 weeks gestation; acute abruption may present with an acute onset of vaginal bleeding, back pain, abdominal pain, uterine contractions, uterine tenderness, and a nonreassuring FHR pattern; chronic abruption may present with intermittent bleeding, retroplacental hematoma, IUGR, oligohydramnios, or preeclampsia; risk factors for placenta abruption include multifetal gestations, multiparity, advanced maternal age, prior abruption, smoking, cocaine, abdominal trauma, chronic hypertension, preeclampsia, eclampsia, PROM, polyhydramnios, and low birth weight; DIC may be a complication of placental abruption, but DIC may also be seen in other pregnancy-related complications (eg, uterine rupture, placenta previa, placenta accreta, eclampsia, severe preeclampsia, HELLP syndrome, septic abortion, amniotic fluid embolism).

- **Ultraviolet A (UVA) radiation** has a longer wavelength compared to UVB radiation. UVA radiation can be divided into long-wavelength UVA1 (340 to 400 nm) and short-wavelength UVA2 (320 to 340 nm). UVA radiation is able to penetrate deeper into the skin affecting the dermis. An easy way to remember that UVA goes deeper into the skin than UVB is that "UVA gets an A+ while UVB gets a B for penetration." UVA radiation appears to be the principal player in the photoaging process, but it may still contribute to and initiate the development of skin cancers.

- Sunburns are principally caused by UVB radiation, but UVA2 can also cause sunburns.

- Psoralen plus UVA therapy (PUVA) used to treat skin disorders such as psoriasis can increase the risk of developing melanoma and nonmelanoma skin cancer, particularly SCC.

- Tanning beds, which primarily emit UVA radiation, have been implicated in increasing the risk of cutaneous SCC, BCC, and melanoma.

- **Lipoxygenase pathway:** Membrane phospholipids → Enzyme phospholipase $A_2$ (PLA$_2$) releases arachidonic acid from the membrane lipid → Enzyme 5-lipoxygenase converts arachidonic acid to leukotriene precursors (HPETEs) → Final products: LTB$_4$ (neutrophil chemotaxis), LTC$_4$ (bronchoconstriction), LTD$_4$ (bronchoconstriction), LTE$_4$ (bronchoconstriction).

- Corticosteroids inhibit the synthesis of COX-2 enzyme and inhibit the enzyme PLA$_2$.

- **Spina bifida aperta**—Also referred to as open spinal dysraphism; "aperta" in Latin means opening; herniation and exposure of the spinal cord and meninges (myelomeningocele) is the most severe form; protrusion of the meninges through an abnormal vertebral opening (meningocele).

- **Palmar grasp**—Placing a finger under the baby's toes causes the toes to curl toward the finger. Present at birth, and disappears by 9 months.

- **Uterine rupture**—Life-threatening pregnancy complication; consider uterine rupture in a patient with a nonreassuring FHR pattern, fetal bradycardia, decelerations (variable, late, or prolonged), uterine contraction abnormalities, ± abdominal pain (ie, may be masked by analgesics), variable vaginal bleeding, loss of fetal station, and maternal hemodynamic instability secondary to intraabdominal hemorrhage; higher risk of uterine rupture in a scarred uterus (eg, prior C-section, uterine surgery, myomectomy) compared to an unscarred uterus; type of prior uterine incision confers a risk of uterine rupture (classic vertical incision [higher risk] > low vertical > low transverse [lower risk]); risk factors for a uterine rupture in the unscarred uterus includes multiple gestation, grand multiparity, malpresentation, abnormal placentation (eg, placenta accreta, increta, or percreta), labor dystocia, macrosomia, uterine overdistension (eg, polyhydramnios), bicornuate uterus, connective tissue disorders, advanced maternal age, injudicious use of uterotonic agents, and trauma.

- **Cyclooxygenase pathway:** Membrane phospholipids → Enzyme phospholipase $A_2$ (PLA$_2$) releases arachidonic acid from the membrane lipid → Enzyme cyclooxygenase (COX-1, COX-2) converts arachidonic acid to prostaglandin precursors (PGG$_2$, PGH$_2$) → Final products: PGE$_2$ (↑ uterine contractions, relaxes smooth muscle of the cervix, induces fever, ↑ sensitivity to pain), PGI$_2$/prostacyclin (↓ platelet aggregation, ↓ uterine tone, vasodilatation), TXA2/thromboxane (↑ platelet aggregation, vasoconstriction).

- NSAIDs, including aspirin, inhibit cyclooxygenase enzymes (COX-1 and COX-2).

- **Patient Safety**—Root cause analysis is an assessment to identify the root cause of the underlying problems that may lead to an adverse outcome (eg, sentinel event). The analysis tries to correct the faulty process or systems in place, rather than an individual. The goal is to reduce similar occurrences in the future and to improve outcomes for patients.

- **Trunk incurvation (Galant reflex)**—While the baby is in the prone position, the examiner strokes along one side of the spine and the baby will move the pelvis toward the side of the stimulus. Present at birth, and disappears by 6 months.

- **Patient Safety**—Use pressure-relieving bedding materials to prevent pressure ulcers.

- Contraindications to MMR vaccine include pregnancy, current febrile illness with fever >101.3°F (38.5°C), active untreated TB, anaphylactic reaction to neomycin, hypersensitivity to gelatin, blood issues (eg, blood dyscrasias, lymphoma, leukemia, malignancy affecting bone marrow or lymphatic system), patients on immunosuppressive therapy (including high-dose steroids), patients with AIDS, patients with HIV who are severely immunocompromised, and family history of immunodeficiency (until recipient of the vaccine shows immune competence). Breastfeeding, positive PPD, PPD test given at the same time as the MMR vaccine, egg allergy, and immunodeficient family member, asymptomatic or mild symptomatic HIV infection are not contraindications to the MMR vaccine.

- **Celecoxib** is a COX-2 inhibitor that provides antipyretic, analgesic, and anti-inflammatory properties. Features of COX-2 inhibitors include a ↓ in gastroduodenal ulcers, ↓ risk of GI bleeding, sulfonamide allergy, and they do not inhibit platelet aggregation. Since COX-2 inhibitors do not inhibit the COX-1 enzyme, COX-1 can provide gastric cytoprotection.

- IV drug users may develop infective endocarditis (IE). The most common cause of IE in IV drug users is *Staphylococcus aureus*, but others may include Streptococci and Enterococci. Most cases of IE due to IV drug use are a right-sided IE. It should be noted that a murmur may not be detectable, but it is possible that deep inspiration (↑ blood to right ventricle) may accentuate a right-sided murmur (see Table 3-6).

- **Craniosynostosis** is the premature fusion of one or more cranial sutures. Premature fusion of the sagittal suture (scaphocephaly or dolichocephaly) can cause the head to be elongated resulting in a narrow face. Premature fusion of the unilateral coronal suture (anterior plagiocephaly) can result in flattening of the forehead with eyebrow elevation on the affected side. Premature fusion of bilateral coronal sutures (brachycephaly) can result in a short, wide, boxlike head.

- **Microcephaly**—A head circumference that is more than 2 standard deviations below the mean for age and gender.

- Average head circumference at birth is 35 cm.

- **Compensated metabolic acidosis:** For every 1 mEq/L fall in $HCO_3^-$, there is a respiratory compensation of a fall of 1.25 mm Hg of $pCO_2$.

- **Compensated metabolic alkalosis:** For every 1 mEq/L elevation in $HCO_3^-$, there is a respiratory compensation of a raise of 0.75 mm Hg of $pCO_2$.

- **Compensated acute respiratory acidosis:** For every 1 mm Hg elevation in $pCO_2$, there is a bicarbonate compensation of a raise of 0.1 mEq/L $HCO_3^-$.

- **Compensated chronic respiratory acidosis:** For every 1 mm Hg elevation in $pCO_2$, there is a bicarbonate compensation of a raise of 0.4 mEq/L $HCO_3^-$.

- **Compensated acute respiratory alkalosis:** For every 1 mm Hg fall in $pCO_2$, there is a bicarbonate compensation of a fall of 0.2 mEq/L $HCO_3^-$.

- A useful guideline in estimating the average plasma glucose is to assume that a HbA1c of 6.0% is equivalent to 120 mg/dL and that with an increase in each percentage point of the HbA1c, there is a rise of 30 mg/dL in the average glucose. For example, a HbA1c of 9.0% is equivalent to an average glucose of 210 mg/dL (ie, 120 mg/dL + 90 mg/dL = 210 mg/dL).

- **Blood group A:** A antigen on cell; anti-B in plasma; may receive blood from A and O; may give blood to A and AB.

- **Blood group B:** B antigen on cell; anti-A in plasma; may receive blood from B and O; may give blood to B and AB.

- **Blood group AB:** Universal recipient; A and B antigen on cell; no anti-A or anti-B in plasma (ie, reason for being the universal recipient); may receive blood from A, B, AB, or O; may give blood to AB only (ie, because A and B antigen on cell).

- **Blood group O:** Universal donor; no A or B antigen on cell (ie, reason for being the universal donor); anti-A and anti-B in plasma; may receive blood from O only (ie, because anti-A and anti-B in plasma); may give blood to A, B, AB, or O; remember that "O" are good "d-**O**-n-o-r-s."

- Vaccines contraindicated in pregnancy include varicella, MMR, live attenuated influenza vaccine (LAIV), and zoster vaccine.

- **Patient Safety**—Practice proper hand hygiene with the use of antiseptic soap or alcohol-based gels. Remember it is still important to clean your hands before and after wearing gloves.

- **Macrocephaly**—A head circumference that is more than 2 standard deviations above the mean for age and gender.

- **Saw palmetto toxicity**—Hypertension, headache, nausea, diarrhea, constipation, urinary retention.

- **Opioid intoxication**—CNS depression, bradycardia, hypotension, depressed respirations, hypothermia, hyporeflexia, miosis, ↓ bowel sounds, euphoria followed by apathy, slurred speech.

- NSAIDs (including aspirin) have the triple A's (**A**ntipyretic, **A**nalgesic, **A**nti-inflammatory properties).

- Acetaminophen has antipyretic and analgesic effect, but has little to no anti-inflammatory properties.

- Zileuton is seen in the treatment of asthma and serves to inhibit the 5-lipoxygenase enzyme.

- Zafirlukast is seen in the treatment of asthma and serves as a leukotriene receptor antagonist.

- Montelukast is seen in the treatment of asthma and allergic rhinitis; it serves as a leukotriene receptor antagonist.

- World Health Organization (WHO) analgesic ladder: Mild pain (non-opioid ± adjuvant) → Mild to Moderate pain (weak opioid ± non-opioid ± adjuvant) → Moderate to Severe pain (stronger opioid ± non-opioid ± adjuvant).

- Non-opioids—Acetaminophen, aspirin, and NSAIDs.

- Weak opioids—Codeine, hydrocodone, tramadol, and propoxyphene.

- Stronger opioids—Morphine, fentanyl, hydromorphone, oxycodone, methadone, and levorphanol.

- **Inhalant intoxication**—Toluene (eg, glues, paint thinners, marker pens, adhesives, acrylic paints, gasoline), nitrous oxide (eg, whipping cream canisters), hydrocarbons (eg, lighter fluid, aerosol propellants, propane, degreasers, dry-cleaning fluids, spot removers, Freons), euphoria, violent behavior, slurred speech, disorientation, ataxia, hallucinations, diplopia, headache, abdominal cramps, nausea, vomiting, eczematoid dermatitis ("glue-sniffer's rash"), arrhythmias, generalized muscle weakness, ↓ reflexes, hand tremor, nystagmus, mydriasis, unusual chemical odor on the breath.

- **Compensated chronic respiratory alkalosis:** For every 1 mm Hg fall in $pCO_2$, there is a bicarbonate compensation of a fall of 0.4 mEq/L $HCO_3^-$. (Note the ratios for all the compensations. For example, in this case, if there is a fall of 10 mm Hg in $pCO_2$, then there should be a fall of 4 mEq/L $HCO_3^-$. In another example, if there is a raise of 10 mm Hg in $pCO_2$ in acute respiratory acidosis, then there should be a compensatory raise of 1 mEq/L $HCO_3^-$.)

- **Amphetamine intoxication**—Agitation, paranoia, tachycardia, hypertension, tachypnea, hyperthermia, hyperreflexia, mydriasis, perspiration, hypervigilance, euphoria.

- **Amphetamine withdrawal**—Hypersomnia, fatigue, ↑ appetite, irritability, delayed depression.

- **Methaqualone intoxication**—"Quaaludes," drowsiness, ataxia, sexual arousal, slurred speech, headache.

- **First generation cephalosporins**—Cefazolin (parenteral), cephalexin (oral); **MOA**—Inhibits bacterial cell wall synthesis by binding to the penicillin binding proteins (PBPs); **Clinical use**—Gram-positive coverage (including staphylococci and streptococci, but not enterococci); minimal gram-negative coverage but can cover *Proteus mirabilis*, *E coli*, and *Klebsiella pneumoniae* (acronym PEcK); absent anaerobic coverage; cefazolin is commonly used for perioperative prophylaxis; **Side effects**—Abdominal pain, rash, eosinophilia, penicillin allergy, abnormal LFTs; **Pregnancy drug rating**—Cefazolin (category B), cephalexin (category B).

- **Opioid withdrawal**—Mydriasis, lacrimation, nausea, vomiting, diarrhea, piloerection, insomnia, runny nose, yawning, muscle aches, abdominal cramping.

- **Cannabis intoxication**—Euphoria, impaired perception and motor skills, conjunctival injection, ↑ appetite, dry mouth, decreased short-term memory.

- **Cannabis withdrawal**—Sleep disturbances, irritability, tremors, ↓ appetite, depressed mood, anxiety, headaches, mood swings.

- **Alcohol intoxication**—Slurred speech, mood lability, incoordination, vomiting, stupor, confusion.

- **Alcohol withdrawal**—Tremors, agitation, insomnia, ↑ heart rate, sweating, clammy skin, GI distress, seizures, anxiety, delirium tremens.

- **Benzodiazepine intoxication**—Slurred speech, confusion, ataxia, somnolence, stupor.

- **Benzodiazepine withdrawal**—Anxiety, insomnia, sweating, irritability, nausea, vomiting, tremors, sweating, seizures, psychosis.

- **Phencyclidine (PCP) intoxication**—"Angel dust," belligerence, violence, psychomotor agitation, hallucinations, tachycardia, hypertension, tachypnea, hyperthermia, hyperacusis, nystagmus, muscle rigidity, catatonia.

- **MDMA intoxication**—"Ecstasy," euphoria, excitement, tachycardia, hypertension, tachypnea, hyperthermia, mydriasis, bruxism.

- **Lysergic acid diethylamide (LSD)**—"Acid," hallucinations, tachycardia, hypertension, hyperthermia, mydriasis, anxiety, piloerection.

- **Patient Safety**—Handoffs are the transfer of essential information from one health-care provider to another. A good handoff includes clear language, avoiding abbreviations, updated information, accurate information, tasks for the receiver must be clearly explained, minimize environmental distractions, allow receiver time to review relevant summary, allow opportunity for questions, verify information, denote severity of the patients, and outline contingency plans.

- **Tobacco withdrawal**—Headache, irritability, difficulty concentrating, depressed, ↑ appetite, tobacco cravings, insomnia, restlessness.

- **Macrolides**—Azithromycin, clarithromycin, erythromycin; **MOA**—Protein synthesis inhibitor by binding to the 50S ribosomal subunit; **Clinical use**—Upper respiratory tract infections, *Haemophilus influenzae*, *Moraxella catarrhalis*, *Streptococcus pneumoniae*, *Legionella pneumophila*, *Chlamydophila pneumoniae*, *Mycoplasma pneumoniae*, *Mycobacterium avium* complex (MAC); **Side effects**—GI distress, rash, QT prolongation, torsades de pointes, hearing loss, pyloric stenosis, abnormal LFTs; **Pregnancy drug rating**—Azithromycin (category B), clarithromycin (category C), erythromycin (category B).

- **Lincosamide**—Clindamycin; **MOA**—Protein synthesis inhibitor by binding to the 50S ribosomal subunit; **Clinical use**—PID, acne, anaerobic infections, streptococcal infections, staphylococcal infections; **Side effects**—Diarrhea (including *Clostridium difficile* colitis); **Pregnancy drug rating**—Clindamycin (category B).

- **Second generation cephalosporins**—Cefuroxime (parenteral and oral), cefoxitin (parenteral), cefotetan (parenteral); **MOA**—Inhibits bacterial cell wall synthesis by binding to the penicillin binding proteins (PBPs); **Clinical use**—Weaker activity against gram-positive organisms compared to the first generation, but extended gram-negative and anaerobic coverage; important distinctions in this generation is that cefuroxime has good activity against *H influenzae* and *M catarrhalis* while cefoxitin and cefotetan have good activity against the anaerobe *Bacteroides fragilis*; **Side effects**—Diarrhea, penicillin allergy; **Pregnancy drug rating**—Cefuroxime (category B), cefoxitin (category B), cefotetan (category B).

- **Glycopeptide**—Vancomycin; **MOA**—Inhibits bacterial cell wall synthesis by binding to the D-ala-D-ala portion of the cell wall precursor; **Clinical use**—Invasive gram-positive infections (including MRSA), *Clostridium difficile*-associated diarrhea; **Side effects**—Ototoxic, nephrotoxic, red man syndrome; **Pregnancy drug rating**—Vancomycin (category B in the oral form, and category C in the intravenous form).

- **Third generation cephalosporins**—Ceftriaxone (parenteral), cefotaxime (parenteral), ceftazidime (parenteral); **MOA**—Inhibits bacterial cell wall synthesis by binding to the penicillin binding proteins (PBPs); **Clinical use**—Weaker activity against gram-positive organisms compared to the first generation, but increased activity against gram-negatives that are resistant to other beta-lactams; most third generations can cross the blood brain barrier; ceftriaxone (↓ activity against *P aeruginosa*, used in gonococcal infections, empiric treatment in meningitis, used in community-acquired pneumonia, used in Lyme disease); cefotaxime (↓ activity against *P aeruginosa*, used against penicillin-resistant pneumococci; used in spontaneous bacterial peritonitis); ceftazidime (↑ activity against *P aeruginosa*); **Side effects**—Diarrhea, rash, penicillin allergy, biliary pseudolithiasis (ceftriaxone can lead to ceftriaxone crystal formation or "sludge" in the gallbladder mimicking a gallstone and causing colicky abdominal pain); **Pregnancy drug rating**—Ceftriaxone (category B), cefotaxime (category B), ceftazidime (category B).

- **Aminoglycosides**—Gentamicin, tobramycin, streptomycin, neomycin, amikacin; **MOA**—Protein synthesis inhibitor by binding to the 30S ribosomal subunits; **Clinical use**—Aerobic gram-negative bacilli infection (including *Pseudomonas aeruginosa*), synergistic with beta-lactams to cover gram-positives (streptococci, staphylococci, enterococci), resistant to anaerobic bacteria; **Side effects**—Ototoxic (usually irreversible), nephrotoxic (usually reversible); **Pregnancy drug rating**—Gentamicin (category D), tobramycin (category D), streptomycin (category D), neomycin (category D), amikacin (category D).

- **Metronidazole**: **MOA**—Formation of toxic compounds that interact with the host cell DNA, resulting in DNA strand breakage and eventually into cell death; **Clinical use**—Anaerobic infections, protozoal infections (including amebiasis), *Clostridium difficile*-associated diarrhea, bacterial vaginosis, trichomoniasis, giardiasis, *H pylori*, abscess; **Side effects**—Metallic taste, disulfiram-like reaction with alcohol, GI distress, peripheral neuropathy, headache, urine darkening; **Pregnancy drug rating**—Metronidazole (category B).

- **Synthetic cathinone intoxication**—"Bath salts," violent behavior, agitation, self-mutilation, hallucinations, paranoia, panic attacks, tachycardia, hypertension, hyperthermia, mydriasis, sweating, seizures.

- **Fourth generation cephalosporin**—Cefepime (parenteral); **MOA**—Inhibits bacterial cell wall synthesis by binding to the penicillin binding proteins (PBPs); **Clinical use**—Improved activity against gram-positive organisms that is comparable to the first generation; greater resistance to beta-lactamases produced by gram-negative bacteria; active against streptococci and methicillin-susceptible staphylococci; ↑ activity against *P aeruginosa* that is similar to ceftazidime; used in febrile neutropenia; used in pneumonia (nosocomial and community-acquired); **Side effects**—Diarrhea, rash, penicillin allergy, seizure; **Pregnancy drug rating**—Cefepime (category B).

- **Fluoroquinolones**—Ciprofloxacin, levofloxacin, norfloxacin, ofloxacin, moxifloxacin, gemifloxacin; **MOA**—Fluoroquinolones are direct inhibitors of bacterial DNA synthesis. All fluoroquinolones can inhibit DNA gyrase (topoisomerase II), but gemifloxacin and moxifloxacin can also inhibit topoisomerase IV, which is another important enzyme in DNA replication; **Clinical use**—Broad-spectrum antibiotics with greatest activity against aerobic gram-negative bacilli; fluoroquinolones are used in gram-negative infections (including *E coli*, *H influenzae*, *M catarrhalis*, *Klebsiella* spp, *Legionella* spp, *Salmonella* spp, *Shigella* spp, *P aeruginosa*, *Proteus* spp, *Neisseria meningitidis*, *Neisseria gonorrhoeae*); CDC no longer recommends fluoroquinolones to treat gonococcal disease; only moxifloxacin has additional coverage against anaerobes; fluoroquinolones are used to treat genitourinary infections, community-acquired pneumonia, nosocomial pneumonia, acute exacerbations of chronic bronchitis, skin infections, acute sinusitis, and prostatitis; **Side effects**—GI distress (including *Clostridium difficile*-associated diarrhea), headache, QT prolongation, tendon rupture, tendinitis, rash, hyperglycemia, hypoglycemia, abnormal LFTs; avoid in patients <18 years old because of concerns of cartilage erosions in weight-bearing joints; avoid in pregnant women because safety in pregnancy has not been established; **Pregnancy drug rating**—Ciprofloxacin (category C), levofloxacin (category C), norfloxacin (category C), ofloxacin (category C), moxifloxacin (category C), gemifloxacin (category C).

- **Tetracyclines**—Doxycycline, minocycline, tetracycline, demeclocycline; **MOA**—Protein synthesis inhibitor by binding to the 30S ribosomal subunit at a position that prevents attachment of the aminoacyl-tRNA; **Clinical use**—Broad-spectrum antibiotics; tetracyclines are used against the spirochete *Borrelia burgdorferi* (Lyme disease), gram-negative *Rickettsia rickettsii* (Rocky mountain spotted fever), atypical pathogen *Mycoplasma pneumoniae* (causes mycoplasma pneumonia), obligate intracellular bacteria *Chlamydophila* spp, *Coxiella burnetii* (Q fever), gram-negative *Vibrio cholerae* (cholera), gram-positive rod *Bacillus anthracis* (anthrax), *H pylori* eradication, and *Ureaplasma urealyticum*; **Side effects**—GI distress (including *Clostridium difficile*-associated diarrhea), photosensitivity, hepatotoxicity, discoloration of the teeth and enamel hypoplasia in children <8 years old; avoid in pregnant women and children <8 years old if possible; **Pregnancy drug rating**—Doxycycline (category D), minocycline (category D), tetracycline (category D), demeclocycline (category D).

- Neutropenia is typically defined as an absolute neutrophil count (ANC) of <1500 cells/μL. An ANC <500 cells/μL would be considered severe neutropenia. The percent segmented neutrophils is part of the equation in calculating the ANC (ie, $ANC = WBC \times [PMN\% + Bands\%]/100$). Neutropenia may be seen in the setting of cancer chemotherapy, infection, autoimmune disorders, and drug-induced conditions. When assessing for neutropenia, remember not to just look at segmented neutrophil percentages in the lab report, but look at the **absolute** neutrophil count because it is **absolutely** better. The ANC is usually a component of the standard CBC report.

- **Carbapenems**—Imipenem-cilastatin, meropenem, doripenem, ertapenem; **MOA**—Inhibits bacterial cell wall synthesis by binding to the penicillin binding proteins (PBPs); low susceptibility to beta-lactamases; **Clinical use**—Broad-spectrum antibiotics that cover gram-negatives, gram-positives, and anaerobes; **Side effects**—GI distress, rash, headache, seizures, allergic cross-reactivity with beta-lactam antibiotics (ie, beta-lactam ring found in carbapenems, monobactams, penicillins, and cephalosporins); **Pregnancy drug rating**—Imipenem-cilastatin (category C), meropenem (category B), doripenem (category B), ertapenem (category B).

- Cilastatin is a compound that is usually added to imipenem therapy because imipenem is normally degraded in the kidney (proximal renal tubule) by an enzyme called renal dehydropeptidase I. Cilastatin inhibits renal dehydropeptidase I and thereby prolongs the antibacterial effect of imipenem and also prevents the formation of nephrotoxic metabolites if imipenem was degraded.

- **Monobactam**—Aztreonam; **MOA**—Inhibits bacterial cell wall synthesis by binding to the penicillin binding protein 3 (PBP-3); resistant to beta-lactamases; **Clinical use**—Greatest activity against gram-negative bacteria (including *Enterobacteriaceae* and *P aeruginosa*); no activity against gram-positive bacteria or anaerobes; synergistic with aminoglycosides; used in patients with penicillin allergies; cross-allergenicity with other beta-lactams are unlikely except for ceftazidime (third generation cephalosporin) because ceftazidime and aztreonam both have a shared side chain; **Side effects**—GI distress, rash, abnormal LFTs; **Pregnancy drug rating**—Aztreonam (category B).

- **St. John's wort toxicity**—Nausea.

- **Ephedra (ma huang) toxicity**—Hypertension, tachycardia.

- **Patient Safety**—Appropriate use of prophylaxis (eg, LMWH, pneumatic compression devices) to prevent perioperative venous thromboembolism (VTE).

# Key Lab Values

The key lab values are basic lab values that you should probably know prior to the exam to facilitate your understanding of the question when asked to analyze a set of lab values. Although the Step 3 exam will provide you with the laboratory values and the reference range, searching for the lab value and processing the information can be a multistep process. Knowing a few basic lab values before the exam can improve your efficiency, maintain your rhythm, and allow for a smoother transition into your analytical thinking on the questions. Although memorizing these lab values may require extra storage space in your brain, you can use your short-term memory by memorizing these lab values 1 to 2 days prior to the exam. The payoff may well be worth it. Remember, passing Step 3 reflects the attitude you take during your preparation, and that includes not discounting the small things.

## SERUM

### Electrolytes

Sodium: 135-146 mEq/L

Potassium: 3.5-5.0 mEq/L

Chloride: 95-105 mEq/L

Bicarbonate: 22-28 mEq/L

Calcium (total): 8.4-10.2 mg/dL

Magnesium: 1.5-2.0 mEq/L

Phosphorus: 3.0-4.5 mg/dL

### Liver Analytes

ALT: 10-40 U/L

AST: 15-40 U/L

Alkaline phosphatase (male): 30-100 U/L

Alkaline phosphatase (female): 45-115 U/L

Total bilirubin: 0.1-1.0 mg/dL

Direct bilirubin: 0.0-0.3 mg/dL

### Endocrine Analytes

Fasting glucose: 70-110 mg/dL

2-hour postprandial glucose: <120 mg/dL

TSH: 0.5-5.0 µU/mL

$T_4$: 5-12 µg/dL

T3RU: 25%-35%

### Lipids

Total cholesterol: 150-240 mg/dL

Triglycerides: 35-160 mg/dL

HDL: 30-70 mg/dL

LDL: <160 mg/dL

### Enzymes

Amylase: 25-125 U/L

LDH: 45-90 U/L

### Renal Analytes

BUN: 7-18 mg/dL

Creatinine: 0.6-1.2 mg/dL

### ABG

pH: 7.35-7.45/ $PCO_2$: 33-45/ $PO_2$: 75-105

## HEMATOLOGIC

### CBC

WBC: 4500-11,000/mm$^3$

Hb (male): 13.5-17.5 g/dL

Hct (male): 41%-53%

Hb (female): 12.0-16.0 g/dL

Hct (female): 36%-46%

Platelets: 150,000-400,000/mm$^3$

### Coagulation Analytes

PT: <12 seconds

PTT: <28 seconds

Bleeding time: 2-7 minutes

## URINE

Calcium: 100-300 mg/24 hr

Total proteins: <150 mg/24 hr

Specific gravity: 1.003-1.030

Urine osmolality: 50-1400 mOsmol/kg $H_2O$

## BMI

BMI: 19-25 kg/m$^2$

### Proteins

Total proteins: 6.0-7.8 g/dL

Albumin: 3.5-5.5 g/dL

### Solute Balance

Serum osmolality: 275-295 mOsmol/kg $H_2O$

### Differentials

Bands: 3%-5%

Segmented neutrophils: 54%-62%

Lymphocytes: 25%-33%

# APPENDIX E

# Final Pearls

- This is your last step in the USLME series, so give the test its due diligence so that you can move forward with your life.

- Remember that a systematic, methodical approach to your preparation will usually lead to a higher percentage of passing any examination.

- Be sure to track your progress throughout the course of your preparation and anticipate which chapters or sections of the chapter will be mastered by the end of each rotation (eg, cardiology chapter by the end of the cardiology rotation, EKG review section by the end of the ICU/CCU service).

- Be open-minded when reading the questions. Do not be too rigid and absolute with classic presentations. Sometimes atypical presentations may be integrated with a classic presentation. Other times, there may be associated features presented with the disease (eg, bacterial vaginosis presented with PID).

- Make sure you answer all questions since unanswered questions are considered wrong answers.

- Try not to skip too many questions because there is no guarantee that the next set of questions will be easier or shorter.

- Try generating an answer after reading the question before looking at the option list.

- On long narrative questions, try reading the last line of the question first because then you know what the question is asking. Then, read the question from the beginning. In this approach, you can read with more intention.

- Take ownership of the exam by controlling the pace of each block and the tempo of the exam day. You should be able to know how many blocks you have completed, what CCS case number you are on, and what quarter you are on in the quarter method. Use the dry-erase board provided on the exam to help you with those three elements.

- Consider bundling all literature interpretation questions toward the end of each block. In this approach, you maintain good rhythm with the other multiple-choice questions.

- Although it is nice to answer questions with "silver-bullet" knowledge (ie, you are 100% sure of answering the question correctly), do not underestimate the power of deductive reasoning. Eliminating clearly wrong answers on the multiple-choice questions based on facts and medical concepts will increase your percentage of answering the question correctly.

- Good test takers can always spot key pieces of information. The pieces of information can then be collectively integrated to formulate the diagnosis and then make good management decisions.

- Remember to keep track of your time on the test (quarter method).

- Give each question an "equal opportunity" in terms of time.

- **Caveat 1**—Do not underestimate the exam.

- **Caveat 2**—Never spend too much time on any one question since some questions could be experimental or piloted questions (ie, consider ambiguous questions as land mines since they can damage your time).

- **Caveat 3**—Time can creep up on you when you least expect it, or it may occur at the end of the day when you are mentally exhausted.

- **Caveat 4**—You cannot expect to pass if you don't put in the time.

- One of the key elements to making sound clinical judgments is to always weigh pertinent facts carefully before making a decision.

- If you read this book and understand the majority of the medical information, then your clinical judgment should be sharper and you should have enough firepower to do well on the exam.

- Remember that it is easy to know a lot if you understand a lot. Once you know a lot, then you have the tools to think with more depth and think critically.

- The more depth you have in your knowledge base, the better you can position yourself at making sound clinical judgment.

- Try to extract the essence of each chapter (not just purely memorizing information) because you ultimately want to sharpen your clinical judgment.

- Once you have read this book and extracted the information from each chapter, try to make sense out of it on a global perspective by interrelating the chapters (ie, connecting points). This is when you tap into sound clinical judgment.

- In your final review prior to the exam, you should be able to go through the book and know all the connecting points without hesitation.

- Consider taking the examination on consecutive days or within 2 to 3 days after day 1. In this respect, you should feel more comfortable going into part 2 of the exam because you already know what to expect. If you prolong the latency period (eg, 1 month later), you might feel a little bit on edge going into part 2 of the exam.

- Between day 1 and day 2, make sure you have time to decompress to get ready for part 2. It is not recommended to look up answers to the questions you remember. If you do, you might second-guess yourself on part 2 and you may shatter your confidence. You need to go into part 2 with a positive mind frame. Remember that the evaluation process is a sum total and not on several questions you remember.

- Take inventory of your clinical judgment skills. Clinicians use their clinical judgment on a day-to-day basis, but they may not be aware of how strong or weak their skills are.

- Do your best to get a good night's rest the day before the exam. If you don't, however, that is okay. It is completely normal and part of the process of taking examinations. Know that the time and effort you put into your preparation cannot be stolen. You will still be able to function at a high level and make good decisions on the exam.

- **On the CCS**, practice the CCS component of the exam with each chapter review. You will be amazed to discover something new each time.

- **On the CCS**, never blow off any CCS cases on the actual exam. Even if you don't know how to manage a patient on the CCS exam, you can always work up the patient based on a pertinent history, physical exam, and updated lab reports. Remember that a thorough approach based on your clinical judgment may not necessarily deduct from your score.

- **On the CCS**, be aware of CCS cases in which you have to defer from further testing and treatment that would not be considered the standard of care. For example, you do not want to do further testing or treatment on a patient with a terminal illness. If you do further testing or treatment, that would be considered an aggressive approach and you will certainly have a low score.

- **On the CCS**, the initial vital signs are a clue to whether the patient is stable or unstable and whether or not the management decisions need to be done expeditiously.

- **On the CCS**, remember to always "bridge" your therapy. Think about what needs to be treated acutely (eg, pain) and what needs to treated in the long term (eg, prevention).

- **On the CCS**, remember to appropriately monitor your patients (eg, pulse oximetry, continuous cardiac monitoring, continuous blood pressure monitoring, pertinent physical exams after treatment, urine output, vital signs, ICU, fetal monitor, PFTs, neuro checks).

- **On the CCS**, if you ever feel overwhelmed with any CCS cases, hit the "refresh" button in your mind by (1) composing yourself, (2) quickly reading the case introduction, (3) identifying key aspects of the initial history, (4) glancing at the vital signs, and (5) asking yourself, "What are the necessary steps in managing this patient?"

# Index

Note: Page numbers followed by *f* indicate figures; page numbers followed by *t* indicate tables.

## A

Null hypothesis (H$_0$), 15
Number needed to harm (NNH), 15
Number needed to treat (NNT), 15
Nursemaid's elbow, 205-206
NWTS (National Wilms' Tumor Study), 279
NYHA (New York Heart Association), 82t
NYHA (New York Heart Association) functional
      classification, 31-32

## O

Observational analytic studies, 13
Obsessive-compulsive disorder (OCD), 229-230
Obsessive-compulsive personality disorder (OCPD), 236t
Obstetrics, 159-191
   antepartum logistics, 160-161t
   breastfeeding, 185-186t
   case study (ectopic pregnancy), 188-191
   cesarean section, 181, 184t
   chromosomal abnormalities, 163t
   CMV, 167-168
   delivery of the baby, 180
   environmental factors, 164
   FDA pregnancy categories, 165t
   fetal heart rate and activity, 181
   HSV, 168
   intrapartum surveillance, 180t
   keywords review, 159-160
   maternal physiologic changes, 160t
   mental health concerns, 187t
   neonatal chlamydial conjunctivitis and pneumonia, 166
   neonatal gonococcal conjunctivitis, 164-166
   parvovirus B19, 169-170
   perinatal infections, 164-168
   postpartum fever, 185, 187t
   PPROM, 181, 184
   pregnancy concerns. See Pregnancy concerns
   prenatal risk assessment, 164, 164t
   prenatal testing and procedures, 161-162t, 161t
   pubic diastasis, 186-188
   single gene disorders, 162, 162t
   syphilis, 170
   TORCH infections, 166
   toxoplasmosis, 167
   varicella, 168-169
Obstructive bronchiolitis, 245
OCB (oligoclonal banding), 141
OCD (obsessive-compulsive disorder), 229-230
OCPD (obsessive-compulsive personality disorder), 236t
OCT (optical coherence tomography), 196
Octreotide, 66
Odds ratio (OR), 14, 317
Odynophagia, 213
Ofloxacin, 335
OGTT (oral glucose tolerance test), 174
Olanzapine, 68t
Oligoclonal banding (OCB), 141
Oligomenorrhea, 108
Olsalazine, 100
Omalizumab, 244t
OME (otitis media with effusion), 216, 217
Omeprazole, 45
Ondansetron, 215
Open-angle glaucoma, 197-199
Open pneumothorax, 262, 263
Open reduction, 203
Open reduction internal fixation (ORIF), 205

Open stone surgery, 277
Ophthalmology, 193-202
   amblyopia, 200
   cataract, 195
   chalazion, 200-201
   conjunctivitis, 201-202
   corneal abrasion, 194
   glaucoma, 197-199
   hordeolum, 201
   inflammatory conditions, 200-202
   keywords review, 193
   macular degeneration, 196-197
   retinal detachment, 195-196
Opioid intoxication, 332
Opioid withdrawal, 333
Opioids, 332
Opsonization, 2
Optical coherence tomography (OCT), 196
Optotype, 193
OR (odds ratio), 14
Oral antidiabetic agents, 82t
Oral glucose challenge test, 174
Oral glucose tolerance test (OGTT), 174
Organ donation, 90
ORIF (open reduction internal fixation), 205
Orthodromic AVRT, 62
Orthopedics, 203-212
   ACL injuries, 208
   case study (carpal tunnel syndrome), 210-212
   clavicle fractures, 204-205
   hip disorders, 207t
   idiopathic scoliosis, 204
   keywords review, 203
   nursemaid's elbow, 205-206
   osteosarcoma, 208-209
   scaphoid fractures, 206
Oscillopsia, 140
Osteogenic sarcoma, 208
Osteoporosis, 282-283
Osteosarcoma, 208-209
Ostium primum defect, 39
Ostium secundum defect, 39
Otalgia, 213
Otitis media with effusion (OME), 216, 217
Otolaryngology, 213-224
   croup, 220-222
   ear disorders, 214-218
   keywords review, 213
   mouth and throat disorders, 220-224
   peritonsillar abscess, 222
   sinusitis, 218-220
Ovarian function cessation, 120
Ovarian torsion, 108-109
Overactive letdown, 186t
Overexcretors, 284t, 285
Oxiconazole, 51

## P

P-mitrale, 29
P-value, 15
P wave, 29, 36, 57, 58, 59, 61
Pachymetry, 198
PAD (peripheral arterial disease), 21t, 298-300
Paget's disease of the breast, 117, 117t, 119
Pain disorder, 234-235
Palilalia, 226

Perinatal infections, 164-168
Peripheral arterial disease (PAD), 21*t*, 298-300
Peritonsillar abscess (PTA), 222
Peritonsillar cellulitis, 222
Persistent motor or vocal tic disorder, 239-240
Personality disorders, 235-236*t*
Perthes maneuver, 301
PFO (patent foramen ovale), 38
PFT (pulmonary function testing), 244, 248
PHACES syndrome, 49
Phalen test, 212
Phase 0 clinical trials, 325
Phase 1 clinical trials, 325
Phase 2 clinical trials, 325
Phase 3 clinical trials, 326
Phase 4 clinical trials, 326
Phencyclidine (PCP) intoxication, 333
Phenoxybenzamine, 78
Phenytoin, 3
Pheochromocytoma, 19*t*, 78-79
Phlebolith, 277
Phlegmasia alba dolens, 295
Phlegmasia cerulea dolens, 295
Phlegmon, 93
Photopsia, 193, 195
Physician-assisted suicide, 90
Physician's responsibilities/rights, 90
Physiologic (normal) split, 18
PICA (posterior inferior cerebellar artery), 144, 144*f*
PID (pelvic inflammatory disease), 309, 321
Pigeon beans, 138
Pigmented BCC, 53*f*, 54
Pioglitazone, 82*t*
PION (posterior ischemic optic neuropathy), 296
PIP (proximal interphalangeal) joints, 288
Pirbuterol, 244*t*
Pituitary disorders, 66-68
Pituitary gigantism, 66, 67
Pityriasis versicolor, 50
Pivot shift test, 208
Placenta abruption, 330
Placenta accreta, 330
Placenta increta, 330
Placenta percreta, 330
Placenta previa, 330
Placental alpha microglobulin-1 protein assay, 184
Plantar grasp, 329
Plaque, 47
Plasma-derived vWF concentrates, 132
Plugged ducts, 185*t*
Plummer-Vinson syndrome, 127
Plummer's disease, 69*t*
PM (polymyositis), 259, 286-288, 293
PMBV (percutaneous mitral balloon valvotomy), 30
PML (progressive multifocal leukoencephalopathy), 142
PMN (polymorphonuclear), 284*t*
PMR (polymyalgia rheumatica), 291-294, 296
Pneumococcal conjugate vaccine (PCV13), 216
Pneumothorax (PTX), 261-264
PNL (percutaneous nephrolithotomy), 271*t*, 277
POAG (primary open-angle glaucoma), 197
POC (products of conception), 171*t*
Podagra, 281, 283
Poikilocytosis, 126
Polyarteritis nodosa (PAN), 300-301
Polycystic ovarian syndrome (PCOS), 121-123

Polycythemia vera (PV), 318
Polymenorrhea, 108
Polymorphonuclear (PMN), 284*t*
Polymyalgia rheumatica (PMR), 291-294, 296
Polymyositis (PM), 259, 286-288, 293
Polymyxin-trimethoprim eye drops, 201
Pontiac fever, 256*t*
Pontine hemorrhage, 149
Positive end-expiratory pressure (PEEP), 242
Positive predictive value (PPV), 12
Post-infarct pericarditis, 45
Post-term, 160
Posterior cerebral artery (PCA), 144, 144*f*
Posterior inferior cerebellar artery (PICA), 144, 144*f*
Posterior ischemic optic neuropathy (PION), 296
Posterior vitreous detachment (PVD), 196
Postpartum blues, 187*t*
Postpartum depression, 187*t*
Postpartum fever, 185, 187*t*
Postpartum psychosis, 187*t*
Posttraumatic stress disorder (PTSD), 228
Potassium iodide, 70
Potter syndrome, 274
Pott's disease, 252
"Powder-burn" lesion, 121
Power, 15
PPD (purified protein derivative), 252
PPIs (proton pump inhibitors), 45, 94
PPROM (preterm premature rupture of membranes), 181, 184
PPV (positive predictive value), 12
PR interval, 57
Prazosin, 22
Prednisolone, 244*t*, 290
Prednisone, 96, 244*t*, 285, 300
Preeclampsia, 177-178
Pregestational diabetes, 175
Pregnancy associated plasma protein A (PAPP-A), 164
Pregnancy concerns, 170-180
    cervical incompetence, 172
    dermatoses of pregnancy, 172, 173*t*
    eclampsia, 178-179
    gestational diabetes, 173-175
    HELLP syndrome, 179-180
    preeclampsia, 177-178
    pregestational diabetes, 175
    rhesus incompatibility, 176-177
    spontaneous abortion, 170-172
    vaccines, 332
Prehn sign, 317
Premature rupture of membranes (PROM), 181
Prenatal risk assessment, 164, 164*t*
Prenatal testing and procedures, 161-162*t*, 161*t*
Presbycusis, 214
Pressure disorder (hypertension), 18-22
Preterm, 160
Preterm premature rupture of membranes (PPROM), 181, 184
Pretibial myxedema, 65
Prevalence, 12
Primary aldosteronism, 19*t*
Primary amenorrhea, 108
Primary biliary cirrhosis (PBC), 24*t*
Primary dysmenorrhea, 108
Primary hyperparathyroidism, 19*t*
Primary open-angle glaucoma (POAG), 197
Primary prevention, 328
Primary progressive MS, 141

Quinsy, 222
Quiz. *See* Rapid-fire clinical judgments

# R

*r* (correlation coefficient), 16
RA (rheumatoid arthritis), 288-291, 293
Rabies, 315
Radiation ablation, 70
Radioactive iodine (RAI), 69*t*
Radioactive iodine uptake (RAIU), 69*t*, 70
RADT (rapid antigen detection test), 223
RAE (right atrial enlargement), 58
RAI (radioactive iodine), 69*t*
RAIU (radioactive iodine uptake), 69*t*, 70
Raloxifene, 119, 120, 282
Randomized controlled trial (RCT), 13
Ranibizumab, 197
Ranitidine, 8
Ranke complex, 254
Rapid antigen detection test (RADT), 223
Rapid-fire clinical judgments, 313-323
Rapid plasma reagin (RPR), 170
RAS (renal artery stenosis), 21*t*
RBBB (right bundle branch block), 18, 39, 40
RBC (red blood cell), 128
RCA (right coronary artery), 26*t*
RCC (renal cell carcinoma), 273
RDW (red cell volume distribution width), 128
Rebleeding, 157
Receiver operating characteristic (ROC) curve, 329
Recombinant factor VIIa (rFVIIa), 149
Recombinant products, 131
Recurrent corneal erosion syndrome, 194
Recurrent croup, 221
Red blood cell (RBC), 128
Red cell volume distribution width (RDW), 128
Regadenoson, 28
Relapsing-remitting MS (RRMS), 140-141
Relative risk (RR), 14
Relative risk reduction (RRR), 14-15
Reliability, 12
Renal analytes, 338
Renal and genitourinary, 269-280
    hereditary disorders, 272-275
    key findings review, 269-270
    kidney disease, 272-275
    nephrolithiasis, 271*t*, 275-278
    urinary crystals, 271*t*, 272*f*
    urine dipstick, 269-270
    urine inspection, 269
    urine sediment (microscopic exam), 270
    Wilms' tumor, 279-280
Renal artery stenosis (RAS), 21*t*
Renal cell carcinoma (RCC), 273
Renal failure, 73*t*
Renal osteodystrophy, 65
Renovascular hypertension, 19*t*
Repaglinide, 82*t*
Reperfusion therapy, 26
Reportable diseases, 89
Reportable events, 90
Reserpine, 68*t*
Residual volume (RV), 242, 245
Resistant hypertension, 20
Respiratory syncytial virus (RSV), 256*t*, 258-259
Reticular veins, 302

Reticulocyte production index (RPI), 126
Retinal detachment, 195-196
Retinal pigment epithelium (RPE), 195
Retinoblastoma, 195
Retrospective study, 13
Rett's disorder, 237*t*
Reye's syndrome, 298
rFVIIa, 149
Rh(D) antigens, 176
Rh(D) negative mother, 176
Rh(D) positive, 176
Rhegmatogenous retinal detachment, 195
Rheumatic fever, 307
Rheumatoid arthritis (RA), 288-291, 293
Rheumatology, 281-294
    case study (polymyalgia rheumatica), 291-294
    crystal-induced arthropathies, 283-286
    dermatomyositis and polymyositis, 286-288
    gout, 283-286
    inclusion body myositis, 288
    inflammatory disorders, 288-291
    inflammatory myopathies, 286-288
    keywords review, 281
    osteoporosis, 282-283
    pseudogout, 286
    rheumatoid arthritis, 288-291
Rhesus incompatibility, 176-177
Rhinosinusitis, 218-220
RhoGAM, 171, 176, 191
RICE, 208
Rifampin (RIF), 252, 253, 255
Right atrial enlargement (RAE), 58
Right bundle branch block (RBBB), 18, 39, 40
Right coronary artery (RCA), 26*t*
Right ventricular hypertrophy (RVH), 30, 41, 58
Rinne test, 214
RIPE, 252
Risedronate, 282
Risk, 14-15
Risk difference, 14
Risk ratio, 14
Risperidone, 68*t*
Risser sign, 204
Ristocetin, 133
Rituximab, 290
ROC curve, 329
Rodent ulcer, 53, 53*f*
Roflumilast, 247
Romano-Ward syndrome, 63
Romberg's test, 140
Root cause analysis, 331
Root reflex, 329
Rosenbach's sign, 35
Rosette test, 176
Rosiglitazone, 82*t*
Rosuvastatin, 24*t*
Rotterdam criteria, 122
Rouleaux, 126
RPE (retinal pigment epithelium), 195
RPI (reticulocyte production index), 126
RPR (rapid plasma reagin), 170
RR (relative risk), 14
RRMS (relapsing-remitting MS), 140-141
RRR (relative risk reduction), 14-15
RSV (respiratory syncytial virus), 256*t*, 258-259
rtPA (alteplase), 250

Spider veins, 302
Spina bifida aperta, 331
Spina bifida occulta, 327
Spinal cord compression, 133
Spinal disease, 142-143
Spinal epidural hematoma, 153
Spiramycin, 167
Spirometry, 244, 246
Spironolactone, 21t
Splenectomy, 130
Splenic rupture, 320
Spondylolisthesis, 140
Spondylolysis, 140
Spondylosis, 140
Spontaneous abortion, 170-172
spp (species), 256t
Spur cells, 125
Squamous cell carcinoma (SCC), 51-53
Squamous cell carcinoma in situ, 52, 52f
SSEP (somatosensory EP), 141
SSP (secondary spontaneous pneumothorax), 261
SSRIs. *See* Selective serotonin reuptake inhibitors (SSRIs)
St. John's wort toxicity, 335
ST elevation myocardial infarction (STEMI), 21t, 25-28
*Staphylococcus aureus,* 256t, 258
*Staphylococcus epidermidis,* 258
*Staphylococcus saprophyticus,* 258
Startle reflex, 329
Statin-induced transaminase elevations, 24
Statins, 24t, 25
Statistics. *See* Biostatistics
Steatorrhea, 97
STEMI (ST elevation myocardial infarction), 21t, 25-28
Stereopsis, 200
Stereotypy, 226
Steroid-dependent colitis, 100
Steroids, 286. *See also* Glucocorticoids
Stevens-Johnson syndrome (SJS), 308
Stimulants, 239
Stone passage facilitators, 277
Stones, 271t, 272f, 275-278
STP (superficial thrombophlebitis), 302
Strabismus, 200
Streptococci, 258
*Streptococcus agalactiae,* 258
*Streptococcus bovis,* 258
*Streptococcus pneumoniae,* 256t, 258
*Streptococcus pyogenes,* 222, 223, 258
*Streptococcus viridans,* 258
Streptokinase, 250
Streptomycin, 334
String sign, 95
Stroke, 143
Struma ovarii thyrotoxicosis, 69t
Struvite stones, 271t, 278
Student quiz. *See* Rapid-fire clinical judgments
Study design, 13
Stye, 201
Subacute lymphocytic thyroiditis, 69t
Subacute thyroiditis, 69t
Subarachnoid hemorrhage (SAH), 154-158
Subarachnoid stroke, 143
Subdural hematoma (SDH), 152f, 153
Subhyaloid retinal hemorrhage, 157
Submucous myoma, 109f
Subpulmonic VSD, 40

Sucking chest wound, 262
Sudden cardiac arrest (SCA), 33
Sudden cardiac death (SCD), 33, 37
Sulconazole, 51
Sulfacetamide, 138
Sulfadiazine, 167
Sulfasalazine
    5-ASA agent, 100
    RA, 289
    reduction in immunoglobulins, 3
Sulfonylureas, 82t
Superficial BCC, 53, 53f
Superficial spreading melanoma, 54, 55f
Superficial thrombophlebitis (STP), 302
Superficial venous system, 301
Superior cerebellar artery (SCA), 144, 144f
Superior vena cava (SVC) syndrome, 313
Supination-flexion technique, 206
Suppositories, 100
Sutures, 329
SVC syndrome, 259, 313
Swan-neck deformity, 281
"Swiss cheese," 40
Symmetrical hearing impairment, 214
Syncope, 37
Syndrome of inappropriate antidiuretic hormone secretion (SIADH), 259
Synovial fluid analysis, 284t
Synthetic cathinone intoxication, 334
Syphilis, 170
Systematic review, 13
Systemic lupus erythematosus (SLE), 304

**T**
$T_3$, 71
$T_3$ resin uptake (T3RU), 71
$T_4$, 71
$T_H1$ cells, 2
$T_H2$ cells, 2
T-score, 283
Tabes dorsalis, 160, 170
Tachycardia, 57
Tactile aphasia, 140
Takayasu arteritis, 296
Tamoxifen, 119, 283
Tamsulosin, 277
Tangential speech, 226
Tanner stages, 326, 327
Target cell, 126
Tazarotene, 48
TB (tuberculosis), 251-255
TB meningitis CSF, 328
TBG (thyroxine-binding globulin), 71
TBII (thyrotropin-binding inhibitory immunoglobulin), 69t, 70
Td vaccine, 316
Tdap vaccine, 316
T1DM (type 1 diabetes mellitus), 79-81, 81t
T2DM (type 2 diabetes mellitus), 81-83, 81t
Tear-shaped RBC, 126
TEE. *See* Transesophageal echocardiography (TEE)
TEF (tracheoesophageal fistula), 163t
Telangiectasias, 302
Telangiectatic (vascular) osteosarcoma, 209
Temporal arteritis, 293
TEN (toxic epidermal necrolysis), 308
Tension pneumothorax, 263-264
Teratogens, 165t

Transthoracic echocardiography (TTE) (*Continued*)
  mitral stenosis, 29
    TIA, 148
    VSD, 41
Transvaginal ultrasound (TVUS), 110
Trastuzumab, 120
Traube's sign, 35
Trauma- and stressor-related disorders, 228-229
Traumatic pneumothorax, 261
TRH (thyrotropin-releasing hormone), 67, 72*t*
Triamcinolone, 285, 286
Triamcinolone acetonide, 244*t*
*Trichomonas vaginalis,* 114, 115
Trichomoniasis, 114-115
Trichotillomania, 226
Tricuspid regurgitation, 17, 18
Tricuspid stenosis, 17, 18
Triglyceride (TG), 24*t*
Triiodothyronine, 71
Triple phosphate, 272*f*
Triple screen, 164
Trismus, 213
Trisomy 13, 163*t*, 164*t*
Trisomy 18, 163*t*, 164*t*
Trisomy 21, 163*t*, 164*t*
Troponins, 27, 44, 250
Trousseau's sign, 75
Trousseau's syndrome, 259
T3RU (T₃ resin uptake), 71
True TIA, 147
Trunk incurvation (Galant reflex), 331
Truthfulness, 87
TS (transient synovitis), 207*t*
TSH (thyroid-stimulating hormone), 72*t*
TSI (thyroid-stimulating immunoglobulin), 69*t*, 70
TSST-1 (toxic shock syndrome toxin - 1), 223
TST (tuberculin skin test), 252
TT vaccine, 316
TTE. *See* Transthoracic echocardiography (TTE)
Tuberculin skin test (TST), 252
Tuberculosis (TB), 251-255
Tubo-ovarian abscess (TOA), 321
Turner's syndrome, 163*t*
TV (tidal volume), 242
TVUS (transvaginal ultrasound), 110
Tympanic membrane (TM), 216
Tympanic membrane (TM) perforation, 217-218
Tympanocentesis, 217
Type 1 diabetes mellitus (T1DM), 79-81, 81*t*
Type 2 diabetes mellitus (T2DM), 81-83, 81*t*
Type I error, 15
Type II error, 15
TZ (transformation zone), 111

**U**
UA (unstable angina), 21*t*
UAE (uterine artery embolization), 110
UC (ulcerative colitis), 96*t*, 97-101
uE3, 164
UFH (unfractionated heparin), 250
Uhthoff sign, 140
Ulcerative colitis (UC), 96*t*, 97-101, 301
Ultrasound (US), 69*t*, 161*t*, 164*t*
Ultraviolet A (UVA) radiation, 331
Ultraviolet B (UVB) radiation, 330

Uncompensated metabolic acidosis, 326
Uncompensated metabolic alkalosis, 326
Uncompensated respiratory acidosis, 326
Uncompensated respiratory alkalosis, 326
Unconjugated estriol (uE3), 164
Underexcretors, 284*t*, 285
Unfractionated heparin (UFH), 250
"Unhappy triad," 208
Unstable angina (UA), 21*t*
UPEP (urine protein electrophoresis), 134
URI (upper respiratory infection), 207*t*
Upper GI series, 96
Upper respiratory infection (UPI), 207*t*
Urease, 278
Ureteroscopy (URS), 277
Urgent cerclage, 172
Uric acid stones, 271*t*, 272*f*
Urinary antigen test, 259
Urinary crystals, 271*t*, 272*f*
Urine dipstick, 269-270
Urine inspection, 269
Urine pH, 269
Urine protein electrophoresis (UPEP), 134
Urine sediment (microscopic exam), 270
Urobilinogen, 270
Urokinase, 250
URS (ureteroscopy), 277
US (ultrasound), 69*t*, 161*t*, 164*t*
USMLE step 3 tips/pointers, 339-340
US Preventive Services Task Force (USPSTF), 23, 111, 318
USPSTF (US Preventive Services Task Force), 23, 111, 318
Uterine artery embolization (UAE), 110
Uterine fibroids, 109*f*
Uterine rupture, 331
UVB radiation, 330

**V**
V/Q scan, 249-250, 251
V sign, 287
v wave, 18
Vaccination (immunization) schedule, 236, 325
VAD (vincristine, adriamycin, or dexamethasone), 134
Validity, 12
Valproic acid, 3
Valsartan, 21*t*
Valvular disorders, 28-30
Vancomycin, 334
Variable deceleration, 181, 183*f*
Varicella, 168-169
Varicella pneumonia, 169
Varicella-zoster immune globulin (VariZIG), 169
Varicella-zoster virus (VZV), 169
Varicocele, 308
Varivax, 169
VariZIG, 169
Vasa previa, 330
Vascular claudication, 143
Vascular disorders, 295-302
  giant cell arteritis, 296-297
  infantile hemangioma, 48-49
  Kawasaki disease, 297-298
  keywords review, 295
  peripheral arterial disease, 298-300
  polyarteritis nodosa, 300-301
  varicose veins, 301-302